NCLEX

American Nursing Review for NCLEX-PN

PN

NCLEX

American Nursing Review for NCLEX-PN

PN

Leona A. Mourad, RN, MSN, ONC

SPRINGHOUSE CORPORATION
SPRINGHOUSE, PENNSYLVANIA

STAFF

Executive Director, Editorial
Stanley Loeb

Director of Trade and Textbooks
Minnie B. Rose, RN, BSN, MEd

Art Director
John Hubbard

Drug Information Editor
George J. Blake, RPh, MS

Editors
Kathy Goldberg, Diane Labus

Copy Editor
Mary Hohenhaus Hardy

Designers
Stephanie Peters (associate art director),
Lorraine Carbo

Art Production
Robert Perry (manager), Donald Knauss, Tom Robbins, Robert Wieder

Typography
David Kosten (director), Diane Paluba (manager), Elizabeth Bergman, Joyce Rossi Biletz, Phyllis Marron, Jim Phillips, Robin Rantz, Valerie L. Rosenberger

Manufacturing
Deborah Meiris (manager), T.A. Landis, Jennifer Suter

The clinical procedures described and recommended in this publication are based on research and consultation with nursing, medical, and legal authorities. To the best of our knowledge, these procedures reflect currently accepted practice; nevertheless, they can't be considered absolute and universal recommendations. For individual application, all recommendations must be considered in light of the patient's clinical condition and, before administration of new or infrequently used drugs, in light of the latest package-insert information. The author and the publisher disclaim responsibility for any adverse effects resulting directly or indirectly from the suggested procedures, from any undetected errors, or from the reader's misunderstanding of the text.

© 1992 by Springhouse Corporation, 1111 Bethlehem Pike, Springhouse, PA 19477. All rights reserved. Reproduction in whole or part by any means whatsoever without written permission of the publisher is prohibited by law. Authorization to photocopy any items for internal or personal use, or the internal or personal use of specific clients, is granted by Springhouse Corporation for users registered with the Copyright Clearance Center (CCC) Transactional Reporting Service, provided that the base fee of $00.00 per copy plus $.75 per page is paid directly to CCC, 27 Congress St., Salem, MA 01970. For those organizations that have been granted a license by CCC, a separate system of payment has been arranged. The fee code for users of the Transactional Reporting Service is 0874343968/92 $00.00 + $.75.
Printed in the United States of America.

PNCLEX-011091

Library of Congress Cataloging-in-Publication Data
Mourad, Leona A.
American nursing review for NCLEX-PN/Leona A. Mourad.
    p.   cm.
  Includes bibliographical references and index.
    1. Practical nursing—Examinations, questions, etc.   I.
Title.
    [DNLM: 1. Nursing, Practical—examination questions.
WY 18 M929a]
RT62.M68 1992
610.73'076—dc20
DNLM/DLC
ISBN 0-87434-396-8
                      91-5133
                      CIP

CONTENTS

Contributors xi
Preface xii

Part I: Pretest

Instructions 3
Questions 3
Answers and rationales 11
Pretest self-diagnostic analysis 17

Part II: Taking NCLEX-PN

Introduction 20
NCLEX-PN test plan 20
Strategies for success 23

Part III: Nursing principles and general nursing procedures

Introduction 29

Nursing principles

Classification of human needs 29
Normal growth and development throughout the life cycle 30
Health and physical assessment guide 37
Legal principles of nursing practice 42
Therapeutic communication 45
Grief and loss 49
Basic nutrition 51
Rehabilitation 66
Inflammation 68
Shock 70
Acid-base balance 74
Fluids and electrolytes 78
Immobility 82

General nursing procedures

Assisting with ambulation 85
Changing a sterile dressing 86
Irrigating a wound 87
Applying a pressure dressing 88
Applying a wet-to-dry dressing 88
Removing sutures or staples 89

Contents *(continued)*

Applying heat and cold 90
Using a heat lamp 91
Collecting specimens 92
Washing the hands 94
Shaving a patient 95

Part IV: Review of clinical nursing

Perioperative nursing

Introduction 98
Preoperative care 98
Intraoperative care 101
Postoperative care 101

Maternity nursing

Introduction 108
Anatomy and physiology of the female reproductive system 108

Prenatal (antepartal) period 111
First trimester 111
Second trimester 118
Third trimester 120

Intrapartal period 124
Labor and delivery 124

Postpartal period 137
Breast-feeding 139
Washing the perineal area 143
Administering a sitz bath 144
Performing a postpartal maternal assessment 145
Assessing the newborn 145
Bathing the newborn 147

Pediatric nursing

Introduction 150

Infant (birth to age 1) 150
Gastroenteritis 150
Congenital heart disease 153
Meningitis 158
Toddler (age 1 to 3) 162
Laryngotracheobronchitis 162
Acetaminophen intoxication 163

Preschooler (age 3 to 6) 166
Acute lymphocytic leukemia 166
School-age child (age 6 to 12) 169
Nephrosis 169
Rheumatic fever 171
Type I diabetes mellitus 173
Adolescent (age 12 to 19) 175
Scoliosis 175
Caring for a child in a Croupette 177
Assisting with bone marrow aspiration or biopsy 178
Teaching insulin self-administration 179

Adult medical-surgical nursing

Introduction 186

Cardiovascular system 186
Anatomy and physiology 186
Congestive heart failure 191
Myocardial infarction 192
Hypertension 194
Arteriosclerosis 195
Applying and monitoring rotating tourniquets 198
Assisting with an electrocardiogram 199
Performing basic cardiopulmonary resuscitation 200
Applying elastic stockings 202

Respiratory system 208
Anatomy and physiology 208
Lobar pneumonia 210
Pulmonary edema 212
Lung cancer 213
Chronic obstructive pulmonary disease 216
Pulmonary tuberculosis 217
Caring for the patient with a chest tube 222
Teaching deep-breathing and coughing exercises 224
Performing postural drainage 225
Administering intermittent positive-pressure breathing treatments 227
Assisting with incentive spirometry 228
Administering oxygen 228
Assisting with thoracentesis 229
Performing tracheal suctioning 230
Providing tracheostomy care 232
Caring for a patient requiring mechanical ventilation 233

Contents *(continued)*

Musculoskeletal system 238
Anatomy and physiology 238
Patient in a cast (fracture of the tibia and fibula) 241
Patient in traction (fracture of the femur) 244
Fracture of the femoral neck 247
Osteoarthritis 253
Rheumatoid arthritis 256
Performing neurovascular checks 263
Assisting with cast application 264
Assisting with cast removal 267
Teaching about skin care after cast removal 268
Applying a sling 268
Assisting with application of balanced-suspension skeletal traction for a
    fractured femur 269
Teaching a patient to use crutches, a cane, or a walker 272

Gastrointestinal system 282
Anatomy and physiology 282
Gastrointestinal ulcer 288
Obstruction of the small intestine 292
Colon cancer... 296
Inserting a nasogastric tube 300
Inserting a Miller-Abbott intestinal tube 302
Inserting a Cantor intestinal tube 303
Maintaining a gastrointestinal tube 305
Removing a nasogastric, Miller-Abbott, or Cantor tube 306
Providing tube feedings 307
Providing gastrostomy or jejunostomy tube feedings 310
Providing jejunal tube feedings 311
Assisting with paracentesis 312
Providing ileostomy care 314
Providing colostomy care 317
Administering a cleansing enema 321
Applying an abdominal binder 323
Inserting a rectal tube 325
Removing a rectal tube 326
Listening for bowel sounds 327
Assisting with proctoscopy 328

Neurologic system 333
Anatomy and physiology 333
Head injury and increased intracranial pressure 338
Cerebrovascular accident 341
Epilepsy 346
Brain tumor 350

Parkinson's disease 352
Performing neurologic checks 357
Placing a patient on a CircOlectric bed 360
Turning a patient on a CircOlectric bed 361
Turning a patient on a Stryker Wedge Frame bed 363
Positioning a patient in bed 365
Assisting with lumbar puncture 368

Genitourinary system 373
Anatomy and physiology 373
Glomerulonephritis 375
Benign prostatic hyperplasia 377
Kidney or bladder tumor 380
Dialysis 383
Inserting a urinary catheter 387
Caring for an indwelling urinary catheter 388
Removing an indwelling urinary catheter 389
Caring for a nephrostomy tube 390
Applying a condom catheter 390
Caring for an arteriovenous shunt 391
Measuring fluid intake and output 393
Measuring urine specific gravity 394
Applying a T-binder 395

Endocrine system 397
Anatomy and physiology 397
Hyperthyroidism 399
Hypothyroidism 401
Cushing's syndrome 403
Addison's disease 405
Type II diabetes mellitus 407
Teaching blood glucose self-monitoring 412
Assisting with the glucose tolerance test 413
Assisting with the radioactive iodine uptake test 414
Collecting 24-hour urine specimens 415

Integumentary system 420
Anatomy and physiology 420
Third-degree burn 421
Caring for pressure ulcers 429

Immune system 432
Anatomy and physiology 432
Acquired immunodeficiency syndrome 435

Contents *(continued)*

Oncology nursing 439
Malignant cell development 439
Ovarian cancer and chemotherapy 441
Lung cancer and radiation therapy 445
Breast cancer and mastectomy 449
Starting an I.V line 455
Caring for a peripheral venous catheter 458
Providing oral hygiene 459
Changing a central line dressing 461

Psychiatric nursing
Introduction 469
Anxiety disorder 471
Bipolar mood disorder—manic phase 474
Depression 476
Alcohol abuse 478
Alzheimer's disease 482
Schizophrenia 485
Anorexia nervosa 487

Part V: Appendices

Appendix 1: Recommended daily dietary allowances 498
Appendix 2: Healthful weights 500
Appendix 3: Sample meal planning exchange lists 501
Appendix 4: Normal values for common laboratory tests ... 504
Appendix 5: Drug administration, calculations, and equivalents 505
Appendix 6: Precautions to take when administering drugs 507
Appendix 7: NANDA nursing diagnostic categories 508
Appendix 8: NCLEX-PN dates and state boards of nursing 509
Appendix 9: Canadian examination information 512
Appendix 10: Selected references 513

Part VI: Practice test

Introduction 516
Sample computer report for the NLN Practice Test 519
NLN Practice Test for PN Licensure 521

Index 534

CONTRIBUTORS

EXECUTIVE CLINICAL EDITOR

Leona A. Mourad, RN, MSN, ONC
Associate Professor Emeritus
Ohio State University
Columbus, Ohio

CONTRIBUTING AUTHORS

Sondra B. Baird, RN, MEd, MSN
Instructor
School of Nursing
Abington Memorial Hospital
Abington, Pa.

F. William Balkie, RN, MBA, CRNA
President
American Nursing Review
Martinsville, N.J.

Carol J. Bininger, RN, PhD
Associate Professor
Ohio State University
Columbus, Ohio

Marcia G. Bower, RN,C, MSN
Level 1 Coordinator
School of Nursing
Abington Memorial Hospital
Abington, Pa.

Mary S. Breese, MA, RD, LD
Assistant Professor Emeritus
Ohio State University,
Columbus, Ohio

Margery G. Garbin, RN, PhD
Senior Vice President
National League for Nursing
New York

Phyllis A. Healy, RN, PhD
Associate Professor
University of Southern Maine
Portland, Maine

Carole E. Kingsbury, RN, EdD
Test Consultant
National League for Nursing
New York

Cecilia Kinsel, RN,C, PhD
Professor
San Antonio College
San Antonio, Tex.

Leona A. Mourad, RN, MSN, ONC
Associate Professor Emeritus
Ohio State University
Columbus, Ohio

Carol Patterson, RN, MSN
Instructor
Raritan Valley Community College
Raritan, N.J.

Carol L. Schaffer, RN, JD
Director
Cleveland Clinic Home Care Services
Cleveland

MaryAnn Troiano, RN, MSN
Adjunct Clinical Instructor
College of Staten Island
Staten Island, N.Y.

CONTENT CONSULTANTS

Sharon Bell, RN, MA
Director
Columbus School of Practical Nursing
Columbus, Ohio

Marilyn Burkart, RN, MSN
Director
Practical Nurse Council
National League for Nursing
New York

BOOK CONSULTANTS

F. William Balkie, RN, MBA, CRNA
President
American Nursing Review
Martinsville, N.J.

Jenkin V. Williams
Executive Vice President
American Nursing Review
Martinsville, N.J.

PREFACE

Practical and vocational nursing practice is an important and respected component of the health care system. Practical and vocational nurses work in all clinical areas of patient care and in all health care settings.

The growing complexity of nursing care has added a technical dimension to practical and vocational nursing that did not exist even a short time ago. Practical and vocational nurses, who are entering the health care system in increasing numbers, typically must assume a greater role in the delivery of care at the technical level. Recent job analyses of practical and vocational nursing practice support this trend toward increasing technical responsibility.

To enter practical nursing, graduates of practical nursing education programs must pass the National Council of State Boards of Nursing Licensure Examination for Practical Nurses (NCLEX-PN). Recent reorganization of this examination resulted in a new test plan first used in 1990.

The purpose of NCLEX-PN (known as the state boards) is to ensure that the practical nurse is competent to practice entry-level technical nursing. Nurses graduating from PN programs must be prepared—both educationally and emotionally—to succeed on this important test. A well-planned study program can prove crucial to their success. *American Nursing Review for NCLEX-PN* has been written and designed so that nurses who use it in the recommended way can be confident of their knowledge of basic nursing—and ready to pass NCLEX-PN.

A note about some basic terms used in this book: *Licensed practical nurse* (LPN) and *licensed vocational nurse* (LVN) are synonymous; which term is used depends on the state in which the nurse practices. In most states, *licensed practical nurse* denotes practical nursing practice. Therefore, we use that term in this book—with the understanding that it applies as well to licensed vocational nurses or vocational nursing practice. (In Canada, licensed practical nurses commonly are referred to as nursing assistants.)

Adopting a strategy for success

To prepare for NCLEX-PN, educators recommend the proven strategy of establishing a baseline of current nursing knowledge and an understanding of how NCLEX-PN is constructed and scored. Knowing how to answer test questions successfully and conducting a comprehensive review of nursing content learned in school enhance the strategy for success. Taking a posttest to measure the results of the study program completes the strategy.

American Nursing Review for NCLEX-PN has all the elements you need to carry out this strategy. By studying this book carefully and taking the pretest and posttest, you will become confident that you have what it takes to pass the examination.

Previewing the book format

This book was developed from the same model as the nationally acclaimed *American Nursing Review for NCLEX-RN,* America's most popular study tool for NCLEX-RN. It includes only essential information, avoiding duplication of information to help you conserve your time. The book is divided into six major parts. To enhance effective study, each part progresses from simple, basic concepts to more complex, technical concepts.

Part I is a pretest developed by the National League for Nursing (NLN). It includes 60 questions, all at the same level of difficulty as NCLEX-PN, covering all clinical areas and all phases of the nursing process. By taking the pretest, you can determine the level of your knowledge about current nursing. To detect any weak areas, complete the score sheet at the end of the pretest; these areas merit extra attention during your study program.

Part II explains the new NCLEX-PN test plan, from which each examination is developed, then offers proven strategies for preparing for the examination and answering questions in the NCLEX style. By reading this part and learning how the test is developed and which categories it evaluates, you will gain added confidence and feel less anxious at test time.

Part III focuses on basic scientific, legal, and humanistic principles and general nursing procedures that apply to all patients in any clinical setting. Because this part contains foundation material that you must be familiar with before proceeding further, you should review it early in your study program.

Part IV is a review of clinical nursing that follows the successful format of *American Nursing Review for NCLEX-RN*. Its case-study approach will help you build familiarity with care plans, situation-type questions, and NCLEX-PN. Organized by clinical area, it starts with perioperative nursing and proceeds through maternity, pediatric, adult medical-surgical, and psychiatric nursing. It presents case studies describing common health problems, using the nursing process as the organizing element. To cover basic pathophysiology, each case study begins with an overview of the patient's specific health problem.

The perioperative nursing section covers patient care during the preoperative, intra-operative, and postoperative periods. It reviews routine care and describes how to prevent and manage postoperative complications.

The maternity nursing section reviews the anatomy and physiology of the female reproductive system, then presents a case study of a normal pregnancy that follows a patient through the three trimesters and labor and delivery. Illustrations enhance the content, as do discussions of pregnancy complications, newborn care, and common procedures in maternity nursing. A chart highlights important information about drugs used in maternity nursing; be sure to study this chart carefully, focusing on the side effects of each drug and related nursing considerations.

The pediatric nursing section reviews the pediatric health conditions that a beginning practical nurse is likely to encounter, then discusses common pediatric nursing procedures. Familiarity with normal growth and development (discussed in Part III) will help you make the best use of this section.

The adult medical-surgical nursing section, organized by body system, reviews the health problems likely to be covered on NCLEX-PN. For each body system, it presents anatomical illustrations, a review of basic anatomy and physiology, and a glossary. Case studies familiarize you with commonly encountered diseases and disorders. Nursing procedures relevant to each body system appear in chart form; a rationale accompanies each procedure step and an asterisk (*) denotes key steps. A drug chart presents the actions, dosages, side effects, and nursing considerations for commonly administered drugs. Make sure you are familiar with all the drugs in these charts, because NCLEX-PN poses questions about many of them. (Be aware that the drug charts in this book present general information about the drugs most likely to be included in NCLEX-PN questions—not about all drugs that may be prescribed. Also keep in mind that only those people authorized to prescribe drugs may do so. For specific information on drug administration and related nursing care, consult medication package inserts.)

The section on psychiatric nursing—the last clinical area covered—focuses on the most common psychiatric disorders for which a practical nurse may provide nursing care. Although few questions on NCLEX-PN relate specifically to mental health, many require knowledge of the principles of psychiatric nursing practice—especially therapeutic communication.

Part V presents appendices covering normal laboratory values; instructions on simple drug dosage calculations; nutrition charts (useful for a quick check or to reinforce learned material); NANDA-approved nursing diagnoses; NCLEX-PN test dates through the end of the century; addresses of state boards of nursing for each U.S. state and provincial nursing associations for each Canadian province; and a list of general references.

Part VI is the posttest—the NLN Practice Test for PN Licensure. Designed by the NLN, this test mirrors the NCLEX-PN test plan. To ensure test reliability and validity as a predictor of success on NCLEX-PN, this test has been administered experimentally to more than 800 practical nursing students. We recommend that you take the Practice Test at the end of your study program for NCLEX-PN. When you return the answer sheet (along with the specified fee), you will receive a report of your score, a prediction of how you will perform on NCLEX-PN, and a list of references for further study of any weak areas. To allow time for any additional study you may need, be sure to complete the Practice Test well before taking NCLEX-PN.

American Nursing Review for NCLEX-PN contains all the information you will need to prepare successfully for NCLEX-PN. (If you encounter unfamiliar information, consult a more comprehensive textbook for additional study.) We are confident you will regard it as a valuable study tool—and will continue to use it as a reference long after you have received your PN license.

Congratulations on choosing nursing as a career, and good luck on NCLEX-PN.

F. William Balkie, RN, MBA, CRNA
President, American Nursing Review

Jenkin Vaughn Williams
Executive Vice President

Part I

Pretest

Part I

Pretest

Instructions 3

Questions 3

Answers and rationales 11

Pretest self-diagnostic analysis 17

Instructions

Select a quiet room where you will not be disturbed. Set the timer for 120 minutes.

The pretest consists of a series of situations appearing in **bold** type, followed by questions pertaining to the situations; each question is followed by four possible answers. Read each question and all possible answers carefully, then select the one best answer. Remember, **each question has only one correct answer.**

Completely blacken the circle in front of the answer you've selected, using a #2 lead pencil. Do not use check marks, X's, or lines. If you change your answer, be sure to erase the old answer completely. (NCLEX-PN is scored electronically. Incomplete erasures may cause both answers to be scored, in which case you will receive no credit for that question.)

If you have trouble understanding a question or are not sure of the answer, place a small mark next to the question number and go back to it after you've completed the test, if you have time. You won't be penalized for guessing because your test results reflect correct answers only.

On the pretest, the number 1, 2, 3, or 4 appears next to each possible answer to a question. These numbers won't appear in NCLEX-PN. They are included on the pretest to help identify the correct answer and the rationale.

This test	**NCLEX-PN**
○ **1.** Atonic.	○ Atonic.
○ **2.** Dystonic.	○ Dystonic.
○ **3.** Hypotonic.	○ Hypotonic.
○ **4.** Hypertonic.	○ Hypertonic.

After you've completed the test and your time is up, check your responses against the correct answers provided at the end of the pretest. The number of the correct answer appears in parentheses ( ), along with the rationale for the correct answer and reasons (when appropriate) why other possible answers are incorrect. Your score on the pretest is the total number of questions answered correctly. Complete the *Pretest self-diagnostic analysis* worksheet (see page 17).

Questions

Mrs. Jennie Clark, age 42, comes to the clinic complaining of increased white vaginal discharge between her menstrual periods. She will undergo a pelvic examination and is scheduled for diagnostic tests, including a cone biopsy.

1. Before Mrs. Clark's pelvic examination, the practical nurse should tell her to
○ 1. empty her bladder.
○ 2. take a vaginal douche.
○ 3. drink a quart of water.
○ 4. check her temperature.

2. Which statement by Mrs. Clark would indicate that she has a correct understanding of the cone biopsy?
○ 1. "My cervix will be observed after being stained with an iodine solution."
○ 2. "The inside of my uterus will be scraped to obtain a tissue specimen."

○ 3. "A special instrument will be inserted through my abdomen to obtain a specimen of the uterine muscle."
○ 4. "A piece of tissue from my cervix will be removed for examination."

Because of the diagnostic test results, Mrs. Clark is admitted to the hospital and has a total abdominal hysterectomy. After a short stay in the recovery room, she is returned to her room.

3. Which of these positions should Mrs. Clark **avoid** during the immediate postoperative period?
○ 1. High Fowler's.
○ 2. Lateral recumbent.
○ 3. Supine.
○ 4. Side-lying.

Mr. John Larson, age 40, visits his physician with gastrointestinal (GI) complaints. The physician orders diagnostic studies, including an upper GI series.

4. Mr. Larson receives instructions about the upper GI series. Which statement would indicate that he understands the instructions?
○ 1. "I will have a special instrument passed through my mouth into my stomach."
○ 2. "I will take several tablets the night before the test."
○ 3. "I will drink a radiopaque fluid while X-rays are taken."
○ 4. "I will be given a radioactive substance before a scan is taken."

5. Which of these findings would indicate that Mr. Larson has an intestinal obstruction?
○ 1. Fecal-smelling vomitus.
○ 2. Loose mucoid stools.
○ 3. Sharp epigastric pain.
○ 4. Fruity breath odor.

Tests reveal that Mr. Larson has an obstruction of the small bowel. A Miller-Abbott tube is to be inserted. He is scheduled for surgery.

6. Mr. Larson asks the practical nurse, "Why do I need this tube?" The nurse's response should include which statement about the Miller-Abbott tube?
○ 1. "It makes it easier to obtain gastric contents for examination."
○ 2. "It is used to prevent secretion of amylase in the intestines."
○ 3. "It will alter acid production in the stomach."
○ 4. "It is used to remove retained intestinal contents."

7. Because Mr. Larson has a Miller-Abbott tube, which of these measures should the practical nurse plan to take?
○ 1. Taping the tube to Mr. Larson's forehead.
○ 2. Irrigating the tube with saline solution at specified times.
○ 3. Connecting the tube to high intermittent suction.
○ 4. Maintaining Mr. Larson in semi-Fowler's position.

Mr. Larson has a small bowel resection for adhesions. After a short stay in the recovery room, he returns to his room. He has a wound (Penrose) drain and a nasogastric tube attached to low intermittent suction.

8. During the immediate postoperative period, which nursing diagnosis should take priority in Mr. Larson's care?
○ 1. Ineffective breathing pattern.
○ 2. Fluid volume deficit.
○ 3. Altered nutrition.
○ 4. Diarrhea.

9. On the second postoperative day, the practical nurse makes several observations. Which one suggests that Mr. Larson has a postoperative complication?
○ 1. Serous wound drainage.
○ 2. Weakness when ambulating.
○ 3. Abdominal distention.
○ 4. Muscle soreness.

Mr. Larson's condition improves. Before discharge, he receives instructions about a high-fiber diet.

10. Mr. Larson would show a correct understanding of his prescribed diet if he selects which of these foods for a high-fiber content?
○ 1. Cheese.
○ 2. White bread.
○ 3. Grapefruit.
○ 4. Broccoli.

Mrs. Janet Doral, age 23, suspects she is pregnant. She calls the prenatal clinic and makes an appointment for a pregnancy test.

11. Mrs. Doral has the pregnancy test. The presence of which of these hormones would confirm her pregnancy?
○ 1. Human chorionic gonadotropin.
○ 2. Progesterone.
○ 3. Follicle stimulating hormone (FSH).
○ 4. Luteinizing hormone (LH).

Mrs. Doral's pregnancy is confirmed; she is 8 weeks pregnant. This is her second pregnancy.

12. During the first trimester, which discomfort of pregnancy is Mrs. Doral most likely to experience?
○ 1. Shortness of breath.
○ 2. Dependent edema.
○ 3. Candidiasis.
○ 4. Urinary frequency.

13. After Mrs. Doral tells the practical nurse that she has nausea in the morning, she receives instructions for minimizing nausea. Which statement by Mrs. Doral indicates that she understands the instructions?
○ 1. "I will avoid drinking hot fluids with breakfast."
○ 2. "I will eat dry crackers before getting out of bed in the morning."
○ 3. "I will not drink fluids within an hour of bedtime."
○ 4. "I will have a protein snack, such as cheese, shortly before going to bed."

14. Which of these instructions about nutrition during a normal pregnancy should the practical nurse be sure to give Mrs. Doral?
○ 1. "You should avoid salt whenever possible, so do not use any salt in your cooking."
○ 2. "Limiting the amount of carbohydrate, such as bread, in your diet will improve your protein metabolism."
○ 3. "Peanut butter is a good source of protein to include in your diet."
○ 4. "You should avoid fats in your diet until after the delivery."

Mrs. Doral attends the prenatal clinic when she is 19 weeks pregnant.

15. While Mrs. Doral is on the examining table, she states that she is experiencing quickening. Which action should the practical nurse take?
○ 1. Inform the charge nurse of Mrs. Doral's complaint.
○ 2. Turn Mrs. Doral onto her left side.
○ 3. Reassure Mrs. Doral that quickening is normal.
○ 4. Remind Mrs. Doral that she may have bloody show now.

Mrs. Doral's pregnancy progresses well. At 38 weeks' gestation, she calls the prenatal clinic and states that her membranes have ruptured and she has not had any contractions. She is told to go to the clinic to determine the status of her membranes.

16. To confirm that Mrs. Doral's membranes have ruptured, the practical nurse should test the amniotic fluid for
○ 1. glucose.
○ 2. pH.
○ 3. color.
○ 4. albumin.

Mrs. Doral is admitted to the hospital and progresses to active labor. Her labor proceeds smoothly, and she delivers a girl.

17. Immediately after the neonate's birth, which of these goals takes priority?
○ 1. Clear her airway.
○ 2. Determine her Apgar scores.
○ 3. Initiate her identification.
○ 4. Maintain her body temperature.

Judy Watkins, age 2 months, is brought to the hospital by her mother because she has been vomiting her formula and passing watery green stools. Judy is admitted to the pediatric unit with a diagnosis of infectious diarrhea and dehydration. An I.V. infusion is started in a scalp vein; she is to have no oral intake.

18. During Judy's admission, which of the following actions should the practical nurse take first?
○ 1. Obtaining a specimen of Judy's stool.
○ 2. Measuring Judy's axillary temperature.
○ 3. Placing Judy on isolation precautions.
○ 4. Testing the specific gravity of Judy's urine.

19. Because Judy is dehydrated, the practical nurse would expect her to have which manifestation?
○ 1. Pulse of 100 beats/minute.
○ 2. Absence of tears when crying.
○ 3. Distended neck veins.
○ 4. Bulging anterior fontanel.

20. After noticing a slight swelling at the insertion site of Judy's I.V. line, the practical nurse should take which action?
○ 1. Stop the infusion.
○ 2. Place a warm soak on the area.
○ 3. Nothing; this is a normal finding.
○ 4. Report this finding to the nurse in charge.

21. The skin over Judy's buttocks appears red. Which measure most likely would prevent further excoriation?
○ 1. Exposing the area to air.
○ 2. Applying baby lotion to the area.
○ 3. Using disposable diapers only.
○ 4. Washing the area with warm water only.

Judy's condition improves.

22. Because of the usual way in which infants such as Judy contract infectious diarrhea, the practical nurse should make sure Mrs. Watkins receives instructions in which of these areas before discharge?
○ 1. Introducing solid foods to Judy's diet.
○ 2. Preparing and storing infant formula.
○ 3. Schedule of infant immunizations.
○ 4. Importance of well-baby checkups.

Cindy Davis, age 5, is admitted to the hospital with a tentative diagnosis of acute lymphocytic leukemia (ALL).

23. A common sign of leukemia in children is
○ 1. maculopapular rash.
○ 2. low-grade fever.
○ 3. photosensitivity.
○ 4. polydipsia.

24. Cindy is scheduled for a bone marrow aspiration. Which of the following approaches is the most effective way for the practical nurse to prepare Cindy for this procedure?
○ 1. Use a doll to show Cindy what will happen during the procedure.
○ 2. Tell Cindy a story about a little girl who had the procedure.
○ 3. Discuss the procedure with Cindy's parents and let them explain it to her.
○ 4. Find out from Cindy's parents if she knows anyone who has had this procedure.

The diagnosis of ALL is confirmed. Cindy is placed on a treatment regimen that includes prednisone (Liquid Pred), vincristine sulfate (Oncovin), and L-asparaginase (Elspar).

25. When Cindy's parents are informed of their daughter's diagnosis, they become angry and hostile toward the medical and nursing staff. The practical nurse should take which action when dealing with Cindy's parents?
○ 1. Tell them that their behavior is not helping Cindy.
○ 2. Help them cope with their feelings.
○ 3. Limit their visiting time with Cindy.
○ 4. Inform them that everything possible is being done to restore Cindy's health.

26. Cindy's platelet count is 20,000/mm³. Based on this information, the practical nurse should include which measure in her plan of care?
○ 1. Provide her with a diet high in iron.
○ 2. Use a hypoallergenic soap on her skin.
○ 3. Change her position every 2 hours.
○ 4. Check her for ecchymosis.

27. Cindy is scheduled to receive a blood transfusion. During the transfusion, she should be observed for signs and symptoms of a transfusion reaction, which include
○ 1. dizziness.
○ 2. chills.
○ 3. hypothermia.
○ 4. hyperreflexia.

28. Because Cindy is receiving vincristine sulfate, the practical nurse frequently should make which assessment?
○ 1. Quality of her pedal pulses.
○ 2. Character of her gait.
○ 3. Amount of glucose in her urine.
○ 4. Regularity of her respiratory rate.

Cindy is being prepared for discharge. She will continue the medication regimen in the outpatient clinic.

29. The practical nurse will know that Cindy's mother understands the teaching about prednisone if she makes which statement?
○ 1. "I will be sure to count Cindy's pulse every day."
○ 2. "Cindy won't be able to eat her favorite oatmeal for breakfast anymore."
○ 3. "I will keep Cindy away from people with colds."
○ 4. "Cindy will rest in bed every afternoon."

Mr. Vincent Taylor, age 72, is admitted to the hospital with symptoms of left-sided congestive heart failure. The physician orders digoxin (Lanoxin), 0.25 mg daily, and a low-sodium diet.

30. The practical nurse should expect Mr. Taylor to have which of these findings associated with left-sided heart failure?
○ 1. Tingling sensation in the fingers.
○ 2. Fluid in the lungs.
○ 3. Abdominal distention.
○ 4. Engorged neck veins.

31. Mr. Taylor is to be maintained on bed rest. Bed rest is ordered mainly for which purpose?
○ 1. To improve the heart's pumping action.
○ 2. To enhance oxygenation of the body tissues.
○ 3. To decrease blood volume throughout the body.
○ 4. To reduce the heart's work load.

32. Mr. Taylor receives instructions on foods with a low sodium content. The practical nurse will know that he understands these instructions if he selects which food as having the lowest sodium content?
○ 1. Tomato soup.
○ 2. Broiled lobster.
○ 3. Tapioca pudding.
○ 4. Fresh string beans.

33. Which of these measures must the practical nurse take when administering digoxin to Mr. Taylor?
○ 1. Give him the medication with a glass of orange juice.
○ 2. Check him for signs of hypokalemia before giving the medication.
○ 3. Instruct him to place the medication under his tongue.
○ 4. Withhold the medication if his pulse is less than 60 beats/minute.

34. The practical nurse should observe Mr. Turner for side effects of digoxin, which include
○ 1. blurred vision.
○ 2. hand tremors.
○ 3. urine retention.
○ 4. hearing loss.

Mrs. Marion David, age 78, is admitted to the hospital after developing signs and symptoms of a cerebrovascular accident (CVA). She is unconscious on admission. An I.V. infusion is started and a central venous pressure (CVP) line is inserted. Mrs. David has a history of hypertension.

35. When Mrs. David is admitted to the medical unit, the practical nurse should give priority to which goal?
○ 1. Preventing skin breakdown.
○ 2. Promoting urinary elimination.
○ 3. Maintaining a patent airway.
○ 4. Preserving muscle function.

36. The physician prescribes an I.V. infusion of 1,000 ml of 5% dextrose in water every 12 hours for Mrs. David. The I.V. setup delivers 15 gtt/ml. Approximately how many drops should be administered each minute?
○ 1. 18.
○ 2. 21.
○ 3. 24.
○ 4. 27.

After 24 hours, Mrs. David becomes fully conscious. A computerized tomography scan reveals a hemorrhage in the left midcerebral artery.

37. When assessing Mrs. David, the practical nurse most likely would expect which of the following findings?
○ 1. Paresthesia.
○ 2. Amnesia.
○ 3. Paraplegia.
○ 4. Hemiplegia.

38. Because Mrs. David has a history of hypertension, which finding would the practical nurse anticipate?
○ 1. A CVP of 8 cm H_2O.
○ 2. A pulse pressure of 40 mm Hg.
○ 3. A diastolic blood pressure of 96 mm Hg.
○ 4. A systolic blood pressure of 134 mm Hg.

Mrs. David's condition stabilizes. Her orders include clonidine hydrochloride (Catapres) and diet as tolerated.

39. Because Mrs. David is receiving clonidine hydrochloride, the practical nurse should take which action?
○ 1. Have Mrs. David change her position slowly.
○ 2. Give Mrs. David the medication before her meals.
○ 3. Encourage Mrs. David to increase her intake of orange juice.
○ 4. Offer Mrs. David a cup of tea with meals.

40. While visiting Mrs. David, her husband asks the practical nurse, "Why does my wife have a splint on her hand?" The practical nurse replies that the splint is necessary to prevent
○ 1. injury to the hand.
○ 2. deformity of the hand.
○ 3. muscle wasting in the hand.
○ 4. edema from developing in the hand.

Mr. Martin Pollard, age 56, is admitted to the hospital with severe signs and symptoms of pulmonary emphysema. He is scheduled for pulmonary function tests. His history reveals that he has smoked two packs of cigarettes a day for 30 years.

41. Because Mr. Pollard has emphysema, the practical nurse would expect him to have which of these signs?
○ 1. Persistent hoarseness.
○ 2. Inspiratory stridor.
○ 3. Night sweats.
○ 4. Barrel chest.

42. Mr. Pollard has trouble coughing up sputum; therefore, the practical nurse is to suction him through his nose. Which of these steps describes an **incorrect** suctioning technique?
○ 1. Lubricating the catheter with sterile water before passing it through the nose.
○ 2. Applying suction when withdrawing the catheter from the nose.
○ 3. Suctioning for no more than 20 seconds at a time.
○ 4. Rotating the catheter when withdrawing it.

43. Mr. Pollard is to receive oxygen by nasal cannula. Which measure would be appropriate for the practical nurse to take?
○ 1. Maintaining the oxygen flow rate at no more than 3 liters/minute.
○ 2. Increasing the oxygen flow rate up to 6 liters/minute, if required.
○ 3. Teaching Mr. Pollard to adjust the oxygen flow rate as needed.
○ 4. Changing Mr. Pollard's oxygen tubing every shift.

44. As the practical nurse assists Mr. Pollard with his breathing exercises, he says, "I don't feel any better. Why should I bother learning how to do these exercises?" The practical nurse should take which action?
○ 1. Tell Mr. Pollard that the physician ordered the exercises.
○ 2. Encourage Mr. Pollard to express his feelings.
○ 3. Ask Mr. Pollard if he would like to do the exercises at another time.
○ 4. Inform the physician of Mr. Pollard's statements.

45. When preparing Mr. Pollard for discharge, the practical nurse reminds him that he will have to stop smoking. Mr. Pollard replies angrily, "Who are you to tell me what to do? I'm older than you." Which response by the practical nurse would be appropriate?
○ 1. "I am giving you this information in your best interest."
○ 2. "You have the right to make your own decisions."
○ 3. "I do not mean to be disrespectful."
○ 4. "If you do not want to take the medical advice, you can do whatever you wish."

Brad Miller, age 18 months, is admitted to the hospital with a fractured femur of the right leg after falling down a flight of stairs. He is placed in Bryant's traction.

46. The practical nurse makes the following observations of Brad and his traction. Which one necessitates intervention?
○ 1. The weights are hanging freely over the foot of the crib.
○ 2. Brad's buttocks are resting on the crib mattress.
○ 3. The ropes are resting in the pulley grooves.
○ 4. Brad's legs are flexed at a 90-degree angle to his body.

47. Because Brad is in Bryant's traction, the practical nurse should include which measure in his care?
○ 1. Bathing him with a bland soap daily.
○ 2. Testing his urine for acetone once each shift.
○ 3. Checking the warmth and color of his toes every 2 hours.
○ 4. Keeping the side rails of his crib padded.

48. Brad must be observed for signs of a head injury because of the way in which his leg injury occurred. Signs of increased intracranial pressure (ICP) in a child of Brad's age include
○ 1. increasing irritability.
○ 2. tachycardia.
○ 3. narrowing pulse pressure.
○ 4. pinpoint pupils.

49. Brad will receive a regular diet. When feeding Brad, the practical nurse should use which approach?
○ 1. Adjust Brad's traction so that he can be turned to one side.
○ 2. Release Brad from traction so that he can sit upright.
○ 3. Ask Brad's mother about his favorite eating position.
○ 4. Maintain Brad in proper traction alignment.

50. To help prevent Brad from developing a common complication of immobility while in traction, the practical nurse should include which of these measures in his plan of care?
○ 1. Provide Brad with a high-fiber diet.
○ 2. Keep a soft light glowing in the corner of Brad's room.
○ 3. Measure Brad's abdominal girth routinely.
○ 4. Put Brad's legs through range-of-motion exercises during every shift.

Ms. Teresa Scott, age 26, is admitted to the hospital with acute pyelonephritis. A urine specimen is to be obtained for routine analysis. The physician's orders include gentamicin sulfate (Garamycin).

51. When assessing Ms. Scott for risk factors of pyelonephritis, the practical nurse should ask her which question?
○ 1. "Do you get cystitis frequently?"
○ 2. "Have you had a sore throat lately?"
○ 3. "Do you hold your urine for a long time before voiding?"
○ 4. "Have you taken any analgesics recently?"

52. Because Ms. Scott has pyelonephritis, the practical nurse would expect her urine to
○ 1. appear cloudy.
○ 2. contain a high level of glucose.
○ 3. show evidence of acetone.
○ 4. have an increased volume.

53. Because Ms. Scott is receiving gentamicin sulfate, the practical nurse should take which measure?
○ 1. Maintain her on bed rest.
○ 2. Decrease her intake of milk products.
○ 3. Increase her fluid intake.
○ 4. Check her urine for protein.

Mrs. Elizabeth Monroe, age 25, is admitted to the labor unit in early labor.

54. When planning care for Mrs. Monroe during the first phase of labor, the practical nurse should encourage Mrs. Monroe to
○ 1. lie on her left side.
○ 2. ambulate.
○ 3. accept pain medication.
○ 4. initiate breathing techniques immediately.

Mrs. Monroe's cervix is dilated 9 cm. She is connected to an external electronic fetal monitor.

55. Which observation concerning the fetal monitor tracing necessitates immediate intervention?
○ 1. Consistent variability of the baseline fetal heart rate.
○ 2. A change in the fetal heart rate that mirrors the uterine contraction.
○ 3. A deceleration of the fetal heart rate with delayed recovery after a uterine contraction.
○ 4. An acceleration of the fetal heart rate of 15 beats/minute lasting 15 seconds.

Mrs. Monroe's labor progresses, and she delivers a boy. After a brief stay in the postpartal recovery room, she is transferred to the postpartal unit. She expresses a wish to breast-feed.

56. Mrs. Monroe receives instructions on breast-feeding. Which statement indicates that she understands the instructions?
○ 1. "I should pull my baby's mouth from my nipple gently to detach him from my breast."
○ 2. "I should use cold compresses to relieve any breast discomfort between feedings."
○ 3. "I should clean my nipples with soap and water gently after each feeding."
○ 4. "I should alternate breasts when I start each feeding."

57. Mrs. Monroe's postpartal care should include periodic assessment for thrombophlebitis by determining if she has
○ 1. a discrepancy in the blood pressure readings of her legs.
○ 2. pain when her feet are dorsiflexed.
○ 3. limited range of motion of her legs.
○ 4. pitting edema in her lower extremities.

Mrs. Anna Barker, age 67, is admitted to the hospital after falling at home. X-rays confirm a fractured right hip. She is placed in Buck's traction and scheduled for an open reduction and internal fixation.

58. While Mrs. Barker is in Buck's traction, which measure should the practical nurse take?
○ 1. Maintain the head of Mrs. Barker's bed at a 45-degree angle.
○ 2. Ensure that Mrs. Barker's right heel touches the bed.
○ 3. Remove the weights when bathing Mrs. Barker's lower extremities.
○ 4. Allow the weights to hang freely at the foot of Mrs. Barker's bed.

59. On Mrs. Barker's admission to the hospital, which observation would represent an abnormal finding?
○ 1. Blood pressure of 112/78 mm Hg.
○ 2. Hemoglobin concentration of 10.2 g/dl.
○ 3. Blood urea nitrogen level of 18 mg/dl.
○ 4. Heart rate of 96 beats/minute.

60. Before surgery, Mrs. Barker receives promethazine hydrochloride (Phenergan) for which purpose?
○ 1. To provide sedation.
○ 2. To inhibit oral secretions.
○ 3. To prevent bleeding problems.
○ 4. To enhance wound healing.

The surgeon performs an open reduction and internal fixation of Mrs. Barker's right hip. After a short stay in the recovery room, Mrs. Barker is returned to her room. Her orders include a clear liquid diet after she becomes fully conscious.

61. After surgery, the practical nurse should maintain Mrs. Barker's affected leg in which position?
○ 1. External rotation.
○ 2. Abduction.
○ 3. Flexion.
○ 4. Hyperextension.

62. Because Mrs. Barker is to receive a clear liquid diet, the practical nurse should offer her which beverage?
○ 1. Coffee.
○ 2. Skim milk.
○ 3. Tea.
○ 4. Orange juice.

Mrs. Barker progresses well and receives instructions about self-care. She has learned to use a walker.

63. Which statement by Mrs. Barker indicates that she needs additional teaching about self-care?
○ 1. "I will wear slippers when walking around the house."
○ 2. "I will limit the number of times I use the stairs in my house."
○ 3. "I will eat a high-fiber diet."
○ 4. "I will continue to do my leg exercises several times a day."

Stop. This is the end of the pretest.

Answers and rationales

The question number appears in **bold** type. The number of the correct answer appears in parentheses ( ) immediately after the question number. Rationales for correct answers and, when appropriate, incorrect answers follow.

To help you evaluate your knowledge base and application of nursing behaviors, each question has been classified as follows:

NP = Phase of the nursing process
CN = Client need.

At the end of this section you'll find the *Pretest self-diagnostic analysis* worksheet, page 17. In the boxes at the top, next to "QUESTION NUMBER," write the numbers of questions you answered incorrectly. Beneath each question number, place check marks in the appropriate boxes corresponding to the reason you answered incorrectly (test-taking skill) as well as the category of patient need and nursing process. Then enter the total number of checks on each line in the "TOTALS" box in the far right column of the worksheet. You now have an individualized profile of weak areas requiring further study (or special attention, if you're taking a review course). By undertaking further study, you'll be totally confident of your success on the day you take NCLEX-PN.

1. (1) Before a pelvic examination, the patient should void to empty her bladder. The procedures in answers 2, 3, and 4 are not necessary before a pelvic examination.
NP: Implementation
CN: Safe, effective care environment

2. (4) A cone-shaped piece of tissue will be removed from the cervix to be examined for suspicious cells. Answers 1, 2, and 3 are incorrect. Schiller's iodine test involves staining the cervix with an iodine solution. In dilatation and curettage, the uterus is scraped. A laparoscopy involves insertion of a fiberoptic instrument into the peritoneal cavity.
NP: Evaluation
CN: Safe, effective care environment

3. (1) To prevent pelvic congestion, the client should not be placed in a high Fowler's position. Answers 2, 3, and 4 are desirable positions that do not contribute to pelvic congestion.
NP: Planning
CN: Physiologic integrity

4. (3) The client having an upper GI series has X-rays of the stomach taken after swallowing barium, a radiopaque substance. Answers 1, 2, and 4 are incorrect because they do not relate to a GI series. A gastroscopy involves passage of a gastroscope through the mouth into the stomach to observe the gastric mucosa. A client takes radiopaque tablets the evening before a gallbladder series. Scans are taken after a radioactive substance is given.
NP: Evaluation
CN: Safe, effective care environment

5. (1) The client with an intestinal obstruction usually has nausea and vomiting; vomiting may be violent and the vomitus may have a fecal odor. Answer 2 is incorrect because the obstruction prevents passage of gas or stools. Answer 3 is incorrect because the client usually reports crampy abdominal pain, not sharp epigastric pain. Answer 4 is incorrect because fruity breath odor is associated with ketoacidosis, and breath odor does not reflect bowel function.
NP: Data collection
CN: Physiologic integrity

6. (4) Miller-Abbott tubes are used for intestinal suction to remove GI contents backed up from an obstruction. Answers 1, 2, and 3 have no bearing on the purpose of the Miller-Abbott tube.
NP: Implementation
CN: Safe, effective care environment

7. (2) To help advance the tube along the obstructed intestine, the physician may want to irrigate it. Answers 1, 3, and 4 are incorrect measures to take relative to a Miller-Abbott tube. Because the tube will be advanced, it should not be secured to the client (answer 1). The tube is connected to low, not high, suction (answer 3). The client should be repositioned frequently to facilitate the tube's passage, not kept in semi-Fowler's position (answer 4).
NP: Implementation
CN: Physiologic integrity

8. (1) An ineffective breathing pattern is a dangerous complication that can occur in a client recovering from general anesthesia. Fluid volume deficit (answer 2) may cause a problem, but it does not take priority over ineffective breathing pattern. Answers 3 and 4 do not represent immediate postoperative problems.
NP: Planning
CN: Safe, effective care environment

9. (3) Postoperative persistent abdominal distention may indicate a serious condition, such as paralytic ileus. Answers 1, 2, and 4 describe expected outcomes following surgery. Serous wound drainage (answer 1) is expected with a Penrose drain; postoperative clients commonly complain of weakness (answer 2); and muscle soreness (answer 4) usually results from positioning during surgery.
NP: Data collection
CN: Physiologic integrity

10. (4) One cup of cooked broccoli contains a moderate amount of total dietary fiber. Answers 1, 2, and 3 are incorrect because cheese, white bread, and grapefruit contain smaller amounts of total dietary fiber.
NP: Evaluation
CN: Physiologic integrity

11. (1) Human chorionic gonadotropin is produced by the placenta and appears in maternal blood or urine 10 to 12 days after conception. Answers 2, 3, and 4 are incorrect because progesterone, FSH, and LH are hormones of the menstrual cycle. (Progesterone is an important hormone of pregnancy as well.)
NP: Data collection
CN: Health promotion and maintenance

12. (4) Urinary frequency is common during both early and late pregnancy because of bladder compression by the uterus. Answers 1, 2, and 3 do not describe common discomforts of the first trimester.
NP: Data collection
CN: Health promotion and maintenance

13. (2) Eating dry crackers immediately before getting out of bed helps to control nausea. Answers 1, 3, and 4 do not minimize nausea.
NP: Evaluation
CN: Health promotion and maintenance

14. (3) Nuts are good sources of protein. Answers 1, 2, and 4 are incorrect because fats, carbohydrates, and salt are important to the diet of a pregnant woman.
NP: Implementation
CN: Health promotion and maintenance

15. (3) Quickening is the pregnant woman's first awareness of fetal movement. Answers 1, 2, and 4 describe inappropriate actions relative to quickening.
NP: Implementation
CN: Health promotion and maintenance

16. (2) The nitrazine test differentiates amniotic fluid, which is alkaline, from urine or vaginal secretions, which are acidic. Answers 1, 3, and 4 are not indicators of membrane rupture.
NP: Data collection
CN: Health promotion and maintenance

17. (1) Establishing a patent airway takes priority. Answers 2, 3, and 4 are important but are not priorities.
NP: Planning
CN: Health promotion and maintenance

18. (3) Infectious diarrhea is highly contagious, and all persons on the pediatric unit should be protected from exposure. Therefore, placing the client on isolation precautions is the first action the practical nurse should take. Answers 1 and 2 are actions to take after isolating the client. Answer 4 also may be required.
NP: Planning
CN: Safe, effective care environment

19. (2) In a child of this age (2 months), absence of tears when crying indicates dehydration. A pulse rate of 100 beats/minute (answer 1) is within normal limits, whereas dehydration causes a rapid pulse rate (above 160 beats/minute in an infant of 2 months). Distended neck veins (answer 3) and bulging fontanels (answer 4) are signs of overhydration.
NP: Data collection
CN: Physiologic integrity

20. (4) Swelling is a possible sign of infiltration of fluids at the I.V. insertion site. The nurse in charge should be informed of this finding so that a decision can be made about further actions. Answers 1, 2, and 3 are not appropriate measures.
NP: Implementation
CN: Safe, effective care environment

21. (1) Exposure to air allows the skin to dry and heal. Bacteria grow best in a warm, moist environment, which is encouraged by the actions described in answers 2 and 3. Answer 4 will not remove the offending bacteria.
NP: Implementation
CN: Physiologic integrity

22. (2) Infants in this age-group most commonly contract infectious diarrhea through improper preparation, handling, or storage of infant formula. Answers 1, 3, and 4 are important topics to discuss with mothers of young infants but do not relate directly to preventing infectious diarrhea.
NP: Implementation
CN: Health promotion and maintenance

23. (2) Most children with ALL have a low-grade fever. Answers 1, 3, and 4 are not common signs of leukemia.
NP: Data collection
CN: Physiologic integrity

24. (1) Typically, the cognitive development of a five-year-old child is at the preoperational level; the child has trouble understanding anything beyond her own experience. Using a doll provides a near-life experience, giving her both an understanding and a sense of control. Answers 2, 3, and 4 require abstract thinking, which the child is too young to accomplish.
NP: Implementation
CN: Safe, effective care environment

25. (2) Parents of a child with a catastrophic illness typically feel guilty about the child's illness and wonder whether any action they took (or failed to take) might have caused it. To cope with their guilt feelings, they may become angry at those around them—particularly health care providers. At this time, they need help in dealing with their feelings. Answers 1 and 3 serve only to chastise them, not help them. Answer 4 does not respond to their needs.
NP: Planning
CN: Psychosocial integrity

26. (4) A normal platelet count for a child age 5 ranges from 150,000 to 400,000/mm³. Leukemia typically causes an extremely low platelet count, predisposing the child to hemorrhage. The child should be checked frequently for signs of hemorrhage, including ecchymosis. The measures described in answers 1, 2, and 3 are not associated with a low platelet count.
NP: Data collection
CN: Physiologic integrity

27. (2) Chills are a classic sign of a transfusion reaction. Answers 1, 3, and 4 are not associated with transfusion reactions.
NP: Data collection
CN: Physiologic integrity

28. (2) Neurotoxicity is a side effect of vincristine sulfate and commonly manifests as ataxia. Answers 1, 3, and 4 do not reflect neurotoxicity.
NP: Evaluation
CN: Physiologic integrity

29. (3) Prednisone increases the child's susceptibility to infections, as does leukemia. Keeping infected people away from the child is a good preventive measure. Answers 1, 2, and 4 describe unnecessary limitations or activities.
NP: Evaluation
CN: Physiologic integrity

30. (2) When the left side of the heart fails, fluid accumulates in the lungs, causing dyspnea. Answers 1, 3, and 4 are signs of right-sided heart failure.
NP: Data collection
CN: Physiologic integrity

31. (4) Bed rest reduces tissue demands for oxygen and decreases the heart's work load. Answer 1 is incorrect because digitalis is used to improve the heart's pumping ability. Answer 2 is incorrect because oxygen therapy is used to enhance oxygenation of the body's tissues. Answer 3 is incorrect because diuretics are prescribed to decrease the blood volume.
NP: Planning
CN: Physiologic integrity

32. (4) Vegetables have a low sodium content. Answers 1, 2, and 3 are incorrect because these foods each have more than 150 mg of sodium in an average portion and should be avoided by a client on a sodium-restricted diet.
NP: Evaluation
CN: Physiologic integrity

33. (4) Before administering digoxin (or another digitalis preparation), the practical nurse must take the client's apical pulse for a full minute. If the pulse rate is below 60 or above 120 beats/minute, the practical nurse should withhold the medication and inform the charge nurse. Answer 1 is incorrect because digoxin does not have to be taken with food or beverages. Answer 2 is incorrect because although digoxin may affect serum potassium levels, these levels should be monitored routinely, negating the need for daily checks for hypokalemia. Answer 3 is incorrect because the sublingual route is not an appropriate administration route for a digitalis preparation.
NP: Planning
CN: Physiologic integrity

34. (1) Side effects of digoxin include nausea, vomiting, anorexia, and visual disturbances, such as blurred or yellow vision. Answers 2, 3, and 4 are not among the known side effects of digoxin.
NP: Evaluation
CN: Physiologic integrity

35. (3) When a client is comatose or unconscious, maintaining a patent airway is a priority. Although answers 1, 2, and 4 are goals in caring for a comatose client, they are not priorities.
NP: Planning
CN: Physiologic integrity

36. (2) 1,000 ml in 12 hours equals 84 ml/hour, or 1.4 ml/minute. 1.4 × 15 = 21 gtt/min. Answers 1, 3, and 4 are calculated incorrectly.
NP: Implementation
CN: Physiologic integrity

37. (4) Hemiplegia—loss of function on one side of the body—occurs in clients who have had a CVA involving a hemorrhage in the left midcerebral artery. Answers 1, 2, and 3 do not result from damage to the midcerebral artery.
NP: Data collection
CN: Physiologic integrity

38. (3) A diastolic pressure above 90 mm Hg or a persistent systolic pressure above 140 mm Hg indicates hypertension. Answer 1 is incorrect because normal CVP is 4 to 10 cm H_2O. Answer 2 is incorrect because normal pulse pressure is 40 to 50 mm Hg. Answer 4 is incorrect because a systolic pressure of 134 mm Hg is within the normal range.
NP: Data collection
CN: Physiologic integrity

39. (1) A client receiving an antihypertensive medication should change position slowly to prevent postural hypotension. Answer 2 is incorrect because clonidine hydrochloride can be taken before or after meals. Answer 3 is incorrect because no therapeutic justification exists for taking this drug with orange juice. Answer 4 is incorrect because overuse of tea and other stimulants should be discouraged.
NP: Implementation
CN: Physiologic integrity

40. (2) Fingers of the affected hand should be extended and the hand and wrist placed in a functional position to prevent deformity. Answers 1, 3, and 4 are not primary reasons for splinting the hand.
NP: Implementation
CN: Physiologic integrity

41. (4) The client with emphysema develops an enlarged, or barrel, chest from trapping of air, loss of lung elasticity, and breakdown of alveolar walls. Persistent hoarseness (answer 1) occurs in laryngitis; inspiratory stridor (answer 2) results from partial obstruction of the larynx or trachea; and night sweats (answer 3) occur in clients with tuberculosis.
NP: Data collection
CN: Physiologic integrity

42. (3) Suctioning should not exceed 10 to 12 seconds; suctioning for 20 seconds would make the client hypoxic. Answers 1, 2, and 4 describe correct suctioning techniques.
NP: Implementation
CN: Safe, effective care environment

43. (1) A client with emphysema who requires oxygen should receive a maximum of 2 to 3 liters/minute. Therefore, answers 2, 3, and 4 are incorrect.
NP: Implementation
CN: Safe, effective care environment

44. (2) Clients who are upset with their regimen should be given the opportunity to ventilate their feelings. Answers 1, 3, and 4 do not respond to the client's feelings.
NP: Implementation
CN: Psychosocial integrity

45. (3) When a client becomes angry and resents a younger health care provider's advice to give up a lifelong habit, the practical nurse should apologize, assuring the client that the intent was not to ridicule or belittle. Answers 1, 2, and 4 would antagonize the client rather than reduce his anger.
NP: Implementation
CN: Psychosocial integrity

46. (2) Proper countertraction occurs when the child's buttocks are raised approximately 2″ (5.1 cm) above the mattress. Answers 1, 3, and 4 do not require intervention; answers 1 and 3 describe proper traction apparatus, and answer 4 describes the correct alignment for a child in Bryant's traction.
NP: Evaluation
CN: Safe, effective care environment

47. (3) Bryant's traction is applied with elastic bandages; bandages that are wrapped too tightly may impair circulation. Warm toes with good color indicate adequate circulation. Answers 1, 2, and 4 are irrelevant to Bryant's traction.
NP: Implementation
CN: Physiologic integrity

48. (1) In a child Brad's age, increasing irritability suggests that the headache is associated with ICP. Answers 2, 3, and 4 describe findings opposite those expected in a child with ICP.
NP: Data collection
CN: Physiologic integrity

49. (4) For Bryant's traction to be effective, it must be continuous, with the child in proper traction alignment. Answers 1 and 2 would interfere with proper traction. Answer 3 is inappropriate because even if the practical nurse knows Brad's favorite feeding position, Brad would have to be fed while in proper traction alignment.
NP: Implementation
CN: Safe, effective care environment

50. (1) Constipation is a common complication of immobility; a high-fiber diet helps prevent constipation. Answers 2 and 3 would not prevent a complication of immobility. Range-of-motion exercises (answer 4) would be impossible without interrupting traction.
NP: Planning
CN: Physiologic integrity

51. (1) Pyelonephritis is a complication of a lower urinary tract infection, such as cystitis or urethritis. Answers 2, 3, and 4 may reveal information about other renal problems but would not elicit information relevant to pyelonephritis.
NP: Data collection
CN: Physiologic integrity

52. (1) Signs of pyelonephritis may include hematuria, cloudy urine, and pus in the urine (pyuria). Answers 2, 3, and 4 are not associated with pyelonephritis.
NP: Data collection
CN: Physiologic integrity

53. (3) Clients receiving gentamicin sulfate should have an increased fluid intake and maintain good hydration to prevent chemical irritation of the renal tubules. Answers 1 and 2 are incorrect because activity and dairy foods need not be limited. Answer 4 is incorrect because creatinine clearance — not protein in the urine — should be determined.
NP: Planning
CN: Physiologic integrity

54. (2) During the first phase of labor, ambulation helps stimulate labor. Answers 1 and 3 are incorrect because lying down and taking pain medications may slow early labor. Answer 4 is incorrect because breathing techniques should begin only after the client can no longer talk through her contractions.
NP: Planning
CN: Health promotion and maintenance

55. (3) A decrease in the fetal heart rate after the start of a uterine contraction with a delayed recovery indicates fetal hypoxia and necessitates immediate intervention. Answer 1 is incorrect because an irregular baseline fetal heart rate and occasional short accelerations are normal. Answer 2 is a sign of fetal head compression, which is normal during this phase of labor. Answer 4 is incorrect because an acceleration of the fetal heart rate of 15 beats/minute lasting 15 seconds is normal.
NP: Implementation
CN: Health promotion and maintenance

56. (4) Alternating the breasts with each breast-feeding promotes emptying of milk from each breast. Answer 1 is incorrect because pulling the baby from the breast before suction is broken can cause nipple trauma. Answer 2 is incorrect because warm — not cold — compresses should be used. Answer 3 is incorrect because soap and water will dry the nipple.
NP: Evaluation
CN: Health promotion and maintenance

57. (2) Pain elicited by dorsiflexing the foot (positive Homan's sign) indicates thrombophlebitis. Answers 1, 3, and 4 are incorrect because blood pressure discrepancies of the legs, dependent edema, and limited range of motion do not indicate thrombophlebitis.
NP: Data collection
CN: Health promotion and maintenance

58. (4) Weights on a traction apparatus should hang freely and unobstructed. Answer 1 is incorrect because the head of the bed should be elevated no more than 30 degrees. Answer 2 is incorrect because the affected heel should be raised off the bed. Answer 3 is incorrect because the weights should not be removed from traction.
NP: Planning
CN: Physiologic integrity

59. (2) A normal hemoglobin concentration for a woman is 12 to 16 g/dl. Answer 1 is incorrect because a blood pressure of 112/78 mm Hg is within the normal range. Answer 3 is incorrect because a normal blood urea nitrogen level is 10 to 20 mg/dl. Answer 4 is incorrect because a normal heart rate ranges from 60 to 100 beats/minute.
NP: Data collection
CN: Physiologic integrity

60. (1) Promethazine hydrochloride is an antihistamine with prominent sedative effects. Answers 2, 3, and 4 are not indications for promethazine hydrochloride.
NP: Planning
CN: Safe, effective care environment

61. (2) A client who has had surgery for a fractured hip should have an abduction splint or pillows placed between the legs to separate them. Answers 1, 3, and 4 are incorrect positions.
NP: Implementation
CN: Physiologic integrity

62. (3) A clear liquid diet allows only tea, broth, gelatin dessert, and other "clear" liquids. Answers 1, 2, and 4 are not clear liquids.
NP: Implementation
CN: Physiologic integrity

63. (1) Loose-fitting bedroom slippers may cause the client to trip and fall. Answers 2, 3, and 4 are expected self-care activities for a client with a hip fracture.
NP: Evaluation
CN: Physiologic integrity

Pretest self-diagnostic analysis

QUESTION NUMBER																											TOTALS
Test-taking skills																											
1. Misread question																											
2. Missed important point																											
3. Forgot fact or concept																											
4. Applied wrong fact or concept																											
5. Drew wrong conclusion																											
6. Incorrectly evaluated distractors																											
7. Mistakenly filled in wrong circle																											
8. Read into question																											
9. Guessed wrong																											
10. Misunderstood question																											
Client need																											
1. Safe, effective care environment																											
2. Physiologic integrity																											
3. Psychosocial integrity																											
4. Health promotion and maintenance																											
Nursing process																											
1. Collecting data																											
2. Planning																											
3. Implementing																											
4. Evaluating																											

Part II

Taking NCLEX-PN

Part II

Taking NCLEX-PN

Introduction 20

NCLEX-PN test plan 20

Strategies for success 23

Introduction

Entry into the practice of practical/vocational nursing (LPN, LVN) in the United States and its territories is regulated by licensing authorities in each jurisdiction. Candidates for licensure must pass a written examination that measures the competencies needed by practical nurses to practice safe, effective nursing. Jurisdictions holding membership in the National Council of State Boards of Nursing (NCSBN) use the National Council Licensure Examination for Practical Nurses (NCLEX-PN). A candidate wishing to take the examination must apply to the state in which the candidate intends to practice.

NCLEX-PN is administered twice each year, in April and October. The examination consists of approximately 240 multiple-choice items. A completely new examination is developed for each test date. Most test items appear as case situations, similar to the items in the Pretest and the National League for Nursing (NLN) Practice Test for PN Licensure in this book. Because most test items require the examinee to apply nursing knowledge in patient care situations, answering correctly requires more than simple recall of facts.

Examinees can expect to see their results 6 to 8 weeks after taking the test. Results are reported to the examinee as *Pass* or *Fail*. Failed candidates receive a graph of their performance, which shows how far short it fell of the passing mark.

NCLEX-PN test plan

NCLEX-PN questions follow a test plan, or blueprint, that organizes the content into two broad categories and specifies the percentage of items to be included in each category. The two categories are nursing process (four steps) and client needs (four types). Each question on the test matches one step of the nursing process and one type of client need.

Nursing process

The phrase *nursing process* refers to a method of applying the art and science of nursing to caring for individuals and groups of clients. NCLEX-PN measures four steps of the nursing process—collecting data (assessment), planning, implementing, and evaluating. The test emphasizes care of clients with commonly occurring health problems having predictable outcomes. The outline below shows the percentage of test items in each category, as well as examples of specific nursing behaviors associated with each step of the nursing process, according to the latest (1989) NCSBN Test Plan of the NCLEX-PN.

A. Collecting data (30% of the test): Contribute to the development of a data base by gathering objective and subjective information about the client.
• Observe the physiologic, psychosocial, health, and safety needs of the client.
• Collect information from the client, significant others, health team members, and records.
• Determine the need for more information.
• Communicate findings of data collected.
B. Planning (20% of the test): Contribute to setting goals of care to meet the client's needs.
• Contribute to developing a nursing care plan for the client with health needs.
• Assist in formulating goals.

• Participate in identifying the client's needs and nursing measures required to achieve goals.
• Communicate needs that may necessitate changes in the care plan.
• Communicate with the client, significant others, and health team members in planning nursing care.

C. Implementing (30% of the test): Initiate and complete actions necessary to accomplish the defined goals.
• Perform basic therapeutic and preventive nursing measures by following a plan of care to achieve established client goals.
• Provide a safe and effective care environment.
• Assist the client, significant others, and health care members to understand the client's plan of care.
• Record client information and report it to other health team members.

D. Evaluating (20% of the test): Participate in determining the extent to which nursing care has achieved its goals.
• Participate in evaluating the effectiveness of the client's nursing care.
• Assist in evaluating the client's response to nursing care and in making appropriate alterations.
• Evaluate the extent to which identified outcomes of the care plan have been achieved.
• Record and describe the client's responses to therapy and care.

Client needs

In the second content category of the NCLEX-PN test plan, client health needs fall into four groups: (1) safe, effective care environment; (2) physiologic integrity; (3) psychosocial integrity; and (4) health promotion and maintenance. This classification resulted from an analysis of a large-scale job survey of nursing practice (Kane and Colton, 1988). Also based on this analysis, each type of patient need is assigned a weight (percentage of items) for representation on the total test. The breakdown below shows the percentage of test items in each category, with examples of specific nursing behaviors associated with each step of the nursing process, in accordance with the latest (1989) NCSBN Test Plan of NCLEX-PN.

Safe, effective care environment (24% to 30% of the test). The practical nurse assists in meeting the client's needs by promoting environmental safety, coordinated and goal-oriented care, and safe and effective treatments and procedures.

Physiologic integrity (42% to 48% of the test). The practical nurse assists in meeting the physiologic integrity needs of the client with common health problems that occur throughout the life cycle and have predictable outcomes by providing basic care, reducing risk potential, and promoting mobility and comfort.

Psychosocial integrity (7% to 13% of the test). The practical nurse assists in meeting the client's needs for psychosocial integrity by promoting coping skills and psychosocial adaptation.

Health promotion and maintenance (15% to 21% of the test). The practical nurse assists in meeting the client's needs throughout the life cycle by promoting continued growth and development, self-care, integrity of support systems, and prevention and early treatment of disease.

Sample questions

The following sample questions illustrate how test items are written and coded according to the nursing process (NP) and client needs (CN) categories. The correct answer is indicated by an asterisk (*).

Mary Watkins, age 76, is admitted to the hospital with degenerative osteoarthritis. She is scheduled for a left hip replacement.

1. Because Mrs. Watkins will receive an antibiotic postoperatively, the practical nurse must obtain her
1. current weight.
2. resting blood pressure.
3. cardiac status.
*4. allergy history.
NP: Collecting data
CN: Safe, effective care environment

2. Mrs. Watkins undergoes the left hip replacement. On the second postoperative day, she tells the practical nurse that she has some tenderness in her left calf. The practical nurse should take which action?
1. Compare the reflexes of Mrs. Watkins' left leg with those of her right leg.
*2. Find out if Mrs. Watkins has pain when she dorsiflexes her left foot.
3. Determine if Mrs. Watkins has a left popliteal pulse.
4. Measure how high Mrs. Watkins can raise her left leg before the muscles tighten.
NP: Collecting data
CN: Physiologic integrity

John Perry, age 64, is admitted to the medical unit with a myocardial infarction. He is given a stat dose of morphine sulfate for chest pain. His orders include bed rest, morphine sulfate 10 mg S.C. q 3 h, and oxygen by nasal cannula, 3 liters/minute.

3. Besides controlling pain, which of these goals should take priority in planning Mr. Perry's care at the time of his admission?
*1. Minimizing his energy expenditure.
2. Increasing his urine output.
3. Improving his understanding of the disease process.
4. Decreasing his cholesterol level.
NP: Planning
CN: Physiologic integrity

4. Mr. Perry complains of chest pain. The practical nurse determines that he received morphine sulfate 2 hours ago. Which of these actions should the practical nurse take next?
1. Increase the oxygen to 5 liters/minute.
2. Lower the head of Mr. Perry's bed.
3. Offer Mr. Perry a carbonated beverage.
*4. Notify the nurse in charge.
NP: Implementing
CN: Safe, effective care environment

Annette Davis is admitted to the hospital during her thirty-ninth week of pregnancy. Her labor progresses normally, and she delivers a girl. Mrs. Davis is transferred to the postpartum unit and Baby Girl Davis is transferred to the nursery. Mrs. Davis plans to breast-feed her baby.

5. Which of these behaviors most strongly indicates that Mrs. Davis is bonding with her baby?

1. She changes the baby's diaper when wet.
*2. She holds the baby close to her during and after breast-feeding.
3. She gives the baby her mother's name.
4. She frequently talks to her friends about the baby.
NP: Collecting data
CN: Psychosocial integrity

6. Mrs. Davis and her baby are about to be discharged when Mrs. Davis makes the following comments to the nurse. Which one indicates that she needs instruction?
1. "I expect that I will have some pink vaginal discharge for about 10 days."
2. "I'm going to express my milk once in a while so that someone else can feed the baby when I'm out for a few hours."
*3. "I won't have to worry about getting pregnant while I'm breast-feeding."
4. "I expect to resume swimming after I've been home for a couple of months."
NP: Evaluation
CN: Health promotion and maintenance

Strategies for success

Preparing for the examination

Graduation from a practical nursing program is one important step toward realizing your career goal of becoming a licensed practical nurse. However, to practice as an LPN, you first must pass the PN licensure examination (NCLEX-PN).

Examination readiness involves three areas of preparedness: intellectual, physical, and emotional. Become test-wise. On an intellectual level, prepare for the test by conducting a thorough overall review of basic nursing skills and knowledge. If you plan to study on your own, work in an organized fashion, using a schedule. If you plan to take a review course, listen carefully to the material presented, question the instructor, and participate actively. Pay attention to content that seems unclear, and devote special attention to areas in which you identify a weakness. To evaluate your weak areas and your need for further study, take the Pretest and NLN Practice Test for PN Licensure in this book.

Because physical and emotional preparedness also influence test performance, these are important factors in success. Be sure you have completed the procedures for filing the required application and paying the appropriate test fee. To avoid last-minute searching, keep all the necessary papers, such as your examination permit, in a safe place. If possible, visit the examination site sometime before you take the NCLEX-PN. That way, you'll know the route and how much time you'll need to get there. Investigate nearby parking and restaurant facilities. If you'll need overnight accommodations, arrange them well in advance.

The night before the examination, gather everything you'll need, such as your examination permit, a watch, gum, candy, and tissues. Plan to take a sweater with you in case the temperature of the testing room fluctuates. (You don't want to worry about how hot or cold you are when you should be concentrating on the test questions.) Get a good night's rest and eat a nourishing breakfast.

Plan to arrive at the examination site early. If you can select a seat, select one toward the front and center of the room to be sure you can hear—and carefully follow—the examiner's instructions.

After distributing the test, the examiner usually reads the directions aloud. Read the directions carefully together with the examiner, and follow them exactly. If you have questions about the directions, ask the examiner before the test begins. Like any examinee, you may feel somewhat anxious about taking NCLEX-PN, because the test is important for entry into practice. Mild anxiety, which increases alertness and attentiveness, can improve your test performance. Excess anxiety, on the other hand, can have a negative effect. Fortunately, by applying some simple practices, you can reduce excess anxiety. For instance, try a simple relaxation technique, such as rhythmic breathing or progressive muscle relaxation.

As you take the sample tests in this book, practice relaxation exercises and positive imagery. Tell yourself that you are a competent nurse, and picture yourself answering questions successfully. Avoid becoming distracted by the behavior of others around you, especially examinees who manifest extreme anxiety. By keeping your anxiety under control, you will concentrate better on the test items. The good feelings that accompany tension reduction will boost your confidence.

Ensuring a positive outcome

Examinations of nursing knowledge most commonly present a patient situation followed by several questions about appropriate nursing actions in the situation described. Taking practice tests and learning specific strategies to deal with multiple-choice test items will help you to select the best response.

First, read the patient situation carefully to get a clear picture of the situation. Next, read the question (stem) with equal care. Pay particular attention to key words in the stem, such as *first, best, highest priority,* and *most important.* For example, suppose a question asks what the nurse should do *first* in a particular situation. You probably will find two or three answers or options that the nurse should do promptly. However, the question asks which one to do *first,* so you must make a judgment.

Avoid reading into the test item something that isn't there, but don't overlook what *is* there. The information you see is your *only* information. Base your answer solely on this information—no more, no less. Take care not to jump to a false conclusion just because something sounds familiar.

Read all four options carefully before making a selection. If you choose the first option as the correct one without reading the others, you'll deny yourself the chance to evaluate the other options—one of which might be an even better response. Consider how each option completes the question or statement, asking yourself if that choice seems reasonable. As you read the stem, decide which option most closely resembles your response. If you don't find among the choices the answer you think is correct, remember that you're looking for the **best answer among those given**—perhaps not the best *possible* answer, but your best choice among the available options.

What if two responses seem equally good? Compare them. How do they differ? Because you can select only one, you must reread both. If you still can't discriminate, make an educated guess from the two most likely choices (you won't lose points for guessing). Also note the question number so that you can reevaluate the response later, if you have time. Don't waste time trying to "overthink" the question.

With the most difficult questions—those for which you have no idea of the correct answer—first take a deep breath. Then remind yourself that you have a wealth of information about nursing that may help you with the answer. Try to transfer your knowledge about a similar situation to the situation in the question. Take, for example, a question about chest tubes—a subject you think you know nothing about. Instead of giving up on the question, think about other tubes that you *do* know something about (such as urinary or nasogastric tubes). Then consider the common principles that apply to all drainage tubes—for example, they should be patent. Does knowledge of this principle help you to select the correct answer? At the least, it may help you to eliminate some incorrect options. Also, when you encounter a difficult question, keep in mind that you don't have to answer every question correctly to pass the examination.

If you develop a mental block or forget the relevant nursing knowledge or principle, note the question number and proceed to the next item. You may find that a later item stimulates recall, allowing you to return to this unanswered question and select an appropriate response.

If you change an answer, be sure to erase carefully, because the test will be scored with an electronic scanning machine that can't determine the intended answer when erasures show. Before turning in your test materials, also check that you have completely filled in all requested information.

Like most other standardized tests, NCLEX-PN is timed. Pace yourself accordingly, using your wristwatch. For a standardized test, allot an average of 1 minute to answer each question. Some questions will take only a few seconds to read and answer; others will take longer. (To prepare yourself for performance pressure on test day, pace yourself as you practice taking the sample tests in this book.) Don't be tempted to reflect for 5 minutes on a difficult item; instead, move along, answer those questions you can, and return later to the more complex items.

Be sure to use all the time allotted. Don't be distracted by examinees around you who finish the test and leave the room ahead of you. Remember — those who finish early don't necessarily answer the questions correctly; in fact, they may leave early in frustration because they *can't* answer the questions, and expect to fail the test.

If you have time remaining at the end of the test, go back and reexamine any unanswered questions. If you can't decide how to respond to a particular question and have time to review it, read the stem and then the first option. Repeat this process with each remaining option. This allows you to evaluate each option specifically by formulating a complete statement from the stem and the options.

Do not expect glaring flaws in the writing of test items. Whereas tests written by your teachers in school may contain one response that is much longer or shorter than the others, NCLEX-PN presents uniformly written and carefully edited options.

NCLEX-PN is an integrated test, which means that it's *not* divided according to content areas. Therefore, expect to shift your focus from a patient of one age, diagnosis, and nursing care need to another patient of a different age, diagnosis, and nursing care need. This test design reflects the competent nurse's ability to meet the needs of different patients in various settings.

The National Council of State Boards of Nursing has designed the examination format carefully. Basic beliefs about human beings and nursing — such as the right of each patient to expect safe, high-quality nursing care — are intrinsic to the NCLEX-PN test plan. Items included in NCLEX-PN relate to today's nursing practice and reflect health care problems seen in hospitals, nursing homes, and other settings.

The concepts integrated throughout NCLEX-PN include those emphasized throughout your nursing education as essential to sound nursing practice. These concepts include basic human needs, health problems, and the effects of age and culture on health care. NCLEX-PN also tests your knowledge of nutrition, pharmacology, and therapeutic communication.

Taking the practice tests in this book gives you the opportunity to test your nursing skills, apply test-taking strategies, and recall and apply nursing knowledge to various patient situations. The tests do not contain a deliberate pattern of correct responses or a hidden trick that makes one response more correct than the others.

By taking the NLN Practice Test for PN Licensure at the end of this book and by applying productive test-taking strategies, you'll gain confidence in your ability to perform successfully on NCLEX-PN. Remember to draw on your memory resources, view yourself positively, and use relaxation techniques if you feel yourself becoming tense.

Part III

Nursing principles and general nursing procedures

Part III

Nursing principles and general nursing procedures

Introduction 29

Nursing principles

Classification of human needs 29

Normal growth and development throughout the life cycle 30

Health and physical assessment guide 37

Legal principles of nursing practice 42

Therapeutic communication 45

Grief and loss 49

Basic nutrition 51

Rehabilitation 66

Inflammation 68

Shock 70

Acid-base balance 74

Fluids and electrolytes 78

Immobility 82

General nursing procedures

Assisting with ambulation 85

Changing a sterile dressing 86

Irrigating a wound 87

Nursing principles and general nursing procedures *(continued)*

Applying a pressure dressing 88

Applying a wet-to-dry dressing 88

Removing sutures or staples 89

Applying heat and cold 90

Using a heat lamp 91

Collecting specimens 92

Washing the hands 94

Shaving a patient 95

Introduction

Practical nurses increasingly must perform technologically complex patient-care tasks. Consequently, a firm foundation in the principles underlying data collection and nursing interventions has become more important than ever. NCLEX-PN evaluates the practical nurse's ability to apply basic principles in caring for patients and performing nursing procedures.

Part III of *American Nursing Review for NCLEX-PN* has two sections: nursing principles and general nursing procedures. Careful study of each section will ensure a solid basis for successful study of the rest of the book.

The first section reviews the humanistic and scientific principles that a practical nurse must understand thoroughly to provide good nursing care with confidence. It begins by reviewing human needs, then discusses fundamental principles underlying patient care in all clinical situations. Pay special attention to therapeutic communication, growth and development, nutrition, acid-base balance, fluids and electrolytes, and immobility. A strong foundation in these subjects and the ability to apply the principles discussed will increase your confidence when taking the examination. Consider legal principles another subject for close study, because it also serves as the basis for test questions.

The second section of Part III discusses nursing procedures commonly carried out on all patients—regardless of age, sex, or clinical setting—that all beginning practical nurses must know how to perform. It explains the purpose of each procedure and presents relevant precautions and nursing considerations.

NURSING PRINCIPLES

Classification of human needs

I. **Introduction**
   A. A theory developed in 1954 by A.H. Maslow proposes that certain needs are basic and must be met before higher-level needs can be met
   B. Unmet needs motivate a person to perform activities to meet these needs
   C. Need levels commonly exist simultaneously and in varying degrees. Higher-level needs may arise before lower-level needs are met completely

II. **Need categories**
   A. *Primary needs* are those that are vital to continuing existence (survival). They include:
      1. oxygen
      2. water
      3. nutrition
      4. elimination
      5. physiologic homeostasis (maintenance of a steady internal environment of the body)
      6. rest and sleep
      7. avoidance of pain
      8. sex (basic but not essential for survival)

B. *Secondary needs* are social needs. They include:
1. security
2. social approval
3. affiliation (belonging to a group or groups)
4. status (standing in the community)
5. knowledge acquisition
6. achievement

III. **Hierarchy of needs**
A. Lower-level needs, such as survival needs, must be met before higher-level needs, such as self-actualization
B. The hierarchy of needs proceeds from the lowest-level to the highest-level needs:
1. physiologic (bodily needs)
2. safety and security
3. belonging and affection
4. esteem and self-respect
5. self-actualization (self-fulfillment, aesthetic needs)

Normal growth and development throughout the life cycle

The practice of nursing requires a thorough understanding of how people grow and develop physically, socially, and morally. Normal growth and development is a dynamic process that proceeds in a predictable way.

Development falls into two major categories—physical-motor and social-play. Usually, it is described in terms of age ranges. This section presents the main accomplishments expected for physical-motor and social-play development. Because development during the first year is so rapid, the ranges are short (encompassing months). As a person matures, changes occur more slowly, so the age ranges are longer (encompassing decades). Although arbitrary, these ranges are accepted widely and can contribute to an understanding of the major developmental milestones. You can expect to find questions on NCLEX-PN that will draw on your knowledge of development and expected age achievements throughout the life cycle.

1 month

Physical-motor development
• Regains lost birth weight (usually weighs 7 to 8 lb [3.2 to 3.6 kg])
• Shows head lag when moved from a lying to sitting position
• Clenches hand when touched by a rattle
• Lifts and turns the head when prone
• Pushes with the toes
• Stares at surroundings
• Becomes quiet upon hearing a voice
Social-play development
• Sleeps 20 hours/day
• Cries when hungry or displeased

2 months

Physical-motor development
• Posterior fontanel closes
• Holds the head in midline position
• Turns the head toward sounds

Social-play development
- Begins smiling in response to pleasurable stimulation
- Shows differentiated crying

3 months

Physical-motor development
- Shows decreased head lag
- Looks at own hands
- Pulls at blankets or clothing

Social-play development
- Coos and babbles
- Cries less frequently
- Recognizes familiar faces and objects

4 months

Physical-motor development
- Moro, tonic neck, and rooting reflexes disappear
- Begins eye-hand coordination
- Balances the head when sitting upright
- Begins to drool
- Turns from back to side
- Lifts the head and shoulders when placed on the abdomen

Social-play development
- Laughs aloud
- Enjoys social interaction
- Seeks attention by fussing
- Sleeps through the night

5 months

Physical-motor development
- Head lag disappears
- Grasps objects voluntarily
- Supports the head when in a sitting position
- Bears weight on the feet when held in a standing position
- Turns from the abdomen to the back

Social-play development
- Squeals
- Smiles at own mirror image
- Tries to hold a bottle
- Has rapid mood swings
- Discovers own body parts

6 months

Physical-motor development
- Birth weight doubles
- Begins teething, as the two lower central incisors erupt
- Grasps and pulls the feet to the mouth
- Sits in a high chair with the back straight
- Turns from the back to the abdomen

Social-play development
- Starts to imitate sounds
- Enjoys hearing own voice
- Cries when interrupted from play
- Awakens in a happy mood

7 months

Physical-motor development
- Begins crawling, using the upper body and dragging the legs
- Bears weight on the feet

- Bounces when held in a standing position
- Bangs a cube on a table
- Transfers objects from one hand to the other
- Shows taste preferences

Social-play development
- Begins to show fear of strangers
- Plays "peekaboo"
- May bite to show aggressiveness

8 months

Physical-motor development
- Sits unsupported
- Shows pincer grasp using the index finger and thumb
- Releases objects at will

Social-play development
- Amuses self more independently and for longer periods
- Responds to the word "no" but does not know its meaning
- Dislikes holding still during dressing and diaper changes
- Becomes anxious when separated from the mother

9 months

Physical-motor development
- Crawls
- Rises to a standing position when supported
- Shows hand preference

Social-play development
- Understands the meaning of "no"
- Tries to imitate sounds
- Fears going to bed and being left alone

10 months

Physical-motor development
- Begins stepping motions when standing
- Sits by falling down after standing
- Maintains balance easily when sitting
- Begins crude release of objects

Social-play development
- Says "mama" and "dada" with appropriate meaning
- Knows own name
- Feeds self crackers and cookies

11 months

Physical-motor development
- Walks by holding on to furniture
- Makes marks on paper with a crayon
- Drops objects purposefully

Social-play development
- Imitates spoken sounds
- Enjoys playing with an empty dish and spoon after meals
- Understands simple directions

1 year

Physical-motor development
- Birth weight triples
- Birth length doubles
- Head circumference equals chest circumference
- Has six teeth
- Walks if someone holds one hand
- Turns many book pages at a time

Social-play development
- Shows such emotions as anger, fear, jealousy, and affection
- Plays with food
- Recognizes objects by name
- Enjoys familiar settings
- Fears new situations
- May become attached to a "security" blanket

1½ years

Physical-motor development
- Abdomen protrudes
- Anterior fontanel closes completely
- Climbs on furniture and stairs
- Throws a ball overhand
- Uses a spoon without rotation
- Shows sphincter control

Social-play development
- Has a vocabulary of roughly 10 words
- Begins temper tantrums
- Has rapid attention shifts
- Shows marked egocentrism

2 years

Physical-motor development
- Chest circumference exceeds head circumference
- Builds a tower of six cubes
- Shows readiness for bowel and bladder training
- Runs with a wide stance
- Kicks a ball

Social-play development
- Talks incessantly in short sentences
- Shows an increasing attention span
- Dislikes sharing with other children

2½ years

Physical-motor development
- Has all deciduous teeth
- Throws a ball
- Jumps in place
- Walks up and down stairs
- Controls the bowel and bladder during the day

Social-play development
- Knows own first and last name
- Can name one color
- May stutter
- Has trouble making decisions

3 years

Physical-motor development
- Controls the bowel and bladder during the night
- Rides a tricycle
- Climbs stairs using alternate feet
- Builds a tower of nine or more blocks
- Can copy a drawing of a circle and name the object

Social-play development
- Talks continuously in three- to four-word sentences
- Asks questions

• Shows parallel and associative play (group play in similar activities with rigid structure)
• Likes to help adults around the house

4 years

Physical-motor development
• Pulse and respiratory rates decrease slightly
• Catches a ball
• Walks down stairs using alternate feet
• Uses scissors successfully
• Copies a drawing of a square
Social-play development
• Asks questions incessantly
• Knows simple songs
• Shows off
• Is independent
• Uses associative play
• Has many fantasies and fears

5 years

Physical-motor development
• Pulse and respiratory rates continue to decrease
• Loses deciduous teeth
• Establishes hand dominance
• Jumps rope
• Walks backward
• Ties shoelaces
Social-play development
• Fears decrease
• Can name four or more colors
• Shows responsibility
• Develops social manners
• Continues with associative play

6 to 8 years

Physical-motor development
• Growth slows
• Permanent teeth erupt
• May insist on performing basic hygiene alone
Social-play development
• Is more willing to share and cooperate
• Likes to win at games
• Participates in the family group
• May be jealous of a younger sibling

9 to 11 years

Physical-motor development
• Is very active
• Shows improved motor coordination
• May become obese
Social-play development
• Is ashamed of poor school grades
• Shows an interest in boy-girl relationships from afar
• Is self-critical

12 to 14 years

Physical-motor development
- Growth increase peaks (a girl's growth is roughly 2 years ahead of a boy's)
- Shows continuing improvement in coordination
- Is preoccupied with continuing bodily changes

Social-play development
- Tries out various roles
- Develops close friendships with members of the opposite sex
- Values group activities
- Has wide mood swings

15 to 17 years

Physical-motor development
- Females achieve physical maturity by age 17
- May experiment sexually

Social-play development
- Values acceptance by peers
- Shows creativity
- Worries about school work
- Shows marked self-centeredness
- Reaches a low point in relationship with parents; may clash with parents

18 to 20 years

Physical-motor development
- Males achieve physical maturity by age 20
- Sexual identity becomes irreversible

Social-play development
- Forms stable relationships
- Develops life goals
- Shows more consistent emotions
- Has fewer conflicts with family
- May desire emancipation from parents

20 to 30 years

Physical-motor development
- Attains maximum physical strength, muscular efficiency, and physiologic reserve
- Must maintain strength through exercise and proper nutrition
- May reach less than desirable body weight (based on insurance actuary standards); proportion of body fat may increase
- Achieves complete skeletal growth by about age 25, although vertebral growth may add ⅛″ to ¼″ (3 to 5 mm) to height up to age 30
- Begins to lose skin moisture and may develop "laugh" lines
- May have an increased cholesterol level after age 21

Social-play development
- Reaches peak productivity
- Develops an outward-looking attitude with new interests
- Maintains learning abilities
- Shows much interest in sex
- Develops care interests
- Builds friendships and relationships with the opposite sex
- Forms intimate relationships; may marry
- Achieves mature social and civic responsibilities
- Must make adjustments on attaining parenthood to incorporate children into the family structure
- May adopt an optional life-style, such as single or communal living, single parenthood, couple without children, or homosexuality

PRINCIPLES AND PROCEDURES

30 to 40 years

Physical-motor development
• Begins to experience decreased physical strength and physiologic reserve
• May gain weight and have trouble losing it
• May acquire more noticeable body fat, with a protruding abdomen, bulging at the waist and hips, and sagging of the posterior arms and thighs
• Continues to lose skin moisture; may develop more pronounced wrinkles
• May show receding hair line at the forehead; may become bald
• Varies nutritional intake, although requirements for protein, iron, calcium and fluids remain constant
• Women begin to lose calcium from bones after age 30, men at a later age
• Maintains high sex drive but performance may be less than satisfactory at times
• Maintains high level of learning and creativity
• Usually maintains constant productivity
• May lose sleep over worry about family, children, or work status
Social-play development
• Identifies self as successful at attaining life goals
• Values work relationships, but also values free time for personal interests and activities
• May view choice of career or vocation as a source of self-esteem
• May experience a crisis after a divorce or illness of a spouse or child
• If part of a working couple, may reduce parent-child interaction and child-rearing time
• Attempts to build a nest egg by saving money; may spend less on material things (except for house and lot)

40 to 65 years

Physical-motor development
• Continues to show declining physical and muscular strength; without proper exercise, nutrition, and rest, may lose as much as one-third of normal body functions by age 60 or 65
• May develop one or more chronic conditions affecting the muscles or joints (such as stiffness, pain, arthritis), lungs (such as bronchitis or emphysema), cardiovascular system (such as myocardial infarction, hypertension, heart failure, peripheral vascular problems, arteriosclerosis), or another condition
• Hair may turn gray and baldness may increase
• May require increased dental care to maintain teeth in good condition; may require dentures
• May have blurred vision; becomes farsighted, necessitating eyeglasses, contact lenses, or bifocals
• Shows less acute hearing; may become deaf
• Women may experience menopause; with loss of estrogen, osteoporosis may develop more rapidly
• Men may experience a milder mid-life crisis
• May experience neurosis, depression, psychotic episodes, or neurologic changes (such as Parkinson's disease, Alzheimer's disease, cerebrovascular accident, and gradual memory loss)
• More likely to develop a severe or life-threatening illnesses (such as cancer, congestive heart failure, emphysema, or myocardial infarction)
• May experience sexual problems from reduced hormonal stimulation, decreased vaginal secretions, prostatic hypertrophy, or alcohol abuse
• Must reduce nutritional intake to maintain optimal health as physical activity decreases

Social-play development
• Reevaluates life goals and achievements
• May feel pronounced stress from attempting to meet the needs of children and elderly parents
• May experience "empty nest" syndrome as children leave home for education, careers, or marriage
• May lose job because of decreased productivity or age discrimination
• Strives to maintain a positive physical appearance despite wrinkling, sagging, or other changes; may have plastic surgery
• May experience a severe life crisis if a spouse becomes ill or dies, causing prolonged grief and depression; may withdraw gradually from family and friends
• May choose early retirement

65 years and over

Physical-motor development
• Shows continuing decline in physical function and strength; may experience bilateral deafness, cataracts, or glaucoma
• May have reduced mobility from arthritis, peripheral neuropathy, osteoporosis, back pain, or fractures
• May develop diabetes
• Has an increased risk of cancer, especially of the brain, colon, prostate, and breast
• Reduced sensitivity to taste may impair appetite or enjoyment of foods, causing loss of weight and muscle strength
• Must exercise to maintain muscle strength and body functions
• May experience constipation and urinary incontinence, causing embarrassment
• Men may experience prostatic hyperplasia with nocturia and decreased urine stream

Social-play development
• Will probably retire, necessitating adjustments to living on a fixed income and the constant presence of a spouse
• May worry about medical expenses
• May become increasingly disengaged socially or become withdrawn
• May suffer prolonged grief, depression, and loneliness from the death of friends or relatives
• Has an increased interest in travel and hobbies
• May engage in volunteer activities
• May require admission to a nursing care facility if unable to care for self

Health and physical assessment guide

I. **Health history**
   A. Definition: a statement of the patient's overall health
   B. Components
      1. Age
      2. Sex
      3. Childhood diseases and immunizations (in an adult, any immunizations against influenza, cholera, or hepatitis B)
      4. Illnesses as an adolescent or adult
      5. Mental or psychiatric illnesses and type of treatment received
      6. Operations
      7. Injuries, including specific organs or tissues involved

8. Hospitalizations, including date and purpose
9. Medication history
   a. Names and dosages of current prescription medications
   b. Names and dosages of current over-the-counter medications
10. Typical diet, including any limitations (such as low-cholesterol, low-salt, or diabetic diet)
11. Exercise (such as walking, jogging, aerobics, stretching or strengthening exercises, or weightlifting)
12. Alcohol intake
13. Tobacco history
    a. Number of cigarettes or cigars the patient smokes daily
    b. Use of smokeless tobacco (such as chewing tobacco or snuff)
14. Sleep and rest patterns, including naps
15. Family history
    a. Current status (alive or dead) of grandparents, parents, and siblings
    b. Current health condition or cause of death of grandparents, parents, and siblings
16. Use of any prostheses (such as eyeglasses, contact lenses, prosthetic limbs or joints, implants, or breast prostheses)
17. Allergies or idiosyncratic reactions to drugs, plants, or other substances
18. Seizures, headaches, dizziness, throbbing or tenseness in the temples or back of the neck
19. Vomiting (type and amount or frequency)
20. Activity tolerance: amount of activity the patient can tolerate before experiencing pain, weakness, fatigue, shortness of breath, or calf cramps
21. Voiding pattern
    a. Incontinence
    b. Nocturia
    c. Urinary urgency
    d. Urinary frequency
    e. Burning on urination
22. Bowel elimination pattern
    a. Constipation or diarrhea
    b. Rectal pain
    c. Hemorrhoids
23. Menstrual history (in a female patient)
    a. Number of pregnancies
    b. Number of births
    c. Number of miscarriages
    d. Number of abortions
24. Living situation
    a. Own or rent
    b. Type of building (for example, ranch-style or split-level house, high-rise apartment, ground-floor or upper-floor apartment)
    c. Wheelchair access or an elevator (as appropriate)
25. Life-style
    a. Occupation
    b. Leisure activities
26. Relationships with family and friends
27. Patient's perception of current health status

      28. Other data (record religion only if the patient volunteers this
         information)

II.   **Physical assessment**

    A. General overview (patient's apparent health status)
      1. Signs of discomfort, pain, or distress
      2. Mood
      3. Facial expressions
      4. Level of alertness or awareness
      5. Appropriateness of responses
      6. Motor functions (such as gait and ability to walk)
    B. Vital signs, weight, and height
      1. Blood pressure in both arms, measured with the patient lying down,
         sitting up, and standing (if possible)
      2. Pulse
        a. Radial pulse rate
        b. Pulse characteristics (such as firm, weak, or thready)
      3. Respirations
        a. Respiratory rate, depth, and rhythm
        b. Wheezing or stridor
      4. Temperature (measured orally or rectally with a digital or electronic
         thermometer; axillary temperature is questionable and should be
         used only as a last resort)
      5. Height and weight (estimated or measured from a bed scale if the
         patient is ill)
    C. Skin
      1. Color
      2. Moisture level
      3. Presence of any lumps, bumps, rashes, petechiae, masses, or vitiligo
         (white patches)
      4. Presence and location of any infection
    D. Nails
      1. Shape
      2. Length
      3. Presence of cracks or creases
    E. Hair
      1. Amount
      2. Texture
      3. Moisture level
      4. Any recent hair loss
    F. Eyes
      1. Visual acuity
      2. Peripheral vision
      3. Blurring
      4. Use of eyeglasses, contact lenses, or a prosthesis
      5. Presence of any eye inflammation or discharge
      6. Drainage or bleeding from the eyes
    G. Ears
      1. Hearing acuity
      2. Presence of cerumen (ear wax)
      3. Condition of the tympanic membrane (ear drum)
      4. Equilibrium (reflects the function of cranial nerve VIII)
      5. Drainage or bleeding from the ears
    H. Nose
      1. Presence of polyps or discharge

2. Olfactory sensitivity
3. Palpable abnormalities of the sinus areas and nose
4. Drainage or bleeding from the nose

I. Mouth, palate, and pharynx
1. Herpes lesions (cold sores or fever blisters) on the mouth and lips
2. Cracks on the lips or at the corners of the mouth
3. Open lesions on the tongue or lips
4. Condition of the mucous membranes, gums, teeth, tongue, and palate
5. Uvula movement
6. Sensitivity to sweet, sour, acidic, and salty tastes
7. Ability to swallow
8. Normal gag reflex
9. Speech clarity
10. Drainage or bleeding from the mouth

J. Neck: Palpation
1. Lymph nodes
   a. Posterior auricular
   b. Occipital
   c. Preauricular
   d. Tonsillary
   e. Submaxillary
   f. Submental
   g. Submandibular
   h. Superficial cervical
   i. Posterior cervical
   j. Supraclavicular
2. Thyroid gland and trachea

K. Breasts and axillae
1. Inspection
   a. Breast symmetry (including size)
   b. Indentations
   c. Nipple discharge
2. Palpation for lumps

L. Thorax and lungs
1. Inspection
   a. Equality and depth of thoracic rise and fall during inhalation and exhalation
   b. Shape and equality of ribs
2. Percussion and auscultation of breath sounds
3. Cough
   a. Sputum production
   b. Sputum color

M. Back
1. Inspection
   a. Shoulders
      (1) Equal height
      (2) Winging of shoulder blades
   b. Vertebral column
      (1) Normal curvatures
      (2) Presence of abnormal curvatures, such as a lateral curvature (scoliosis)
      (3) Vertebral column positioned in the center of the back
      (4) Convex curve of the thoracic vertebrae

(5) Concave curve of the cervical and lumbar vertebrae

(6) Presence of an abnormal hump (gibbus) of the thoracic vertebrae

   c. Equal height of the hips

2. Palpation of the back for tender or sore areas

N. Heart

1. Inspection of the chest for heaves and palpitations

2. Examination for a thrill (racing or pounding of the heart) by placing the palm over the patient's heart

3. Auscultation of the apical heart beat

O. Abdomen

1. Inspection

   a. Midline position of the umbilicus

   b. Umbilicus type ("inny" or "outy")

   c. Presence of scars, masses, bulges, rashes, moles, or bruises

2. Palpation for tenderness or pain

3. Auscultation for bowel sounds in all four abdominal quadrants

4. Palpation

   a. Presence of a hernia in the groin

   b. Any lymph node enlargement in the groin

P. Genitalia

1. Inspection

   a. Lesions

   b. Drainage from the penis (in a male)

   c. Drainage in the external perineal area and vagina (in a female)

2. Palpation of the scrotum for masses (in a male)

Q. Upper and lower extremities: Inspection

1. Rashes

2. Lesions

3. Edema

4. Equality of size

R. Motor function

1. Range of motion of all joints

2. Muscle tone

3. Strength of grip

4. Ability to contract all muscles

5. Coordinated movements

6. Gait

7. Stepping reflexes

S. Sensory function

1. Ability to distinguish sharp from dull pressure

2. Ability to locate the source of pressure

3. Presence of numbness and tingling

T. Neurologic status

1. Level of consciousness

2. Orientation to time, place, and person

3. Mood

4. Cognitive function

5. Presence of any tics or tremors

U. Secondary sex characteristics

1. Depth of voice

2. Hair distribution

3. Fat deposits

Legal principles of nursing practice

I.   **Nurse practice act**
   A. Description
      1. The nurse practice act of each state defines the legal scope of nursing practice within the state
      2. Most nurse practice acts are written broadly, covering a variety of evolving practice situations; they do not address most specific nursing actions
      3. Nurse practice acts define unprofessional conduct and list violations that can lead to disciplinary or other action
      4. The nurse practice act should be regarded as a source of specific information about state law regarding nursing practice; the state board of nursing serves as a source of information about whether a particular nursing activity falls within the realm of the nurse practice act
   B. Nurse's responsibility
      1. The nurse must stay abreast of current standards of practice
      2. The nurse is responsible for understanding current standards within the context of the more broadly stated law of the particular state

II.   **Torts**
   A. Description
      1. Torts are civil or private wrongs to a person or property (except breach of contract) for which an injured party (plaintiff) can claim damages in court
      2. The plaintiff who can demonstrate proof of a wrong through evidence can obtain a legal remedy
      3. A tort may be unintentional, intentional, or quasi-intentional
   B. Unintentional tort
      1. An unintentional tort is an act that fails to meet a duty owed to a person and causes injury to that person
      2. Negligence, one type of unintentional tort, is failure to discharge one's duty by using reasonable care
         a. To determine if negligence has occurred, the nurse-defendant's actions are weighed against the standard of care expected—what a reasonably prudent nurse would have done under similar circumstances. To judge nursing care, the court may consider expert testimony, publications, textbooks, and professional education in addition to written standards of nursing practice
         b. To prove negligence, a patient-plaintiff must prove the following:
            (1) The nurse owed the plaintiff a duty that a reasonable and prudent nurse would render
            (2) A breach of duty occurred, either by omission (failure to perform the duty) or commission (unreasonable performance of the duty)
            (3) The breach of duty is related to the injury, referred to as *proximate cause,* and defined variously by state laws
               (a) "But for" (the plaintiff would not have been injured but for the nurse's breach of duty)
               (b) Substantial factor (the nurse's breach of duty was a substantial factor in the injury)

                (c) Forseeability (the nurse's breach of duty foreseeably led to and caused the plaintiff's injury)

           (4) The defendant owes the plaintiff compensatory damages, which are determined on the basis of a physical or psychological injury whose monetary value has been substantiated

      c. To avoid or defend against a charge of negligence, the nurse should follow basic guidelines

        (1) Know what duty is owed to a patient

        (2) Know the standard of care

        (3) Deliver care consistent with the standard of care

        (4) Document care rendered that reflects conformance with the standard of care

        (5) Follow policies and procedures

    3. Malpractice, the second type of unintentional tort, is negligence in the practice of one's profession

      a. The elements of malpractice are identical to those of negligence, except that the duty owed is a professional one and involves special knowledge and skill

      b. The application of malpractice to nurses differs from one state to the next

        (1) Some states apply an ordinary standard

        (2) Others apply a professional standard when the nurse's act requires special knowledge and skill

C. Intentional tort

  1. An intentional tort is defined as a direct invasion of a person's legal rights

  2. Intentional torts include assault, battery, and false imprisonment

    a. *Assault* is an imminent threat of harmful or offensive body contact with another person; for example, a nurse who draws up an injection in front of a patient who has requested not to receive it may be committing assault because the patient fears the nurse will administer the unwanted injection

    b. *Battery* refers to physical contact with another person without that person's consent; for example, a nurse administers an injection despite the patient's request not to receive it

    c. *False imprisonment* is the unlawful restraint of a person against his or her will; for example, a nurse places a patient in restraints despite lack of basis for using restraints (such as patient protection)

D. Quasi-intentional tort

  1. A quasi-intentional tort is an act that interferes with a person's intangible interests, such as privacy or reputation

  2. Types of quasi-intentional torts include invasion of privacy and defamation (slander or libel)

    a. Invasion of privacy and breach of confidentiality may occur when a nurse discloses confidential information about a patient to others without the patient's consent

    b. Defamation is an injury to a plaintiff's reputation in the community as a result of a false statement

      (1) Defamation can be written (libel) or spoken (slander)

      (2) Truth is an absolute defense against defamation

III. Informed consent

A. Description

1. Informed consent—a patient right—refers to permission obtained from a patient to perform a specific procedure or treatment
2. The nurse's role in informed consent is to ensure that the patient has all the knowledge necessary to give informed consent and has signed a consent form

B. Elements of informed consent

1. Informed consent must be voluntary, based on adequate knowledge, and competent
2. Consent is voluntary when the patient has a real choice whether to agree to the procedure or treatment
3. Consent is based on adequate knowledge under the following conditions:
   a. The patient has received a description of the procedure or treatment
   b. The patient has received an explanation of risks and benefits of the procedure or treatment
   c. The patient has received an explanation of appropriate alternative procedures or treatments
   d. The patient has received an explanation of the consequences of not having the procedure or treatment
4. Consent is competent when the patient is an adult of sound mind and is capable legally and mentally of making a decision that will affect physical well-being
   a. For a minor (someone below the legal age of competence), only the parent or legal guardian legally can consent to treatment; however, exceptions to the presumption of a minor's incompetence exist
   b. An adult above the legal age of competence can lose the legal capacity to consent only through a formal judicial process— usually on the basis of medical and psychiatric testimony. For an incompetent adult, consent must be obtained from a court-appointed guardian

C. Exceptions to the need to obtain informed consent

1. Consent is implied in life-threatening emergencies
2. Consent can be waived if the physician believes that informing a patient fully would harm the patient's health or well-being (physician's therapeutic privilege)

IV. Documentation

A. Importance

1. Documentation promotes continuity of care and communication among disciplines
2. It also serves as legal proof of the quality of care provided

B. General guidelines

1. Some basic principles apply to documentation of nursing care
2. Documentation should be focused on treatments, occurrences, and patient responses to procedures and treatments
3. Documentation must be clear, concise, and accurate
4. Documentation errors must be obvious and unobscured; for example, an error should be crossed out with a single line only, then initialed to indicate the error and change

C. Incident reports
   1. Description
      a. An incident report describes an action that happened that is inconsistent with normal and orderly hospital routine, and the follow-up care provided
      b. The nurse should treat incident reports as other documentation tools by writing them accurately and including them in the patient's record
      c. The state board of nursing should be consulted for legal interpretation of incident reporting requirements for a particular state (NCLEX-PN limits test questions to the general principles of incident reports)
   2. Purpose
      a. Incident reports serve as risk-management tools
      b. Incident reports sometimes are considered quality assurance records (if so, they may not be introduced in a trial in most states)

Therapeutic communication

Communication can help or harm a patient. By using therapeutic communication, a method of verbal and nonverbal communications, the nurse helps preserve the patient's self-esteem and promotes emotional and spiritual well-being. Therapeutic communication can influence a patient consciously or lead a patient to a better understanding. The charts below provide general guidelines and specific techniques that ensure therapeutic communication, describe behaviors that block therapeutic communication, and demonstrate how to substitute helpful remarks for harmful ones.

Ensuring therapeutic communication

General guidelines

The following guidelines help establish a framework for therapeutic communication. For each guideline, an example and rationale appear.

GUIDELINE	EXAMPLE	RATIONALE
Ask for a description first, thoughts second, and feelings last.	1. "What did the biopsy show?" 2. "What thoughts do you have about that?" 3. "How do you feel about that?"	Descriptions are less threatening than thoughts and feelings; asking for a description first helps ease the patient into exploring the situation.
Ask about the significance of the event.	"What does having cancer mean to you?"	This allows accurate assessment of the patient's needs based on what the patient says.
Ask for more information instead of assuming you know what the patient is experiencing or assuming the patient would respond the same way you would.	Patient: "They tell me I'm dying." Nurse: "You must feel bad." Patient: "They tell me I'm dying." Nurse: "Tell me more about that." Patient: "I just found out I have cancer." Nurse: "What does that mean to you?"	The nurse who makes a faulty assumption will end up with incorrect information. By asking for further information, the nurse has a better chance of discovering more about the patient's perspective.
Check out your impressions.	The patient avoids eye contact with the nurse. The nurse says, "I'm wondering what's going on. You haven't looked at me all day."	Checking out impressions is a healthy, mature communication method that clarifies the meaning of the patient's behavior and prevents the nurse from making wrong assumptions.
Ask open-ended questions rather than questions that require a simple "yes" or "no."	"What were you told about _____?" "Who told you you're dying?" "Tell me about the pain." "How do you think we could best work together?"	Using open-ended questions, the nurse can gather more information and involve the patient actively in care.
Focus on people rather than things.	Patient: "My sister Edith gave me this new gown. Isn't it pretty?" Nurse: "Yes, it is. Tell me about you and Edith."	Focusing on people yields information about the patient's social supports and may provide clues about how the patient has dealt with similar situations in the past.
Ask for specifics and avoid generalities.	Patient: "The doctors here are so cold." Nurse: "Tell me about one time you saw a doctor being cold."	Asking for specifics helps the patient focus on a particular experience and reactions to that experience rather than getting caught up in a general reaction that is harder to work with.
Use "I" statements.	Patient: "The nurses here are all so busy." Nurse: "I know I feel very rushed. I'd appreciate your telling me how that affects you."	"I" statements acknowledge that you can't speak for anyone but yourself and show that you're willing to take responsibility for your own behavior.

Adapted with permission from J. Karshmer (1982). Rules of thumb: Hints for the psychiatric nursing student. *Journal of Psychiatric Nursing and Mental Health Services,* 20(3), 24-28.

Ensuring therapeutic communication *(continued)*

Specific techniques

The specific techniques presented here, along with corresponding descriptions and examples, are crucial to therapeutic communication.

TECHNIQUE	DESCRIPTION	EXAMPLE
Maintaining silence	Remain silent to allow the patient time to gather thoughts and sort through feelings.	The patient doesn't respond verbally when asked how she feels about impending breast surgery. The nurse then remains silent, focusing attention on the patient.
Suggesting	Make suggestions in a tentative way to help the patient consider additional options.	Patient:"I don't know what to do." Nurse: "Have you ever thought about ...?" "Would you consider ...?" "What do you think might happen if ...?"
Restating	Repeat what the patient has just said to show that you were listening and encourage the patient to say more.	Patient: "I'm not sure if I should take chemotherapy." Nurse: "You're not sure about taking chemotherapy."
Clarifying	Ask for more information to avoid confusion or misinterpretation.	Patient: "It's such a mystery to me." Nurse: "I'm not sure what you're talking about." Patient: "This medicine is no good." Nurse: "What do you mean?"
Using broad openings	Make a general statement designed to obtain information.	"Tell me about your weekend." "How did it go yesterday?" "Anything special on your mind?"
Focusing	Help the patient talk about a specific issue or topic.	Patient: "I hate having cancer." Nurse: "Tell me more." (If the patient changes the subject and talks about other things, the nurse can say, "I'd like you to say more about hating having cancer.")

(continued)

Ensuring therapeutic communication *(continued)*

Blocks to therapeutic communication

Without realizing the effects, the nurse may behave in a way that discourages therapeutic communication. This chart describes such behaviors and explains why the nurse should avoid them.

BEHAVIOR	EXPLANATION
Assuming a closed body stance (crossed arms and legs)	This stance conveys defensiveness and nonacceptance, which may make the patient feel uncomfortable about burdening you with problems or concerns.
Placing hands on the hips or pointing a finger while talking	This may make the patient feel put down, scolded, or intimidated.
Failing to look at the patient while talking	This conveys disinterest, lack of self-confidence, and unwillingness to get involved.
Standing over the patient rather than communicating at eye level	This intimidates the patient.
Talking over the intercom rather than going to the patient's room	This makes the patient feel unimportant and depersonalized and prevents you from establishing or maintaining rapport.
Using strong language (profanity) or speaking in a raised voice	This may offend, threaten, or intimidate the patient.
Giving advice or telling the patient what to do	This prevents the patient from arriving at conclusions independently and promotes dependence on others to solve problems.
Following your agenda instead of the patient's (such as by not listening to the patient or by changing the subject)	This is demeaning, making the patient feel unimportant and misunderstood, and gives the impression that you're uncomfortable with the patient's concerns.
Using cliches ("You have one of the best doctors," "It's normal to be scared about your surgery," "Lots of other people have gotten through this. You can too," or "You shouldn't worry, everything will be just fine.")	Cliches make the patient feel alone, unheard, discounted, and misunderstood.
Asking many "why" questions	This may put pressure on the patient to make up an answer to save face, or cause the patient to feel stupid if a satisfactory answer doesn't come to mind.

Ensuring therapeutic communication (continued)

Comparing helpful and harmful remarks

The nurse should choose helpful remarks and avoid harmful remarks when interacting with patients. The chart below offers helpful remarks to substitute for harmful ones.

HELPFUL REMARK	HARMFUL REMARK
"I'd like to hear your thoughts (feelings) about _____."	"This is what you need to do." "I'm tired of hearing you talk about..."
"I can see you're upset. Tell me about that."	"Why are you so upset?" "You're acting like a baby." "You must really be sad (mad, happy, etc.)."
"I'd like to talk with you about your upper GI test."	"Here's a pamphlet about the test you're scheduled for. If you don't understand something, let me know."
"I can understand that."	"I know exactly how you feel."
"What's your understanding of what was said?"	"What the doctor said was..."
"What would help you to understand the procedure better?"	"I've already explained this to you three times. Why can't you understand?"

Grief and loss

Grief is a healthy response to loss, promoting the acceptance of loss. It occurs in people who have a chronic or terminal illness, have undergone mutilating surgery, or have experienced the death of a loved one. Bowlby developed a concept of grief that encompasses three distinct phases. For a description of each phase and corresponding nursing implementations, see the chart on page 50.

Caring for the patient experiencing grief

When caring for a patient who has experienced a loss, the nurse should consider the phase of grief, as described by Bowlby. The chart below describes typical reactions during each phase of grief, along with nursing implementations and rationales.

TYPICAL REACTIONS	NURSING IMPLEMENTATIONS AND RATIONALES
Phase 1	

• Shock
• Disbelief
• Guilt
• Anger (directed inward or at others)
• Crying
	• Do not pressure the patient to talk about the loss prematurely.
	   Pressuring the patient to talk about the loss could force recognition of the loss prematurely. Before talking about the loss, the patient must get used to it.
	• Allow the patient to express anger.
	   Expression of anger releases tension; allowing it conveys the nurse's acceptance of the patient's pain.
	• Spend time with the patient; you needn't say anything special relating to the loss.
	   The nurse's mere presence is comforting and conveys a willingness to share the patient's grief.

Phase 2	

• Restlessness
• Disorganization
• Poor appetite
• Fatigue
• Weakness
• Feelings of loneliness and helplessness
• Recurrent thoughts of the lost person or object
• Sighing
• Disinterest in previously satisfying activities
• Dwelling in the past
	• Allow the patient to talk about the loss.
	   Talking about the loss helps the patient come to grips with it.
	• Assist the patient with activities of daily living, as needed.
	   Assistance conveys understanding and acceptance of the patient's lack of energy.
	• Offer food in small portions rather than full meals.
	   Large amounts of food can be overwhelming; the patient is more likely to eat when food is presented in small portions.
	• Initiate discussion of the loss.
	   The patient probably needs to talk about the loss and prefers that others not avoid the topic. By initiating discussion, the nurse relieves the patient of the burden of deciding whether it's an acceptable discussion topic.
	• Help the patient participate in activities.
	   Participation decreases feelings of loneliness and helplessness.

Phase 3	

• Planning for the future
• Ability to think about the lost person or object without emotional pain
• Ability to form new relationships
	• Discuss the lost person or object spontaneously with the patient.
	   This acknowledges the importance of the lost person or object to the patient.
	• Support the patient's new-found interests.
	   This promote's the patient's efforts to develop a life without the lost person or object.

Adapted with permission from G. Stuart and S. Surdeen (1987). *Principles and Practice of Psychiatric Nursing*. St. Louis: Mosby, pp. 453-454.

Basic nutrition

I. **Purpose of foods and fluids**
    A. To provide the body with nutrients needed to maintain life
    B. To prevent disease and malnutrition
    C. To sustain the ability to perform work

II. **Recommended dietary allowances**
    A. Description
       1. Recommended dietary allowances (RDAs) were established by the Food and Nutrition Board of the National Research Council
       2. They specify levels of essential nutrients that are adequate to meet the nutritional needs of nearly all healthy people in the United States
          a. RDAs reflect minimal needs plus a safety factor that allows for individual variations
          b. RDAs have not been established for all vitamins and minerals
       3. RDAs are based on average weights and heights for various sex and age categories
          a. They include categories for pregnant and lactating females
          b. For elderly people, RDAs for calories, thiamine, riboflavin, and niacin are slightly lower than for younger adults because they are based on total caloric intake
       4. RDAs are revised periodically to reflect new research data (for the 1990 revision, see Appendix 1)
    B. Purpose
       1. RDAs help prevent nutrient deficiency disease in healthy adults and promote normal growth in infants and children
       2. They were designed to help plan and evaluate diets for groups of people over an extended period
       3. Over time, intake of less than two-thirds of an RDA may lead to a nutrient deficiency
       4. RDAs may not be adequate for people suffering serious illness, traumatic stress, and certain other conditions

III. **U.S. Recommended Dietary Allowances**
    A. Description
       1. U.S. Recommended Dietary Allowances (USRDAs) are a condensed version of the RDAs
       2. Usually, they reflect the highest RDA in all age and sex categories for a given nutrient
          a. For example, the USRDA for iron is 15 mg, which is the RDA for adult females during the reproductive years
          b. Therefore, a food that provides 50% of the RDA for iron actually provides *more* than 50% of the RDA for a male, whose RDA for iron is 12 mg
    B. Purpose
       1. USRDAs serve as a guide for food product labeling
       2. They are used for labeling of food products that have added nutrients or make nutritional claims

IV. **Essential nutrients**
    A. General information
       1. To function normally, the body requires a constant supply of energy from food, expressed in terms of kilocalories (kcal), or calories

2. The three basic fuel nutrients that provide energy for metabolism are carbohydrates, proteins, and fats
3. Micronutrients, fluid, and electrolytes also are essential to the diet

B. Calories
1. One calorie is the amount of energy (heat) needed to raise the temperature of 1 kg of water 1° C
2. Calories provide energy for muscle contraction, synthesis of chemical compounds, and transport of nutrients across cell membranes
3. Excess calories are stored in the form of body fat to be used for energy during fasting. If caloric intake exceeds caloric needs for a prolonged period, excess fat results in obesity
   a. Caloric needs depend on age, sex, height, weight, physical activity level, and climate
   b. The only accurate way to determine caloric needs (other than through direct calorimetry measurements) is to determine how many calories a person expends to maintain an ideal body weight over time

C. Carbohydrates
1. Carbohydrates yield 4 calories/g
2. They make up the largest portion of the average diet
3. Types of carbohydrates include digestible and indigestible carbohydrates (see *Classifying carbohydrates*, page 60)
   a. Digestible carbohydrates provide the body with energy and an immediate glucose source. Although some excess carbohydrate can be stored in the body as glycogen, most digestible carbohydrate is converted and stored as fat
   b. Indigestible carbohydrates (such as fiber) are derived from plant cell structures and cannot be broken down by digestive enzymes
      (1) Insoluble fiber (called dietary fiber) helps maintain normal gastrointestinal peristalsis
      (2) Soluble fiber decreases the digestion and absorption rates of such nutrients as cholesterol and fat-soluble vitamins

D. Proteins
1. Proteins yield 4 calories/g
2. They consist of amino acids
   a. About half of the amino acids are essential — not synthesized by the body — and must be supplied by the diet
   b. The amount of essential amino acids in a protein determines whether the protein is complete or incomplete
      (1) Complete proteins (usually from animal sources) contain all the essential amino acids needed to sustain life and growth
      (2) Partially incomplete proteins (usually from plant sources) contain the essential amino acids needed to sustain life but not to support growth
      (3) Incomplete proteins (usually from plant sources) do not contain the essential amino acids needed to sustain life or growth
   c. An adequate diet must supply the essential amino acids plus enough other amino acids to allow for synthesis of nonessential amino acids, maintain adequate tissue protein, and allow synthesis of structural and functional proteins (such as hormones and enzymes)
3. Proteins can be converted and utilized for energy if insufficient calories are consumed

4. The need for protein increases when the need for hormones and enzymes increases, such as during periods of stress, trauma, healing, and growth

5. The RDA for protein is 0.8 g/kg of ideal weight for adults

E. Fats (lipids)
 1. Fats yield 9 calories/g
 2. They supply a concentrated source of calories and essential fatty acids (linoleic and linolenic acids)
 3. Fats are classified as simple, compound, or derived lipids
    a. Simple lipids include fatty acids and glycerides
       (1) Fatty acids are classified as saturated, monounsaturated, or polyunsaturated
           (a) Essential fatty acids are fatty acids that cannot be synthesized by the body
           (b) They are required for normal growth and cell structure formation
           (c) Essential fatty acids serve as precursors for prostaglandins and other hormonelike compounds
           (d) Found in vegetable oils, essential fatty acids are polyunsaturated
       (2) Glycerides include monoglycerides, diglycerides, and triglycerides (the latter account for most dietary fats)
    b. Compound lipids include phospholipids and lipoproteins
    c. Derived lipids include cholesterol and other sterols
       (1) Cholesterol provides no calories
       (2) It is used in cell membranes and is an important bile component
       (3) Because the body synthesizes adequate cholesterol to meet metabolic needs, it need not be included in the diet
 4. No RDA exists for fat; dietary fat requirements depend on caloric needs

F. Micronutrients
 1. Micronutrients include vitamins and minerals
 2. These substances are needed by the body in minute amounts (For information on the major food sources, functions, and deficiency symptoms of vitamins and minerals with established RDAs, see *Guide to vitamins and minerals,* pages 60 to 61)

G. Fluids and electrolytes
 1. Fluids and electrolytes are essential to maintaining life
 2. Fluid and electrolyte balance reflects a delicate metabolic mechanism controlled by many factors (See "Acid-base balance," pages 74 to 78, and "Fluids and electrolytes," pages 78 to 82)
 3. Fluids (body water) are obtained from foods and beverages
    a. Fluids are a byproduct of carbohydrate, protein, and fat metabolism
    b. Typically, they account for slightly more than half of the body weight
 4. Electrolytes also are obtained from foods and beverages; the three major electrolytes are sodium, chloride, and potassium

V. Daily nutritional requirements
A. Adequate diet
 1. A nutritionally adequate diet contains foods in sufficient amounts and variety to supply the RDA of each nutrient
 2. It also contains enough calories to maintain an ideal body weight

PRINCIPLES AND
PROCEDURES

B. Basic four food groups
   1. The basic four food groups are a tool for food selection that help ensure a nutritionally adequate diet (For details on these groups, see *Guidelines for healthful eating,* page 62)
   2. By eating the recommended number of daily servings from each food group, the average person can obtain adequate proteins, vitamins, and minerals
      a. A person who needs more calories can obtain them from additional servings from these food groups, plus fats, oils, sugar, and alcohol
      b. To obtain the 2 to 4 liters of fluid required daily, a person should supplement fluid in foods and beverages with water

VI. **Other considerations**
   A. Convenience foods and combination dishes
      1. These products (such as casseroles), which contain more than one food group, are not included in the basic four food groups
      2. Their nutrient value can be determined from their ingredients, as shown on the label
         a. Many food labels specify the grams of carbohydrate, protein, and fat provided
         b. Food labels also typically include USRDAs for vitamins and minerals
   B. Nutrient enrichment and fortification
      1. Nutrient enrichment and fortification are governmental concerns
      2. These methods help more people obtain a nutritionally adequate diet from processed foods
      3. Fortified foods include milk fortified with vitamin D and juices fortified with vitamin C or calcium
      4. Enriched foods include breads, cereals, and pasta products enriched with B-vitamins and iron
   C. Desirable weight
      1. Experts disagree as to what constitutes an ideal or desirable body weight
      2. Various formulas can be used to calculate ideal weight
      3. The weight tables published by the Metropolitan Life Insurance Company commonly are used as ranges for weight related to body structure and height (see Appendix 2)
         a. These tables were revised in 1983
         b. However, many nutritionists use the original tables published in 1959 in the belief that they represent more desirable weights than those in the revised tables

VII. **Nutritional guidelines**
   A. Origins
      1. To help the public interpret current research on eating patterns, various agencies and organizations have published guidelines and standards specifying the components of a healthful diet (see *Recommendations for a healthful weight and diet,* pages 62 and 63)
      2. These efforts were spurred by public interest in the health aspects of nutrition
   B. Specific guidelines
      1. The U.S Department of Agriculture (USDA) and U.S. Department of Health and Human Services (USDHH) published the third edition of *Nutrition and Your Health: Dietary Guidelines for Americans* in 1990

a. These guidelines indicate which foods Americans should eat more of to ensure a healthful diet

b. They also specify foods to eat in moderation

2. The American Heart Association (AHA) published *An Eating Plan for Healthy Americans* in 1985

   a. These guidelines are more specific about recommended intake of fat, cholesterol, and salt

   b. AHA recommends limiting protein to 15% of total calories

3. The National Cancer Institute (NCI) published *Diet, Nutrition, and Cancer Prevention* in 1987

   a. These guidelines recommend increased intake of fiber and decreased intake of fat, salt, and alcohol (associated with a higher cancer incidence)

   b. Unlike other organizations, NCI does not specify recommended cholesterol intake

4. The National Academy of Science (NAS) published *Diet and Health: Implication for Reducing Chronic Disease Risk* in 1989

   a. These guidelines recommend an adequate calcium intake and an optimal fluoride intake during the growth years.

   b. They also advise Americans to avoid dietary supplements in excess of RDAs during any one day

VIII. Nutritional deficiencies and related problems

A. Protein-energy malnutrition (PEM)

1. This deficiency, which results from a drastic decrease in food intake, causes starvation or semistarvation

2. PEM can be primary or secondary

   a. Primary PEM is most common in developing countries lacking sufficient food

   b. Secondary PEM stems from an inability to ingest, digest, absorb, or utilize food. It is most common in patients with acute illness, anorexia nervosa, or terminal cancer

3. To avoid the consequences of PEM (such as poor wound healing or intolerance of chemotherapy or radiation therapy), many hospitals have established nutritional support services or teams

   a. Such personnel are devoted solely to alternative feeding methods, such as tube feedings and total parenteral nutrition (TPN)

   b. If the patient can eat and absorb nutrients via the gastrointestinal tract, oral intake should supplement TPN or other alternative feeding methods to maintain gastrointestinal integrity and stimulate digestive enzyme secretion

B. Iron-deficiency anemia

1. This disorder is characterized by a decreased hemoglobin level, depletion of iron stores, and pale red blood cells

2. In the United States, it most often results from inadequate iron intake or blood loss

3. Iron-deficiency anemia is most common in infants, teenage girls, and menstruating or pregnant females

4. Iron should be consumed in a readily absorbable form

   a. It is absorbed poorly from the gastrointestinal tract

   b. Heme iron (such as in meat) is absorbed better than nonheme iron (such as in leafy green vegetables)

   c. Because ascorbic acid enhances iron absorption, iron supplements and iron-containing foods should be taken with ascorbic acid

　　　　5. Iron-deficiency anemia typically is treated with oral iron supplementation

C. Osteoporosis
　　1. This condition is characterized by decreased bone density
　　　　a. It results from accelerated calcium resorption (loss) from the bones
　　　　b. The bones become porous, fragile, and fracture-prone
　　2. Osteoporosis mainly affects postmenopausal women
　　　　a. In some cases, calcium and estrogen therapy are prescribed for postmenopausal women to slow the calcium resorption rate
　　　　b. To help prevent osteoporosis, elderly people should maintain adequate calcium intake, get enough exercise, and avoid excessive intake of fiber and alcohol
　　3. Adequate fluoride intake may help prevent osteoporosis, as suggested by lower incidence of osteoporosis in high-fluoride areas
　　4. Because bone mass peaks at about age 25, the RDA for calcium (1,200 mg) is highest for ages 11 through 24

IX.　Special dietary considerations
A. Cardiovascular disease
　　1. A fat-restricted diet typically is recommended for patients with an elevated serum cholesterol or triglyceride level because they are at risk for coronary heart disease (CHD)
　　　　a. The goal of the fat-restricted diet is to lower the level of serum lipids (such as cholesterol) to within an acceptable range
　　　　　　(1) The National Cholesterol Education Program has established categories for serum cholesterol levels
　　　　　　　　(a) A level below 200 mg/dl is desirable
　　　　　　　　(b) A level of 200 to 239 mg/dl indicates a borderline risk for CHD
　　　　　　　　(c) A level above 240 mg/dl indicates a high risk for CHD
　　　　　　(2) Patients with serum cholesterol levels above 200 mg/dl may be placed on the modified-fat diet recommended by the National Cholesterol Education Program
　　　　　　(3) Certain dietary and life-style changes reduce the level of serum low-density lipoproteins (associated with CHD) while raising the level of serum high-density lipoproteins (which may protect against CHD)
　　　　　　(4) To reduce the serum cholesterol level, experts recommend the following measures:
　　　　　　　　(a) Decrease saturated fat intake to 10% of total calories
　　　　　　　　(b) Decrease cholesterol intake to 300 mg/day
　　　　　　　　(c) Increase intake of polyunsaturated and monounsaturated fats to 10% of total calories
　　　　　　　　(d) Increase intake of soluble fiber
　　　　　　　　(e) Increase exercise levels
　　　　　　　　(f) Maintain an ideal weight
　　　　b. Patients with elevated serum triglyceride levels also should reduce consumption of alcohol and simple carbohydrates (such as table sugar) because these substances may elevate triglyceride levels (For information on foods to avoid and to increase on a fat-restricted diet, see *Food lists for fat-modified diets,* page 64)
　　2. A sodium-restricted diet usually is recommended for patients with decreased cardiac function resulting in fluid retention (edema), such as from congestive heart failure

a. The major source of dietary sodium is sodium chloride (table salt)

b. Foods, food additives, and preservatives contain varying amounts of sodium
   (1) Highly processed foods typically contain more sodium than homemade foods
   (2) Animal products have a higher sodium content than vegetables, fruits, and grains. However, sodium may be added to processed cereals, breads, and canned vegetables

c. Sodium-restricted diets fall into four categories
   (1) For the most liberal category, which allows 4,000 mg/day sodium, the patient must avoid only those foods listed in *Foods to avoid on a sodium-restricted diet,* page 64
   (2) For the second category, which allows 2,000 mg/day sodium, the patient must substitute salt-free bread, butter, and margarine for their salt-containing counterparts
   (3) The third category allows 1,000 mg/day sodium
      (a) It includes all the restrictions of the first two categories
      (b) It also restricts intake of milk, eggs, meat, and fish
      (c) This diet rarely is used outside a health care facility
   (4) The most restrictive diet category allows only 500 mg/day sodium
      (a) It includes all the restrictions of the first three categories
      (b) The patient also must substitute low-sodium milk for regular milk
      (c) This diet rarely is used outside a health care facility

d. Some patients with hypertension must restrict sodium intake
   (1) Only a small percentage of hypertensive patients are salt sensitive
   (2) In these patients, weight reduction is the most effective dietary measure to lower blood pressure

B. Diabetes mellitus
   1. The goal of the diabetic diet is to normalize the blood glucose level to the extent possible by following these guidelines:
      a. Consume a nutritionally adequate diet
      b. Avoid sucrose
      c. Attain or maintain ideal weight
      d. Maintain a consistent meal schedule by eating approximately the same amount of food at the same time each day
   2. Typically, the diabetic diet is divided into meals and snacks to supply an even food intake throughout the day
      a. Patients with insulin-dependent (Type I) diabetes may eat three meals, a midmorning or midafternoon snack, and a bedtime snack
         (1) The midmorning and midafternoon snack provide extra glucose and are especially important for the patient who takes a split or mixed dose of regular and intermediate-acting insulins
         (2) The bedtime snack is essential to cover the insulin that takes effect during sleep
      b. Patients with non-insulin-dependent (Type II) diabetes, who typically are overweight, usually are not permitted to have snacks because they must limit calories (however, the patient taking an oral hypoglycemic agent usually needs a small bedtime snack)

3. To help the diabetic patient plan meals, the American Diabetes Association and the American Dietetic Association have developed exchange lists
   a. Exchange lists are lists of foods with similar carbohydrate, protein, and fat content
   b. They are used to plan menus from the calculated diet prescription
   c. Using these lists, the patient can substitute one food for any other food in the same list without altering nutrient intake (however, the foods may differ in vitamin and mineral content)
   d. Exchange lists allow diabetic patients to eat a variety of foods while consuming approximately the same amount of food at the same time each day
4. To develop a diet order (prescription) for a diabetic patient, the appropriate calorie allowance is determined
   a. The calorie allowance is based on the patient's age, height, weight, and activity level
      (1) The patient who must lose weight usually is allowed 10 calories/lb of ideal weight
      (2) The patient who must maintain current weight usually is permitted 20 calories/lb of ideal weight
      (3) The patient who must gain weight usually is allowed 30 calories/lb of ideal weight
   b. Carbohydrate, protein, and fat allowances are calculated according to recommendations of the American Diabetes Association
      (1) Proteins should account for 12% to 20% of calories
      (2) Fats should account for 30% of calories
      (3) Carbohydrates should account for 50% to 60% of calories
   c. The diet prescription is translated into numbers of exchanges and used to develop a meal plan based on the patient's eating habits (For a typical day's menu for a patient on a 1,500-calorie/day diet, see *Meal plan based on a typical 1,500-calorie diet,* page 65)
5. Other dietary considerations for diabetic patients include the following:
   a. Because these patients are predisposed to atherosclerosis, they should eat foods that improve serum glucose control, such as those low in fats (particularly saturated fat) and high in complex carbohydrates and dietary fiber
   b. Use of special (dietetic) food products is discouraged as expensive and unnecessary. However, beverages containing artificial sweeteners are acceptable and add variety to the diet
   c. Sucrose consumed in small amounts does not increase blood glucose levels in the stable diabetic patient. However, most authorities recommend that diabetic patients avoid sucrose because it has the potential to increase the blood glucose level
   d. Diabetic patients should avoid alcohol because it provides only "empty" calories (those without nutritional value)
   e. Food labeling allows easier incorporation of convenience foods into the diabetic diet

C. Renal disease
1. The dietary goal for the patient with renal disease is to tailor food and fluid intake to the kidneys' ability to retain or excrete metabolic end products

2. The patient may need to modify intake of protein, sodium, phosphate, potassium, and fluid
   a. Protein restriction is necessary because the patient typically retains urea, the major product of protein metabolism
      (1) Because most people consume more protein than they need, reducing protein intake to match the RDA (0.8 g/kg of ideal weight) is relatively easy
      (2) If protein reduction does not achieve nitrogen balance, further protein restriction is needed
      (3) The patient should restrict intake of incomplete proteins severely because they cause urea production and do not provide essential amino acids. To do this, the patient typically must eat special low-protein breads and cereals
      (4) To prevent the use of protein as an energy source, the patient on a protein-modified diet must consume adequate calories
   b. Sodium restriction by the patient with renal disease depends on the kidneys' ability to excrete sodium and water
   c. Phosphate restriction is necessary because renal disease typically causes phosphate retention
      (1) Most patients need reduce dietary phosphate only slightly
      (2) Eliminating milk and milk products usually is sufficient
   d. Potassium restriction is needed if the patient cannot eliminate potassium; the patient should limit consumption of potassium-rich foods (see *Potassium-rich foods,* page 65)
   e. Fluids are restricted to the amount of daily urine output, plus 200 ml for insensible losses
3. Dietary restrictions during dialysis usually are less stringent because dialysis removes waste products, helping to maintain nitrogen, fluid, and electrolyte balance

PRINCIPLES AND PROCEDURES

Nutritional concepts and nursing considerations

The charts presented on the next few pages will enhance your understanding of important nutritional concepts and help you provide better nursing care for the patient with special nutritional concerns.

Classifying carbohydrates

Carbohydrates provide energy for metabolism through digestion and conversion to simple sugars. Some types of carbohydrates are indigestible (referred to as dietary fiber).

CLASS	TYPE	SOURCES
Digestible	• Complex sugars • Simple sugars	• Polysaccharides in starches • Monosaccharides and disaccharides in fruits, vegetables, milk, and sucrose (table sugar)
Indigestible (insoluble)	• Cellulose • Hemicellulose • Lignin	• Bran portion of grains • Bran cereals, whole grains • Structural fibers in various fruits and vegetables
Indigestible (soluble)	• Pectins • Gums • Mucilages	• Most fruits • Oatmeal, legumes • Seeds, seaweeds, psyllium hydrophilic mucilloids (such as Metamucil)

Adapted with permission from J.L. Salvin (1987). Dietary fiber: Classification, chemical analysis, and food sources. *Journal of the American Dietary Association,* 87:1164.

Guide to vitamins and minerals

This table describes the major functions of vitamins and minerals, lists selected findings in vitamin or mineral deficiency, and presents selected food sources of vitamins and minerals.

VITAMIN OR MINERAL	FUNCTIONS	DEFICIENCY FINDINGS	FOOD SOURCES
Vitamins			
Vitamin A	Helps eye adapt to darkness; promotes normal epithelial tissue and bone growth	Night blindness; dry, hard epithelial tissues	Dairy products, organ meats, deep green and yellow vegetables
Vitamin B_1 (thiamine)	Coenzyme for carbohydrate metabolism; helps maintain a healthy nervous system	Polyneuritis, poor appetite	Pork, whole-grain or enriched cereals
Vitamin B_2 (riboflavin)	Coenzyme for carbohydrate and fat metabolism; promotes healthy skin and eyes	Cracks at the corners of mouth; sore mouth and gums	Milk, meat, fish, whole-grain or enriched cereals
Vitamin B_6 (pyridoxine)	Coenzyme for protein and amino acid metabolism	Malaise, depression, decreased glucose tolerance	Meat, poultry, fish
Vitamin B_{12}	Coenzyme for carbohydrate, protein, and fat metabolism; maintains normal red blood cells	Pernicious anemia, anorexia, weight loss	Meat, dairy products, eggs, yeast
Vitamin C	Antioxidant; promotes collagen formation	Bleeding gums, capillary wall rupture, poor wound healing	Citrus fruits, green leafy vegetables, potatoes

Nutritional concepts and nursing considerations *(continued)*

Guide to vitamins and minerals *(continued)*

VITAMIN OR MINERAL	FUNCTIONS	DEFICIENCY FINDINGS	FOOD SOURCES
Vitamins *(continued)*			
Vitamin D	Promotes normal growth and maintenance of bones and teeth	Rickets (children), osteomalacia (adults)	Fish, eggs, liver, fortified milk
Vitamin E	Antioxidant; maintains cell membranes	Muscle weakness; delivery of premature or low-birth-weight neonate	Polyunsaturated fatty acids, oils, nuts, legumes
Vitamin K	Promotes synthesis of blood-clotting factors	Impaired blood clotting	Leafy deep-green vegetables
Folate	Promotes amino acid metabolism; maintains normal red blood cells	Megaloblastic anemia, decreased mental function	Dark-green vegetables, beef, eggs, whole-grain cereals
Niacin	Coenzyme for carbohydrate, protein, and fat metabolism; promotes healthy skin and nerves	Dermatitis, glossitis, poor appetite	Meat, poultry, fish, whole-grain or enriched cereals
Minerals			
Calcium	Maintains strong bones and teeth	Decreased bone strength and density	Milk and dairy products
Iodine	Promotes thyroid hormone synthesis	Goiter (thyroid gland enlargement)	Seafood, iodized salt
Iron	Promotes hemoglobin and energy production	Iron-deficiency anemia	Meat, eggs, whole-grain breads and cereals
Magnesium	Promotes muscle and nerve function	Neuromuscular changes	Cereals, nuts, legumes
Phosphorus	Promotes energy production	Disruption of many metabolic processes	Meats, poultry, fish, dairy products, whole grains, legumes
Selenium	Promotes normal growth and human reproduction	Growth retardation	Seafood, meat
Zinc	Promotes wound healing; maintains appetite and taste	Poor wound healing, diarrhea, anorexia	Meat, seafood

(continued)

PRINCIPLES AND PROCEDURES

Nutritional concepts and nursing considerations *(continued)*

Guidelines for healthful eating

To ensure optimal health, the daily diet should include a wide variety of foods from the basic four food groups, eaten in moderation. This chart provides basic guidelines.

FOOD GROUP	NUTRIENTS SUPPLIED	RECOMMENDED DAILY INTAKE
Milk group	Protein, riboflavin, calcium, and others	Adults: 2 servings Children: 3 servings Adolescents, pregnant, and breast-feeding women: 4 servings
Meat group	Protein, niacin, iron, vitamin B_1, and others	All ages: 2 servings Pregnant women: 3 servings
Vegetables and fruits group	Vitamin A, vitamin C, and others	4 servings
Grain group	Carbohydrate, vitamin B_1, iron, niacin	4 servings
Combination foods (containing foods from more than one food group)	Depends on constituent foods	Depends on constituent foods
Other foods, which contain many calories but few nutrients, should not replace foods from the four basic food groups as nutrient sources. These foods include: condiments (barbecue sauce, catsup, mustard, olives, pickles, salt, soy sauce), chips and	related products (corn chips, popcorn, potato chips, pretzels, tortilla chips), fats and oils (butter, coffee whitener, cream, gravy, cream sauce, lard, margarine, mayonnaise, oil, salad dressing, shortening, sour cream), sweets (brownies, cakes,	candy, cookies, doughnuts, honey, jam, jelly, pies, sugar, sweet rolls, syrup), alcohol (beer, gin, rum, vodka, whiskey, wine), and other beverages (coffee, fruit-flavored drinks, soft drinks, tea).

Adapted with permission from the National Dairy Council. *Guide to good eating* (5th ed.). Rosemont, Ill. 1989, 1991.

Recommendations for a healthful weight and diet

This chart compares the recommendations of several agencies and organizations for weight and intake of fat, cholesterol, sodium, carbohydrates, and alcohol. (For an explanation of the abbreviations used here, see the abbreviation key.)

FACTOR	AGENCY OR ORGANIZATION	RECOMMENDATIONS
Weight	USDA/USDHHS	Maintain a healthful weight.
	AHA	Attain and maintain desirable weight.
	NCI	Avoid obesity.
	NAS	Maintain appropriate weight.

Nutritional concepts and nursing considerations *(continued)*

Recommendations for a healthful weight and diet *(continued)*

FACTOR	AGENCY OR ORGANIZATION	RECOMMENDATIONS
Fat	USDA/USDHHS	Eat a diet low in fat and saturated fat.
	AHA	Decrease intake of total fats to 30% of calories and saturated fats to less than 10% of calories; increase intake of polyunsaturated fats to 10% of calories.
	NCI	Decrease intake of total fats to 30% of total calories.
	NAS	Reduce intake of total fats to 30% of calories or less.
Cholesterol	USDA/USDHHS	Eat a diet low in cholesterol.
	AHA	Reduce daily cholesterol intake to less than 100 mg/1,000 calories (not to exceed 300 mg).
	NCI	Not specified.
	NAS	Reduce daily cholesterol intake to 300 mg or less.
Sodium (salt)	USDA/USDHHS	Use salt and sodium in moderation.
	AHA	Decrease sodium intake to 1 g/1,000 calories (not to exceed 3 g).
	NCI	Minimize consumption of salt-cured, salt-pickled, and smoked foods.
	NAS	Limit daily sodium intake to 6 g or less.
Carbohydrates	USDA/USDHHS	Eat a diet that includes plenty of fruits, vegetables, and grains. Use sugars only in moderation.
	AHA	Decrease intake of simple sugars. Increase intake of fruits, vegetables, and cereals to 50% or 55% of calories.
	NCI	Increase intake of fiber to 20 or 30 g/day (not to exceed 35 g).
	NAS	Consume six or more daily servings of complex carbohydrates and starch. Consume five or more daily servings of fruits and vegetables (preferably those rich in vitamins A and C).
Alcohol	USDA/USDHHS	If you drink alcoholic beverages, do so only in moderation.
	AHA	Limit alcohol consumption to 15% of calories (not to exceed 50 ml of alcohol daily).
	NCI	Consume alcoholic beverages in moderation, if at all.
	NAS	Limit daily alcohol consumption to less than two servings.

Abbreviation key:
USDA: *U.S. Department of Agriculture*
USDHHS: *U.S. Department of Health and Human Services*

AHA: *American Heart Association*
NCI: *National Cancer Institute*
NAS: *National Academy of Science*

(continued)

Nutritional concepts and nursing considerations *(continued)*

Food lists for fat-modified diets

Except as permitted by a physician, patients on fat-modified diets should avoid the foods in the left column below. They may eat the foods in the right column according to the physician's orders or guidelines.

RESTRICTED FOODS	ALLOWABLE FOODS
Animal products high in saturated fat or cholesterol Fatty meats, organ meats Spareribs, pork sausage, bacon Hard cheese, processed cheese Luncheon meats, wieners Whole milk, butter, lard Coffee cream, sour cream Eggs, ice cream	**Vegetable products high in monounsaturated fat** Olive oil Rapeseed oil (canola oil) **Vegetable products high in polyunsaturated fat** Corn, safflower, and sunflower oils
Vegetable products high in saturated fat Coconut oil Palm oil, palm kernel oil Cocoa butter	**Good dietary fiber sources** Bran cereals, oatmeal Dried peas, beans, lentils, legumes Corn, lima beans, and other vegetables Berries and other fruits Whole grain, rye breads

Foods to avoid on a sodium-restricted diet

Patients who must restrict their sodium intake should avoid the foods listed below (except when the label on a packaged or processed food item shows a reduced sodium content). Some labels list the sodium content in milligrams. Others use the terms below, designated by the Food and Drug Administration and the U.S. Department of Agriculture.
Low sodium: containing 140 mg sodium/serving or less
Very low sodium: containing 35 mg sodium/serving or less
Sodium free: containing less than 5 mg sodium/serving

CATEGORY	RESTRICTED FOODS
Meats, cheeses, entrees	• All processed meats, such as chicken or turkey roll, ham, or Canadian bacon • Luncheon meats, frankfurters, corned or dried beef • Canned or dried fish and meats • Frozen entrees and TV dinners • Processed cheese and cheese spreads • Packaged Italian, Mexican, or Oriental foods
Vegetables and fruits	• Sauerkraut, pickles, olives • Canned vegetables, frozen vegetables in cream or cheese sauce
Breads and cereals	• Salted crackers, snack crackers • Packaged breading and stuffing mixes
Fats	• Salt pork • Bacon grease
Soups	• Canned soup, broth, bouillon, consommé • Dried or instant soup mixes
Snack foods	• Salted crackers, pretzels, potato and corn chips • Cheese puffs, fried pork rinds, salted nuts
Seasonings and flavorings	• Chili sauce, soy sauce, steak sauce, barbecue sauce • Cooking wine and sherry • Canned or instant gravy and sauce mixes • Salt, meat tenderizers, celery and onion salt, seasoned salt

Nutritional concepts and nursing considerations *(continued)*

Meal plan based on a typical 1,500-calorie diet

Exchange lists, developed jointly by the American Diabetes Association and the American Dietetic Association, help the diabetic patient plan meals. The meal plan below shows how exchanges can be used to plan a daily menu for a diabetic patient on a 1,500 calorie/day diet.

	FOOD	NUMBER OF EXCHANGES
Breakfast	½ grapefruit	1 fruit exchange
	½ cup oatmeal	1 bread exchange
	1 slice toast	1 bread exchange
	1 tsp margarine	1 fat exchange
	1 cup skim milk	1 skim milk exchange
Lunch	Sandwich: 2 slices bread	2 bread exchanges
	2 oz ham	2 meat exchanges
	2 tsp margarine	2 fat exchanges
	1 tsp mustard	Free
	½ cup tomato juice	1 vegetable exchange
	1 small apple	1 fruit exchange
Dinner	2 oz hamburger	2 meat exchanges
	1 cup potatoes	2 bread exchanges
	1 cup carrots	2 vegetable exchanges
	2 tsp margarine	2 fat exchanges
	1 cup watermelon	1 fruit exchange
	coffee	Free
Bedtime	1 cup skim milk	1 skim milk exchange
	2 graham crackers	1 bread exchange

Potassium-rich foods

The table below lists good food sources of potassium.

Fruits and fruit juices	**Vegetables and vegetable juices**	**Other foods**
Apricots	Artichokes	Chocolate
Avocados	Carrots (raw)	Dried peas and beans
Bananas	Collard greens	Molasses
Cantaloupe	Dandelion greens	Nuts
Dried fruit (such as raisins)	Potatoes (white and sweet)	
Honeydew	Spinach	
Nectarines	Tomatoes	
Orange juice	Tomato juice	
Oranges	Winter squash	
Peaches (fresh)		
Prune juice		
Prunes		
Tangelos		

Rehabilitation

I. **Definition: restoration of a patient to normal or near-normal functions after a disabling injury or illness**
II. **Goals**
    A. To preserve the patient's remaining functions
    B. To help the patient regain or improve mobility
    C. To prevent additional loss of function or ability
    D. To help the patient function at home and within society
III. **Indications for rehabilitation**
    A. Injury or illness causing paralysis
    B. Cerebrovascular accident (stroke)
    C. Amputation
    D. Multiple injury
    E. Loss of normal speech necessitating speech therapy
    F. Muscle atrophy necessitating exercises
IV. **Factors influencing rehabilitation**
    A. Age: may affect the patient's ability to understand and participate in rehabilitative activities
    B. Injury severity: dictates length of rehabilitation needed
    C. Educational level: may influence the patient's ability to understand and participate in rehabilitation
    D. Financial or insurance status
    E. Type of treatment required
        1. Immediate (acute) care
        2. Long-term care
    F. Availability of appropriate rehabilitation facilities
    G. Legislation protecting the rights of patients needing rehabilitation and authorizing removal of barriers or discrimination
V. **Rehabilitative modalities, services, and supplies**
    A. Assistance with activities of daily living (ADLs) to help the patient relearn or perform daily activities:
        1. bathing
        2. eating
        3. dressing
        4. using the toilet
        5. transferring oneself
        6. speaking or communicating
    B. Repetitive exercises to increase muscle tone, strength, or precision
        1. Active exercises: exercises performed independently by the patient
        2. Active-assisted exercises: exercises performed by the patient with therapist assistance
        3. Resistive-active exercises: exercises performed by the patient with resistance provided by weights, ropes, and pulleys
        4. Passive exercises: exercises performed on the patient by the therapist without the patient's active participation
        5. Special or selective exercises: exercises designed to meet the patient's special needs

C. Heat or cold application to treat injured tissues
 1. Heat
   a. May be moist or dry
   b. Examples
     (1) Hot or warm soaks (packs)
     (2) Whirlpool bath
     (3) Warm bath
     (4) Diathermy
 2. Cold: may be applied via an ice bag or an ice/slush bath (to immerse a body part)
D. Ultrasound treatments to reach deeper muscles and joints
E. Occupational therapy
 1. Assists the patient with home management
 2. Trains the patient how to use special utensils or equipment needed to perform ADLs
F. Physical therapy to help restore movement
 1. Specialized muscle retraining
 2. Substitution of other muscles
G. Speech therapy
 1. Helps the patient relearn speech
 2. Teaches the patient how to use alternative speech methods, such as speech-amplifying or mechanical devices
H. Nutritional or dietary counseling
 1. Helps the patient make dietary modifications
 2. Teaches the patient how to prepare food
 3. Provides special instructions on eating methods
I. Sexual counseling
 1. Helps the patient learn about alternative positions and techniques for sex
 2. Helps the patient cope with feelings about altered sexual function
J. Self-catheterization program
K. Bladder or bowel training programs
L. Social services
 1. Helps the patient with financial assistance
 2. Helps the patient with living arrangements and other matters
M. Recreational therapy to provide diversionary activities
N. Devices to shape or hold a weakened body part
 1. Splints
 2. Pads
 3. Special molds
O. Prostheses to replace a deformed or missing part
P. Ambulatory aids to increase mobility
 1. Walkers
 2. Crutches
 3. Canes
 4. Wheelchairs
 5. Braces
 6. Parallel bars
Q. Special utensils adapted to the patient's needs
 1. Reachers
 2. Silverware
 3. Pots and pans

VI. **Psychophysiologic factors affecting rehabilitative goal achievement**
   A. Patient's response to the injury or illness
   B. Patient's stress responses and coping mechanisms
   C. Patient's potential for regaining function
   D. Patient's adaptation to residual functions or disabilities
VII. **Rehabilitation team members**
   A. Physicians
      1. Internists
      2. Surgeons
      3. Orthopedic specialists
      4. Neurologists
      5. Neurosurgeons
      6. Physiatrists
      7. Plastic surgeons
      8. Vascular surgeons
      9. Psychiatrists
      10. Psychologists
      11. Dentists
      12. Radiologists
   B. Nurses
      1. Clinical nurse specialists
      2. Registered nurses
      3. Licensed practical nurses
      4. Nursing students
   C. Pharmacists and pharmacy technicians
   D. Dietitians
   E. Physical therapists
   F. Occupational therapists
   G. Nursing assistants or aides
   H. Social workers
   I. Speech therapists
   J. Recreational therapists
   K. Vocational guidance counselors
   L. Sex counselors
   M. Prosthetists or orthotists
   N. Dental hygienists
   O. Medical supply and equipment counselors
   P. Financial advisors
   Q. Ministers, priests, rabbis, or other religious or spiritual counselors
   R. Educational counselors
   S. Infection control specialists

Inflammation

I.   **Introduction**
   A. Occurs as a response of the body to injury
   B. Also may result from pathogenic (disease-producing) organisms
II. **Cardinal signs of inflammation**
   A. Local signs at the cell injury site
      1. Redness (rubor) from dilation of arteries, which brings more blood
         to the injury site

2. Heat (calor) from increased metabolism and increased blood at the injury site
3. Pain (dolor) from release of irritating chemicals and pressure on nerve endings from edema or injury
4. Swelling (tumor) from increased capillary permeability with accumulation of interstitial fluid at the injury site
5. Loss of function from the injury itself or from multiple changes in the inflamed area
6. Other changes related to the inflammatory response
   a. Migration of leukocytes (white blood cells) to the injury site
   b. Phagocytosis: engulfment and digestion of irritants
   c. Surrounding (walling off) of the inflamed area by leukocytes to stop the spread of inflammation
   d. Exudate formation (from fluid accumulation in the inflamed area) to dilute irritants and draw antibodies to aid tissue defense. Exudate may be:
      (1) serous (clear)
      (2) purulent (containing pus)
      (3) sanguineous (containing blood)
      (4) a combination of the above
   e. Increased size (hypertrophy) or decreased size (atrophy) of inflamed cells
   f. Spread of inflammation from local extension into contiguous tissues, signalled by red streaks radiating along blood vessels
B. Systemic signs
   1. Redness, such as flushing of the face, neck, or other areas
   2. Heat (fever) as the body increases its temperature to make the environment unfavorable for pathogens
   3. Pain, such as headache, joint aches, and backache
   4. Generalized edema
   5. Loss of function, such as weakness, malaise, or fatigue

III. **Factors affecting inflammation**
A. Blood supply
B. Number of leukocytes at the injury site (to keep the inflammation localized and kill pathogens)
C. Nutritional status (availability of iron, proteins, vitamins A, C, and D, and various minerals for cell repair and regeneration)
D. Foreign material in the inflamed area (such as dirt or debris) which may prevent healing or cause localized infection
E. Age (healing slows with advancing age)

IV. **Restoration (healing) of inflammation**
A. Resolution
   1. Total remission of signs and symptoms
   2. No residual evidence of inflammation
B. Repair
   1. Generation of new cells to replace those lost during inflammation
   2. Similarity of new cells to the normal cells lost
C. Scar formation: organization of fibrous connective tissue to form scars or granulation tissue

V. **Complications of inflammation**
A. Infection from excessive pathogens at the injury site or an inadequate inflammatory response

    B. Contractures
      1. Characterized by shortening or tightening of tissues
      2. Cause deformity from excess scarring
    C. Strictures
      1. Characterized by narrowing of the lumen of a hollow organ, such as the esophagus or intestine
      2. Result from scar tissue
    D. Adhesions
      1. Characterized by a band of scar tissue that binds together two anatomical surfaces that normally are separate
      2. May cause functional changes, pain, or other problems
    E. Hernia: outward bulging of tissue
    F. Keloids: excess or overgrowth of scar tissue
    G. Granulomas: accumulation of scar tissue within scar tissue (such as a keloid or neuroma)

  VI. **Nursing considerations**
    A. Monitoring
      1. Vital signs, noting any elevated temperature, spiking temperature, or increased pulse or respiratory rate
      2. Injury site, noting the presence and amount of any drainage (which should decrease as inflammation resolves)
      3. Contents from other openings or orifices, noting such abnormalities as cloudy urine, yellow sputum, diarrhea, or vomiting
      4. Patient complaints of fatigue, malaise, anorexia, and pain—all signs of inflammation
    B. Assessing for redness, swelling, pain, and tenderness in the inflamed area
    C. Reporting any complaints of burning on urination, pain on respiration, productive cough with yellow sputum, or increased pain or drainage from the inflamed area
    D. Documenting all findings on the patient's chart

Shock

  I. **Introduction**
    A. A state of acute circulatory failure characterized by inadequate cellular perfusion and decreased oxygenation from reduced circulating blood volume
    B. May cause cellular death from impaired perfusion, which reduces cellular oxygenation

  II. **Causes**
    A. Heart (pump) failure
    B. Blood volume depletion (as from hemorrhage or dehydration)
    C. Changes in blood vessel responses causing vasodilation or vasoconstriction

  III. **Classification**
    A. Anaphylactic shock
      1. This is an antigen-antibody reaction causing massive vasodilation

2. Underlying causes include:
   a. drug allergy
   b. transfusion reaction
   c. insect sting
B. Hypovolemic shock
   1. This form of shock occurs when circulating fluid volume decreases
   2. The underlying cause is excessive loss of body fluids, such as from hemorrhage, burns, severe vomiting, or diarrhea
C. Cardiogenic shock
   1. This form of shock occurs when the left ventricle of the heart fails, leading to circulatory collapse
   2. Underlying causes include:
      a. myocardial infarction
      b. cardiac arrest
D. Neurogenic shock
   1. This form of shock takes place when the sympathetic nervous system is interrupted, resulting in massive vasodilation
   2. Underlying causes include:
      a. spinal cord injury
      b. spinal anesthesia
      c. damage to the medulla oblongata
E. Septic shock
   1. This form of shock results from release of toxins (poisons) from certain bacteria (especially gram-positive and gram-negative organisms), causing massive vasodilation
   2. Septic shock is fatal in half the cases
   3. Underlying causes include:
      a. gram-negative sepsis (such as from *Pseudomonas, Klebsiella, Proteus* and *Escherichia coli* organisms)
      b. gram-positive sepsis (such as from *Staphylococcus* and *Streptococcus* organisms)

IV. **Nursing considerations**
A. General guidelines
   1. The patient requires prompt action to prevent death
   2. Treatment is guided by certain basic principles, regardless of the cause of shock
   3. The general implementations described below may need to be augmented by others, depending on the specific type of shock
B. General implementations
   1. Position the patient to maintain an open airway
   2. Maintain the patient on bed rest to decrease oxygen demands
   3. Administer oxygen, if ordered, by the prescribed method (nasal catheter, cannula, or mechanical ventilator)
   4. Monitor vital signs frequently (as often as every 5 to 15 minutes)
   5. Monitor the patient's level of consciousness hourly and perform all neurologic checks
   6. Monitor the patient's skin color to determine adequacy of perfusion
   7. Place the patient in a modified Trendelenburg position (with the head of the bed raised 20 to 30 degrees and the foot raised to 45 degrees); this position helps to keep vital organs perfused (elevating the head and feet increases venous return)
   8. Monitor fluid replacement closely to restore blood volume, increase perfusion, and help maintain blood pressure at desirable levels

9. Administer plasma, packed red blood cells, albumin or dextran (Macrodex), as ordered, to increase blood volume and blood pressure
10. Turn or reposition the patient every 2 hours to prevent pressure ulcers or problems caused by immobility
11. Maintain strict aseptic technique to prevent infection (a weakened patient is more likely to develop infection)
12. Administer ordered medications properly and on schedule to maintain adequate blood drug levels
13. Listen to bowel sounds to determine if perfusion is adequate; check for abdominal pain or distention
14. Monitor cardiac functions on a cardiac monitor; report any abnormal rhythms or contractions
15. Monitor fluid intake and output and urine specific gravity hourly to determine the adequacy of fluid replacement and renal perfusion
16. Monitor laboratory data for signs of acid-base imbalance, anoxia, and other abnormalities
17. If possible, provide long, uninterrupted rest periods to allow the patient to rest and avoid exhaustion. Optimally, the patient should be allowed to rest uninterrupted for at least 90 minutes
18. Monitor central venous pressure readings to determine the adequacy of fluid replacement and cardiac function
19. Keep the patient covered lightly to prevent chilling
20. Provide emotional support to the patient and family
21. Observe for possible complications, such as congestive heart failure, pneumonia, renal failure, pulmonary edema, metabolic acidosis, and progressive vascular clotting
22. Record all findings promptly and accurately on flow sheets or nursing sheets

C. Anaphylactic shock
  1. Assess the patient for:
     a. wheezing
     b. dyspnea
     c. bronchospasm (as evidenced by gasping, inability to speak, and anxiety)
     d. redness near the site of an insect bite
     e. rash or hives
     f. vocal changes (from tightness of the throat)
  2. Carry out the following implementations:
     a. administering epinephrine (Adrenalin) in a 1:1,000 dilution, 0.1 to 0.3 ml subcutaneously, as ordered
        (1) Epinephrine dilates the bronchi and constricts arterioles and capillaries
        (2) Because epinephrine increases the heart rate, observe the patient for tachycardia and nervousness
     b. administering an antihistamine (such as diphenhydramine [Benadryl] or brompheniramine [Dimetane]), as ordered
        (1) Antihistamines relieve bronchospasm, hives, itching, and other allergic reactions
        (2) Because antihistamines may cause drowsiness and muscle incoordination, caution the patient not to drive, use heavy equipment or tools, or ingest alcohol or other depressant substances

  c. administering corticosteroids, as ordered, to decrease inflammation and improve microcirculation

  d. administering oxygen, if ordered, to correct impaired tissue perfusion

 D. Hypovolemic shock

  1. Assess the patient for:

   a. low blood pressure

   b. decreased urine output

   c. restlessness

   d. decreased central venous pressure

   e. increased pulse and respiratory rates

  2. Carry out the following implementations:

   a. replacing blood volume, as ordered, by administering fluids,
blood products, or volume expanders

   b. administering oxygen, if ordered, to correct impaired tissue perfusion

 E. Cardiogenic shock

  1. Assess the patient for:

   a. vital signs

   b. evidence of heart failure, pulmonary edema, myocardial infarction, or cardiac arrest

  2. Carry out the following implementations:

   a. administering vasodilatory drugs (such as dopamine [Intropin]
or sodium nitroprusside [Nipride]) to decrease peripheral resistance, thereby reducing the work load of the heart

   b. administering oxygen, if ordered, to correct impaired tissue perfusion

   c. performing cardiopulmonary resuscitation, if pulse and respirations are absent (see "Performing basic cardiopulmonary resuscitation," page 199)

 F. Neurogenic shock

  1. Assess the patient for:

   a. hypotension (which may be pronounced)

   b. change in the level of consciousness and mental function

   c. slow pulse (bradycardia)

   d. low body temperature

  2. Carry out the following implementations:

   a. administering vasopressors, such as epinephrine, as ordered, to
counteract massive vasodilation

   b. monitoring vital signs every 5 minutes initially after vasopressor
administration, then every 15 minutes until the patient is stable

   c. administering steroids, as ordered, to protect the lysosomal
membrane from leaking destructive enzymes

   d. administering oxygen, as ordered, to correct impaired tissue
perfusion

 G. Septic shock

  1. Assess the patient for:

   a. chills

   b. fever

   c. spiking temperature (shaking chills and high fevers commonly
precede a sudden drop in blood pressure, skin color changes,
and late shock)

   d. disorientation, restlessness, and confusion (from inadequate cerebral perfusion)

    e. skin color changes (a grayish cast with gram-negative sepsis and redness with gram-positive sepsis)

    f. possible infection sources (such as peritonitis), instrumentation (such as cystoscopy), toxic shock syndrome from tampon use, or food poisoning

2. Carry out the following implementations:

    a. ensuring prompt treatment to prevent death

    b. monitoring the patient closely for signs of infection that may signal deeper septic shock (described above) and reporting these signs immediately to prevent shock from developing or progressing further

    c. administering oxygen immediately, as ordered, to counter anoxia

    d. initiating I.V therapy promptly, as ordered, to keep the vein open

    e. administering antibiotics, as ordered, to combat infection, such as gentamycin (Garamicin) for gram-negative sepsis or nafcillin (Nafcil), ampicillin (Amcill), or erythromycin for gram-positive sepsis

    f. administering steroids, as ordered, to reduce inflammation

Acid-base balance

  I. **Definition: relationship of the body's hydrogen (H) ion concentration to hydroxyl (OH) ion concentration**

  II. **General information**

    A. Reflects the ratio of acids to bases in the body (relationship of carbonic acid to bicarbonate)

    B. Exists when the body produces and excretes acids and bases to maintain a normal acid-base ratio of 1:20 (1 part carbonic acid to 20 parts bicarbonate)

    C. Is influenced by many factors

    D. Is altered by various diseases

  III. **Determination of acid-base status**

    A. Made from arterial blood gas samples

    B. Depends on several values

      1. Blood pH

        a. Normal values range from 7.35 to 7.45 — slightly alkaline, or basic

        b. A neutral pH (one that is neither acidic or alkaline) is 7

      2. Partial pressure of arterial carbon dioxide ($PaCO_2$): normally ranges from 35 to 45 mm Hg

      3. Partial pressure of arterial oxygen (PaO_2): normally measures 90 ± 10 mm Hg

      4. Serum bicarbonate: normally ranges from 21 to 29 mEq/liter (25 ± 4 mEq/liter)

  IV. **Acid-base regulation**

    A. Performed by blood buffers, respiratory buffers, and kidney buffers, all working in concert

B. Description
  1. Blood buffers
      a. These buffers work continuously to help maintain acid-base balance
          (1) In response to a change in pH, hemoglobin in red blood cells shifts chloride ions in or out of the cell walls
          (2) Each chloride ion leaving the cell is replaced by a bicarbonate ion
          (3) The kidneys excrete or absorb bicarbonate to help maintain a normal acid-base balance
      b. In response to a change in pH, plasma proteins act as buffers by attracting or releasing hydrogen ions
      c. Bicarbonate attempts to maintain blood pH between 7.35 and 7.45, with a ratio of 20 parts bicarbonate to 1 part carbonic acid
  2. Respiratory buffers
      a. The lungs react to a change in pH within 1 to 3 minutes by increasing or decreasing the respiratory rate to retain or eliminate carbon dioxide (CO_2)
          (1) CO_2, an acidic molecule, dissolves in water in the blood, forming carbonic acid ($CO_2 + H_2O = H_2CO_3$, or carbonic acid)
          (2) Increased CO_2 levels, which are equivalent to increased hydrogen ions, reduce the blood pH
      b. When the blood pH drops below normal, the respiratory center in the medulla triggers slower or more shallow breathing, reducing CO_2 elimination; consequently, the blood pH level rises
      c. When the blood pH level rises above normal, breathing becomes deeper and the respiratory center increases CO_2 elimination; consequently, the blood pH decreases
  3. Kidney (metabolic) buffers
      a. These buffers help normalize the blood pH by increasing or decreasing the amount of bicarbonate ions in extracellular fluid
      b. This buffer system takes longer than the respiratory buffers—from a few hours to several days
      c. The kidneys regulate *metabolic* acid-base balance in several ways
          (1) They excrete or absorb hydrogen ions as needed; hydrogen ions make more acids
          (2) They form more carbonic acid to lower the blood pH, or more ammonia (NH_3) to raise the blood pH (ammonia is alkaline)

V. **Types of acid-base imbalances**
A. Acidosis
  1. Is characterized by a blood pH below 7.35
  2. Results from an increased hydrogen ion concentration or a decreased H_2CO_3 level
  3. May be respiratory or metabolic
      a. Respiratory acidosis occurs when CO_2 accumulates
      b. Causes include conditions that impede CO_2 excretion by the lungs:
          (1) oversedation
          (2) chronic obstructive pulmonary disease such as emphysema, asthma, or bronchitis

          (3) brain injury

          (4) chest-wall injury

          (5) airway obstruction

          (6) hypoventilation

          (7) improper ventilatory settings

          (8) pneumonia

      c. *Metabolic acidosis* occurs when the kidneys cannot clear excess acids

          (1) Bicarbonate decreases or retention of hydrogen ions increases

          (2) Causes include:

            (a) diabetic ketoacidosis (from excess ketones caused by lack of insulin)

            (b) renal failure (from phosphate and sulfate retention)

            (c) severe diarrhea (from excessive loss of bicarbonate and sodium ions)

            (d) excessive exercising leading to increased lactic acid levels

            (e) intake of large doses of ammonium chloride (an acidifying drug)

B. Alkalosis

  1. Is characterized by a decreased hydrogen ion concentration or an abnormal bicarbonate (HCO_3^-) elevation

  2. May be respiratory or metabolic

      a. *Respiratory alkalosis* occurs when the level of CO_2 in the blood decreases

          (1) Physiologic causes include:

            (a) hyperventilation (such as from pain or anxiety)

            (b) sepsis

          (2) Mechanical causes include:

            (a) incorrect mechanical ventilator settings

            (b) mechanical ventilator malfunction

      b. *Metabolic alkalosis* occurs when the HCO_3^- level increases

          (1) It may also result from a decreased hydrogen ion concentration

          (2) Causes include:

            (a) excess intake of antacids or bicarbonate (used to treat indigestion or ulcers)

            (b) excessive vomiting (causing loss of hydrochloric acid)

            (c) irrigation of a nasogastric (NG) tube using plain water instead of normal saline solution (causing loss of hydrogen or chloride ions)

            (d) NG tube suctioning

VI. Nursing care

A. Respiratory acidosis

  1. Assessment

      a. Observe the patient for slow, shallow respirations, drowsiness, headache, confusion, or coma

      b. Check for hyperventilation (rapid, deep breathing), reflecting the lungs' attempt to excrete excess CO_2

      c. Evaluate the patient for periodic apnea, reflecting CO_2 narcosis (CO_2 insensitivity of the respiratory center)

2. Implementations
   a. Instruct the patient to perform deep-breathing exercises hourly to decrease the CO_2 level
   b. Obtain an order for incentive spirometry to increase ventilation and help reduce the $PaCO_2$ level
   c. Suction the patient, as ordered and needed, to clear the airway
   d. Administer only 1 to 2 liters of oxygen (if ordered) to prevent $PaCO_2$ narcosis
   e. Observe and monitor the patient's level of consciousness
   f. Reposition an unconscious patient every 2 hours
   g. Monitor the patient for headache or confusion
   h. Offer support and encourage the patient to cooperate with treatments
   i. Check vital signs and record all patient responses to implementations
   j. Listen to breath sounds in all lung lobes

B. Respiratory alkalosis
   1. Assessment
      a. Observe the patient for hyperventilation and increased respiratory depth
      b. Evaluate for muscle twitching, numbness, or tingling of fingers or toes
      c. Note any gasping for breath or seizures (caused by lack of circulating ionized calcium needed for muscle contractions)
   2. Implementations
      a. Instruct the patient to breathe only through the nose with the lips closed to prevent hyperventilation and excess CO_2 elimination
      b. Instruct the patient to breathe into a paper bag to increase CO_2 retention
      c. Administer a sedative, if ordered, to depress the respiratory center and decrease the respiratory rate
      d. Provide emotional support to reduce patient anxiety and promote well-being

C. Metabolic acidosis
   1. Assessment
      a. Evaluate the patient for headache, drowsiness, disorientation, or coma, caused by central nervous system depression
      b. Note any signs or symptoms of dehydration (in a patient with diarrhea)
      c. Check for rapid, deep breathing (Kussmaul's respirations), caused by CO_2 excess
      d. Evaluate the patient for cardiac arrhythmias related to excess serum potassium levels (reflecting potassium displacement by hydrogen ions and subsequent potassium entry into the bloodstream)
      e. Check for a fruity breath odor, resulting from the lungs' attempt to excrete ketones
   2. Implementations
      a. Administer medications, as ordered
         (1) Administer insulin, as ordered, if metabolic acidosis stems from diabetic ketoacidosis (lowers acid levels by aiding movement of carbohydrates into cells to metabolize ketones)

PRINCIPLES AND PROCEDURES

      (2) Administer sodium bicarbonate, as ordered, to increase base and improve the ratio of bicarbonate to CO_2

      (3) Administer sodium lactate, as ordered, to restore acid-base balance because this substance metabolizes to bicarbonate in the liver

  b. Monitor the patient's blood glucose level hourly for a return to normal (80 to 120 mg/dl)

  c. Monitor apical pulses for arrhythmias caused by high serum potassium levels

  d. Monitor vital signs, as ordered

  e. Monitor fluid intake and output frequently

  f. Check the level of consciousness hourly

  g. Monitor laboratory data to assess therapeutic effectiveness and alerting the physician to any data suggesting that treatment should be continued or changed

  h. Transfer the patient for dialysis, if ordered, if acidosis stems from renal failure

D. Metabolic alkalosis

  1. Assessment

    a. Check for agitation, irritability, disorientation, seizures, or coma, caused by cerebral overstimulation from high alkaline levels

    b. Evaluate for restlessness, twitching, numbness or tingling of the fingers and toes, resulting from lack of ionized calcium

    c. Note any apnea, caused by the lungs' attempt to retain CO_2 to restore a normal acid-base ratio

    d. Observe for an irregular apical pulse or cardiac arrhythmia, caused by hydrogen, chloride, or potassium loss

  2. Implementations

    a. Discourage the patient from self-medicating with antacids

    b. Use normal saline solution to irrigate NG tubes to prevent hydrogen and chloride ion loss

    c. Provide ordered fluid and electrolyte replacements to restore fluids and electrolytes

    d. Monitor laboratory values for return to normal or evidence that further treatment is needed

    e. Allow the patient to engage in activity as indicated (may need to enforce bed rest initially, followed by activity as tolerated)

Fluids and electrolytes

I.   **General information**

A. Fluids (body water) make up 45% to 60% of the total body weight

  1. Fluids are contained inside cells (intracellular fluid), between cells (interstitial fluid), and in the plasma (intravascular fluid)

  2. Interstitial and intravascular fluids are called extracellular fluids

B. Electrolytes are ions that carry a positive or negative charge and dissolve in solutions

  1. Sodium, potassium, and calcium—three of the body's major electrolytes—carry a positive charge (thus, they are called cations)

       a. Sodium
          (1) Governs the movement of fluid into or out of cells
          (2) Relates closely to the body's fluid level
       b. Potassium
          (1) Helps regulate neuromuscular excitability
          (2) Helps govern muscle contraction
       c. Calcium
          (1) Is a component of extracellular fluid and soft-tissue cells
          (2) Is required for such body functions as nerve impulse transmission, muscle contraction, cardiac function, and blood coagulation
    2. Chloride, bicarbonate, sulfate, and phosphate carry a negative charge; thus, they are called anions
    3. Electrolyte concentration in solution is stated as milliequivalents per liter (mEq/liter)

II. Mechanisms of fluid and electrolyte movement into and out of cells

    A. *Osmosis* involves movement of pure solvents (such as water) from an area of lower solute concentration to an area of greater solute concentration
       1. Movement occurs across a membrane that is permeable to the solvent but impermeable to solid molecules
       2. This results in equal concentrations of solution on each side of the membrane
    B. *Diffusion* involves movement of such substances as electrolytes (solutes) from an area of greater concentration to an area of lower concentration
    C. *Active transport* involves movement of substances across the cell membrane by means of chemical activity that permits entry of larger molecules than otherwise could enter the cell
       1. Penetration by large molecules disturbs the cell's internal equilibrium
       2. In response, the cell releases materials through its membrane

III. Fluid imbalance

    A. Fluid excess (fluid overload, or hypervolemia) occurs when the body's fluid level is excessive
    B. Fluid deficit (dehydration, or hypovolemia) occurs when the body's fluid level is insufficient

IV. Electrolyte imbalances

    A. Sodium imbalance is characterized by an abnormally high or low serum sodium level
       1. The normal serum sodium level is 135 to 145 mEq/liter
       2. Sodium excess (hypernatremia) results from:
          a. excessive intake or administration of sodium chloride (salt)
          b. dehydration
          c. diarrhea with greater loss of fluid than sodium
          d. excessive perspiration
          e. fever
       3. Sodium deficiency (hyponatremia) results from:
          a. diuretic administration
          b. lack of dietary sodium
          c. renal disease
          d. vomiting
          e. fluid replacement with water only
          f. use of water instead of normal saline solution to irrigate tubes

B. Potassium imbalance is characterized by an abnormally high or low serum potassium level
   1. The normal serum potassium level ranges from 3.5 to 5 mEq/liter
   2. Potassium excess (hyperkalemia) results from:
      a. renal disease (which impedes potassium excretion)
      b. burn injury (from cell destruction that frees intracellular potassium)
      c. crush injuries (from release of intracellular potassium)
      d. diabetic ketoacidosis (from intracellular potassium displacement by hydrogen ions)
   3. Potassium deficiency (hypokalemia) results from:
      a. use of diuretics
      b. insufficient potassium intake
      c. administration of corticosteroids (which cause sodium retention and potassium excretion)
      d. vomiting or diarrhea
      e. fasting
C. Calcium imbalance is characterized by an abnormally high or low serum calcium level
   1. Total serum calcium levels normally range from 4.5 to 5.5 mEq/liter
   2. Calcium excess (hypercalcemia) results from:
      a. prolonged immobilization (from loss of calcium from bones)
      b. excess vitamin D intake
      c. hyperparathyroidism
      d. parathyroid gland tumor
   3. Calcium deficiency (hypocalcemia) results from:
      a. parathyroid gland removal
      b. decreased vitamin D intake
      c. excessive intake of antacids containing magnesium or aluminum

V. **Nursing care**
   A. For fluid excess:
      1. Assess the patient for tachycardia (rapid heart rate), neck vein distention, high blood pressure, flushed skin, and edema
      2. Carry out the following implementations:
         a. slowing or discontinuing the I.V. solutions, as ordered
         b. decreasing the patient's oral fluid intake
         c. administering diuretics, as ordered, to promote fluid excretion
   B. For fluid deficit:
      1. Assess the patient for thirst, reduced skin turgor (sluggish return of the skin to the usual shape and position when pinched); cracked or dry lips; decreased urine output (under 30 ml/hour); weight loss; and dark, concentrated urine
      2. Carry out the following implementations:
         a. administering I.V. solutions, as ordered, to replace fluids
         b. increasing oral fluid intake, as ordered, to replace fluids
   C. For hypernatremia:
      1. Assess the patient for weight gain; pitting edema; increased blood pressure; dyspnea; thirst; dry, sticky mucous membranes; and seizures
      2. Carry out the following implementations:
         a. increasing fluid intake (to reduce the sodium content of extracellular fluid)
         b. providing a sodium-restricted diet

      c. weighing the patient daily

      d. measuring vital signs

D. For hyponatremia:

  1. Assess the patient for weakness, restlessness, delirium, abdominal cramps, decreased urine output, decreased blood pressure, and seizures

  2. Carry out the following implementations:

      a. administering I.V. solutions containing sodium to replace fluids

      b. teaching the patient about sodium loss during diuretic administration

      c. using normal saline solution to irrigate tubes or give enemas

      d. using caution when giving tap-water enemas because this procedure may cause sodium loss

      e. documenting fluid intake and output accurately

      f. restricting the patient's fluid intake (to increase the serum sodium level)

E. For hyperkalemia:

  1. Assess the patient for weak, flaccid muscles; dizziness; electrocardiograph changes; cardiac arrhythmias, including ventricular fibrillation; and cardiac arrest (if the serum potassium level approaches 7 to 8 mEq/liter)

  2. Carry out the following implementations:

      a. restricting potassium intake if the patient has renal disease

      b. administering sodium polystyrene sulfonate (Kayexalate), a resin that exchanges potassium for nonabsorbable sodium ions, as ordered

      c. administering agents that increase urinary potassium excretion, such as thiazide diuretics, as ordered

      d. assisting with renal dialysis, as ordered and needed

      e. forcing fluids (unless the patient has renal disease) to increase urine output and flush out excess potassium

F. For hypokalemia:

  1. Assess the patient for muscle weakness, decreased reflexes, low blood pressure, fatigue, paralytic ileus, cardiac arrhythmias, and weak pulse

  2. Carry out the following implementations:

      a. instructing the patient to eat potassium-rich foods, such as watermelon, cantaloupe, potatoes, bananas, orange juice, and dried fruits

      b. administering an oral potassium supplement, as ordered, followed by water (to eliminate the supplement's unpleasant taste)

      c. administering I.V. potassium replacement slowly, as ordered

        (1) Ensuring that potassium in the I.V. solution does not exceed 40 mEq/liter

        (2) Observing the I.V. site for infiltration (potassium administration can cause phlebitis)

      d. administering a potassium replacement, as ordered, to help prevent digitalis toxicity (in a patient receiving digitalis)

G. For hypercalcemia:

  1. Assess the patient for decreased muscle tone, tiredness, flank pain associated with kidney stones, bone pain, nausea, vomiting, and cardiac arrest

2. Carry out the following implementations:
   a. providing a diet abundant in acid ash foods (such as fish, meat, eggs, corn, and prunes) to acidify the urine and keep calcium-based kidney stones in solution in urine
   b. limiting the patient's calcium intake by restricting milk and milk products
   c. monitoring for digitalis toxicity caused by high calcium levels (in patients receiving digitalis)

H. For hypocalcemia:
   1. Assess the patient for abdominal cramps, muscle cramps, muscle twitching, tetany with tingling in the fingers or around the lips and laryngospasm, a positive Chvostek's sign (cheek spasm and eyelid twitching when the facial nerve is tapped just in front of the ear), and a positive Trousseau's sign (spasm of the fingers and forearm after blood pressure cuff inflation)
   2. Carry out the following implementations:
      a. administering ordered I.V. calcium replacements slowly
      b. instructing the patient to increase vitamin D intake by consuming plenty of milk and dairy products (vitamin D is needed for calcium absorption)

Immobility

I. **Definition: a decrease in the ability to move all or part of the body**
II. **Causes**
   A. Anoxia (loss of oxygen to cells, leading to cellular death or altered cell function)
   B. Degenerative conditions, such as joint disease
   C. Infectious agents, which may cause temporary immobility (such as toxic shock syndrome resulting from staphylococci)
   D. Medications
      1. Certain sedatives
      2. Anesthetics
      3. Poisons
   E. Severe anxiety
   F. Medical treatments, which may cause temporary immobility (such as those requiring bed rest or application of a cast or splint)
   G. Trauma that cuts a nerve, nerve pathways, or muscle fibers to or from affected tissues, which can cause paraplegia or quadriplegia
III. **Classification**
   A. Immobility resulting from loss of motor function
      1. Quadriplegia: paralysis of all extremities
      2. Paraplegia: paralysis of the legs
      3. Hemiplegia: paralysis of one side of the body
   B. Immobility resulting from loss of sensory function
      1. Blindness
      2. Deafness
      3. Hemianopsia: blindness or defective vision in half of the visual field of one or both eyes
      4. Agnosia: inability to recognize an object or thing
      5. Anesthesia: loss of touch and pain sensation

6. Proprioceptive loss: lack of awareness of one's position in space
7. Aphasia: defect or loss of language function
    a. Motor (expressive) aphasia is the inability to speak intended words
    b. Sensory (receptive) aphasia is the inability to understand words

IV. Nursing considerations
A. Major nursing goals
    1. Helping to preserve the function of unaffected tissues
    2. Promoting maximal function of affected tissues
B. Complications of immobility (by body system)
    1. Musculoskeletal complications: muscle atrophy, muscle spasms, contractions
    2. Neurologic complications: paralysis, anesthesia, altered pain perceptions (with acute or chronic pain syndromes)
    3. Respiratory complications: anoxia, atelectasis, pneumonia
    4. Cardiovascular complications: arrhythmia, tachycardia, phlebitis, thrombus, embolism
    5. Integumentary complications: pressure ulcers
    6. Gastrointestinal complications: nausea, vomiting, abdominal distention, diarrhea, constipation
    7. Genitourinary complications: urinary tract infections, renal or bladder calculi
    8. Endocrine complications: osteoporosis, weight loss, fever
    9. Psychological complications: grief, anxiety, altered role performance
C. Nursing care to prevent complications
    1. Musculoskeletal complications
        a. Perform range-of-motion exercises
        b. Perform muscle-setting exercises
        c. Handle the patient's tissues and joints gently
        d. Administer muscle-relaxant medications, as ordered
        e. Reposition the patient frequently
    2. Neurologic complications
        a. Perform neurologic checks
        b. Administer sedatives or pain medications, as ordered
        c. Use blankets, special mattresses, or pads to reduce pressure on tissues with deficient sensation
    3. Respiratory complications
        a. Encourage breathing exercises
        b. Help the patient perform breathing exercises with a spirometer or mechanical ventilator, as ordered
        c. Suction, as needed
    4. Cardiovascular complications
        a. Monitor vital signs carefully
        b. Encourage the patient to move muscles and joints and perform exercises
        c. Apply elastic hosiery and elevate the legs, as ordered
        d. Check capillary refill periodically
        e. Administer oxygen, as ordered
        f. Monitor I.V. infusion sites carefully for signs of phlebitis
        g. Note any patient complaints of soreness in the calves to detect thrombophlebitis
        h. Monitor laboratory data for abnormal hemoglobin, hematocrit, and electrolyte values

5. Integumentary complications
   a. Massage around bony prominences
   b. Turn the patient every 2 hours as needed
   c. Use mattresses and pads to lessen pressure on bony prominences that can impair circulation
6. Gastrointestinal complications
   a. Perform thorough oral hygiene
   b. Assist the patient with feeding
   c. Provide a wholesome diet with a high fiber content to prevent constipation
   d. Administer I.V. fluids, as ordered (up to 3,000 ml/24 hours)
   e. Measure fluid intake and output
   f. Administer a rectal suppository or perform rectal stimulation, if needed
   g. Listen for bowel sounds in all abdominal quadrants
7. Genitourinary complications
   a. Monitor urine output
   b. Note any patient complaints of urinary burning, frequency, and urgency or flank pain (which may indicate kidney stones)
   c. Note any complaints of chills or fever
8. Endocrine complications
   a. Weigh the patient daily
   b. Perform active and passive exercises (if the patient is able)
   c. Monitor laboratory data for abnormal results
9. Psychological complications
   a. Assist the patient to cope with grief
   b. Help the patient adapt to losses and changes in life-style and employment

GENERAL NURSING PROCEDURES

Assisting with ambulation

Purpose

To help the patient get out of bed and walk; to help the patient walk using an ambulatory aid, such as a cane, crutch, or walker

Steps

1. Raise the head of the bed to high Fowler's position to help the patient out of bed and allow vascular adjustment to the position change.
2. Place the patient's robe and nonskid slippers or shoes within easy reach.
3. Lower the bed to the lowest position.
4. Help the patient to a sitting position on the edge of the bed, with feet on the floor. Ask how the patient feels, and check the pulse. If this is the patient's first time out of bed after prolonged bed rest, measure blood pressure and compare it to previous readings.
5. If the patient's pulse and blood pressure are acceptable, help the patient put on the robe and assume a standing position. Stand directly in front of the patient with your hands under the patient's arms and the patient's hands on your shoulders. To keep the patient's knees extended and prevent them from buckling, place your knees in front of the patient's knees. Have the patient stand still briefly to allow blood pressure to stabilize; ask how the patient feels.
6. Grasp the patient around the waist, or have the patient hold onto your forearm with elbow bent as you help the patient walk. (Or you may place your arm around the patient's waist to lend support.) If the patient is weak, ask for help so one nurse is on either side of the patient; or tie a belt around the patient's waist to hold the patient.
7. If the patient cannot be disconnected from an I.V. line, have an assistant bring the I.V. tubing or pole along as you walk with the patient, or have the patient grasp the I.V. pole for support and push the pole along while walking (if the patient's condition permits).

8. After every few steps, have the patient stop, then ask how the patient feels. If this is the patient's first time up, walk only a short distance (such as to a chair in the room) to avoid tiring the patient.
9. Check the path ahead for obstructions or hazards, such as loose tile, loose cord, or puddles.
10. When ambulation ends, help the patient into a chair (if the patient's condition allows) or help the patient back into bed.
11. If this is the patient's first time up, measure pulse and blood pressure when the patient returns to bed.
12. Document the ambulation, noting the distance walked and the patient's response.

Precautions and nursing considerations

• For 1 or 2 days before ambulation is scheduled to begin, have the patient perform muscle-toning exercises to increase muscle strength.
• Before ambulation begins, determine the patient's need for help by assessing for:
  factors that promote ambulation—alertness, adequate muscle mass and strength, presence of both legs (or prostheses), younger age, short period of bed rest.
  factors that impede ambulation—musculoskeletal or neurologic disease, paraplegia or hemiplegia, impaired balance, bone disease (such as osteomyelitis or fracture), age 65 or older, chronic illness, prolonged bed rest, presence of tubing or drainage systems, medications that can cause weakness or confusion, defective vision, defective hearing (unless the patient has a hearing aid).
• If necessary, seek help from another person to ensure safe ambulation.
• Keep a long towel or belt handy to wrap around the patient's waist to keep the patient from falling. (For more information on assisting with ambulation, see "Teaching a patient to use crutches, a cane, or a walker," pages 272 and 273.)

Changing a sterile dressing

Purpose
To support the natural wound-healing process, prevent the spread of disease-causing organisms, promote a return to normal function (homeostasis), and prevent additional injury

Steps
1. Assess the wound for signs of healing.
2. Check the physician's order for type of wound care, dressing change, and type of dressing needed.
3. Gather needed supplies: sterile solution, sterile dressings of various sizes, sterile gloves, clean disposable gloves, plastic bag, tape or ties, swabs with antiseptic, adhesive remover, and sterile drape (towel).
4. Explain the procedure to the patient, then position the patient comfortably. Close the curtain and door for privacy.
5. Wash your hands.
6. Place the plastic bag within easy reach.
7. Put on the clean disposable gloves.
8. Open the ties on the soiled dressing, or loosen the adhesive tape. Remove the dressing, touching only its outer surface.
9. Holding the dressing out of the patient's sight, observe it for appearance and amount of drainage, then discard it in the plastic bag.
10. Remove the gloves and discard them in the plastic bag.
11. Open the sterile dressing tray or sterile dressings and place them on the sterile drape on the overbed table.
12. Open the sterile swabs or sterile solution, if ordered. (Typically, the physician orders povidone-iodine [Betadine] swabs, saline solution, or hydrogen peroxide.)
13. Put on the sterile gloves.
14. Closely inspect the wound for appearance, noting such signs of inflammation as redness, edema, drainage, and open areas. Note any patient complaints of local pain or tenderness.

15. If the wound contains excess drainage, wipe the wound site, working from clean to contaminated areas.
16. Using antiseptic swabs, clean the wound by stroking the swab from the wound to the outer skin. Use a separate swab for each stroke, and swab until you have cleaned the entire wound.
17. Using a swab, clean around any drains in the wound area.
18. Apply a dry sterile dressing to the wound. (To fit a gauze dressing around a drain, you may need to cut the dressing using sterile scissors.)
19. If the dressing is small, apply an ABD pad over it as an outer cover.
20. Apply tape over the dressing and secure the dressing with Montgomery straps or ties, as needed. (An abdominal binder may be used to hold the dressing.)
21. Remove the gloves and discard them in the plastic bag. Also discard any opened and unused supplies.
22. Close the solution bottles and replace them in the patient's cupboard or stand, if appropriate.
23. Replace the patient's gown and help the patient to a comfortable position.
24. Discard the plastic bag in the correct receptacle in the utility room.
25. Wash your hands.
26. Document the dressing change on the patient's chart, noting the type and amount of drainage, wound condition, and any patient complaints related to the wound.

Precautions and nursing considerations
• Before beginning, make sure you understand the principles of sterile technique (including wound healing and pathogen transfer) and know which dressing must be used for the type of wound present.
• Make sure you can recognize the signs and symptoms of inflammation and infection to detect these conditions promptly.

Irrigating a wound

Purpose
To flush the wound of drainage and debris and to promote wound healing and formation of granulation tissue

Steps
1. Check the physician's order for the type of solution specified (usually half-strength hydrogen peroxide and normal saline solution).

2. Gather needed supplies, as described in "Changing a sterile dressing," plus a sterile basin for the irrigating solution, a syringe to hold the solution and flush the wound, and a linen-saver (protective) pad.

3. Follow steps 4 to 11 under "Changing a sterile dressing."

4. Open the sterile basin and place it on a sterile field. Pour the correct amount of solution into the basin. Open the syringe wrapper and place the syringe on the sterile field.

5. Put on the sterile gloves.

6. Closely inspect the wound for appearance, noting such signs of inflammation as redness, edema, drainage, and open areas.

7. Place the clean basin or extra dressings at the patient's side or at the base of the wound to catch the irrigating solution and drainage.

8. Fill the syringe with irrigating solution and gently flush the wound, working from clean to contaminated areas. Use care to avoid splashing the solution on the patient or yourself.

9. Continue to flush the wound until it is free of drainage. If the wound extends under the skin, a catheter may be needed to insert solution into deeper wound areas.

10. Remove the basin and soaked dressings from the wound. If the gloves have become contaminated, replace them with a new pair.

11. Clean the wound of excess drainage, then swab the wound area as needed, using antiseptic swabs.

12. If the wound is to be packed with sterile gauze, use the forceps in the dressing set to pack gauze into deeper areas. Pack the gauze loosely but thoroughly so it fills the entire area.

13. Apply a dry sterile dressing over the wound, as needed.

14. Cover the dressing with tape, Montgomery straps, or ties, as needed.

15. Discard the irrigating solution in the bathroom after inspecting the drainage.

16. Gather all soiled supplies and discard them in the plastic bag.

17. Remove the gloves and discard them in the plastic bag.

18. Replace lids to the solutions and place the solutions where they can be used with the next patient.

19. Help the patient to a comfortable position.

20. Discard all soiled materials in appropriate refuse receptacles in the utility room.

21. Wash your hands.

22. Document the wound irrigation, wound condition, type and amount of drainage, signs or symptoms of continuing infection or healing, and other pertinent data.

Precautions and nursing considerations
• Before beginning, assess the wound. Make sure you understand the principles of sterile technique, including wound healing and pathogen transfer, and that you know which dressing must be used for the specific type of wound.

• Make sure you are familiar with the signs and symptoms of inflammation and infection so you can detect these conditions promptly.

Applying a pressure dressing

Purpose
To control sudden or unexpected excessive bleeding, to support underlying tissues, or to support a skin graft. When applied to the site of a partial-thickness skin graft, a pressure dressing (called a stent in this case) is used to reduce the risk of edema and hold the graft in place. Usually, the stent is secured with long threads tied diagonally over fluffed dressings piled over the graft.

Steps
To control bleeding:
1. If you are the first person to notice excessive bleeding, stay with the patient and call for help orally or with the signal light.
2. Try to locate the bleeding site, then apply direct pressure to the site with a towel, dressing, or your hand to control blood loss.
3. Maintain direct pressure on the bleeding site until and after help arrives.
4. Ask another nurse to check the patient's vital signs while you continue to apply pressure.

5. Notify the physician as soon as possible; surgery may be required.
6. Document all actions on the patient's chart.
To support a partial-thickness skin graft:
1. Apply a pressure dressing (stent) to the graft by fluffing up soft, stretchy cotton (such as Kerlex), placing it over the graft, and securing the cotton in place by tying preplaced cotton threads diagonally across it.
2. Make sure the ties are snug so that they hold the cotton securely in place when pressure is applied to the graft.

Precautions and nursing considerations
• When applying a pressure dressing to stop bleeding, make sure to apply pressure continuously over the bleeding site.
• When applying a stent to support a skin graft, take care not to obstruct arterial and capillary flow by tying the ties too tightly.
• Do not change a stent dressing without a physician's order.

Applying a wet-to-dry dressing

Purpose
To help remove debris from a wound; to increase or promote wound healing

Steps
1. Read the physician's order for the wet-to-dry dressing and the type of solution needed.
2. Gather needed supplies: sterile scissors, forceps, sterile 4″ × 3″ pads, fine-mesh gauze strips, sterile drape, sterile basin for the solution, irrigating solution, clean disposable gloves, sterile gloves, tape or Montgomery straps, linen-saver pad, and plastic bag for soiled dressings.
3. Explain the procedure to the patient and position the patient comfortably. Close the curtain and door for privacy.
4. Position the plastic bag for easy access. Expose the wound and place the linen-saver pad under the wound area.
5. Wash your hands and put on the clean disposable gloves.

6. Remove the ties or tape from the dressing and lift the dressing off with the forceps or your fingers. To aid removal, pull the dressing gently; *do not* moisten the dressing. The dressing may be soiled with drainage or it may be dry and virtually unsoiled.
7. Assess drainage for type and amount.
8. Discard the dressing in the plastic bag.
9. Remove the gloves and discard them in the plastic bag.
10. Prepare sterile supplies. Place the basin in the sterile field and pour the irrigating solution into the basin.
11. Put on the sterile gloves.
12. Inspect the wound for color, drainage, and presence of drains or sutures.
13. As needed, clean any drainage or debris from the wound area.
14. Dampen a fine-mesh gauze strip (depending on institutional policy, you may use one to three strips).
15. Place the dampened gauze strip over the wound

and press it into the wound surface firmly to cover all areas.

16. Cover the gauze strip with dry, fine-mesh gauze strips or a dry 4″ × 3″ pad, according to institutional policy. The dressing must dry between changes, so do not make it heavy or thick.

17. Apply tape or tie with Montgomery straps.

18. Help the patient to a comfortable position.

19. Discard the supplies in the plastic bag, remove the gloves, and discard the bag and gloves in the proper receptacle in the utility room.

20. Wash your hands.

21. Document the procedure in the patient's chart, noting wound condition and the type and amount of drainage.

Precautions and nursing considerations

• Do not dampen a wet-to-dry dressing so much that it cannot dry in 2 to 4 hours. An excessively wet dressing causes skin maceration and increases bacterial growth.

• Make sure to follow medical and surgical asepsis guidelines.

PRINCIPLES AND PROCEDURES

Removing sutures or staples

Purpose

To promote complete wound healing and prevent infection

Steps

1. Read the physician's order for suture or staple removal.

2. Gather needed supplies: sterile scissors/forceps set or sterile staple extractor, plastic disposable bag, sterile antiseptic swabs, 4″ × 3″ pad, butterfly adhesive strips, sterile gloves, and clean disposable gloves.

3. Explain the procedure to the patient and position the patient comfortably, with the wound exposed. Close the curtain and door for privacy.

4. Position the plastic bag for easy access.

5. Wash your hands.

6. Open the sterile package and antiseptic swabs.

7. Put on the clean disposable gloves and remove any dressing.

8. Inspect the wound for healing.

9. Remove and discard the disposable gloves. Put on the sterile gloves.

10. Clean the sutures or staples with the antiseptic swabs. Discard the swabs in the plastic bag.

11. For *staples,* remove the staples by placing the staple extractor tips in the center of each staple. Close the extractor handles so the ends of the staple come out of the incision. Discard staples in the plastic bag.

For *intermittent sutures,* grasp one end of the suture with the forceps and snip the suture close to the skin near the knot. Remove the entire knot and suture in one stroke. Discard all sutures on the 4″ × 3″ pad (placed near the incision). If ordered, remove only every other suture. (The remaining sutures may be removed a day or more later.)

For *continuous sutures,* snip the first suture close to the skin at the end distal to the knot. Remove the first spiral with a smooth, gentle motion. Continue in this manner until the entire suture line has been removed.

12. For either sutures or staples, if a slight separation appears, place a butterfly strip over the area.

13. Clean the suture or staple line, as needed.

14. Apply a 4″ × 3″ pad to the site, or leave the area open to air.

15. Help the patient to a comfortable position.

16. Remove the gloves.

17. Discard the supplies in the plastic bag and discard the bag and gloves in the proper receptacle in the utility room.

18. Wash your hands.

19. Document the procedure in the patient's chart, noting the wound condition.

Precautions and nursing considerations

• Institutional policy may dictate which personnel are permitted to remove sutures or staples.

• Practice this procedure under supervision before performing it alone.

Applying heat and cold

Purpose
• Heat application: To improve blood flow (by vasodilation), reduce venous congestion, decrease pain and soreness, and remove cellular waste (by increased circulation)
• Cold application: To decrease blood flow (by vasoconstriction), decrease edema (by vasoconstriction), reduce pain and soreness (by decreasing pressure on nerve endings), decrease tissue oxygen needs, increase blood clotting at the involved site, and reduce inflammation

Steps
1. Prepare the proper heat or cold appliance according to the physician's order.
  Heat may be applied by heating pad, sitz bath, warm tub immersion, aquathermic pad (a pad containing water heated to a specific temperature), warm moist compress, hot water bottle, or heat lamp. (For instructions on administering heat lamp treatments, see "Using a heat lamp.")
  Cold may be applied by ice bag, ice collar, ice cap, or cold compress.
2. After filling a water bottle, ice bag, or ice collar, remove any air inside the container. (Air acts as an insulator, preventing the full effects of heat or cold.)
3. Place a cover over the appliance to protect the patient's skin. (Temperature extremes can cause burns.)
4. Check the temperature of the appliance; a compress applied directly to the skin should have a moderate temperature. With a heating pad or aquathermic pad, check the thermostat for proper function. If the patient will be immersed in warm tub water, check water temperature first; stay with the patient during the treatment.
5. Place the heat or cold appliance on the involved area, and record the time.

6. During the treatment, check the patient frequently, noting the condition of the skin at the involved site.
7. Instruct the patient not to adjust the temperature or thermostat of the appliance but to call the nurse for help if the appliance is uncomfortably hot or cold. Make sure the call light is within easy reach.
8. If the patient has a motor or sensory deficit and cannot move away from a temperature source or sense temperature changes, remain with the patient during the treatment.
9. After the prescribed time, remove the appliance.
10. Document the time, the patient's response, and condition of the skin in the patient's chart.

Precautions and nursing considerations
• Make sure you understand the specific purpose of heat or cold application for each patient and are familiar with the effects of heat and cold.
• Verify that the appliance is at the specified temperature before treatment begins:
very hot: 105° to 115° F (41° to 46° C)
hot: 98° to 105° F (37° to 41° C)
warm: 93° to 98° F (34° to 37° C)
tepid: 80° to 93° F (27° to 34° C)
cool: 65° to 80° F (18° to 27° C)
cold: 50° to 65° F (10° to 18° C)
• Do not apply heat or cold directly without using a protective cover (such as a hot water bottle, a heating pad, or an ice bag or cap).
• Short periods of heat or cold application are well tolerated, but prolonged exposure can cause tissue injury.
• Certain conditions increase the risk of injury from heat or cold application—for example, advanced age, confusion, unconsciousness, an open wound, marked edema, peripheral vascular conditions (including arteriosclerosis and diabetes), and spinal cord injury.

Using a heat lamp

Purpose
To promote drying of a draining or weeping wound or to increase circulation to injured tissues (a heat lamp emits dry heat, which is less likely than moist heat to injure tissues because it does not penetrate as deeply)

Steps
1. Read the physician's order for the heat lamp treatment and area to be treated.
2. Inspect the injured area for injury type and depth, stasis, and pressure ulcers.
3. Explain the procedure to the patient and position the patient comfortably, with the injured area exposed fully. Close the curtain and door for privacy.
4. Assess the injured area for sensitivity to pain and temperature changes by using touch, pin prick, or warm water. Insensitivity contraindicates heat lamp treatment because it may cause added injury.
5. To prevent burning, place the heat lamp a safe distance away from the injured area. With a 40- to 60-watt bulb, place it 24″ (61 cm) away; with a 60- to 75-watt bulb, 30″ (76 cm) away.
6. Turn the heat lamp on. Place your hand over the injured area to determine whether the light is directed properly.
7. During the treatment, check the patient every 5 minutes to inspect the skin, observe the patient's position, and ask if the patient feels any burning sensation.
8. If the patient reports a burning sensation, stop the treatment. Otherwise, continue the treatment for 20 minutes.
9. After the treatment, move the heat lamp to a safe area in the room where the bulb cannot break accidentally.
10. Help the patient to a comfortable position and open the curtain.
11. Wash your hands.
12. Document the heat lamp application in the patient's chart, noting skin color in the injured area and condition of injured tissues before and after treatment.

Precautions and nursing considerations
• Make sure you understand the effects of heat on injured tissues.
• Verify that the heat lamp has a light source (usually a 40- to 75-watt bulb) enclosed in an adjustable neck lamp.
• Do not use an infrared heat lamp because it directs heat in a beam that does not scatter and may further injure weakened tissues.

PRINCIPLES AND PROCEDURES

Collecting specimens

Purpose

To permit laboratory analysis of a midstream urine specimen, sputum specimen, stool specimen, or wound drainage specimen for presence or absence of disease-producing organisms or type and amount of organisms present

Steps

Midstream urine specimen

1. Assess the patient's ability to understand instructions and walk to the bathroom.

2. Gather sterile specimen supplies: a tray with sterile cotton balls, sterile specimen container, antiseptic in a container (bottle), and sterile gloves.

3. If the patient can understand instructions and collect the specimen independently, provide thorough instructions (as described below) and allow the patient to collect the specimen. When collecting the specimen yourself, first open the tray, pour antiseptic over the cotton balls, and clean the patient's genital area.

4. For a male patient, clean the end of the penis with gloved fingers by moving a moistened cotton ball in a circular motion from the center to the outer edges of the penile tip. After urination starts, place the specimen container under the urine stream and collect 30 ml of urine. Place the lid on the specimen container to avoid spills or contamination.

5. For a female patient, put on gloves, spread the labia with the thumb and index finger, and clean the perineal area with a moistened cotton ball, working from front to back. Use one cotton ball with each stroke to clean the right side, left side, then the center of the perineal area. After urination starts, place the specimen container under the urine stream and collect about 30 ml of urine. Place the lid on the container.

6. The patient may finish voiding in the toilet.

7. Remove the gloves and discard them appropriately.

8. Wash your hands.

9. Label the specimen and attach the proper requisition form.

10. Send the specimen to the laboratory.

11. Document the time and type of specimen collected on the patient's chart.

Sputum specimen

1. Check the physician's order for the type of specimen needed, such as cytologic specimen (cells), culture (specific organisms), or acid-fast bacilli (for possible tuberculosis). With a culture, sensitivity tests may be performed to determine antibiotic sensitivity.

2. Instruct the patient about specimen collection and its purpose. If the specimen will be collected at this time, close the curtain and door for privacy. If collection will take place later, provide appropriate instructions for the patient to collect it at the specified time.

3. Assess the patient's ability to cough deeply and expectorate.

4. Supply a specimen container with lid and tissues.

5. Have the patient take three or four deep breaths and exhale thoroughly.

6. Open the specimen container and place the lid with the inner surface facing upward to prevent contamination.

7. Ask the patient to cough deeply (more than just clearing the throat) and to expectorate into the container—without touching the inside of the container to the face or lips.

8. Instruct the patient to repeat the deep breaths and coughing until adequate sputum has been collected (about ½ to 1 tsp, if possible).

9. Close the sputum container and offer tissues, if needed.

10. Help the patient to a comfortable position.

11. Label the specimen container and attach a laboratory requisition slip.

12. Open the curtain in the patient's room.

13. Send the specimen to the laboratory immediately.

14. Document the time and type of specimen collected on the patient's chart, noting sputum color, odor, and other characteristics (such as thickness or presence of mucus or blood).

Stool specimen

1. Check the physician's order for the specific type of analysis to be performed.

2. Gather needed supplies: stool specimen container, tongue blades, and clean disposable gloves. Take these items to the patient's room.

3. Tell the patient to notify you when the urge to defecate occurs.

4. When the patient reports the urge to defecate, instruct the patient to void first. As appropriate, save or discard the urine. (The stool specimen should not mix with urine or toilet water.)

5. Have the patient defecate into a bedside commode, specimen hat, or bedpan.

6. Put on disposable gloves. Using tongue blades, collect the stool specimen—approximately 1″ of formed stool or 1 tbsp of liquid stool.

7. If the specimen will be analyzed for culture, remove a sterile swab from the plastic tube (inside the specimen container), gather a small piece of stool on the swab, and replace the swab in the tube. Then place the lid on the stool specimen container.

8. Attach a label and laboratory requisition slip to the specimen.

9. Help the patient to a comfortable position.

10. Dispose of the remaining stool in the toilet and clean the commode, specimen hat, or bedpan.

11. Wash your hands.

12. Send the specimen to the laboratory immediately.

13. Document the time and type of specimen collected on the patient's chart, noting stool appearance and odor, as appropriate.

Wound drainage specimen

1. Check the physician's order for the purpose of the specimen (usually culture and sensitivity).

2. Gather needed supplies: two culture tubes with cotton-tipped swab and transport medium in the tip, sterile gloves, clean disposable gloves, sterile dressing materials, and disposable plastic bag.

3. Explain the procedure to the patient. If the specimen will be gathered at this time, close the curtain and door to ensure privacy and prevent drafts.

4. Open the disposable plastic bag and place it within easy reach.

5. Put on the disposable gloves.

6. Remove the soiled dressing from the wound. Observe it for type, color, odor, and amount of drainage, then discard it in the plastic bag. Remove the disposable gloves and discard them in the plastic bag.

7. Put on the sterile gloves.

8. Clean the area around the wound with an antiseptic swab to remove exudate.

9. Open one culture tube and insert the tip of the cotton swab into the drainage area around the wound. Rotate gently to collect enough drainage for the culture.

10. Replace the cotton applicator in the culture tube.

11. Crush the ampule of culture medium at the tip of the culture tube and push the applicator into the fluid.

12. Collect a second specimen in the second culture tube to ensure enough material for analysis.

13. Clean the wound and apply a new dressing (see "Changing a sterile dressing," page 86).

14. Attach labels to the culture tubes, noting the drainage site, and attach laboratory requisition slips.

15. Wash your hands.

16. Send the specimen to the laboratory immediately.

17. Document the time, number of culture tubes collected, wound condition, and amount, type, and character of drainage on the patient's chart.

Precautions and nursing considerations

• Make sure to collect enough material for the desired test or analysis.

• Label the specimens correctly to ensure proper identification and patient care.

• To prevent contamination causing inaccurate test results, use aseptic technique when collecting specimens.

• Keep in mind that specimen collection may cause the patient embarrassment or discomfort.

Washing the hands

Purpose

To remove dirt and microorganisms from the hands, fingers, and beneath the nails

Steps

1. Assemble needed supplies near a source of warm running water: soap in containers (may be liquid soap with an antimicrobial agent), nail file, paper towels, and a disposal container.

2. Use the nail file to remove dirt beneath the nails and to file the nails, if needed. Remove any false nails; if institutional policy dictates, remove nail polish. (Short nails help prevent injury to the self or other persons. You should not wear false nails because microorganisms or debris may be trapped between the false and real nails. Nail polish harbors microorganisms and may chip, flake, and drop onto clean areas.)

3. Remove any rings with stone settings, which may harbor microorganisms. (However, you may wear a plain wedding band.) If you are wearing a watch, remove it or slide it up the forearm to allow thorough washing and drying of hands.

4. Inspect the fingers and hands for skin breaks, such as cuts and hangnails. Skin breaks may harbor microorganisms that could transfer to patients or cause infection in the nurse. If you have open sores on the hands or fingers, wear gloves or request reassignment to nonpatient contact.

5. Turn on the water and adjust the flow so the water is warm and runs slowly. (Warm water causes less depletion of protective oils than hot water.)

6. Hold your hands under the running water to wet them thoroughly. To allow the water to flow by gravity from less contaminated (soiled) areas to more contaminated areas, keep the hands lower than the elbows.

7. Apply soap to your hands. With liquid soap, use about 1 tsp; with bar soap, rub the bar between your hands firmly to create a lather. Rinse the bar before returning it to the sink.

8. Rub your hands with firm, circular movements to create the friction needed to remove microorganisms. Wash your fingers by interlacing them, and wash the backs of the hands, palms, and wrists. Continue for 15 for 30 seconds. (If your hands are especially soiled, continue this step for 1 minute.)

9. Rinse all soap from your hands by holding them under running water, keeping the fingers lower than the wrists to aid removal of debris and organisms.

10. Dry your hands thoroughly with a paper towel or clean cloth towel. Discard the damp towel in the proper container.

11. Stop the water flow. If the sink has hand-operated faucet handles, turn the handles with a towel so your hand does not touch the handles. (Handles are considered soiled or contaminated.)

Precautions and nursing considerations

• If you have open sores on your hands or fingers, wear gloves or request reassignment to nonpatient contact.

• Keep your hands lower than forearm level when washing them so that soiled water does not run up the forearms.

• Dry your hands thoroughly to prevent chafing, which can lead to skin cracks or openings.

Shaving a patient

Purpose
To promote patient comfort and a positive self-image by shaving the facial hair of a patient who cannot shave himself.

Steps
1. Wash your hands to help prevent the spread of microorganisms.

2. Find out if the patient prefers a razor or an electric shaver. Assess for restrictions against use of a safety razor.

3. Assemble needed supplies: safety razor or electric shaver, shaving cream or soap, basin of warm water, clean disposable gloves, mirror (if available), towel and washcloth, and aftershave powder or lotion (if available).

4. Place or assist the patient to an appropriate position:
• high Fowler's position behind the overbed table (this position promotes patient participation)
• seated in a chair behind the overbed table
• supine with the head of the bed elevated, if the patient is unconscious or otherwise cannot participate (this position is convenient for the nurse).

5. Shave the patient. When using a safety razor, first apply a warm, moist washcloth to the face to soften the hair. Lather the face with soap or shaving cream. Then hold the skin taut with the nondominant hand (to allow a closer shave), and move the razor in the direction of hair growth. Finally, rinse the face with a warm, moist washcloth.

When using an electric razor, hold the skin taut with the nondominant hand and move the razor in the direction of hair growth.

6. Apply aftershave powder or lotion, as desired, to soothe the skin.

7. Document the procedure.

Precautions and nursing considerations
• Because of the increased risk for bleeding, use an electric razor instead of a safety razor if the patient has a decreased platelet count or is receiving anticoagulant therapy.
• Encourage the patient to participate, if possible. (For instance, he may be able to perform many of the steps independently.)

PRINCIPLES AND PROCEDURES

Part IV

Review of clinical nursing

Perioperative nursing

Maternity nursing

Pediatric nursing

Adult medical-surgical nursing

Psychiatric nursing

Perioperative nursing

Introduction 98

Preoperative period

Preoperative care 98

Intraoperative period

Intraoperative care 101

Postoperative period

Postoperative care 101

Introduction

This section reviews nursing care during the perioperative period—the operative portion of the patient's surgical experience. Perioperative care encompasses the preoperative, intraoperative, and postoperative phases.

To provide effective, compassionate care during each phase, the nurse must possess specific knowledge and skills. Perioperative care is demanding and arduous. Typically, the patient is frightened, anxious, and confused. If this is the patient's first surgical experience, he may feel that his life is in the nurse's hands. The nurse, in return, must ensure the best possible care.

Besides discussing routine preoperative data collection, this section covers patient teaching, and general comfort measures to relieve anxiety. Then it describes nursing responsibilities during the intraoperative phase—the time the patient spends in the surgical suite and operating room. The nurse working in either of these intraoperative areas has special responsibilities and must undergo special training. However, all nurses must understand basic intraoperative nursing responsibilities; NCLEX-PN may include questions about these topics. Turning to the postoperative phase, which begins when the patient leaves the operating room, the text highlights important nursing functions, emphasizing assessment and comfort measures. It includes charts that describe postoperative positioning, ambulation, body alignment, and postoperative problems and complications. You can expect to find questions on these topics on NCLEX-PN.

PREOPERATIVE PERIOD

Preoperative care

I. **Introduction**
   A. Activities and preparations that take place before the patient is transferred to the surgical suite
   B. Required before an operation, a special examination, or administration of a general or regional anesthetic
   C. Occurs in an ambulatory surgery setting or in the patient's room on a nursing unit
II. **Assessment**
   A. Preadmission
      1. In many cases, personal data are collected on admission forms sent to and returned by the patient before admission to the hospital or ambulatory care unit
      2. Laboratory studies, including complete blood counts, bleeding and clotting studies, and urinalysis, may be conducted during the patient's last preadmission visit to the physician or on an outpatient basis
      3. An electrocardiogram may be performed on an outpatient basis
   B. Admission
      1. On admission, additional laboratory studies (such as fasting blood glucose analysis, blood urea nitrogen and creatinine levels, and blood typing and cross matching) may be done

    2. A chest X-ray also may be performed

C. Preoperative
1. Before surgery, collect the following data:
   a. patient's current medical condition
   b. purpose of upcoming surgery or examination
   c. past surgeries and possible complications
   d. current medications and dosages
      (1) Prescription medications
      (2) Over-the-counter medications
   e. smoking habits and tobacco use
   f. use of alcohol and illicit drugs (such as heroin or cocaine)
   g. current health problems
      (1) Cardiovascular conditions, such as angina, myocardial infarction, hypertension, or congestive heart failure
      (2) Bleeding or coagulation problems
      (3) Respiratory infections
      (4) Renal disease or urinary tract infections
      (5) Diabetes
      (6) Liver disease
      (7) Neurologic disease
      (8) Vascular problems that may cause emboli or thrombi (clots)
      (9) Asthma or emphysema
   h. allergies
   i. mobility status
      (1) Gait
      (2) Muscle strength and coordination
      (3) Range of motion
      (4) Use of an aid, such as a cane or crutches
   j. vital signs, temperature, weight, and height
   k. general appearance, skin color, energy level, alertness, and ability to understand and answer questions
   l. vision (use of glasses or contact lenses)
   m. hearing (use of a hearing aid)
   n. nutritional status, including special dietary needs
   o. psychological status
      (1) Coping behaviors
      (2) Family and social supports
      (3) Anxiety or concerns about upcoming surgery
      (4) Language barriers
   p. financial status, including availability of health insurance or worker's compensation
2. Make sure the patient has signed an operative permit and an informed consent form

III. Patient teaching

A. General preoperative teaching
1. Teach the patient about required laboratory studies and diagnostic examinations
2. Explain that the patient must restrict foods and fluids for at least 8 hours before surgery
3. Inform the patient that an enema, a suppository, or other bowel preparation may be required
4. Teach the patient about preoperative hygiene, such as a shower or bath and skin preparation (both on the nursing unit and in the operative suite)

5. Explain that anesthesia personnel will visit the patient
6. Provide other appropriate information, such as the need for special braces, appliances, or antiembolism stockings
7. Teach the patient about preoperative medications
8. Teach the patient about special treatments required, such as antibiotics, I.V. therapy, nasogastric tube or urinary catheter insertion, or intermittent positive pressure breathing
9. Clarify the sequence of events to anticipate
   a. When the patient will leave the nursing unit
   b. How long the patient will be in the waiting area
   c. How long the operation usually lasts
   d. How long the patient will be in the recovery room
   e. When the patient will return to the nursing unit
B. Special preoperative teaching
   1. Teach the patient how to do deep-breathing exercises (these may or may not include coughing)
   2. Explain how to perform leg and foot exercises
   3. Teach the patient how to use a trapeze
   4. Instruct the patient how to get out of bed properly
   5. Teach the patient how to splint the incision
   6. Explain pain-management techniques
   7. Teach the patient how to use the call light
   8. Inform the patient that the bed has side rails for safety
   9. Teach the patient about urine collection equipment
   10. Teach the patient about fluid intake and output measurements
   11. Explain that the patient's vital signs, dressings, and breath and bowel sounds will be monitored frequently

IV. **Types of surgery**
A. Elective surgery
   1. Elective surgery is surgery that is recommended (such as hernia repair) or required within a short period (such as cataract extraction)
   2. It also includes cosmetic or optional surgery (such as a face-lift or rhinoplasty)
B. Emergency surgery, to make immediate repairs (such as after a gunshot wound)
C. Palliative surgery, to reduce pain (such as by cutting nerves) or to ease a bowel obstruction (such as with a colostomy)
D. Diagnostic surgery, to examine a body region or to identify the cause of a sign or symptom (such as exploratory laparotomy or lymph node biopsy)
E. Curative surgery, to remove a diseased part (such as an appendectomy or total joint replacement)

V. **Suffixes (word endings) used to denote types of surgical procedures**
A. -ectomy: surgical removal of (such as appendectomy)
B. -lysis: surgical breaking up or detachment of (such as neurolysis, or breaking up of adhesions around a nerve)
C. -orrhaphy: surgical repair of (such as herniorrhaphy)
D. -oscopy: surgical inspection of (such as gastroscopy)
E. -ostomy: surgical creation of an artificial permanent opening between two hollow organs or between one or more such viscera and the abdominal wall (such as colostomy)
F. -otomy: surgical incision of (such as tracheotomy)
G. -plasty: reconstruction or repair of (such as rhinoplasty)

INTRAOPERATIVE PERIOD

Intraoperative care

I. **Introduction**
   A. The intraoperative period begins when the patient is placed on the operating room table
   B. It ends when the patient is transferred to the postanesthesia care unit

II. **Nurse's role**
   A. Assigned nursing responsibilities may be highly specialized, such as acting as first assistant
   B. In some cases, however, the nurse has broad responsibilities
      1. Recognizing the patient's potential for skin breakdown
      2. Taking steps to protect bony prominences
      3. Positioning the patient on the table, using good body-alignment principles

POSTOPERATIVE PERIOD

Postoperative care

I. **Postanesthesia recovery care**
   A. Read the physician's progress notes on the operative procedure to learn about:
      1. the patient's preoperative condition
      2. operative procedure planned
      3. operative procedure performed
      4. operative physical findings
      5. complications of surgery
   B. Read the anesthesiologist's record of the operative procedure to learn about:
      1. the patient's vital signs
      2. fluids, blood, plasma expanders, or other substances administered during surgery
      3. estimated blood loss
      4. the patient's tolerance of anesthesia
   C. Check the circulating nurse's record (if available) to learn about the patient's condition and any unusual occurrences, such as:
      1. an inaccurate sponge count that necessitated a sponge search
      2. inadvertent cutting or puncture of a blood vessel, bowel, or bladder
   D. Listen to the report by the nurse from the postanesthesia care unit to learn about:
      1. the operation
      2. the patient's current vital signs
      3. need for oxygen therapy
      4. I.V. solution and I.V. flow rate
      5. whether the patient has a nasogastric tube or urinary catheter
      6. whether any narcotic analgesic was given

    a. Name of analgesic
    b. Dosage
    c. Administration time

7. dressing and wound drains
8. use of external support (such as a knee or joint immobilizer, abduction splint, sling, cast, or other support or prosthesis)
9. whether the patient has voided
10. the patient's present condition (including alertness, nausea, and skin color)

II. **Surgical nursing care**

A. When the patient returns to the nursing unit, record the time of the patient's return

B. Assess the patient by:
  1. measuring vital signs and comparing them with the last recorded vital signs
  2. evaluating the patient's condition and neurologic status
    a. State of alertness (such as awake or drowsy)
    b. Level of consciousness
    c. Ability to move the extremities
  3. noting skin color and characteristics (such as dry, damp, cool, or cold)
  4. inspecting the operative wound, dressing, and drainage tubing or appliance
  5. observing the I.V. infusion
    a. Type of solution
    b. Infusion rate
    c. Amount of infusion remaining
  6. inspecting the I.V. site
  7. evaluating the patient for pain and discomfort
  8. determining the patient's urinary status
    a. Presence of a catheter
    b. Urge to void
    c. Bladder distention
    d. Urine in a drainage bag
  9. evaluating the patient for nausea and vomiting

C. Carry out the following implementations:
  1. placing the patient in a comfortable position, with the head of the bed flat or slightly elevated
  2. placing the call light within reach
  3. connecting any tubing to gravity or suction, as needed
  4. placing an emesis basin and tissues within reach if the patient has nausea or vomiting
  5. reading the physician's postoperative orders before leaving the unit to determine the need for immediate additional care measures (such as reducing the I.V. rate or removing a urinary catheter)
  6. discussing the patient's condition with the family (if present) to assure them of the patient's status
  7. transferring the physician's orders to the patient's Kardex (if not done by the charge nurse or primary care nurse)
  8. completing the patient's Kardex by entering nursing diagnoses and interventions

Postoperative ambulation

Typically, the patient can ambulate on the evening after surgery or on the first postoperative day. However, in some cases, ambulation must be delayed, as this chart explains.

PROCEDURE	WHEN AMBULATION BEGINS
Craniotomy or burr holes	Second postoperative day (if the patient has multiple burr holes)
Cerebral artery anastomosis	Second or third postoperative day (depending on the anastomosis site)
Spinal fusion	Second or third postoperative day
Pelvic exenteration	Third to fifth postoperative day
Coronary artery bypass	First, second, or third postoperative day (depending on the patient's general condition)
Correction of atrial or septal defect	First or second postoperative day

9. providing continuing nursing care
   a. Helping the patient ambulate, as ordered, to prevent complications, increase the patient's sense of well-being, improve gastrointestinal and urinary functions, and promote wound healing
   b. Encouraging deep-breathing exercises every 2 hours and urging the patient to use the appropriate breathing apparatus
   c. Listening to breath sounds in all lung lobes
   d. Administering pain medications or monitoring analgesia via a patient-controlled analgesia (PCA) pump
      (1) Record the amount of medication received (usually every 4 hours)
      (2) Monitor the patient for pain relief at least every 4 hours to improve patient comfort and promote participation in postoperative activities
   e. Giving food and fluids, as ordered
      (1) The patient may receive clear fluids, full liquids, a regular diet, or a special diet
      (2) Note any nausea or vomiting, abdominal distention, constipation, or diarrhea (such as from antibiotic use)
      (3) Monitor bowel sounds in all four abdominal quadrants
   f. Measuring urine output every 8 hours, noting any complaints of urinary burning, urgency, or frequency (possible signs of urinary tract infection)
   g. Encouraging the patient to perform leg and foot exercises every 2 hours
   h. Changing wound dressings, as ordered, noting signs of healing and decreasing inflammation (such as less redness, edema, and soreness)
   i. Recording the amount of drainage in collecting appliances
   j. Observing skin and bony prominences for signs of pressure, color changes, or skin breaks

Postoperative positioning and turning

Usually, the nurse can position the postoperative patient in a low or semi-Fowler's position, and can turn the patient from side to side. However, exceptions apply for patients recovering from certain surgical procedures. The chart below describes proper patient positioning and turning in such cases.

SURGICAL PROCEDURE	POSTOPERATIVE POSITIONING	POSTOPERATIVE TURNING
Pneumonectomy	High Fowler's	Turn the patient to the operative side only (to keep the remaining lung expanded).
Infratentorial craniotomy	Flat	Logroll the patient from side to side.
Hemorrhoidectomy	Flat	As appropriate, turn the patient from side to side and onto the abdomen for comfort.
Total hip replacement	Low Fowler's or flat	Turn the patient to the nonoperative side only, unless the physician's order specifically permits turning to the operative side.
Total knee or shoulder replacement	Low or high Fowler's	Turn the patient to the nonoperative side only.
Spinal fusion with metallic rods or bone grafts	Flat	Turn the patient from side to side.
Cataract removal	Low or high Fowler's	Turn the patient to the nonoperative side only.
Stapedectomy	Low Fowler's	Turn the patient to the nonoperative side only.

    k. Repositioning the patient every 2 to 4 hours
    l. Encouraging fluid intake after I.V. fluids are discontinued
    m. Observing the patient for a positive outlook and desire for discharge (which usually occurs on or about the fourth postoperative day)
    n. Initiating discharge teaching for self-care, as needed
      (1) Teaching topics typically include:
        (a) caring for wounds and indwelling catheters
        (b) medication schedule, dosage, and administration route
        (c) use of nonnarcotic analgesics
        (d) application of antiembolism stockings
        (e) dietary instructions
      (2) Cover other topics as appropriate
    o. Teaching the patient about resuming physical activities, such as work, sexual activities, and driving (according to the physician's orders)
    p. Evaluating for signs and symptoms of postoperative problems or complications (see *Postoperative problems and complications*)

q. Completing discharge charting
   (1) Include the time of discharge, discharge method (ambulatory, wheelchair, or other), place to which the patient is discharged, and the patient's general condition and mood
   (2) Include special instructions or restrictions, if needed

---

Postoperative problems and complications

Postoperative problems are temporary conditions that medications or other interventions can relieve. Postoperative complications are longer-lasting, unexpected developments that require prolonged or varied treatments and may delay or prevent the patient's full recovery. This chart, arranged by body system, lists postoperative problems and complications along with related nursing considerations.

Cardiovascular system

Postoperative problem
- Hypotension

Postoperative complications
- Hemorrhage
- Phlebitis
- Pulmonary embolism
- Shock
- Thrombophlebitis

Nursing considerations

For hemorrhage
- Measure vital signs every 1 to 2 hours, as indicated.

For phlebitis
- Check the I.V. site for redness, pain, and infiltration.

For pulmonary embolism
- Check for such signs and symptoms as chest pain, increased respiratory and pulse rates, blood pressure fluctuations, dyspnea, and a patient sense of danger.

For shock
- Administer I.V. fluids, as ordered, to maintain fluid intake. Check the apical pulse, as indicated. (For other nursing measures, see "Shock," pages 70 to 74.)

For thrombophlebitis
- Note patient complaints of calf pain.
- Check for a positive Homan's sign (calf pain when the foot is dorsiflexed).

Gastrointestinal system

Postoperative problems
- Abdominal distention
- Nausea
- Vomiting
- Hiccoughs

Postoperative complications
- Paralytic ileus
- Parotitis (surgical mumps)

Nursing considerations

In general
- Withhold food and fluids, as ordered (or encourage food and fluid intake, as indicated).

- Provide ice chips.
- Determine if the patient is expelling gas (flatus).
- Administer a suppository.
- Check stools for consistency.
- Encourage or provide oral hygiene to prevent parotitis.
- Encourage ambulation to stimulate bowel function

For nausea
- Administer antiemetic medications, as ordered.

For abdominal distention and paralytic ileus
- Listen to bowel sounds in all abdominal quadrants to detect ileus or distention.

Genitourinary system

Postoperative problem
- Urine retention

Postoperative complications
- Renal failure (urine output may drop below 30 ml/hour after general anesthesia)
- Urinary tract infection

Nursing considerations

For renal failure
- Instruct the patient to void 8 to 10 hours postoperatively.
- Use voiding aids, if necessary, such as immersing the patient's hands in warm water, pouring warm water over the vulva (for a female), having the patient stand to void (for a male patient) or use the bathroom (if permitted), providing privacy during voiding, and inserting a urinary catheter, as ordered, if distention is pronounced and the patient is uncomfortable or cannot void.
- Measure fluid input and output carefully; in an adult, urine output should measure 30 ml/hour.
- Increase fluid intake to enhance renal blood flow.

For urinary tract infection
- Administer antibiotics, as ordered.

(continued)

Postoperative problems and complications *(continued)*

Integumentary system

Postoperative problem
● Wound soreness

Postoperative complications
● Dehiscence (opening of wound edges)
● Evisceration (bulging of internal organs through the incision)
● Hematoma
● Wound infection

Nursing considerations

For dehiscence
● Enforce bedrest.
● Place adhesive wound closures (Steri-strips) over the affected area.
● Instruct the patient not to cough.
● Notify the physician.

For evisceration
● Cover the internal contents with pads soaked in sterile saline solution.
● Notify the physician immediately; surgical repair may be necessary.

For hematoma
● Be aware that the lesion may be opened and drained surgically and a pressure dressing may be applied. As appropriate, measure the amount of drainage.

For wound infection
● With each dressing change, assess the wound for signs of healing or continued infection (such as increased pain, purulent drainage, redness, and edema).
● Note any elevated temperature.

Neurologic system

Postoperative problem
● Persistent pain

Postoperative complication
● Malignant hyperthermia (a life-threatening reaction to anesthesia and lack of liver enzymes)

Nursing considerations

For malignant hyperthermia
● Check vital signs, noting any persistent temperature elevation.
● Note any change in the level of consciousness or lack of alertness with muscle flaccidity.
● The patient may be transferred to the intensive care unit.

Respiratory system

Postoperative problem
● Hypoventilation

Postoperative complications
● Atelectasis
● Pneumonia

Nursing considerations

For atelectasis and pneumonia
● Have the patient breathe deeply every 2 hours.
● Use an appropriate respiratory apparatus to increase the depth of respirations, as ordered.
Use an intermittent positive pressure breathing machine every 4 hours, as ordered.
● Perform vibration and clapping to loosen secretions; assess secretions for amount, color, and odor.

Maternity nursing

Introduction 108

Anatomy and physiology of the female reproductive system 108

Prenatal period

First trimester 111

Second trimester 118

Third trimester 120

Intrapartal period

Labor and delivery 124

Postpartal period

Breast-feeding 139

Selected nursing procedures

Washing the perineal area 143

Administering a sitz bath 144

Performing a postpartal maternal assessment 145

Assessing the newborn 145

Bathing the newborn 147

Introduction

Nursing care during pregnancy—a normal health state—has a psychological as well as a physical dimension. Moreover, having a child is a family affair. To give the experience optimum meaning and value, maternity nursing must be family-centered.

This section reviews the essentials of maternity care that the beginning practical nurse is most likely to provide. It aims to help the nurse gain competence in clinical nursing—the area of maternity nursing that NCLEX-PN evaluates.

This section begins by reviewing the anatomy and physiology of the female reproductive system, highlighting the menstrual cycle. To understand conception and family planning management, all nurses must master these topics. Next comes a series of case studies, based on the nursing process, that describe a patient with a normal pregnancy from the time she first suspects she is pregnant through delivery and the early postpartal period. This section also details nursing procedures commonly performed by maternity nurses, emphasizing safety and nursing management. To promote understanding, it includes charts and illustrations that present abnormal conditions and complications of pregnancy as well as drugs commonly used in maternity care. (NCLEX-PN usually does not include questions on high-risk patients and those with pregnancy complications because they receive care from more experienced nurses in highly specialized units.)

Anatomy and physiology of the female reproductive system

I.   **Anatomy**
  A. External structures
    1. Clitoris: small erectile body beneath the anterior labial commissure
    2. Labia majora
      a. Consist of two folds of cellular adipose tissue on either side of the vaginal opening
      b. Extend from the mons pubis to the perineum
    3. Labia minora: narrow folds of skin between the labia majora and vagina
    4. Mons pubis: pad of fatty tissue over the symphysis pubis
    5. Perineum: skin, muscles, and fascia that support the pelvic floor
    6. Prepuce: fold of labia minora covering the clitoris
    7. Urethral orifice
      a. Is a canal within the vestibule, between the vagina and clitoris
      b. Conveys urine for discharge
  B. Internal structures
    1. Fallopian tubes
      a. Are a pair of tubes, each closely adjoining an ovary, that convey the ovum from the ovary to the uterus
      b. Open medially into the uterus, distally into the abdominal cavity
      c. May serve as a fertilization site

Reviewing the female reproductive system

These illustrations show the major external and internal structures of the female reproductive system.

EXTERNAL STRUCTURES

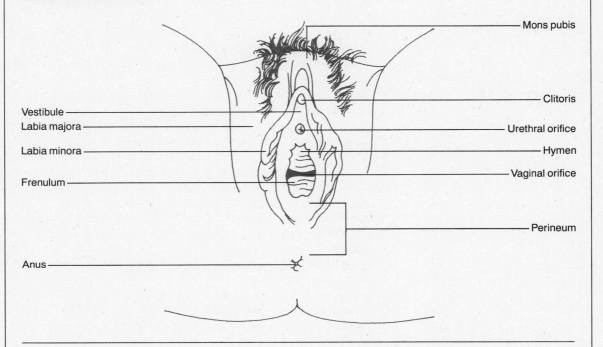

- Mons pubis
- Clitoris
- Urethral orifice
- Hymen
- Vaginal orifice
- Perineum

- Vestibule
- Labia majora
- Labia minora
- Frenulum
- Anus

INTERNAL STRUCTURES

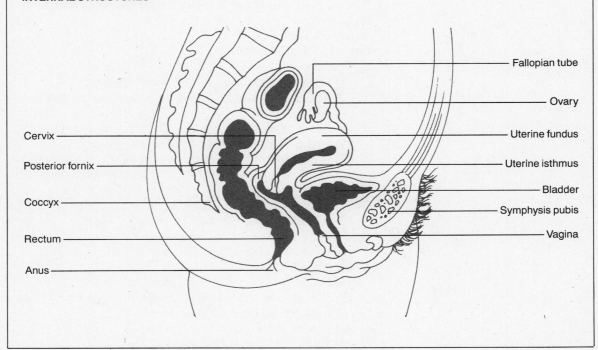

- Fallopian tube
- Ovary
- Uterine fundus
- Uterine isthmus
- Bladder
- Symphysis pubis
- Vagina

- Cervix
- Posterior fornix
- Coccyx
- Rectum
- Anus

MATERNITY NURSING

2. Ovary
   a. Is an almond-shaped body on either side of the pelvic cavity, attached to the uterus and situated near the fallopian tube
   b. Produces and expels ova (eggs)
3. Pelvis
   a. Bony ring between the trunk and thighs
   b. Consists of four bones
      (1) Two hip bones
      (2) Sacrum
      (3) Coccyx
   c. Articulates at the two sacroiliac joints (sacrococcygeal joint and symphysis pubis)
   d. Is lined by fibrocartilage, which softens during pregnancy to allow the pelvis to move during labor
   e. May be measured by internal examination, external examination (pelvimetry), or X-ray pelvimetry
4. Uterus
   a. Is a hollow, muscular, pear-shaped structure in the pelvic cavity between the bladder and rectum
   b. Has three segments—fundus, body, and cervix
   c. Contains and nourishes the embryo or fetus from implantation of a fertilized egg to expulsion of the fetus during delivery
5. Vagina
   a. Is a musculomembranous, dilatable passage situated between the bladder and rectum
   b. Serves as a receptacle for semen and a duct for uterine discharge (during menstruation)
   c. Acts as a passageway through which the fetus is delivered

II. **Physiology**
   A. Normal menstrual cycle
      1. Periodic vaginal discharge of blood, mucus, and epithelium from the nonpregnant uterus
      2. Begins at puberty
      3. Consists of four phases
         a. Proliferative phase
            (1) Occurs on days 5 to 14 of the menstrual cycle
            (2) Is marked by ovarian follicle maturation and estrogen secretion
         b. Ovulation phase
            (1) Occurs on days 10 to 16 of the menstrual cycle
            (2) Is marked by rupture of the ovarian follicle, ovum release, and development of the follicle into the corpus luteum
         c. Secretory phase
            (1) Occurs on days 14 to 28 of the menstrual cycle
            (2) Is marked by development of the corpus luteum within the ovary and progesterone secretion by the corpus luteum to allow ovum implantation in the uterine wall
         d. Menstrual phase
            (1) Occurs on days 1 to 5 of the menstrual cycle
            (2) Is marked by shedding of the endometrium and menstruation onset (unless conception occurs)
            (3) Usually occurs every 27 to 28 days
            (4) Varies from 3 to 7 days' duration

Glossary

Antepartal period (antepartum): period that starts with conception and ends with labor onset

Contraction: involuntary, intermittent shortening or tightening of uterine muscle fibers during labor

Duration of a uterine contraction: elapsed time from the start to the end of one uterine contraction

Embryo: prenatal development stage extending from implantation of the fertilized ovum (about 2 weeks after conception) to the end of the seventh or eighth week

Fetus: unborn offspring from about the eighth week after fertilization until birth

Frequency of uterine contractions: elapsed time from the start of one contraction to the start of the next contraction

Intrapartal period (intrapartum): period encompassing labor and delivery

Newborn: infant during the first 28 days after delivery

Postpartal period (postpartum): period beginning after delivery that lasts approximately 6 weeks

Trimester: one of three periods, each lasting approximately 3 months, into which pregnancy is divided

PRENATAL PERIOD

The prenatal, or antenatal, period extends from conception to the onset of labor. During this time, care of the patient and her fetus focuses on maintaining health and preventing complications. The nurse also must collect data about the family's physiologic, psychological, and sociocultural adaptations to pregnancy and must provide teaching and counseling. The three-part clinical situation that follows focuses on care of the patient and family during the three trimesters of a normal pregnancy.

First trimester

Overview

The first trimester, which starts with conception, is a time of ambivalence, excitement, and apprehension. The patient needs to feel that she is important and welcome, and must be taught about the normal physiologic changes she will experience.

Clinical situation

Mary Ann McGowan, age 23, a married patient, has been receiving care from an infertility specialist for 3 months for help in becoming pregnant. Today, she visits the physician because she is 6 weeks late for her menstrual period and has had extreme fatigue and early-morning nausea and vomiting. If a pregnancy is confirmed, it will be her first.

Assessment

Nursing behaviors	Nursing rationales
1. Assist in taking Mrs. McGowan's health history, beginning with a general health history.	**1.** Pregnancy is a normal health state. Information obtained during the health history interview will be used to plan Mrs. McGowan's care throughout her pregnancy. A general health history helps determine if a patient is at risk for pregnancy complications from such conditions as anemia, diabetes mellitus, cardiac or renal disease, or sexually transmitted disease.
2. Assist in taking Mrs. McGowan's family health history.	**2.** The family health history may suggest or reveal a genetically transmitted disease. If so, this information must be considered in her plan of care, and Mrs. McGowan should receive genetic counseling.
3. Assist in taking Mrs. McGowan's menstrual history.	**3.** The menstrual history helps identify problems and determine the expected date of confinement (EDC). To calculate the EDC, use Nagele's rule: Count backwards 3 months from the first day of the patient's last menstrual period (LMP), then add 1 year and 7 days. Mrs. McGowan's LMP was August 8; therefore, her EDC is May 5.
4. Assist in taking Mrs. McGowan's obstetric history, including her gravida and para status.	**4.** The obstetric history reveals information about previous pregnancies, including delivery method, length of labor, the newborn's size and gestational age, and any complications. *Gravida* refers to the total number of pregnancies a woman has had (including the current pregnancy), regardless of pregnancy outcome. *Para* refers to the number of past pregnancies that produced a viable newborn or had a gestation of at least 20 weeks.
5. Assist the RN with physical assessment of Mrs. McGowan, beginning with vital sign measurement.	**5.** Physical assessment determines Mrs. McGowan's health status, which should be monitored throughout pregnancy for deviations. Vital signs provide baseline data that will be used for comparison as her pregnancy advances.
6. Assist the RN in assessing fundal height.	**6.** Assessment of fundal height indicates approximate weeks of gestation, as follows: • At 12 weeks, the fundus is located at the symphysis pubis. • At 20 to 24 weeks, it is located at the umbilicus. • At 36 weeks, it is located at the xiphoid. • At 40 weeks, the fetus begins to descend in the pelvis (a phenomenon called lightening). This causes the fundus to drop to a position between the xiphoid and umbilicus.

MATERNITY NURSING

7. Assist the RN in assessing Mrs. McGowan's abdomen for striae gravidarum, linea nigra, and diastasis recti abdominis.

7. Striae gravidarum are pinkish or shiny white lines that result from stretching, rupture, and atrophy of deep connective tissue. Linea nigra is a dark line extending from the umbilicus to the symphysis pubis; it results from hormonal changes. Diastasis recti abdominis is a separation of the rectus abdominis muscles that may occur late in pregnancy when tension strains the muscles. (These changes typically occur later in pregnancy.)

8. Assist the RN in assessing Mrs. McGowan for breast tissue enlargement, nipple and areola darkening, and colostrum secretion.

8. Hormonal changes cause the breasts to enlarge, preparing them for lactation. Increased melanotropin darkens the nipples and areolae. Colostrum, the precursor of mature milk, is the first secretion from the breasts after delivery.

9. Assist the RN in assessing Mrs. McGowan for weight gain.

9. Weight gain during pregnancy should be consistent, with no sudden increases, and should total 26 to 30 lb (11.8 to 13.6 kg). During the first trimester, Mrs. McGowan should gain approximately 1 to 2 lb (0.45 to 0.9 kg); during the second and third trimesters, 1 lb/week.

10. Assist the RN in assessing Mrs. McGowan for cardiovascular changes, including increased blood volume, increased pulse rate, and decreased blood pressure.

10. Total blood volume increases about 30% during pregnancy without altering laboratory hematology values. Greater cardiac output and reduced total peripheral resistance cause the pulse rate to increase. Blood pressure drops during the first trimester and remains decreased throughout pregnancy.

11. Assist the RN in assessing Mrs. McGowan for respiratory changes.

11. Shortness of breath occurs in early pregnancy from anemia and in late pregnancy as the enlarging uterus presses against the lungs (causing upward displacement of the diaphragm).

12. Assist the RN in assessing Mrs. McGowan for gastrointestinal (GI) changes.

12. Heartburn, flatulence, and constipation are common because pregnancy interferes with GI motility. High progesterone levels and pressure from the enlarging uterus reduce peristalsis.

13. Assist the RN in assessing Mrs. McGowan for renal changes, such as urinary frequency, urinary stasis, and occasional glucosuria.

13. Urinary frequency, common during the first and third trimesters, results from increased pressure on the bladder from the enlarging uterus. Ureter dilation and stretching contribute to urinary stasis. Pregnant women sometimes excrete glucose.

14. Assist the RN in assessing Mrs. McGowan for

14. Most important endocrine changes during preg-

endocrine changes.

nancy are associated with the placenta and pituitary gland.

15. Assist with the external and internal pelvic examinations.

15. An external pelvic examination can detect vaginal discharge, growths, and other abnormalities. An internal examination is performed to confirm the pregnancy, determine fetal gestational age, identify potential risk factors, and measure the bony pelvis.

16. Evaluate Mrs. McGowan for presumptive signs of pregnancy:
• amenorrhea
• nausea and vomiting
• urinary frequency
• breast changes
• Chadwick's sign
• sleepiness and fatigue
• quickening
• skin pigmentation changes (linea nigra, darkened areolae, and chloasma).

16. Presumptive signs of pregnancy may indicate various conditions besides pregnancy. Although amenorrhea, nausea, vomiting, urinary frequency, and breast changes are normal responses to pregnancy, they also may stem from hormonal imbalance, emotional disturbance, or another disorder. Chadwick's sign is increased pelvic vascularity and a bluish vaginal color. Early in pregnancy, the patient needs more sleep and commonly feels fatigued. Quickening is fetal movement as perceived by the patient. Hormonal changes darken the skin pigmentation; chloasma refers to facial pigmentary changes during pregnancy.

17. Evaluate Mrs. McGowan for probable signs of pregnancy:
• an enlarged uterus
• Hegar's sign
• Braxton-Hicks contractions
• ballottement
• Goodell's sign
• positive pregnancy test.

17. Probable signs of pregnancy usually indicate pregnancy, but may result from other conditions. Uterine enlargement typically signifies a growing fetus, if accompanied by presumptive signs. Hegar's sign refers to softening of the lower uterine segment. Braxton-Hicks contractions are uncoordinated contractions of the enlarging uterus that become more frequent as pregnancy advances. Ballottement is the rebound reflex of the fetus when palpated by the examiner. Goodell's sign is cervical softening, usually occurring during the second month. A positive pregnancy test indicates the presence of human chorionic gonadotropin; however, because this test is not 100% accurate, it is a probable rather than positive sign of pregnancy.

18. Evaluate Mrs. McGowan for positive signs of pregnancy:
• fetal heart tones (FHTs)
• palpation of fetal movement
• fetal skeletal outline on sonogram.

18. Positive signs confirm pregnancy. The examiner can hear FHTs through a Doppler device at 10 to 12 weeks' gestation and through a stethoscope after 16 to 20 weeks. FHTs range from 110 to 160 beats/minute. The examiner can palpate fetal movement at about 20 weeks' gestation. A sonogram can visualize the fetus harmlessly throughout pregnancy. (X-rays in early pregnancy are teratogenic.)

MATERNITY NURSING

19. Ensure that the following tests have been performed:
- hemoglobin, hematocrit, and complete blood count
- routine urinalysis
- blood type and Rh factor
- serology
- acquired immunodeficiency syndrome (AIDS) and hepatitis screening
- urinary chorionic gonadotropin (UCG)
- cervical smears for sexually transmitted diseases (gonococcus, beta-streptococcus, and chlamydia)
- Cooley's anemia and sickle-cell disease tests.

19. Routine laboratory tests contribute to health assessment and establish baseline data for the pregnant patient. They should be repeated periodically throughout pregnancy. Routine urinalysis can rule out kidney infections, glucosuria, and stasis. Determination of blood type and Rh factor helps predict maternal-fetal incompatibilities (such as with an Rh-negative mother). Serologic tests screen for syphilis. AIDS testing is indicated for the patient in a high-risk group; hepatitis screening has been performed routinely on pregnant patients since 1987. A positive UCG test indicates pregnancy. Sexually transmitted diseases put the pregnant patient and her fetus at risk; treatment depends on the specific disease and its stage. Testing for Cooley's anemia and sickle-cell disease is important because these diseases are transmitted genetically. Cooley's anemia may cause a sharp drop in the blood count; sickle-cell disease reduces the blood's oxygen-carrying capacity.

20. Assess the psychosocial status of Mrs. McGowan and her husband by evaluating:
- their psychological adaptation to the first trimester of pregnancy
- Mrs. McGowan's learning needs
- Mrs. McGowan's support systems
- the family's economic status
- the family's living conditions
- the family's ethnic and cultural values, beliefs, and practices.

20. Psychosocial assessment helps anticipate the couple's needs. The major psychological task of the first trimester is accepting the pregnancy. Excitement, ambivalence, or apprehension are normal for both expectant parents. The pregnant patient must be familiar with the normal physiologic changes she will experience so that she can distinguish them from abnormal or unexpected changes. To plan for Mrs. McGowan's care, the nurse must find out which people are close to her emotionally (such as spouse, parents, siblings, and friends) and identify two or three people she can depend on for help during pregnancy. Evaluating the family's economic status helps the nurse plan for their health maintenance care as well as Mrs. McGowan's prenatal care. Adequate living conditions are essential for Mrs. McGowan and her expanding family. Assessing ethnic and cultural factors helps the nurse understand variations in family adaptations to pregnancy; the nurse then can plan individualized care while avoiding inappropriate generalizations within or across various ethnic and cultural groups.

Nursing diagnoses
- Knowledge deficit related to a first pregnancy
- Potential fluid volume deficit related to increased body fluid needs

MATERNITY NURSING

Planning and goals

• The results of Mrs. McGowan's physical and diagnostic examinations will be within normal limits. Her health history will pose no threat to this pregnancy.
• Mrs. McGowan will be able to describe any deviations from a normal pregnancy.
• Mrs. McGowan will express concerns about her pregnancy and its effects on her and her family's psychosocial needs.
• Mrs. McGowan will keep her scheduled prenatal appointments.

Implementation

Nursing behaviors

1. Teach Mrs. McGowan about the danger signs of pregnancy:
• vaginal bleeding
• abrupt fluid escape from the vagina
• swelling of the face or fingers
• severe headaches
• visual disturbances, such as blurred or dimmed vision or dots or flashes of light before the eyes
• abdominal pain
• persistent vomiting
• chills and fever.

2. Explain the importance of avoiding over-the-counter medications and other nonprescribed substances.

3. Teach Mrs. McGowan how to manage nausea and vomiting (morning sickness).

4. Stress the importance of maintaining regular health supervision during pregnancy. A suggested routine includes:
• monthly visits through week 32
• bimonthly visits through week 36
• weekly visits from week 37 until delivery.

5. Give Mrs. McGowan a chance to ask questions and talk about her expectations. Listen attentively as she speaks.

Nursing rationales

1. Danger signs of pregnancy may indicate such complications as spontaneous abortion, abruptio placentae, fluid and electrolyte imbalance, pregnancy-induced hypertension, or infection. Any of these signs should be reported immediately because early detection is crucial to the success of treatment.

2. Many over-the-counter medications are teratogenic, especially when taken during the first trimester—the time when fetal organs are developing.

3. Nausea and vomiting can be managed by eating dry crackers before rising; eating small, frequent, high-protein meals; and avoiding fried and spicy foods.

4. Prenatal care dramatically affects the quality of life and well-being of both patient and fetus. During scheduled prenatal visits, the physician can detect any complications and treat them promptly. Prenatal visits also give the nurse a chance to teach the patient and answer her questions related to pregnancy, labor and delivery, and postpartal and newborn care.

5. This helps establish a positive nurse-patient relationship and allows the nurse to help Mrs. McGowan address problems she may be experiencing, such as familial, financial, or cultural problems.

Evaluation (outcomes)

• Mrs. McGowan's health history, physical, and diagnostic findings are within normal limits.
• Mrs. McGowan describes the danger signs of pregnancy and the importance of reporting them to her physician.
• Mrs. McGowan recognizes the bodily changes that occur in the first trimester of pregnancy.
• Mrs. McGowan identifies sources of emotional and material support to meet her and her family's needs during pregnancy.
• Mrs. McGowan has made an appointment for her next prenatal visit.

Menstrual cycle

The hypothalamus stimulates the anterior pituitary gland to accelerate secretion of the gonadotropic hormones: follicle-stimulating hormone (FSH) and luteinizing hormone (LH). FSH stimulates the ovum to mature. The graffian follicle secretes estrogen; elevated estrogen levels inhibit FSH production. Increased LH levels contribute to ovulation.

Calculation of the fertile period is based on the approximate life of the sperm (72 hours) and the egg (24 hours). The corpus luteum secretes progesterone; elevated progesterone levels inhibit LH production.

If fertilization does not occur, the corpus luteum regresses, estrogen and progesterone levels drop, and menses occurs roughly 14 days after ovulation. If fertilization does occur, the corpus luteum continues to produce progesterone until the placenta is formed.

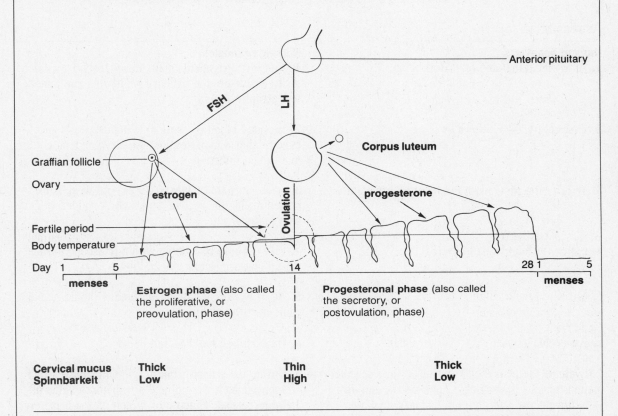

MATERNITY NURSING

Adapted with permission from American Professional Education, Inc. *American nursing review study guide for NCLEX-RN.* Hackensack, NJ. 1986.

Second trimester

Overview

The second trimester, which starts with the fourth month of pregnancy, is a period of relative quiet. Typically, the pregnant woman now accepts the reality of the expected child and focuses on the pregnancy, with thoughts of the expected child dominating. The family may feel left out.

Clinical situation
(continued)

Mary Ann McGowan is in the fifth month of her pregnancy, which has progressed without complications. During her prenatal visit today, she tells the nurse that she has some questions about activity, work, and hygiene.

Assessment

Nursing behaviors	**Nursing rationales**
1. Assess maternal and fetal well-being.	**1.** Routine assessments made during each prenatal visit help ensure the patient's well-being and may detect complications.
2. Assess Mrs. McGowan's vital signs.	**2.** Elevated blood pressure may indicate early pregnancy-induced hypertension. An elevated temperature may signal infection.
3. Weigh Mrs. McGowan and record her weight.	**3.** A weight gain of 1 lb (0.45 kg) per week is expected during the second trimester. A sudden weight gain may indicate fluid retention.
4. Listen for fetal heart tones (FHTs).	**4.** FHTs should be audible with a fetoscope during the second trimester.
5. Measure fundal height.	**5.** At 20 weeks' gestation, the fundus should be palpable near the umbilicus.
6. Assess for quickening (fetal movement).	**6.** Quickening should be felt daily.
7. Evaluate the results of Mrs. McGowan's routine diagnostic tests: hemoglobin, hematocrit, and urinalysis (for glucose and protein).	**7.** During the second trimester, a hemoglobin value of approximately 11 g/dl and a hematocrit value of 35% are normal. Glucose or protein in the urine are abnormal findings that warrant further investigation.
8. Assess Mr. and Mrs. McGowan's psychosocial adaptation to the second trimester.	**8.** The couple should show an awareness that the fetus is a separate being by acknowledging quickening and planning for delivery. Failure to do this reflects dysfunctional adaptation or a need for information.

Nursing diagnoses

• Altered nutrition (more than body requirements) related to additional nutritional needs of the patient and fetus
• Potential altered sexuality patterns related to introspection

Planning and goals
- Mrs. McGowan's second trimester will progress without complications.
- Mrs. McGowan will describe the adaptations to activities of daily living required during the second trimester.
- Mrs. McGowan will ask questions about fetal development during the second trimester.
- Mrs. McGowan will discuss the dietary changes needed during the second trimester.
- Mrs. McGowan will keep her scheduled prenatal visits.

Implementation

Nursing behaviors	Nursing rationales
1. Teach Mrs. McGowan about general health measures and common concerns of pregnancy.	**1.** The second trimester is the ideal time for teaching.
2. Teach Mrs. McGowan about exercises to perform during the second trimester.	**2.** Mrs. McGowan must take safety precautions when exercising, obtain the physician's approval before beginning a new exercise program, and never exercise to the point of fatigue. Walking is the best exercise during pregnancy.
3. Teach Mrs. McGowan about dental care during pregnancy.	**3.** Pregnant women should get regular dental check-ups and avoid X-rays.
4. Provide instructions about bathing.	**4.** The pregnant woman can take daily showers and tub baths. (However, in late pregnancy, she should avoid tub baths because her balance is poor.) She should perform breast care daily but avoid nipple dryness.
5. Teach Mrs. McGowan about clothing and accessories to wear as her pregnancy advances.	**5.** The pregnant woman should wear a supportive bra and low-heeled shoes and avoid restrictive clothing.
6. Teach Mrs. McGowan to avoid douching.	**6.** The pregnant woman should avoid douching unless the physician prescribes it.
7. Provide instructions about immunizations.	**7.** The pregnant woman should not receive live virus immunizations.
8. Provide guidelines for Mrs. McGowan to follow when travelling.	**8.** When travelling by car, the pregnant woman should stop every 2 hours to stretch her legs and walk. Before air travel, she should check any restrictions imposed by the airline or physician. She should not travel in unpressurized airplanes.
9. Provide instructions about alcohol consumption.	**9.** The pregnant woman should not consume alcohol in any form.
10. Advise Mrs. McGowan about smoking.	**10.** The pregnant woman should avoid smoking. Studies indicate that pregnant women who smoke have a greater chance of delivering a low-birth-weight newborn.

MATERNITY NURSING

11. Provide dietary guidelines.

11. Requirements for calories, protein, calcium, and iron increase during pregnancy.

12. Provide instructions about sexual intercourse.

12. Restrictions regarding sexual intercourse vary with the pregnancy state. Recommend various ways to demonstrate love and affection.

13. Teach Mrs. McGowan how to manage constipation.

13. If Mrs. McGowan becomes constipated, she should eat high-fiber foods (such as fruits and vegetables), increase her fluid intake, and get adequate exercise. Warn her never to take laxatives or enemas.

14. Teach Mrs. McGowan how to manage hemorrhoids.

14. The physician may prescribe medications to manage hemorrhoids. Advise Mrs. McGowan to eat a high-fiber diet (as for constipation) and to avoid long periods of sitting.

15. Teach Mrs. McGowan how to manage leg aches and cramps.

15. Mrs. McGowan should extend and elevate her legs and dorsiflex her feet. With the physician's consent, she should increase her calcium intake and decrease her phosphorus intake.

16. Provide instructions on preventing or coping with backache.

16. Good posture is important during pregnancy. Rest periods and pelvic rocking exercises also may help relieve back discomfort.

17. Give Mrs. McGowan a chance to ask questions and talk about her expectations.

17. This helps establish a positive nurse-patient relationship.

18. Schedule Mrs. McGowan's next prenatal visit.

18. During the second trimester, she should make prenatal visits every 4 weeks.

Evaluation (outcomes)

• Mrs. McGowan's pregnancy continues to progress without complications.
• Mrs. McGowan can describe how to maintain her pregnancy by eating a proper diet, getting enough exercise, avoiding common annoyances of pregnancy, and maintaining other good health practices.
• Mrs. McGowan expresses an interest in the developing fetus and her pregnancy status.
• Mrs. McGowan makes an appointment for her next prenatal visit.

Third trimester

Overview

During the third trimester, the pregnant woman begins to prepare for her child's birth. She experiences such physical symptoms as shortness of breath, urinary frequency, fatigue, and constipation. This trimester is marked by great anticipation of the expected child and the desire to experience parenthood. The family begins preparing the home for the new baby.

Clinical situation
(continued)

Mary Ann McGowan is now in the eighth month of her pregnancy, which has progressed without complications. She states that she looks forward to the birth of her baby, and asks how to prepare for labor and delivery.

Assessment

Nursing behaviors

1. Evaluate maternal and fetal well-being.

Nursing rationales

1. Routine assessments performed during each prenatal visit help ensure the patient's general well-being and detect complications of pregnancy.

2. Assess Mr. and Mrs. McGowan's psychosocial status. Find out if they have attended childbirth classes, are prepared for labor and delivery, and are prepared to provide care for their newborn.

2. During the third trimester, both parents should prepare to cope with labor and delivery by asking key questions, attending childbirth classes, preparing the home nursery, and acknowledging that they are going to be parents.

Nursing diagnoses

• Knowledge deficit related to labor and delivery
• Potential for ineffective individual coping related to preparation for labor and delivery

Planning and goals

• Mrs. McGowan and her husband will attend childbirth classes and describe their preparations for labor and delivery.
• Mrs. McGowan and her husband will ask questions that show a desire for information about newborn care.
• Mrs. McGowan will be able to describe the premonitory (warning) signs of labor and state how to respond to them appropriately.
• Mrs. McGowan's pregnancy will continue to term without complications.

Implementation

Nursing behaviors

1. Assist the RN in reviewing with Mr. and Mrs. McGowan the techniques they will use during labor and delivery.

Nursing rationales

1. The more prepared the McGowans are, the less fearful they will be during labor and delivery. Advise them to attend childbirth classes, if they have not done so.

2. Review the premonitory signs of labor:
• lightening
• urinary frequency
• weight loss
• bloody show
• energy spurt
• amniotic membrane rupture
• Braxton-Hicks contractions.

2. When Mrs. McGowan experiences premonitory signs, she should prepare for labor. Lightening refers to fetal descent, which eases breathing. Urinary frequency results from pressure by the uterus on the bladder during lightening. Weight loss, which may amount to 1 to 2 lb (0.45 to 0.9 kg), is caused by hormonal changes. Bloody show (or a pinkish discharge) usually appears when the mucus plug is expelled. An energy spurt may occur as the basal metabolic rate rises. If the amniotic membranes rupture prematurely, Mrs. McGowan should report this to the physician immediately. Braxton-Hicks contractions are irregular uterine contractions that do not cause cervical effacement and dilation.

3. Schedule Mrs. McGowan's next prenatal visit.

3. During the eighth month, she should make prenatal visits every 2 weeks; during the ninth month, every week. After week 36, the physician may perform a weekly internal vaginal examination to evaluate cervical changes.

MATERNITY NURSING

Evaluation (outcomes)

- Mr. and Mrs. McGowan attend childbirth classes.
- Mrs. McGowan describes the premonitory signs of labor and appropriate responses.
- Mrs. McGowan's pregnancy continues to term without complications.

Fetal development

This series of illustrations shows how the fetus develops from week 4 to week 38 of gestation.

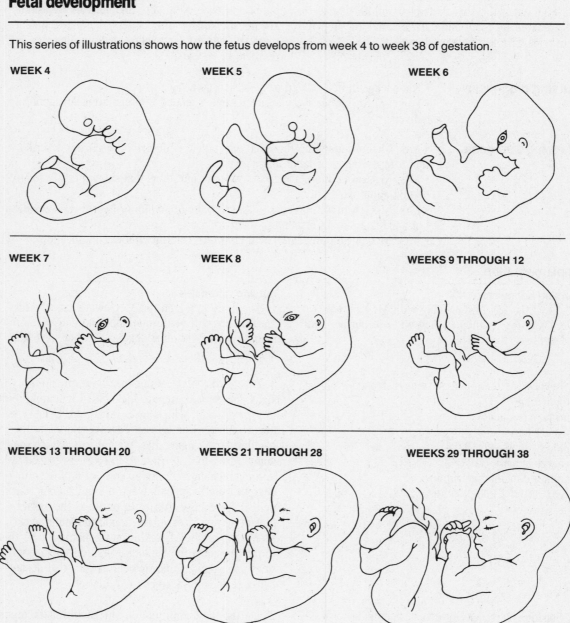

WEEK 4

WEEK 5

WEEK 6

WEEK 7

WEEK 8

WEEKS 9 THROUGH 12

WEEKS 13 THROUGH 20

WEEKS 21 THROUGH 28

WEEKS 29 THROUGH 38

From *Attending Ob/Gyn Patients*. Nursing Photobook Series. Springhouse, Pa. Springhouse Corporation, 1984.

Pregnancy complications

An interplay of physiologic and psychological factors can cause complications during pregnancy. The chart below describes the common hemorrhagic complications that necessitate intervention.

COMPLICATION	CAUSE	NURSING CONSIDERATIONS
Abruptio placentae Premature detachment of the normally situated placenta from the uterine wall; a complication of hypofibrinogenemia. Types of abruptio placentae include total abruptio placentae (complete detachment) and partial abruptio placentae (partial detachment). Signs and symptoms include concealed hemorrhage, overt hemorrhage, or both; pain from uterine distention (caused by bleeding); boardlike abdomen with shock; and signs of fetal distress.	• Multiparity • Pregnancy-induced hypertension • Abdominal trauma • Cocaine use	• Replace lost blood, as ordered. • Administer I.V. fluids, as ordered. • Monitor maternal and fetal condition. • Observe the patient for shock; monitor blood loss. • Explain all procedures thoroughly to the patient. • Enforce bed rest, if the condition is mild. • Help prepare the patient for vaginal or cesarean delivery, as appropriate.
Placenta previa Abnormal placental implantation in the lower uterine segment, over or near the cervical opening, or os. Types of placenta previa include total placenta previa (in which the placenta completely covers the cervical opening), partial placenta previa (in which the placenta partially covers the opening), and placenta previa marginalis (in which the placenta meets the rim of the opening but does not block it). The condition is diagnosed by sonogram. The risk of placenta previa increases with age and multiparity. Signs and symptoms include painless bleeding (hemorrhage) during the third trimester, ranging from slight to massive; abdominal softness (except during contractions); and signs of fetal distress.	• Multiple gestation • Uterine tumor • Molar pregnancy • Reduced vascularity of the upper uterine segment (such as from scarring caused by surgery)	• The patient must be hospitalized. • Enforce bedrest. • Do not perform a pelvic or rectal digital examination. • Tell the patient what is happening and what procedures will be performed. • Monitor maternal and fetal condition. • Prepare the patient for delivery. • The patient risks postoperative and postpartal infection; observe for signs and symptoms of infection. • With total placenta previa, if the patient has frank bleeding, cesarean delivery is necessary. • With partial placenta previa, cesarean delivery usually is necessary. • With placenta previa marginalis, cesarean delivery occasionally is necessary.
Spontaneous abortion Spontaneous termination of pregnancy before the fetus attains viability. Signs and symptoms include vaginal bleeding, lower abdominal pain or cramping, and signs and symptoms of shock. Types of spontaneous abortion include inevitable, incomplete, and threatened. With an inevitable abortion (one that cannot be halted), the cervix is dilated. With an incomplete abortion (in which some products of conception are retained), signs and symptoms include a smaller-than-expected uterus for gestational age and a closed cervical os; cramping and bleeding may be absent. With a threatened abortion, expect signs and symptoms of spontaneous abortion. However, if the fetus is alive and the placenta properly attached, the pregnancy may continue.	• Fetoplacental developmental defects • Psychological factors • Maternal factors (diabetes mellitus, infection, systemic disorders, cocaine use, hypertension, genetic factors) • Closed cervix	• With inevitable abortion, the patient must be hospitalized; enforce bedrest; administer I.V. fluids, as ordered; replace fluids and lost blood, as ordered and necessary; and keep a complete pad count and save all tissue samples. • With incomplete abortion, assist with dilatation and curettage. • With threatened abortion, enforce bedrest; teach the patient to avoid straining, lifting, and carrying; provide a light diet; administer a mild sedative, if ordered; and instruct the patient to abstain from sexual intercourse.

INTRAPARTAL PERIOD

The intrapartal period, which extends from the start of labor through the first hour after delivery, brings the product of conception into the world. Nursing care during this intense period focuses on ensuring the well-being of the patient and fetus to produce a healthy newborn and promoting family adaptation to the childbirth process.

Labor and delivery

Overview

To be an active leader during childbirth, the nurse must understand the physiology of labor and delivery and recognize how sociocultural and personal factors can affect the childbirth experience. The following care plan focuses on the nurse caring for the patient and family during labor and delivery.

Clinical situation

Mary Ann McGowan, age 23, is a primigravid patient who arrives on the labor and delivery unit stating that today is her due date. Her membranes ruptured earlier in the day, and she now has mild contractions every 5 minutes. An examination reveals that her vital signs are stable, fetal heart tones (FHTs) measure 132 beats/minute in the lower right quadrant, and the fetal presenting part is the vertex, at station +1. Her cervix is dilated 4 cm and 100% effaced. The physician's written admission orders include a lower one-third perineal shave, nothing by mouth, and 1,000 ml dextrose 5% in water (D_5W) administered I.V. at a rate of 75 ml/hour.

Assessment

Nursing behaviors

1. Review Mrs. McGowan's prenatal record for important data.

2. Review Mrs. McGowan's prenatal record to determine her age.

3. Review Mrs. McGowan's prenatal record to learn about her gravida and para status.

4. Review Mrs. McGowan's prenatal record to learn about her expected date of confinement (EDC).

5. Review Mrs. McGowan's prenatal record to find out if she had prenatal complications.

Nursing rationales

1. The prenatal record, which includes vital signs, weight gain, FHTs, and fundal heights, shows how the pregnancy has progressed. Such information contributes to baseline assessment data and helps manage labor and delivery.

2. An extreme childbearing age may contribute to labor or delivery complications.

3. Information about previous obstetric history and intrapartal experiences may help predict aspects of the current labor and delivery.

4. EDC provides information about gestational age and may help the nurse anticipate problems.

5. The nurse must consider such complications as diabetes, pregnancy-induced hypertension (PIH), and preeclampsia when planning care during labor and delivery.

6. Review Mrs. McGowan's prenatal record for information about allergies.

6. The nurse should note any food or drug allergies.

7. Review Mrs. McGowan's prenatal record to learn about her prenatal medications.

7. Information about current medications helps the nurse anticipate adverse effects, effects on labor, and interactions with drugs administered during labor and delivery.

8. Review Mrs. McGowan's prenatal record to find out about prenatal laboratory results.

8. Important laboratory data include urinalysis, hemoglobin and hematocrit levels, complete blood counts, and Rh and blood typing.

9. Assist the RN in assessing uterine contractions.

9. During labor, the assessment routine varies with the setting, available equipment, and individual patient needs. To assess contractions and help plan nursing care, identify the stage and phase of labor and evaluate contraction onset, frequency, duration, and intensity.

Mrs. McGowan is in the early phase of the first stage of labor, when contractions should be monitored continuously by an electronic monitor. The fetal monitor continuously records uterine activity and FHTs, and displays this information in various ways: as audible FHTs, as numerical FHTs, and as a strip correlating FHTs with contraction frequency, duration, and strength. With external monitoring, the tocotransducer is placed over the fundus and the transducer is placed over the fetal back. With internal monitoring, the monitoring catheter (pressure transducer) is placed inside the uterus to monitor contractions and an electrode is attached to the fetal scalp to monitor FHTs.

10. Assist the RN in assessing the status of Mrs. McGowan's amniotic membranes.

10. Mrs. McGowan's membranes may be intact, leaking, or ruptured. If she is unsure of her membrane status, vaginal secretions may be tested with nitrazine paper. The paper will turn dark blue if secretions contain amniotic fluid, which is slightly alkaline (pH 7.2). Ferning of secretions also indicates membrane rupture.

11. Assess Mrs. McGowan for bloody show.

11. Bloody show is a premonitory sign that labor has begun.

12. Assess Mrs. McGowan's vital signs on her arrival, then hourly. Take her temperature every 4 hours, unless otherwise indicated.

12. Vital signs provide baseline information and contribute to overall assessment of both patient and fetus during labor.

13. Monitor FHTs by electronic monitor or fetoscope every 15 minutes.

13. The nurse must monitor FHTs routinely and also after membrane rupture, before and after medication administration, and after enema administration.

MATERNITY NURSING

14. Assist the RN in assessing results of the external and internal vaginal examinations.

14. Vaginal examination is done on admission and repeated throughout labor. During the first phase of labor, however, it is done less frequently. Vaginal discharge or lesions noted during the external examination warrant further investigation and may necessitate a change in delivery method. The internal examination reveals fetal presentation, position, and station as well as cervical dilation and effacement. This examination calls for aseptic technique.

15. Assist the RN in assessing laboratory test results, including urinalysis and complete blood count (CBC).

15. Laboratory tests are performed on admission to collect baseline information and identify potential problems. Mrs. McGowan's urine may contain a small amount of glucose but should not contain protein or bacteria. CBC helps identify such problems as anemia, infection, and excessive bleeding or dehydration.

16. Assist the RN in assessing Mr. and Mrs. McGowan's attendance at childbirth classes, knowledge of childbearing, and expectations.

16. Assessing the expectant couple's understanding of the childbirth process and use of coping methods enhances the nurse's effectiveness in providing care.

17. Assess Mr. and Mrs. McGowan's emotional status from verbal and nonverbal signs, such as facial expressions and body language.

17. Changes in emotional status are expected during labor and usually relate to the phases and stages of labor.

18. Assess Mrs. McGowan for other signs, as described in steps 19 to 21.

18. Additional information helps to determine the care she will need.

19. Assess Mrs. McGowan for edema.

19. Edema may indicate PIH or another complication.

20. Assess Mrs. McGowan for a rash.

20. A rash may indicate infection.

21. Assess Mrs. McGowan for an abdominal scar.

21. An abdominal scar may indicate previous uterine surgery.

22. Assess Mrs. McGowan for the time of her most recent food or fluid intake.

22. Intestinal peristalsis decreases during labor. Recent food or fluid intake may cause nausea or vomiting; if Mrs. McGowan requires general anesthesia, this may lead to aspiration.

23. Assess Mrs. McGowan for prostheses, such as dentures, contact lenses, or glasses.

23. All prostheses must be removed before general anesthesia is administered.

24. Find out which infant feeding method Mrs. McGowan has chosen.

24. If she plans to breast-feed, she will need to consume 300 extra calories/day and cannot receive medications after delivery. If she plans to use infant formula, she may receive lactation-suppressant medications.

Nursing diagnoses
- Altered urinary elimination related to increased urinary frequency
- Pain related to labor contractions

Planning and goals
- Mrs. McGowan will express an understanding of the labor and delivery process.
- Mrs. McGowan will respond positively to the support person present.
- Mrs. McGowan will be able to follow directions and assist with the birthing process.
- Mrs. McGowan and her fetus will remain free from complications during labor and delivery.
- Mrs. McGowan and her husband will show positive bonding during the fourth stage of labor.

Implementation

Nursing behaviors	**Nursing rationales**
1. Transcribe and carry out all admission procedures, as ordered.	**1.** The physician's orders are based on the patient's individual needs.
2. If ordered, follow institutional procedures and precautions for a perineal shave and enema administration.	**2.** Removal of perineal hair helps prevent or reduce infection. A perineal shave can vary from a "mini" to full. (Perineal shaves no longer are done routinely.) An enema helps reduce tissue trauma during labor and delivery and promotes comfort.
3. Encourage Mrs. McGowan to void.	**3.** This helps prevent trauma from distention and enhances patient comfort. The nurse should assess Mrs. McGowan's bladder routinely during labor.
4. Withhold oral foods and fluids. Carefully monitor the I.V. solution (used to prevent dehydration), I.V. site, and I.V. flow rate.	**4.** These measures ensure patient safety.
5. Provide comfort measures for Mrs. McGowan.	**5.** Comfort measures help reduce discomfort caused by cervical dilation and effacement and uterine contractions. (Narcotic analgesics are not administered in the early phase of labor because they slow labor progress.)
6. Assist Mrs. McGowan with ambulation, if permitted.	**6.** Ambulation may help reduce discomfort and shorten labor.
7. If Mrs. McGowan is confined to bed, encourage her to lie on her left side, elevate the head of the bed, and provide pillows for support.	**7.** These measures help prevent vena cava syndrome (supine hypotension).
8. Encourage Mrs. McGowan to use the breathing and distraction techniques she has learned.	**8.** Using breathing and distraction techniques during the latent phase of the first stage of labor relaxes the patient.
9. During the pelvic examination, encourage Mrs. McGowan to relax the pelvic floor muscles.	**9.** Relaxing the pelvic floor muscles reduces resistance and increases patient comfort during pelvic examination.

MATERNITY NURSING

10. Provide emotional support by orienting Mrs. McGowan to her room and the unit, providing privacy, explaining procedures, and answering questions. Make sure she knows how to call the nurse for help. Reassess her emotional status frequently.

10. Familiarity with surroundings and the ability to call the nurse for help increase the patient's comfort and sense of security. (Typically, the patient looks to the nurse to answer her questions throughout labor and delivery.) During the latent phase of the first stage of labor, the patient usually is excited, talkative, responsive to suggestions, and slightly anxious.

Clinical situation
(continued)

Active phase of the first stage
Mary Ann McGowan's labor has progressed to the second, or active, phase of the first stage. Her contractions are strong, occur every 3½ minutes, and last 45 seconds. During her last vaginal examination, her cervix was dilated 6 cm and 100% effaced; the vertex was at +1 station. Her membranes ruptured earlier in the day. The physician has ordered meperidine (Demerol) 40 mg I.V. for pain relief, if needed.

Implementation

Nursing behaviors

1. Assist the RN in monitoring Mrs. McGowan's uterine contractions.

2. Monitor Mrs. McGowan's pulse, respirations, and blood pressure every 30 minutes. Take her temperature every 4 hours.

3. Monitor and record FHTs continuously.

4. Assist the RN in performing a vaginal examination, when necessary, to determine cervical dilation.

5. Administer care related to membrane rupture:
• Listen to FHTs.
• Place a dry pad under Mrs. McGowan's buttocks and change it as needed.
• If the membranes rupture after her admission, record the time of rupture and the appearance of the amniotic fluid.
• Confine Mrs. McGowan to bed.

6. Provide comfort measures for Mrs. McGowan:
• Place her in the most comfortable position.
• Provide sacral massage and assist with pelvic rocking to help reduce back discomfort.
• Reinforce positive coping methods.
• Apply a cool, moist cloth to her forehead.
• Administer pain medication, as ordered; keep the side rails up as a safety precaution.

Nursing rationales

1. The nurse must monitor uterine contractions more frequently during the active phase because of changes that occur at this time and to plan appropriate care.

2. Vital sign changes may be the first warning of a potential problem.

3. FHTs may indicate fetal distress or complications.

4. The vaginal examination is conducted during the active phase; however, it should be done as infrequently as possible to prevent infection and discomfort.

5. Membrane rupture may be spontaneous or induced artificially. After it occurs, the nurse should listen to FHTs to detect signs of distress. If the presenting part is not engaged, umbilical cord prolapse may occur. (For details on umbilical cord prolapse, see *Labor complications,* pages 133 and 134.)

6. Patient comfort promotes cooperation during labor and delivery. Sacral massage and pelvic rocking help relieve backache. As active labor continues, increased physical and emotional effort are required; the patient must draw on positive coping methods to deal with discomfort. A cool, moist cloth can be refreshing and provide a psychological boost. Pain medication may be administered during the active phase of labor; FHTs should be checked before and after administration.

7. Provide emotional support for Mrs. McGowan.

7. The patient needs emotional support during the active phase of labor, when labor becomes uncomfortable. Typically, she becomes more serious, self-centered, and anxious.

Clinical situation
(continued)

Transitional phase of the first stage
Mary Ann McGowan has progressed to the transitional phase of the first stage of labor. Her contractions have become strong. She is perspiring profusely, and has just vomited. Her cervix is dilated 8 cm, with the vertex at +1 station. FHTs are within normal limits. She states that she feels the urge to push.

Implementation

Nursing behaviors

1. Monitor and record uterine contraction characteristics.

2. Monitor fetal status by assessing and recording FHTs, using an electronic monitor or fetoscope, every 5 to 15 minutes. Assist the RN in assessing amniotic fluid for meconium.

3. Assist the RN in performing a vaginal examination.

4. Assess for additional signs of transition:
• increase in dark, bloody show
• nausea and vomiting
• perspiration
• skin irritability
• urge to push.

5. Provide comfort measures for Mrs. McGowan:
• Place her in the most comfortable position.
• Reinforce learned coping techniques.
• Place moist cloths on her forehead and lips.
• Place a dry pad under her buttocks.
• Provide sacral massage, if requested.

6. Encourage Mrs. McGowan to blow or pant instead of push when she feels the urge to push.

7. Provide emotional support for Mrs. McGowan and her husband. Stay with them, and offer praise and encouragement.

Nursing rationales

1. During this phase, the nurse must monitor the patient more closely than during active labor and must assess contractions continuously.

2. As labor intensifies, the nurse must assess fetal status more frequently.

3. The RN performs a vaginal examination to assess fetal station, cervical dilation and effacement, and membrane status.

4. These signs are characteristic of the transitional phase.

5. The transitional phase of labor can be extremely demanding. Mrs. McGowan needs reinforcement to perform complicated breathing patterns and distraction techniques. She may appreciate refreshing moist cloths on the forehead and lips. If she has back pain, she may want a sacral massage.

6. Pushing (bearing down) before the cervix is dilated fully may cause cervical edema, obstruction, or laceration. Effective blowing or panting helps prevent pushing. (However, be sure stay alert for hyperventilation.)

7. The transitional phase is the most difficult labor phase and can be overwhelming. Mrs. McGowan needs someone to rely on to help her maintain control and decrease her fear of being alone.

MATERNITY NURSING

Clinical situation
(continued)

Second stage of labor
Mary Ann McGowan has completed the first stage of labor and appears relieved that she can now start to push with her contractions. Perineal bulging is apparent and her cervix is dilated 10 cm.

Implementation

Nursing behaviors

1. Assist the RN in monitoring and recording contractions.

2. Monitor and record fetal status by assessing FHTs continuously or after each contraction and by reassessing for signs of fetal distress.

3. Assist the RN in performing a vaginal examination to determine fetal station.

4. Monitor Mrs. McGowan continuously for other signs and symptoms of the second stage of labor:
• increased bloody show
• urge to push
• uncontrollable leg shaking
• perineal bulging
• crowning
• rectal bulging.

5. Instruct Mrs. McGowan to use her abdominal muscles to push with contractions.

6. Provide comfort measures, and encourage Mrs. McGowan to rest between contractions.

7. When crowning starts, prepare Mrs. McGowan for delivery, as described in steps 8 and 9.

8. Position Mrs. McGowan in the birthing bed, chair, delivery table, or position of choice.

9. Clean Mrs. McGowan's perineum.

10. Assist with delivery by encouraging Mrs. McGowan to pant or blow as the head of the fetus is delivered.

Nursing rationales

1. Contractions must be monitored more closely during the second stage.

2. A pattern of early decelerations may appear, indicating head compression as the fetus proceeds through the birth canal.

3. Determination of fetal station is vital. A primigravid patient usually progresses through the second stage more slowly than a multigravid patient.

4. As the fetus moves through the birth canal, the presenting part puts pressure on surrounding tissues. The patient may experience some or all of these signs and symptoms.

5. Using the abdominal muscles to push helps move the fetus through the birth canal.

6. Comfort measures resemble those used during the transitional phase. The patient needs to rest between contractions to conserve energy.

7. For a primigravid patient, delivery preparations begin when crowning starts; for a multigravid patient, they begin during the transitional phase.

8. If a delivery table with stirrups is used, place both of the patient's legs in the stirrups at the same time. (After delivery, remove them at the same time.) This helps prevent straining of leg muscles.

9. The perineum should be cleaned with antiseptic solution. Be sure to work from clean to soiled areas.

10. Panting or blowing reduces the risk of forceful expulsion of the head.

11. If needed, provide forceps or equipment for episiotomy repair.

11. Forceps (most commonly, low or outlet forceps) may be used during delivery. They are applied when the fetal head is below the ischial spines to lift the head over the perineum. The physician may perform an episiotomy to facilitate delivery and shorten the second stage of labor or to prevent perineal lacerations. (A midline incision is used whenever possible.) Perineal lacerations are classified by degree. First-degree lacerations are the most superficial; third- and fourth-degree lacerations, the most extensive. Third- and fourth-degree lacerations contraindicate rectal medication administration during the postpartal period. (Suspect a cervical laceration in a postpartal patient who has excessive vaginal bleeding and a firm fundus.)

12. Continue to provide emotional support, praise, and encouragement to the McGowans.

12. Typically, the patient gains renewed energy and a sense of control when she is allowed to push, and responds well to encouragement.

13. Allow the McGowans to touch their newborn as soon as possible after delivery.

13. Early family interactions enhance parent-child bonding.

Clinical situation
(continued)

Third and fourth stages of labor
Mary Ann McGowan delivers a 9 lb, 2 oz (4.1 kg) boy without complications. She and her husband are happy and relieved.

Implementation

Nursing behaviors

1. During the third stage, administer oxytocic medications, as ordered. Examples of oxytocic medications include oxytocin (Pitocin), methylergonovine maleate (Methergine), and ergonovine maleate (Ergotrate).

Nursing rationales

1. Placental separation from the uterine wall leads to bleeding. Oxytocics help control bleeding by inducing myometrial contractions and blood vessel constriction.

2. Lower Mrs. McGowan's legs from the stirrups and help her to a comfortable position. Provide her with a blanket if she is chilled.

2. Mrs. McGowan may feel chilled from loss of body heat, weight, and fluids—or simply from excitement.

3. Assist the RN in providing newborn care, as described in steps 4 to 10.

3. Immediate newborn care is performed according to priorities.

4. Maintain a patent airway in the newborn.

4. To clear the airway, suction may be needed. Suction the newborn's mouth first, then the nose, keeping the head in a dependent position for mucus drainage.

5. Gently rub the newborn's back.

5. This stimulates respirations.

Assigning an Apgar score

The Apgar score, assigned at 1 minute and 5 minutes after delivery, is a simple, rapid, and practical way to determine a newborn's condition. A score of 0 to 2 is assigned in five assessment categories—heart rate, respirations, muscle tone, reflex irritability, and color. The higher the score, the better the newborn's condition.
- A score below 4 indicates severe depression calling for immediate care and continuous evaluation.
- A score of 4 to 6 indicates moderate depression necessitating immediate care.
- A score of 7 to 10 means that no special intervention is required.

The chart below shows the criteria for assigning scores in each assessment category.

ASSESSMENT CATEGORY	SCORE 0	SCORE 1	SCORE 2
Heart rate	Absent	Below 100 beats/minute	Above 100 beats/minute
Respirations	Absent	Slow, irregular	Vigorous cry
Muscle tone	Limp, flaccid	Some muscle tone; sluggish return of extremities to a flexed position after extension	Quick return of extremities to a flexed position after extension
Reflex irritability (response to sole stimulation or insertion of a bulb syringe into a nostril)	No response	Some motion, weak cry	Vigorous cry
Color	Completely pale or blue	Bluish hands and feet	Completely pink

6. Assist the RN in assigning the newborn's Apgar score at 1 and 5 minutes after delivery by evaluating five assessment categories—heart rate, respirations, muscle tone, reflex irritability, and color.

6. The Apgar score provides an immediate index of the newborn's status.

7. Keep the newborn warm.

7. An immature temperature-regulating mechanism causes the newborn to take on the environmental temperature. To prevent cold stress, make sure the newborn remains warm.

8. Administer eye prophylaxis to the newborn by applying 1% silver nitrate or an antibiotic ointment.

8. Eye prophylaxis helps prevent blindness resulting from a maternal infection. It should be administered within 1 hour of delivery.

9. Complete the required newborn identification procedures: footprints, fingerprints, and bracelets.

9. Proper identification is a safety consideration.

10. Perform a preliminary cephalocaudal assessment.

10. This brief assessment helps rule out any obvious injuries or anomalies. A more complete assessment, including gestational age assessment, is performed later.

Clinical situation
(continued)

Mary Ann McGowan is moved to the postpartal nursing unit.

MATERNITY NURSING

Implementation

Nursing behaviors

1. Monitor Mrs. McGowan closely during the fourth stage of labor (the first hour after delivery of the placenta).

Nursing rationales

1. Close monitoring during the first hour is crucial to prevent and manage complications.

Labor complications

Various complications can occur during labor. Some may threaten the life of the patient, her fetus, or both. This chart describes the most common complications.

COMPLICATION	CAUSE	NURSING INTERVENTIONS
Intrapartal hemorrhage Abnormal bleeding between the onset of labor and the fourth stage of labor. Hemorrhage can be mild to severe. Signs and symptoms include restlessness, pallor, diaphoresis, stupor, and decreased renal function.	Various maternal or placental factors. Maternal risk factors include hypertension, dystocia, uterine overdistention, diabetes, previous bleeding history, cervical and vaginal lacerations, and uterine rupture. Placental risk factors include placenta previa, abruptio placentae, and retained placental fragments.	• Assess the patient for risk factors. • Observe for restlessness, anxiety, and sudden pain. • Watch for and report any unusual bleeding. • Notify the physician or nurse-midwife of the patient's condition. • Monitor vital signs frequently. • Monitor uterine activity and fetal heart rate (FHR). • Observe for changes in skin color. • Monitor level of consciousness. • Administer oxygen, as ordered. • Help the RN prepare the patient for emergency cesarean delivery, if indicated. • Tell the patient what is happening.
Umbilical cord prolapse Umbilical cord displacement to a level at or below the presenting part. This condition impedes the flow of oxygen to the fetus and can cause serious fetal brain damage or fetal death. Signs and symptoms include cord protrusion from the vagina, meconium-stained amniotic fluid, and meconium passage. Fetal indications of cord prolapse and compression include FHR changes and variable decelerations on the fetal heart monitor. Risk factors for cord prolapse include: • membrane rupture before the presenting part is engaged • breech or transverse presentation • preterm delivery • multiple-gestation pregnancy.	Amniotic membrane rupture	• Manually relieve pressure on the cord by the presenting part by keeping surgically gloved fingers in the vagina continuously until delivery. • Calm the patient and provide emotional support so that she cooperates with her care. Do not leave her unattended. • Make sure a second nurse notifies the physician of the patient's condition or seeks a physician in the delivery-room area. • Have the patient assume a knee-to-chest position, or adjust the bed to Trendelenburg's position. • Administer oxygen, as ordered, to maximize fetal oxygenation. • If the cord protrudes, keep it moist with sterile saline solution. • Assist with emergency cesarean delivery, as appropriate.

(continued)

Labor complications *(continued)*

COMPLICATION	CAUSE	NURSING INTERVENTIONS
Dystocia Abnormal labor or failure of labor progression. Uterine contractions are classified as hypertonic (extremely painful), hypotonic (weak, infrequent, irregular, and ineffective), or dystonic (asymmetrical and ineffective).	Uterine, fetal, or pelvic factors. Uterine factors include uterine muscle inertia or dysfunction. Fetal factors include abnormal presentation or position, certain anomalies, and cephalopelvic disproportion. Pelvic factors include pelvic contraction and maternal pelvic masses. (A full bladder or rectum also may impede labor progress. However, this condition can be corrected easily by allowing and encouraging voiding every 2 hours and by catheterizing or administering an enema, as ordered and necessary.)	• Assist the RN in monitoring contractions for intensity, duration, and frequency. • Assist the RN in monitoring cervical progress and comparing it with normal labor progress. • Assist the RN in monitoring FHR relative to contractions. • Assist the RN in monitoring fetal presentation, position, descent, caput, and molding. • Monitor the patient's vital signs, hydration status, and level of fatigue. • As appropriate, provide comfort measures, such as back rubs, position changes, and cool compresses. • Explain the causes of dystocia and specific interventions to the expectant parents. • Keep the expectant parents informed of labor progress and fetal status. • Allow the expectant parents to participate in decision-making whenever possible.
Fetal distress Response of the fetus to a decreased fetal oxygen supply, as identified from fetal heart tones (FHTs). Signs of fetal distress include fetal hyperactivity, persistent fetal tachycardia or bradycardia, and meconium-stained amniotic fluid.	Maternal or fetal factors. Maternal factors include anemia, hypertension, hypotension, preeclampsia, abruptio placentae, placenta previa, medications (including oxytocics), prolonged contractions, or pressure on the placenta. Fetal factors include a prolapsed, knotted, or nuchal umbilical cord.	• Assist the RN in monitoring FHTs for baseline beat-to-beat variability and periodic changes. • Assist the RN in monitoring FHTs with uterine contractions. • Assist the RN in monitoring the frequency, intensity, and duration of uterine contractions. • Assist the RN in discontinuing oxytocin administration, if needed. • Place the patient in a left lateral position for early and late decelerations. • Administer oxygen at 7 to 8 liters/minute, as ordered and necessary. • Notify the physician of fetal status while the RN stays with the patient. • Prepare the patient for cesarean delivery. • Inform the expectant parents of anticipated or ongoing procedures and labor progress.

2. Monitor Mrs. McGowan's vital signs every 15 minutes.

2. Vital signs reflect the patient's general well-being and may signal possible complications.

3. Perform a postpartal assessment every 15 minutes, as described in steps 4 to 7.

3. Postpartal assessment must be done frequently to assess the patient's immediate response to delivery.

4. Assess the fundus, noting its consistency and position.

4. The fundus should be firm and located in the midline near the umbilicus. If it is not firm, massage it to stimulate contractions and control bleeding.

5. Assess the bladder for distention and encourage Mrs. McGowan to void.

5. The bladder should be observed for filling and the degree to which it displaces the uterus (if appropriate).

6. Assess lochia for amount and color.

6. Lochia should be bright red and heavy during the immediate postpartal period.

7. Assess the perineum for intactness, hematomas, and hemorrhoids.

7. A hematoma may develop from tissue trauma; treatment involves ice application to minimize swelling, then heat application. Evaluate the approximation of any perineal repair. Hemorrhoids may arise from the trauma of labor and delivery.

8. Provide comfort measures for Mrs. McGowan, including a comfortable bed position, hygiene (bathing, linen changes, and bed pads), and rest periods.

8. Promoting comfort contributes to the patient's feeling of well-being.

9. Provide nourishment for Mrs. McGowan.

9. Labor and delivery involve tremendous muscular activity and energy exertion. Afterward, the patient may be hungry and thirsty.

10. Continue to provide emotional support to Mrs. McGowan and her husband.

10. Providing an atmosphere of acceptance and relaxation enhances parent-child attachment and family integration.

Evaluation (outcomes)

• Mrs. McGowan and her newborn progress through labor and delivery without complications; both are healthy.
• Mrs. McGowan responds positively to the nurse's coaching during labor and delivery.
• Mrs. McGowan and her husband participate effectively during labor and delivery.
• Mrs. McGowan and her husband are comfortable and happy with the newborn and display attachment behaviors.

MATERNITY NURSING

Congenital abnormalities

Congenital abnormalities affect thousands of newborns each year. The abnormalities described below are those most frequently encountered by entry-level nurses. (For details on the treatment and nursing management of these conditions, see the section on "Pediatric Nursing.")

CONGENITAL ABNORMALITY	SIGNS AND SYMPTOMS	NURSING INTERVENTIONS
Bladder exstrophy Congenital eversion of the urinary bladder	• Appearance of the bladder and urethra outside the abdominal cavity	• Postoperatively, apply moist dressings to the bladder. • Change the newborn's diapers frequently. • Avoiding placing tight garments over the affected area. • Provide emotional support to the parents.
Cleft lip, cleft palate Readily visible midline fissure or opening in the lip or palate or both	• Difficulty maintaining suction on a nipple • Coughing and choking during feedings • Respiratory distress	• Feed the newborn with a special nipple or special technique. • Keep the newborn upright during feedings. • Keep the affected area clean. • Give postoperative feedings slowly, observing for regurgitation and aspiration. • Encourage the parents to participate in infant feeding and care. • Provide emotional support to the parents.
Clubfoot (talipes) Congenital foot deformity in which the foot is twisted out of position or shape because of a unilateral or bilateral deviation of the metatarsal bones. Talipes equinovarus is the most common form.	• Downward and inward turning of the affected foot (with equinovarus).	• Observe for circulatory impairment after cast application. • Teach the parents how to provide cast care. • Provide emotional support to the child.
Congenital hip dislocation Hip joint malformation in which the head of the femur improperly lies in the acetabulum and slips out on movement	• Asymmetry of the gluteal and thigh folds • Limited hip abduction • Apparent femur shortening (as shown by the level of flexed knees) • Ortolani's sign (audible click during hip abduction and rotation)	• Provide cast care if the newborn is placed in a spica cast. • Position the newborn with legs slightly flexed and abducted. • Use a double diaper. • Provide skin care.
Diaphragmatic hernia Herniation of the abdominal contents into the thoracic cavity	• Protrusion of the abdominal contents through the chest defect • Cyanosis and chest retractions • Small, scaphoid abdomen • Absence of breath sounds on the affected side	• Keep the newborn's head elevated before and after surgery. • Postoperatively, observe chest tube function and position the newborn on the affected side. • Observe and manage the nasogastric or gastrostomy tube. • Monitor for respiratory distress.
Epispadias Congenital anomaly in which the urethra opens on the dorsal surface of the penis	• Appearance of the urinary meatus on the dorsal aspect of the penis	• Monitor the urine flow and urethra opening. • Provide preoperative and postoperative care.

Congenital abnormalities *(continued)*

CONGENITAL ABNORMALITY	SIGNS AND SYMPTOMS	NURSING INTERVENTIONS
Hypospadias Congenital anomaly in which the urinary meatus is located on the underside of the penis. (In a rare corresponding defect in females, the urinary meatus is located in the vagina.)	• Urethra that opens on the ventral surface of the penis, with urine flow directed downward	• Provide preoperative and postoperative care. • Teach the parents how to provide home care.
Imperforate anus Malformation in the anorectal region resulting in a blind rectal pouch or a fistulous connection to the perineum, urethra, bladder, or vagina	• Nonpatent anus (identified initially when a rectal thermometer is inserted) • No meconium passage within 24 hours of delivery	• Observe for distress caused by increasing abdominal distention. • Withhold feedings until the diagnosis is confirmed. • Provide postoperative care, as appropriate. • Provide emotional support to the parents.
Spina bifida (meningomyelocele) Neural tube defect in which part of the meninges and spinal cord protrude through the vertebral column (from failure of the vertebral body to fuse during embryonic development)	• Protrusion of a saclike meningeal portion through a vertebral defect	• Protect the defect from infection by cleaning it and applying a moist sterile dressing. • Position the newborn to keep pressure off the defect. • Position the newborn prone for feedings. • Provide emotional support to the parents.

POSTPARTAL PERIOD

The postpartal period begins with the fourth stage of labor and extends for approximately 6 weeks. During this time, reproductive organs return to a nonpregnant state and various physiologic and psychological changes take place. Both parents must adjust to their new roles.

Postpartal complications

Postpartal complications can be physiologic or psychological. This chart describes the most common postpartal complications, along with interventions that are crucial to patient comfort and safety.

COMPLICATION	CAUSES	NURSING INTERVENTIONS
Parental maladaptation Inability of the new parent to adapt positively to the newborn. The parent manifests negative feelings toward the newborn and has trouble becoming attached to the newborn.	Problems within the couple's relationship, the couple's experiences with previous pregnancies, the couple's attitude toward a new family member, or events that occurred during labor and delivery	• Assess parent-newborn attachment during the acquaintance phase (the period of mutual learning and orientation). • Observe the parents periodically for positive attachment behaviors, such as attraction to the newborn; close physical contact and face-to-face and eye contact with the newborn; nurturing of the newborn; sensitivity to the newborn's needs; and taking pleasure in interacting with the newborn. • Evaluate and report to the RN persistent maladaptive attachment behaviors, such as describing the newborn in negative terms or showing indifference or inattention toward the newborn. • Determine the parents' goals, including their expectations of the newborn. • Assess the parents' learning needs regarding newborn care.
Postpartal depression ("maternity blues") Emotional aftermath of childbirth, usually occurring between the third and tenth day postpartum. Signs and symptoms typically include mild depression, anxiety, irritability, and weepiness lasting from 1 to 2 hours or several days. (Postpartal depression also may take more severe forms.)	May be hard to pinpoint. The condition probably results from the new responsibilities of motherhood or from such physiologic factors as the postpartal decrease in maternal hormone levels. Fatigue and anxiety over the newborn and the patient's concern over her ability to assume the role of mother may contribute to depression.	• Learn how to detect signs and symptoms of postpartal depression. • Discuss signs and symptoms of postpartal depression with the patient. • Allow the patient to cry and express her feelings. • Make sure the patient gets adequate rest and nourishment. • Teach the patient how to care for her newborn; give positive reinforcement and praise as the patient provides newborn care. • Treat each postpartal patient as a unique individual, tailoring nursing care to her needs. • Warn the patient that postpartal depression may arise after discharge and may last for several days. Instruct her to notify the physician if her depression persists.
Postpartal hemorrhage Hemorrhage arising from a site within the reproductive tract. Postpartal hemorrhage may cause cardiovascular collapse and other serious complications, including coagulatory defects.	Various prenatal, antepartal, or intrapartal factors, occurring alone or in combination. Prenatal factors include fibroid uterus, grandmultiparity, previous postpartal hemorrhage from uterine atony, and coagulation defects. Antepartal and intrapartal factors include hypotonic myometrium; general anesthesia; prolonged or rapid labor; labor with vigorous oxytocin stimulation; retention of placental tissues; genital trauma; cervical, vaginal, or perineal lacerations; uterine rupture; operative procedures; and uterine inversion.	• Promote voiding by massaging the uterus frequently and instructing the patient to do this herself. • Determine if the uterus is boggy; as necessary, massage the fundus. • Check lochia for clots or tissue fragments. • Note whether lochia is bright red, dark, or absent and whether uterine size is increasing. • Ensure proper infusion of I.V. fluids. • Assist with oxytocin administration, as ordered and necessary. • Monitor vital signs, especially blood pressure. • Measure urine output; ensure insertion of a urinary catheter, if necessary and ordered. • Count vaginal pads and estimate blood loss. • Observe for signs and symptoms of shock, such as pallor, cyanosis, clamminess, and chills. • Observe for changes in level of consciousness. • Place the patient in Trendelenburg's position. • Administer oxygen by mask at 7 liters/minute, as ordered. • Notify the physician of the patient's condition. • Prepare the patient for surgery.

Breast-feeding

Overview   Infant feeding method is a private matter for the parents to decide. For the new mother, successful feeding is a major concern—one that proves crucial to developing positive feelings about her new role. Guidance from a knowledgeable nurse can help make infant feeding a rewarding experience.

Clinical situation   Mary Ann McGowan and infant Joey, 6 hours old, are rooming-in at the hospital. Two hours ago, Joey accepted and retained 1 oz (30 ml) of glucose 5% in water and showed positive sucking. Mrs. McGowan plans to breast-feed Joey beginning with his next feeding.

Assessment

Nursing behaviors	**Nursing rationales**
1. Assess Mrs. McGowan's condition.	**1.** To breast-feed, Mrs. McGowan must be awake, relatively energetic, and free from pain.
2. Assess Joey's condition.	**2.** Breast-feeding is more likely to succeed when the newborn is alert and awake.

Nursing diagnoses
• Knowledge deficit related to breast-feeding techniques
• Altered maternal nutrition (less than body requirements) related to increased nutritional needs

Planning and goals
• Mrs. McGowan will achieve a basic understanding of the physiology of lactation and breast-feeding techniques.
• Joey will meet his fluid and nutritional needs through breast-feeding.
• Mrs. McGowan will become accustomed to Joey's feeding patterns and behaviors.
• Mrs. McGowan and Joey will share a satisfying breast-feeding experience.

Implementation

Nursing behaviors	**Nursing rationales**
1. Prepare Mrs. McGowan for breast-feeding by instructing her to wash her hands and breasts and by providing privacy and a calm, restful environment.	**1.** Preparation will lower Mrs. McGowan's frustration level and decrease the time Joey must wait to start feeding once he becomes ready to feed. Washing the hands protects Joey from infection. Privacy and a calm, restful environment promote the let-down reflex (necessary to make milk available to the newborn).
2. Teach Mrs. McGowan about comfortable breast-feeding positions, including the side-lying position, sitting position, and football hold. Instruct her to position Joey so that he can breathe and does not pull on the breast.	**2.** Teaching Mrs. McGowan various breast-feeding positions allows her to feel that the position she chooses is right for her. A comfortable position allows both mother and newborn to relax and get acquainted. Changing position helps prevent nipple soreness.

3. Teach Mrs. McGowan about newborn feeding reflexes and show her how to elicit them; help Joey grasp the nipple and areola; holding the breast, squeeze some colostrum (the first form of milk) from the breast to moisten the nipple and to allow Joey to smell the milk and learn to look for feedings.

4. Anticipate Mrs. McGowan's concerns about breast-feeding, as described in steps 5 to 10.

5. Help Mrs. McGowan adjust to Joey's sucking cycle.

6. Teach Mrs. McGowan not to try to breast-feed if Joey is sleepy.

7. If Mrs. McGowan becomes anxious about Joey's lack of milk intake or fears he is rejecting her milk, reassure her that rejection probably is normal. Stress that most newborns lose approximately 5% to 10% of birth weight during the first few days after delivery. Mention that Joey has enough stored body fluids to meet his needs during these days.

8. Teach Mrs. McGowan how to break nipple suction by inserting a finger into Joey's mouth next to the nipple.

9. Teach Mrs. McGowan how and when to burp Joey.

10. Instruct Mrs. McGowan to place Joey on his right side or abdomen after he finishes feeding.

11. Document the instructions given to Mrs. McGowan as well as her and Joey's responses to the feeding.

12. Provide privacy so that Mrs. McGowan can breast-feed alone. Place the call bell nearby in case she has problems.

3. Rooting, sucking, swallowing, and gagging reflexes are present at birth. With proper teaching, Mrs. McGowan can elicit them herself. Joey must grasp both the nipple and areola to trigger the milk flow and prevent nipple abrasion. The smell of milk may be necessary to trigger the chain of events that initiates breast-feeding.

4. Anticipating concerns helps Mrs. McGowan achieve breast-feeding success and independence.

5. There is no right or wrong way for a newborn to suck or feed. Sucking behaviors are individualized and variable; for instance, a newborn may suck, then compress the nipple, then swallow, then rest. Joey should not be forced to adopt a sucking rhythm that is unnatural for him.

6. Newborns feed when they are hungry; many do not breast-feed well for the first few days after delivery.

7. Providing reassurance and teaching about normal milk intake and newborn weight will help ease Mrs. McGowan's fears.

8. Mrs. McGowan must break nipple suction in this manner to prevent Joey from causing nipple damage and pain.

9. Mrs. McGowan can burp Joey before alternating breasts or after the feeding ends.

10. A right side-lying or abdominal position aids stomach emptying and prevents aspiration caused by regurgitation.

11. Documentation promotes continuity of care and identifies areas where further teaching may be required.

12. Mrs. McGowan needs to gain self-confidence in breast-feeding; being alone with the newborn promotes this.

13. Inform Mrs. McGowan about breast-feeding classes given on the unit. Topics discussed typically include breast-feeding schedule, intervals between feedings, length of breast-feeding sessions, ways to encourage milk let-down, and supplementary and complementary feedings.

13. Group classes allow postpartal patients to discuss their feelings with other breast-feeding mothers. The breast-feeding schedule should be self-regulatory or on demand (the newborn cries when hungry). Initially, most breast-feeding newborns feed on demand every 2 to 3 hours. As the mother's milk production increases and the newborn becomes more satisfied and fulfills sucking needs, the interval between feedings increases. The newborn should feed at each breast for 5 to 7 minutes initially, then increase gradually to 10 to 15 minutes on the first breast and as long as desired on the second. To reduce potential let-down problems, Mrs. McGowan can use such self-care measures as taking a warm shower or warm compresses applied to the breasts, drinking a warm liquid, getting adequate rest, and increasing fluid and protein intake. Supplementary feedings (those given instead of breast-feeding) should not begin until lactation is well established; complementary feedings (those given in addition to breast-feeding) may include infant formula, water, or stored breast milk. If Mrs. McGowan plans to give supplementary or complementary feedings, she should learn how to prepare formula.

14. Teach Mrs. McGowan how to perform nipple care by:
• washing the nipples with plain water when showering.
• using nipple cream (Masse) if the breasts are sensitive
• allowing the nipples to air dry
• using absorbent nursing pads or a large handkerchief if the nipples leak.

14. Nipple care reduces nipple soreness and helps prevent discomfort during breast-feeding. Because nipples secrete oil and milk enzymes serve as natural antiseptics, Mrs. McGowan should wash the nipples with plain water only. (Washing the hands is more important to hygiene than washing the nipples.) Cream or lanolin applied lightly to dry nipples relieves friction, which can cause irritation. Cotton bras are recommended to maintain dry nipples. Exposing the nipples to air for short periods toughens them, making them more erect.

15. Teach Mrs. McGowan methods to relieve breast engorgement, including massaging the breasts before feeding and alternately during a feeding, and expressing breast milk manually or by pump during periods when the newborn cannot breast-feed.

15. Breast engorgement during the first few days after delivery interferes with the let-down reflex and causes the newborn's sucking to be choppy instead of rhythmic. Breast massage promotes let-down. If Mrs. McGowan cannot breast-feed, she may need to empty her milk by expressing it. Manual expression is best because it closely resembles the action of the newborn's mouth during breast-feeding. (Alternatively, an electric pump can be used.) Expressed milk can be frozen for later use.

16. Inform Mrs. McGowan about breast-feeding support groups, give her literature on breast-feeding, and provide information about the La Leche League as necessary. Also provide important telephone numbers, such as those of the pediatric nurse practitioner and physician.

16. To enhance long-term breast-feeding success, the breast-feeding patient should continue to receive support and information after discharge.

MATERNITY NURSING

**Evaluation
(outcomes)**

• Mrs. McGowan has a basic understanding of lactation and has begun to breast-feed Joey successfully.
• Joey's nutritional needs are being met.
• Both Mrs. McGowan and Joey are satisfied with breast-feeding.
• Joey's fluid intake and output are normal.

Ensuring safe infant bottle-feeding

By becoming familiar with the information presented here, the nurse can help ensure that a bottle-fed infant receives safe, adequate nourishment.

Infant feeding options

Cultural, social, and psychological factors influence the new mother's choice of infant feeding method. The table below compares common formulas used in bottle-feeding.

FORMULA	CHARACTERISTICS
Commercially prepared formula (Similac, Enfamil, SMA)	• Adequately meets infants' nutritional needs • Typically has a nonfat cow's milk base • Sometimes is "humanized" (with a low electrolyte and whey-casein ratio, similar to that of human milk) • Usually costs more than cow's milk
Cow's milk	• Contains more protein, sodium, and calcium and less carbohydrate than human milk • Has a fat and calorie content and a water-to-solids ratio similar to that of human milk • Is harder to digest than human milk because of its greater curd tension (must be boiled, pasteurized, or homogenized to reduce curd tension)
Milk substitutes Soybean-based formula	• Appropriate for infants who cannot tolerate milk-based formula
Nonfat milk	• Nonfat milk is not recommended for infants under age 1 because it contains excessive protein and inadequate levels of calories, iron, vitamin C, and essential fatty acids.

Formula preparation

Although ready-to-feed formula and disposable bottles are expensive, they are easy to prepare and save time. This chart compares three formula preparation methods.

METHOD	DESCRIPTION
Single-bottle	• This is the simplest preparation method. • Each bottle is prepared individually at the time of use. • The bottle, cap, and nipple must be washed in hot, soapy water, then rinsed thoroughly. • The prepared bottle is given to the infant immediately after preparation. • After the feeding, the bottle, cap, and nipple must be rinsed with cold water.
Terminal sterilization	• A one-day supply of formula is prepared. • The bottles are placed in a pan with water and sterilized for 25 minutes.
Aseptic method	• Equipment and ingredients are boiled, then combined using aseptic technique. • The prepared bottles are placed in the refrigerator. • This is the least common preparation method used today.

Ensuring safe infant bottle-feeding *(continued)*

Bottle-feeding guidelines

Successful newborn feeding is a major concern of the new mother and promotes a positive self-concept. The nurse provides guidance for bottle-feeding and anticipates the mother's needs.

● Inform the patient that a feeding takes 20 to 25 minutes.
● Advise the patient that she should be comfortable and relaxed when bottle-feeding. Instruct her to wash her hands before beginning the feeding.
● Encourage the infant's father to help feed the infant.
● Instruct the patient to hold the infant in a semierect position. (Holding the infant also promotes bonding.)
● Teach the patient to burp the infant frequently, especially in the middle of the feeding and after the feeding ends.
● Instruct the patient to place the infant on the right side or on the abdomen after the feeding to prevent aspiration and regurgitation.

SELECTED NURSING PROCEDURES

The procedures described below commonly are performed by the nurse providing antepartal, intrapartal, postpartal, or newborn care. (Procedure steps preceded by an asterisk are especially important.)

(margin tab) MATERNITY NURSING

Washing the perineal area

Introduction   Cleaning the patient's perineum, vulva, and anal area helps prevent infection of perineal wounds (from dried lochia accumulation) and promotes comfort.

Steps	**Rationales**
1. Gather needed supplies: clean disposable gloves, hip pad or bedpan, cleansing solution, gauze sponge or cotton balls, and clean perineal pad.	**1.** Gathering supplies in advance aids patient comfort.
2. Explain the procedure to the patient.	**2.** Explanations reduce patient anxiety and help the patient gain a sense of control.
3. Wash your hands.	**3.** This helps prevent the spread of infectious micro-organisms.
4. Put on clean disposable gloves.	**4.** Gloves maintain asepsis.
5. Place a hip pad or bedpan under the patient's buttocks.	**5.** This prevents soiling of the bed.
*6. Remove the perineal pad, noting the color, amount, and odor of lochia.	***6.** Inspecting the lochia helps detect infection.

*7. Gently pour a cleansing solution (such as a povidine-iodine mixture [Betadine] or plain tap water) over the perineum. Rinse with tap water.

*7. This helps prevent perineal infection.

8. Dry the perineal area with a gauze sponge or cotton ball. Using a single downward stroke, work from the labia to the perineum.

8. This drying method prevents recontamination.

9. Replace the soiled perineal pad with a fresh one, touching only the outside of the pad and placing the inner aspect of the pad against the vulva.

9. This prevents perineal contamination.

10. Teach the patient how to perform perineal self-care.

10. After discharge, the patient must clean the perineal area after voiding and defecating.

11. Document the procedure in the patient's chart, noting the condition of the perineum.

11. Documentation proves that the procedure was done, assures high-quality care, and provides legal protection.

Administering a sitz bath

Introduction   A sitz bath, in which the patient's hips and buttocks are immersed in water or saline solution, promotes perineal comfort, stimulates perineal circulation, and promotes healing of an episiotomy during the early postpartal period.

Steps

Rationales

1. Gather needed supplies: sitz bath basin, perineal pad, and towel.

1. Gathering supplies in advance aids patient comfort and promotes a smooth procedure.

2. Place the sitz bath basin snugly on the toilet seat.

2. This ensures the basin's stability, helping to prevent the patient from falling off the basin or spilling water.

3. Fill the basin with water and test its temperature, which should be 100° to 110° F (38° to 43.3° C).

3. Testing water temperature prevents burns.

4. Help the patient onto the basin and instruct her to relax her gluteal muscles.

4. Relaxing the gluteal muscles exposes the entire perineum to water.

5. Instruct the patient to remain in the sitz bath for 15 to 20 minutes, three times daily.

5. This duration and frequency promotes healing and comfort while ensuring safety.

6. After the sitz bath, teach the patient to dry the perineum gently and apply a perineal pad.

6. Gentle drying minimizes perineal trauma.

7. Apply an anesthetic or soothing ointment, spray, or medicated pad to the perineum, if ordered.

7. These preparations help prevent infection and promote patient comfort.

8. Document the procedure in the patient's chart.

8. Documentation proves that the procedure was done, assures high-quality care, and provides legal protection.

Performing a postpartal maternal assessment

Introduction   The nurse should perform a physical assessment of the patient shortly after delivery, then several times daily during the next few days to assess for retrogressive changes (involution) of the uterus, vagina, and other genital structures and for progressive changes of the breasts.

Steps	**Rationales**
1. Wash your hands.	**1.** This helps prevent the spread of infectious microorganisms.
2. Assess fundal height and uterine firmness.	**2.** Uterine involution should begin immediately after delivery; a uterus that remains soft is likely to bleed, causing hemorrhage.
3. Assess lochia for color, amount, and odor.	**3.** Lochia should be bright red (lochia rubra) for approximately the first 3 days after delivery, pink to brown (lochia serosa) from day 3 to day 10, and cream colored (lochia alba) from day 10 to 6 weeks postpartum. Lochia should never be excessive or malodorous.
4. Assess the perineum for intactness, hematomas, and hemorrhoids. Observe for approximation of any perineal repair.	**4.** A hematoma may develop from tissue trauma. Hemorrhoids may arise before or after delivery, from the trauma of labor and delivery.
5. Assess the condition of the breasts, checking for heat, edema, and engorgement; evaluate the nipples for fissures, cracks, and soreness.	**5.** The breasts should be soft, filling, smooth, non-tender, and full. They may vary in size and fullness, depending on whether the patient is breast-feeding and on the number of days since delivery.
6. Document all assessment findings.	**6.** Documentation proves that the procedure was done, assures high-quality care, and provides legal protection.

Assessing the newborn

Introduction   Within 24 hours of delivery, the nurse should perform a physical examination of the newborn to evaluate the newborn's general condition, detect any abnormalities, and provide baseline data.

Steps	**Rationales**
1. Wash your hands and put on clean disposable gloves.	**1.** This minimizes the risk of nosocomial infection.
2. Check the newborn's vital signs and blood pressure.	**2.** Vital signs and blood pressure indicate the newborn's overall status; abnormal findings may signal a problem.

3. Measure the newborn's weight and length.

3. This establishes baseline data.

4. Measure head and chest circumference.

4. This provides baseline data that help determine growth.

5. Inspect the head and fontanels for molding, cephalhematoma, abrasion, and unusual pigmentation. Assess the face, eyes, ears, lips, and mouth.

5. This helps detect abnormalities.

6. Assess the clavicles, chest, and abdomen for unusual pigmentation or anomalies.

6. This helps detect asymmetry or anomalies.

7. Inspect the umbilical cord for color and presence of three vessels; smell the cord.

7. The umbilical cord should contain two arteries and one vein; it should be odorless.

8. Inspect and palpate the genitals. In a male, inspect the penis, foreskin, urinary orifice, testes, and scrotum. In a female, inspect the labia majora, which should cover the labia minora. Assess the vaginal orifice and urinary meatus, which should be visible beneath the clitoris; also check for vaginal discharge.

8. This detects any genital ambiguity, permitting early genetic studies, if necessary.

9. Assess the buttocks and anus.

9. The buttocks should have symmetrical folds and be separated by a crease. The anus should be patent; meconium passage should occur within the first 24 hours.

10. Assess the trunk and extremities; evaluate leg and arm flexion and length. Arms and legs should be symmetrical in shape and function. Flexor muscles should have good tone. Inspect for toe webbing, number of digits, palmar creases, and range of motion in joints.

10. This helps detect asymmetry, lack of function, and any anomalies.

11. Assess the spine and back for shape and condition. The spine should be free of masses or abnormal curves.

11. This helps detect abnormalities.

12. Assess the hips for adduction and abduction. The hips should adduct; abduction should exceed 60 degrees.

12. This detects congenital hip anomalies.

13. Assess for the rooting, sucking, Moro, palmar and plantar grasp, tonic neck, Babinski, stepping, and dancing reflexes. Also assess for head lag, prone crawl, trunk incurvation, blinking, sneezing, yawning, and symmetrical function and strength of the extremities. These reflexes and motor functions should be present at birth; head lag should not exceed 45 degrees.

13. This helps detect abnormalities.

14. Document the assessment; notify the RN or physician immediately of any major abnormalities.

14. Documentation permits immediate intervention for any serious condition. It also proves that the procedure was done, assures high-quality care, and provides legal protection.

Bathing the newborn

Introduction

Bathing the newborn helps to ensure hygiene, which helps protect the neonate from infection and skin irritation, and allows the nurse to observe the newborn's characteristics. For the mother, bathing provides a chance to interact with the newborn. Also, after the newborn is discharged, the mother may notice the first signs of eczema, heat rash, or more serious conditions while bathing the newborn.

Steps	**Rationales**
1. Gather needed supplies: basin, sink, or tub; washcloth; bath soap; towel; clean clothes for the newborn.	**1.** Gathering supplies in advance ensures that the nurse will not have to leave the newborn alone to obtain a forgotten item.
2. Fill the basin, sink, or tub with water. Test water temperature by placing your elbow in the water; it should feel comfortable.	**2.** Testing prevents burning. The elbow is a temperature-sensitive area.
*3. Wash each of the newborn's eyes, working from the inner canthus (next to the nose) outward. Use a clean section of the washcloth to clean the second eye. Do not wash across the bridge of the nose.	***3.** This method helps prevent transfer of any infection.
*4. Holding the newborn securely in a football position, wash the scalp with soap, then rinse with water. Dry with a towel.	***4.** This decreases pressure on the newborn's soft fontanels. The football position is secure, reducing the risk of losing a grip on the newborn.
5. Wash the newborn's face with soap. Rinse and dry.	**5.** This removes shedding skin and oils from the face.
6. Wash the newborn's trunk, arms, and legs. Then turn the newborn onto the abdomen and wash the back. Finally, wash the genital area. On all areas, use a gentle motion.	**6.** This ensures cleaning of all areas. Washing gently prevents injury to the newborn's fragile skin.
7. Rinse the newborn with a washcloth and clear water, rinsing the genital area last. (Or you may immerse the newborn in a second tub to rinse.)	**7.** Rinsing removes accumulated dirt, skin, and soap.
8. Pat the newborn completely dry, paying special attention to the neck and inguinal creases.	**8.** This helps prevent infection from moistness.
9. Clean around the umbilical cord stump with alcohol.	**9.** The umbilical area is prone to infection.
10. Dress the newborn in warm clothing.	**10.** The newborn loses heat rapidly and must be kept warm.
11. Document the procedure.	**11.** Documentation permits immediate intervention for any serious condition. It also proves that the procedure was done, assures high-quality care, and provides legal protection.

MATERNITY NURSING

Drugs used in maternity nursing

This chart presents information about drugs commonly prescribed for antepartal and intrapartal patients, including the drug action, dosage, and common side effects. Nursing considerations focus on patient comfort and teaching. When administering any drug to a pregnant patient, be sure to consider the potential effects on the fetus.

DRUG	ACTION	USUAL ADULT DOS-AGE	COMMON SIDE EFFECTS	NURSING CONSIDERATIONS
Oxytocics: oxytocin (Pitocin), ergonovine maleate (Ergotrate), methylergo-novine ma-leate (Methergine)	• Stimulate uterine contractions • Increase uterine muscle tone	I.V.: 10 to 40 units added to 1,000 ml of I.V. solution I.M. injection: 10 units	• Cardiac arrhyth-mias • Nausea and vom-iting • Uterine hyperton-icity • Uterine rupture • Hypertension • Postpartal hemor-rhage • Fetal bradycardia • Neonatal jaundice	• Monitor blood pressure, pulse, and res-pirations every 5 to 10 minutes, or as or-dered. • Assist the RN in assessing uterine con-tractions and uterus status between con-tractions. • Monitor fluid intake and output. • After delivery, monitor for hypertensive episodes and subarachnoid hemor-rhage.
Magnesium sulfate	• Anticonvulsant and central ner-vous system de-pressant; prevents and controls seizures associated with pregnancy-in-duced hyperten-sion • Reduces blood pressure by va-sodilation	4 g in 250 ml D_5W initially; administer by slow I.V. infu-sion (5 ml/30 sec). May fol-low with 4 to 5 g given by I.M. injection. (Dosage schedule var-ies.)	• Pulmonary edema • Respiratory paral-ysis • Reflex loss • Respiratory dis-tress • Cardiac depres-sion • Flushing and sweating • Hypotension • Fetal hyporeflexia	• Maintain strict bed rest. • Monitor fluid intake and output closely. • Monitor vital signs frequently. • Assess for subjective symptoms, such as thirst, hot or cold sensations, and tin-gling. • Check reflexes frequently. • Provide emotional support to the pa-tient and family. • With I.V. administration, onset of drug action is immediate; with I.M. administra-tion, onset occurs in 1 hour.
Vitamins (fat-soluble: A, D, E, and K; water-solu-ble: C, B complex)	• Prevent or treat vitamin deficien-cies in patients who are preg-nant or lactating or who eat inad-equate diets.	Varies with the nature and severity of vitamin de-ficiency	• Nausea and vom-iting • Constipation • Irritability	• Instruct the patient to follow the physi-cian's orders for daily dosage and follow-up therapy. • To prevent hypervitaminosis, avoid ex-cessive use of large-volume parenteral solutions of multivitamin supplements containing fat-soluble vitamins. • Store vitamins in a cool place in light-resistant containers to limit degradation. • Record all vitamin intake at each pre-natal visit. • Toxicity from a vitamin overdose can cause more serious problems than vita-min deficiency.

Pediatric nursing

Introduction 150

Infant (birth to age 1)

Gastroenteritis 150

Congenital heart disease 153

Meningitis 158

Toddler (age 1 to 3)

Laryngotracheobronchitis 162

Acetaminophen intoxication 163

Preschooler (age 3 to 6)

Acute lymphocytic leukemia 166

School-age child (age 6 to 12)

Nephrosis 169

Rheumatic fever 171

Type I diabetes mellitus 173

Adolescent (age 12 to 19)

Scoliosis 175

Selected nursing procedures

Caring for a child in a Croupette 177

Assisting with bone marrow aspiration or biopsy 178

Teaching insulin self-administration 179

PEDIATRIC
NURSING

Introduction

Pediatric nursing requires special knowledge of children's developmental needs and health problems. The nurse must be familiar with the principles basic to both adult and pediatric nursing—then apply these principles carefully to a special population.

Pediatric patients are fragile. Although they may recover from illness more quickly than adults, some deteriorate more rapidly and with fewer apparent symptoms. Infants especially are prone to rapid shifts in physiologic status because of their large skin-surface area relative to body weight; small, narrow passageways; and immunologic immaturity. Children with chronic diseases are at particularly high risk and require the most astute nursing skills.

The nurse providing pediatric care also must attend to the parents' needs. A child's hospitalization causes a crisis for the parents, who feel that they no longer control their child's life. Such feelings—and the corresponding behavior—call for skillful nursing interventions.

This section presents clinical situations based on common pediatric health problems that demonstrate the key principles of pediatric care. Taking a chronological approach, it begins with health problems affecting infants, then progresses to problems affecting toddlers, preschoolers, school-age children, and adolescents.

INFANT (BIRTH TO AGE 1)

Gastroenteritis

Overview

Gastroenteritis is an acute inflammation of the lining of the stomach and intestines. In pediatric patients, the most common sign of gastroenteritis is diarrhea, a disturbance of intestinal motility and fluid absorption that causes abnormal loss of fluids and electrolytes. The condition poses a particular danger to infants.

Acute diarrhea, which may stem from a virus or bacteria, commonly is infectious. In children, rotaviruses are the major viral cause of diarrhea. Common bacterial causes of diarrhea in children include *Shigella, Salmonella,* and staphylococcus organisms. In children under age 2, *Escherichia coli* is the major bacterial cause.

Clinical situation

Mark Garcia, age 4 months, is brought to the hospital by his mother. Mrs. Garcia reports that Mark has had green, foul-smelling, liquid stools of increasing frequency; 1 day before the diarrhea began, he vomited and had a runny nose. Now Mark is listless and refuses to eat. The physician admits him to the hospital.

Assessment

Nursing behaviors
1. Obtain a detailed history from Mrs. Garcia about the onset of Mark's illness, including a description of his behavior and stools. Ask if anyone else in the family has been ill recently.

Nursing rationales
1. The history of Mark's illness contributes to assessment data upon which the physician will make a diagnosis. Also, signs and symptoms may help pinpoint the cause of gastroenteritis. Diarrhea accompanied by respiratory problems commonly results from a rotavirus. Gastroenteritis with a viral or bacterial cause usually has a rapid onset.

Glossary

Agranulocytosis: abnormal blood condition characterized by a sharp drop in the number of granulocytes; results in fever and ulcers of the mouth, rectum, and vagina

Antistreptolysin O titer: antibody level that indicates exposure to streptococcal organisms

Aortic valve: valve that opens from the left ventricle into the aorta

Ascites: accumulation of fluid within the peritoneal cavity

Atrial septal defect: congenital cardiac defect characterized by an abnormal opening between the two atria

Brudzinski's sign: involuntary flexion of the knee and hip when the neck is raised passively; may indicate meningitis (not reliable in infants)

Chest retraction: inward pulling of the sternum and ribs, signalling respiratory distress. It is more obvious in infants and small children because of their soft cartilage.

Coarctation of the aorta: congenital cardiac defect characterized by narrowing of the aorta where it exits the heart

Glucagon: hormone causing rapid conversion of glycogen to glucose in the liver

Hepatotoxicity: property of exerting a destructive effect on liver cells

Hyperglycemia: abnormally high blood glucose level (for example, a consistent blood glucose level above 140 mg/dl for 8 to 12 hours after a meal)

Hypertonic diarrhea: diarrhea in which fluid loss exceeds electrolyte loss

Hypoalbuminemia: abnormal condition characterized by a decreased serum albumin level

Hypoglycemia: abnormally low blood glucose level (for example, a blood glucose level below 60 mg/dl)

Hypotonic diarrhea: diarrhea in which electrolyte loss exceeds fluid loss

Induction chemotherapy: initial chemotherapy administered to induce cancer remission

Isotonic diarrhea: diarrhea in which equal amounts of fluids and electrolytes are lost

Kernig's sign: pain or resistance on leg extension; may indicate meningitis (not reliable in infants)

Ketoacidosis: acidosis accompanied by ketone accumulation resulting from faulty carbohydrate metabolism; a complication of diabetes mellitus

Kyphosis: abnormal condition characterized by increased convexity in the curvature of the thoracic spine (hunched back)

Leukocytosis: abnormal increase in the number of leukocytes (white blood cells)

Lipoatrophy: atrophy (loss) of subcutaneous fat; may occur at the site of repeated insulin injections

Lordosis: forward curvature of the lumbar spine; common in toddlers, contributing to the appearance of a protruding stomach

Maintenance chemotherapy: chemotherapy administered to maintain cancer remission

Meninges: tissues covering the brain and spinal cord

Mitral valve: valve between the left atrium and left ventricle; typically suffers damage from the carditis of rheumatic fever

Nuchal rigidity: involuntary muscle stiffness of the neck, manifested by pain when the head is flexed; a sign of meningitis

Opisthotonos: prolonged muscle spasm causing acute involuntary arching of the back; occurs in severe meningitis

Oxygen saturation: percentage of oxygen carried by hemoglobin molecules

Patent ductus arteriosus (PDA): failure of the fetal ductus arteriosus to close after birth, allowing blood from the aorta to enter the pulmonary artery and recirculate through the lungs

Reinduction chemotherapy: chemotherapy administered when a patient has a cancer relapse

Respiratory syncytial virus: myxovirus causing formation of syncytia (giant cells) in tissue culture; a common cause of acute bronchiolitis, bronchopneumonia, and colds in infants and young children

Stridor: loud inspiratory noise accompanying respiratory distress; indicates upper airway narrowing

Subcutaneous nodules: small, firm bodies that form over bony prominences during rheumatic fever and eventually disappear

Syndrome of inappropriate antidiuretic hormone (SIADH): abnormal condition characterized by excessive release of ADH, causing fluid and electrolyte imbalance; occurs in up to 50% of children with meningitis, markedly decreasing urine output

Tetrad spell: hypoxic episode occurring in a child with tetralogy of Fallot, characterized by hypoxia leading to squatting. Squatting compresses the femoral vein, decreasing blood flow to the right side of the heart and relieving hypoxia

Tetralogy of Fallot: congenital cardiac defect characterized by four defects (ventricular septal defect, overriding aorta, pulmonary stenosis, and right ventricular hypertrophy)

Thrombocytopenia: abnormal blood condition characterized by a decrease in the number of platelets

Transposition of the great vessels: congenital cardiac defect in which the pulmonary artery arises from the left ventricle and the aorta arises from the right ventricle

Ventricular septal defect (VSD): congenital cardiac defect characterized by an opening between the two ventricles

PEDIATRIC NURSING

2. Take baseline vital signs.

2. This is an important part of the admission assessment. Diarrhea and subsequent fluid loss cause increased pulse and respiratory rates and an elevated temperature.

3. Weigh Mark. Ask Mrs. Garcia how much Mark weighed before this illness.

3. Diarrhea commonly is associated with weight loss. If Mark has had a significant weight loss, he may need I.V. fluids.

4. Assess Mark's skin turgor, mucous membranes, and anterior fontanel. Check for signs of electrolyte loss.

4. In a child, significant fluid loss causes poor skin turgor, dry mucous membranes, and a depressed anterior fontanel. Diarrhea typically causes sodium and potassium loss.

5. Assess Mark's perianal area for skin breakdown.

5. Because loose stools have a high bile content and an alkaline pH, they may irritate an infant's skin. Continued exposure to liquid stool contents may exacerbate skin breakdown.

Nursing diagnoses

- Fluid volume deficit related to diarrhea
- Diarrhea

Planning and goals

- Mark's weight will return to normal.
- Mark's fluid intake and output will be equal.
- Mark will regain normal skin integrity.
- Other infants and children on Mark's unit will remain free from gastroenteritis.

Implementation

Nursing behaviors

1. Weigh Mark's soiled diapers and record the output. If possible, separate stool output from urine output for recording. Otherwise, record the total amount in the output column. To ensure proper output measurement, weigh a paper diaper on a gram scale before placing it on Mark; when the diaper is soiled, weigh it again. The discrepancy between the two weights represents output. (One gram in weight equals 1 ml in volume.)

Nursing rationales

1. An infant with diarrhea may have decreased urine output from renal dysfunction caused by prolonged fluid volume deficit. Normal urine output for an infant is at least 1 ml/kg/hour.

2. With each stool specimen, perform ordered diagnostic tests (for example, tests for pH, blood, and reducing substances). Send stools to the laboratory for culture and sensitivity testing, as ordered. If stools contain mucus threads, include some of the threads in the stool specimen to aid diagnosis.

2. Results of stool specimen tests help the physician determine the diagnosis and appropriate treatment. Normally, stool has a neutral or slightly alkaline pH. Bloody stools indicate bowel irritation. Reducing substances indicate inadequate absorption and spilling of sugar in the stool. Stool culture and sensitivity tests guide selection of medication to treat infectious diarrhea.

3. Measure the specific gravity of Mark's urine with a dipstick or urinometer.

3. After fluid resuscitation, Mark's specific gravity should be normal (1.010 to 1.025), unless his renal function is not impaired.

PEDIATRIC NURSING

4. Ensure that Mark receives appropriate parenteral or oral fluids. Evaluate his skin turgor, mucous membranes, anterior fontanel, and urine output for signs of response to fluid therapy. When oral feedings begin, evaluate his response to these.

5. Change Mark's diapers frequently. Clean the perineal area and buttocks carefully with water and mild soap after each soiling. Dry the skin thoroughly before reapplying the diaper; if possible, leave the skin exposed to air and a heat lamp placed at least 18″ (46 cm) away from the skin. Apply a protective ointment, if prescribed. (However, do not use protective ointment before applying a heat lamp.) Avoid taking Mark's temperature rectally.

6. Institute enteric isolation procedures (gloves and a gown). Teach Mark's parents to wash their hands thoroughly before and after handling Mark.

7. Administer prescribed medications, as ordered.

4. To allow the bowels to rest, an infant with severe diarrhea initially must receive parenteral fluids. Once the bowels have rested and diarrhea stools are less frequent, oral feedings can begin gradually. Typically, an oral electrolyte and glucose solution is given first. If Mark can tolerate this, he will be advanced to diluted formula. When he can tolerate solid foods, he may receive the "BRAT" diet — banana, rice cereal, applesauce, and toast.

5. Changing diapers frequently and cleaning the perineal area and buttocks reduce irritation from loose stools. Leaving the skin exposed to air and a heat lamp promotes healing. Taking rectal temperatures can further irritate or tear fragile tissue.

6. Anyone who anticipates contact with Mark's stools should use enteric isolation procedures. Anyone coming into contact with Mark must perform strict hand washing to prevent the spread of gastroenteritis within the hospital.

7. Antibiotics are given to treat the specific bacterial causative agent. Mark will receive parenteral electrolyte replacements until his serum electrolyte values return to normal.

Evaluation (outcomes)

- Mark's weight returns to normal.
- Mark's fluid intake and output are equal.
- Mark regains normal skin integrity.
- Other infants and children on Mark's unit remain free from gastroenteritis.

Congenital heart disease

Overview

Congenital heart disease (CHD) is a collective term for a group of congenital defects occurring in approximately 8 of 1,000 live births. CHD probably results from combined genetic and environmental factors (such as poor maternal prenatal nutrition and maternal exposure to viruses). Up to age 1, CHD is the leading cause of death among children with congenital abnormalities.

Depending on the hemodynamic changes that result, CHD is classified as acyanotic or cyanotic. Acyanotic defects typically lead to congestive heart failure (CHF). The most common acyanotic defects are ventricular septal defect (VSD), atrial septal defect, patent ductus arteriosus, and coarctation of the aorta. Cyanotic defects, such as tetralogy of Fallot and transposition of the great vessels, are less common but carry a worse prognosis. (For details on CHD, see *Common congenital heart defects,* pages 154 and 155.)

PEDIATRIC NURSING

Common congenital heart defects

The chart below describes the pathophysiology of the major acyanotic and cyanotic congenital heart defects.

Major acyanotic defects

Atrial septal defects

An atrial septal defect is an abnormal opening between the right and left atria. Basically, three types of abnormalities result from incorrect development of the atrial septum. An incompetent foramen ovale is the most common defect. The high ostium secundum defect results from abnormal development of the septum secundum. Improper development of the septum primum produces a basal opening known as an ostium primum defect, commonly involving the atrioventricular valves. Generally, left to right shunting of blood occurs in all atrial septal defects.

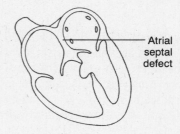
Atrial septal defect

Coarctation of the aorta

Coarctation of the aorta is a narrowing of the aortic lumen, which exists as a preductal or postductal obstruction, depending on the position of the obstruction in relation to the ductus arteriosus. Coarctations exist with great variation in anatomic features.

The lesion obstructs the flow of blood through the aorta, causing an increased left ventricular pressure and work load.

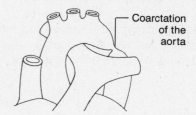
Coarctation of the aorta

Patent ductus arteriosus

The patent ductus arteriosus is a vascular connection that, during fetal life, short-circuits the pulmonary vascular bed and directs blood from the pulmonary artery to the aorta. Functional closure of the ductus normally occurs soon after birth. If the ductus remains patent after birth, the direction of blood flow in the ductus is reversed by the higher pressure in the aorta.

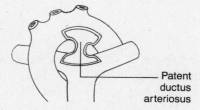
Patent ductus arteriosus

Ventricular septal defects

A ventricular septal defect is an abnormal opening between the right and left ventricle. Ventricular septal defects vary in size and may occur in either the membranous or muscular portion of the ventricular septum. Because of higher pressure in the left ventricle, blood shunts from the left to right ventricle during systole. If pulmonary vascular resistance produces pulmonary hypertension, blood shunting is then reversed (from the right to the left ventricle), with cyanosis resulting.

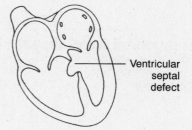
Ventricular septal defect

Common congenital heart defects *(continued)*

Major cyanotic defects

Complete transposition of great vessels

This anomaly is an embryologic defect caused by a straight division of the bulbar trunk without normal spiraling. As a result, the aorta originates from the right ventricle and the pulmonary artery from the left ventricle. An abnormal communication between the two circulations must be present to sustain life.

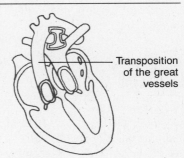

Transposition of the great vessels

Tetralogy of Fallot

Tetralogy of Fallot is a combination of four defects: pulmonary stenosis, ventricular septal defect, overriding aorta, and hypertrophy of the right ventricle. It is the most common defect causing cyanosis in patients surviving beyond age 2.

The severity of symptoms depends on the degree of pulmonary stenosis, the size of the ventricular septal defect, and the degree to which the aorta overrides the septal defect.

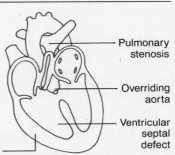
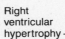

Pulmonary stenosis

Overriding aorta

Ventricular septal defect

Right ventricular hypertrophy

Tricuspid atresia

Tricuspid valvular atresia is characterized by a small right ventricle, a large left ventricle, and, usually, diminished pulmonary circulation. Blood from the right atrium passes through an atrial septal defect into the left atrium, mixes with oxygenated blood returning from the lungs, flows into the left ventricle, and is propelled into the systemic circulation. The lungs may receive blood through one of three routes; a small ventricular septal defect, patent ductus arteriosus, or bronchial vessels.

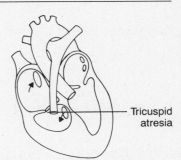

Tricuspid atresia

Truncus arteriosus

Truncus arteriosus is a retention of the embryonic bulbar trunk resulting from the failure of normal septation and division of this trunk into an aorta and pulmonary artery. This single arterial trunk overrides the ventricles and receives blood from them through a ventricular septal defect. The entire pulmonary and systemic circulation is supplied from this common arterial trunk.

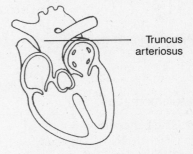

Truncus arteriosus

PEDIATRIC NURSING

Clinical situation

Jimmy Petroc, age 6 weeks, visits the pediatrician for a routine checkup. He now weighs 6 lb, 6 oz (2.9 kg); at birth, he weighed 7 lb, 2 oz (3.2 kg). Jimmy's mother reports that he has had trouble sucking on his bottle for the last 2 weeks and has been vomiting. She also states that he seems more irritable and cries frequently; when he wakes up, his head is wet.

On physical examination, the pediatrician detects a loud, harsh heart murmur, and refers Jimmy to the pediatric cardiologist. The cardiologist suspects Jimmy has VSD and admits him to the hospital for evaluation. Planned diagnostic tests include a chest X-ray, echocardiogram, and cardiac catheterization.

Assessment

Nursing behaviors

1. Obtain a detailed history from Mrs. Petroc, including the onset of Jimmy's illness. Ask her to describe his behavior during feedings.

Nursing rationales

1. The history of the illness helps the physician make a diagnosis. Infants with VSD may be asymptomatic at birth. However, within 6 to 8 weeks, they typically develop signs of CHF (from a left-to-right shunt and subsequent pulmonary overload). Inability to suck is associated with tachycardia (a resting pulse above 160 beats/minute) and tachypnea (a resting respiratory rate above 60 breaths/minute).

2. Take Jimmy's baseline vital signs.

2. Infants with CHF usually have tachycardia and tachypnea. Because they are predisposed to respiratory infections, they may be febrile.

3. Weigh Jimmy. Ask Mrs. Petroc how much Jimmy weighed at birth.

3. Infants with CHF usually lose weight because they cannot ingest enough nutrients.

4. Assess Jimmy for signs of fluid overload.

4. Infants with CHF may have edema in dependent areas, such as the sacrum or periorbital region. A left-to-right shunt causes pulmonary overload and consequent respiratory symptoms.

5. Ask Mrs. Petroc how often she changes Jimmy's diapers.

5. CHF reduces renal blood flow, decreasing urine output.

Nursing diagnoses

• Altered nutrition (less than body requirements) related to inability to ingest adequate nutrients
• Decreased cardiac output related to the structural heart defect

Planning and goals

• Jimmy's weight will return to a normal level.
• Jimmy's pulse and respiratory rates will return to normal.
• Mrs. Petroc will express an understanding of the treatments she must implement for Jimmy at home.

Implementation

Nursing behaviors

1. Begin feeding Jimmy the prescribed formula in small, frequent amounts, as ordered.

Nursing rationales

1. Infants with CHF are less likely to vomit or become tired when given small, frequent feedings. (To increase caloric intake without increasing volume, the physician may prescribe a high-calorie formula.)

PEDIATRIC NURSING

2. Explain to Mrs. Petroc that Jimmy will not receive foods or fluids by mouth for 4 to 6 hours before his cardiac catheterization.

2. Because Jimmy will be sedated for cardiac catheterization, his stomach should be empty to decrease the risk of aspiration.

3. Assist in preparing Jimmy and his parents for cardiac catheterization.

3. Before cardiac catheterization, Jimmy must undergo a chest X-ray and echocardiogram. Catheterization will take several hours; Jimmy's parents need to know where to wait and when the physician will speak to them.

4. After Jimmy's return to the pediatric unit, check his vital signs frequently until he is stable.

4. Cardiac catheterization is an invasive procedure that may cause heart arrhythmias. Also, an infant may suffer hypothermia afterward, so Jimmy may need to be placed on a radiant warmer until his temperature stabilizes. If he bleeds from the catheterization site, he may suffer hypovolemia, causing tachycardia.

5. Check for signs of bleeding at the catheterization site (usually the femoral area in an infant). Measure Jimmy's peripheral pulses and compare pulses in opposite extremities.

5. Jimmy should have a pressure dressing over the catheterization site. His leg should be immobilized for 24 hours to prevent bleeding from the site. Because catheterization may cause a thrombus, which could occlude the peripheral circulation, the temperature, capillary refill, and pulses of both feet and both legs should be checked. (If pulses cannot be palpated manually, use a Doppler device.)

6. When Jimmy awakens, offer him a bottle.

6. Because Jimmy went without oral intake for several hours before the catheterization, he may be at risk for dehydration. Jimmy must be awake and alert enough to suck and swallow properly to avoid choking during feeding.

7. Teach Mrs. Petroc the signs and symptoms of recurring CHF.

7. An infant with CHF may need additional treatment as he grows. If Jimmy begins to have difficulty breathing, decreased sucking ability, or increased irritability, Mrs. Petroc should take him to the physician for evaluation.

8. Administer prescribed medications to Jimmy, as ordered, and teach Mrs. Petroc how to administer them at home.

8. An infant with CHF typically receives digoxin (Lanoxin) and a diuretic, such as furosemide (Lasix). Digoxin slows the heart rate and strengthens the heart; furosemide helps eliminate extra fluid to reduce the heart's work load. Mrs. Petroc needs to know the signs and symptoms of digoxin toxicity in an infant (vomiting, refusal to feed, and diarrhea) as well as those of hypokalemia (from furosemide therapy).

Evaluation (outcomes)

- Jimmy regains at least his birth weight.
- Jimmy's heart and respiratory rates are normal.
- Mrs. Petroc expresses an understanding of how to care for Jimmy at home.
- Mrs. Petroc states that she is comfortable caring for Jimmy.

PEDIATRIC NURSING

Surgical corrections for congenital heart defects

To correct or reduce symptoms of a congenital heart defect, the surgeon may perform one of the procedures described here.

DEFECT	SURGICAL CORRECTION
Patent ductus arteriosus	• Surgical ligation of the ductus arteriosus
Atrial septal defect	• Palliative: Pulmonary artery banding • Corrective: Closure or patching of the defect
Ventricular septal defect	• Palliative: Pulmonary artery banding • Corrective: Closure or patching of the defect
Coarctation of the aorta	• Removal of the narrow aortic portion, with end-to-end anastomosis
Tetralogy of Fallot	• Correction of pulmonary artery stenosis, closure of the ventricular septal defect, and movement of the aorta to the left ventricle
Transposition of the great vessels	• Switching of vessels to correct their anatomic position (Jatene procedure) • Prosthesis insertion to divert systemic venous blood to the mitral valve and pulmonary venous blood to the tricuspid valve (Mustard or Senning operation)

Meningitis

Overview

Meningitis is an infection or inflammation of the meninges (the membranes covering the brain and spinal cord). It most commonly results from bacterial infection. The causative bacterial organisms vary with the patient's age. *Escherichia coli,* group B streptococcus, and staphylococcus organisms typically cause meningitis in infants up to age 2 months. In children age 2 months to 3 years, common causes of meningitis include *Haemophilus influenza* B, *Streptococcus pneumoniae,* and *Neisseria meningitides.*

Clinical situation

Lisa Ching, age 1, is brought to the emergency department by her mother, who reports that Lisa has had a fever and irritability for 3 days. After assessment, Lisa is admitted to the pediatric intensive care unit with a diagnosis of meningitis.

Assessment

Nursing behaviors

1. Obtain a detailed history from Lisa's mother about the onset of illness. Ask if others in the family have been ill recently.

2. Take Lisa's baseline vital signs.

Nursing rationales

1. Among children age 1, *H. influenza* B (HIB) commonly causes meningitis. In older children, HIB may cause only respiratory signs and symptoms. (For recommended ages for HIB and other childhood immunizations, see *Pediatric immunization schedule.*)

2. Children with bacterial meningitis typically have a high temperature.

Pediatric immunization schedule

Immunizations are preventive health measures that involve a primary dose followed by a booster dose. The chart below shows recommended ages for childhood immunizations. (However, these ages are not absolute.)

RECOMMENDED AGE	IMMUNIZATION
2 months	DTP, OPV, Hibtiter
4 months	DTP, OPV, Hibtiter
6 months	DTP, OPV, Hibtiter
15 months	MMR, Hibtiter
18 months	DTP, OPV
4 to 6 years	DTP, OPV
12 years	Second MMR
14 to 16 years	Td

Abbreviation key:
DTP: diphtheria and tetanus toxoids with pertussis vaccine
OPV: oral poliovirus vaccine
MMR: measles, mumps, and rubella viruses (live vaccine)
Hibtiter: *Haemophilus influenzae* vaccine
Td: adult tetanus toxoid and diphtheria vaccine

Adapted with permission from the American Academy of Pediatrics. *Report of the committee on infectious diseases* (22nd ed.). Evanston, IL. 1991.

3. Perform a thorough neurologic assessment, including a neurologic check.

3. Bacterial meningitis causes increased intracranial pressure (ICP), which manifests as a bulging anterior fontanel and irritability. Lisa also may have opisthotonos and nuchal rigidity. (However, because she is only a year old and her cranial bones have not fused completely, she may not have classic signs of increased ICP.)

4. Measure Lisa's frontal occipital circumference (FOC) during initial assessment, then daily.

4. FOC must be measured frequently because meningitis may lead to hydrocephaly in a child Lisa's age.

Nursing diagnoses
- Hyperthermia related to central nervous system (CNS) infection
- Potential for injury related to seizures

Planning and goals
- Lisa will remain free from seizures.
- Lisa will maintain a constant FOC.
- Other infants on the unit will remain free from meningitis.

Implementation

Nursing behaviors
1. Assist the physician with lumbar puncture.

Nursing rationales
1. Lumbar puncture must be done to confirm the diagnosis and identify the causative organism. Blood will be drawn for serum glucose testing to compare with the glucose level in cerebrospinal fluid (CSF). After lumbar puncture, Lisa will receive I.V. antibiotics until results of culture and sensitivity tests arrive (after 72 hours). If the causative organism is sensitive to one or more antibiotics, the physician will order the appropriate antibiotics.

PEDIATRIC NURSING

2. Place Lisa in isolation.

2. Bacterial meningitis is contagious. To protect other children on the unit, Lisa should remain in isolation for at least 24 hours after antibiotic therapy begins.

3. Check the I.V. site frequently.

3. Because Lisa has a CNS infection, antibiotic doses must be high so that the drug can cross the blood-brain barrier. However, high doses can cause marked vein irritation.

4. Record Lisa's vital signs, neurologic check findings, fluid intake and output, FOC, and fontanel status.

4. These findings provide crucial information about Lisa's progress. For instance, low fluid output could indicate the syndrome of inappropriate antidiuretic hormone, which calls for a change in I.V. fluid orders and careful electrolyte evaluation. An increasing FOC could signal hydrocephaly, which warrants surgical intervention.

5. Organize nursing care to prevent overstimulation.

5. Overstimulation of an already irritable child may cause a further ICP increase.

6. Keep Lisa's head elevated.

6. Head elevation reduces ICP. Before a ventriculo-peritoneal (VP) shunt is placed, ICP must decrease. (For more information on the VP shunt, see *Visualizing a ventriculoperitoneal shunt.*)

Clinical situation
(continued)

Lisa undergoes surgery for placement of a VP shunt.

Implementation

Nursing behaviors	**Nursing rationales**
1. Keep Lisa flat for 24 hours after she returns from surgery.	**1.** The VP shunt should cause ICP to decrease; if it decreases too quickly, however, intracranial capillaries may tear.
2. Continue to measure FOC daily.	**2.** Persistent head enlargement may indicate VP shunt malfunction.
3. Inspect and document the appearance of surgical sites on the side of Lisa's head and on the abdominal wall.	**3.** Each surgical site will be covered with a dressing; check the dressings for drainage. Once the dressings are removed, check the incisions for signs of infection. Swelling of the head incision around the VP shunt may signify CSF leakage.
4. Evaluate Lisa's response to the environment.	**4.** Unless Lisa has suffered permanent brain damage from meningitis, she should demonstrate the same developmental skills as before her illness.

PEDIATRIC NURSING

5. Teach Mrs. Ching about the signs and symptoms of increased ICP.

5. Even after Lisa recovers from meningitis, the VP shunt may become obstructed from mucus threads and sticky CSF (caused by glucose). Mrs. Ching should be instructed to call the physician if Lisa begins to vomit, runs a fever, has a bulging anterior fontanel, or shows a change in level of consciousness.

Evaluation (outcomes)

- Lisa has only two seizures while in the hospital.
- Lisa's FOC decreases.
- Lisa's VP shunt functions appropriately.
- Other infants on the unit remain free from meningitis.

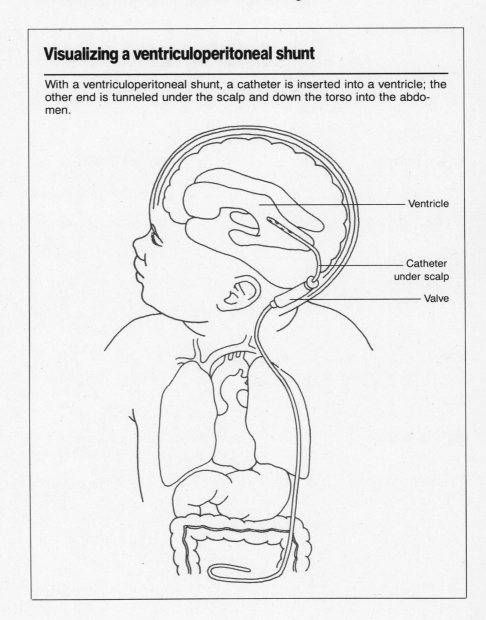

Visualizing a ventriculoperitoneal shunt

With a ventriculoperitoneal shunt, a catheter is inserted into a ventricle; the other end is tunneled under the scalp and down the torso into the abdomen.

Ventricle

Catheter under scalp

Valve

TODDLER (AGE 1 TO 3)

Laryngotracheobronchitis

Overview

Laryngotracheobronchitis (LTB) is an acute inflammation of the larynx, trachea, and bronchus (also called croup). Signs and symptoms include a brassy cough and inspiratory stridor. LTB most commonly results from viral infection, but may stem from bacterial infection. Like other respiratory infections, it causes greater respiratory distress in infants and small children because of their small, narrow airways. Immunologic immaturity also predisposes infants to respiratory infection. The incidence of LTB rises with the pollen count.

Clinical situation

Chelsea Adams, age 2, is brought to the pediatric emergency department crying by her anxious parents in the middle of the night. Mr. and Mrs. Adams report that Chelsea awoke with a brassy cough and seemed frightened; she has had signs and symptoms of an upper respiratory infection. On assessment her rectal temperature measures 100° F (38° C), her pulse is 110 beats/minute, and her respiratory rate is 35 breaths/minute. She appears slightly cyanotic.

Assessment

Nursing behaviors	Nursing rationales
1. Assess and record the degree of Chelsea's respiratory distress.	**1.** If Chelsea develops laryngospasm, she may need emergency intervention for acute respiratory distress.
2. Take Chelsea's baseline vital signs.	**2.** This will help determine the extent of her respiratory distress. (Some medications prescribed for respiratory distress may alter vital signs.)
3. Weigh Chelsea.	**3.** Weight helps determine correct medication dosages. The nurse should weigh Chelsea rather than rely on her parents' memory of her weight from the last physician's visit.
4. Monitor Chelsea's pulse oximetry readings for oxygen saturation level and pulse rate.	**4.** Chelsea may need additional oxygen if her oxygen saturation level falls below 90%. The pulse oximeter also records the pulse, helping to monitor Chelsea for tachycardia.

Nursing diagnoses

• Ineffective airway clearance related to laryngotracheobronchial infection
• Impaired gas exchange related to compromised airway passages

Planning and goals

• Chelsea's vital signs will return to within normal limits.
• Chelsea's cyanosis will resolve.
• Mr. and Mrs. Adams will express an understanding of appropriate home care for Chelsea.

Implementation

Nursing behaviors	**Nursing rationales**
1. Provide supplemental oxygen by mask, nasal cannula, or Croupette, as ordered (if Chelsea is transferred from the emergency department to the hospital's pediatric unit).	**1.** Laryngospasms and fear may cause Chelsea's oxygen saturation level to fall below 90%. Consequently, she will need supplemental oxygen until the medications begin to relieve her airway obstruction.
2. Provide high atmospheric humidity, as ordered.	**2.** Humidity helps liquefy secretions. As appropriate, provide humidity with a Croupette. Suggest that Mr. and Mrs. Adams purchase a cool mist vaporizer for home use to prevent burns from a steam vaporizer. (For information on using a Croupette, see "Caring for a child in a Croupette," pages 177 and 178.)
3. Administer prescribed medications, as ordered.	**3.** The physician may order an emetic, such as syrup of ipecac, to induce vomiting (and thereby disrupt laryngospasms); a bronchodilator given by hand-held nebulizer (such as albuterol [Proventil]), which can provide relief within 10 to 30 minutes; an I.V. bronchodilator (such as aminophylline [Phyllocontin]); and corticosteroids (usually given I.V.) to decrease the inflammatory response.
4. Continue to record Chelsea's vital signs and blood pressure to document her response to treatment.	**4.** If medications do not lower Chelsea's pulse and respiratory rates, she may have to be admitted to the hospital. (A child who fails to respond to emergency treatment after 3 or 4 hours usually is admitted.) Blood pressure should be recorded because bronchodilators may cause hypotension. An increased respiratory rate and increased chest retractions indicate worsening respiratory distress and the need for a tracheostomy.
5. Teach Mr. and Mrs. Adams how to manage a croup attack at home by having Chelsea sit in the bathroom while a hot shower runs full force.	**5.** The humidity produced by a hot shower helps alleviate laryngospasm.

Evaluation (outcomes)

- Chelsea's vital signs are within normal limits.
- Chelsea remains free from cyanosis.
- Mr. and Mrs. Adams express an understanding of how to manage a croup attack at home.

Acetaminophen intoxication

Overview

Toddlers are at risk for ingesting poisonous substances because of their curiosity and advancing motor skills. Unfortunately, some parents fail to "childproof" the home, not realizing that a toddler can gain access to dangerous substances by climbing furniture and opening containers. Acetaminophen (Tylenol), now available in both adult and pediatric strengths, is the most common pharmacologic poisoning agent among children. Acetaminophen ingestion can cause liver toxicity, a serious medical problem.

Clinical situation   Roland Petersen, age 18 months, is brought to the emergency department by his mother, who found him sleeping next to an empty bottle of adult-strength acetaminophen tablets. She states that she checked on Roland 2 hours before finding him asleep; she does not know how many tablets were in the bottle.

Assessment

Nursing behaviors

1. Take Roland's baseline vital signs.

2. Weigh Roland.

3. Assess Roland thoroughly for anorexia, nausea, vomiting, diaphoresis, and malaise.

Nursing rationales

1. Vital signs serve as a basis for later comparison.

2. The physician will determine appropriate treatments based on Roland's weight.

3. A child may be asymptomatic for up to 24 hours after acetaminophen ingestion. Time of symptom onset should be noted.

Nursing diagnoses
- Potential for injury related to hepatotoxicity
- Parental knowledge deficit related to childproofing the home

Planning and goals
- Roland will remain free from signs and symptoms of acetaminophen intoxication.
- Roland will remain free from injury caused by acetaminophen ingestion.
- Mr. and Mrs. Petersen will express an understanding of ways to ensure Roland's future safety at home.

Implementation

Nursing behaviors

1. Assist the physician with interventions to remove acetaminophen from Roland's system.

2. If Roland is awake, administer ipecac, as ordered, and have him drink several glasses of water to induce vomiting. (As ordered, repeat the dose in 20 minutes if he has not vomited.)

3. If Roland ingested the acetaminophen 10 hours ago or less, administer oral charcoal and a cathartic, as ordered. (After 2 hours, gastric lavage will be performed to eliminate the charcoal.)

4. After gastric lavage, administer acetylcysteine (Mucomyst), if ordered.

5. Assist with continuing care for Roland if he is admitted to the hospital.

Nursing rationales

1. Choice of treatment is based on the number of hours since ingestion, amount of acetaminophen ingested, and Roland's serum acetaminophen level.

2. Ipecac is used if the physician suspects acetaminophen is still in the stomach. (If Mrs. Petersen had called the physician from home, she would have been told to administer ipecac there before taking Roland to the hospital.)

3. Charcoal absorbs any acetaminophen remaining in the stomach and prevents it from being processed in the body. The cathartic increases gastrointestinal activity to help eliminate acetaminophen from the body.

4. Acetylcysteine, an antidote for acetaminophen, is given if the child has a toxic serum acetaminophen level.

5. If Roland has absorbed a toxic amount of acetaminophen, he may develop liver failure. To monitor for this complication, frequent laboratory tests of liver function will be done.

PEDIATRIC NURSING

6. Discuss with Mr. and Mrs. Petersen methods to childproof the home, and review normal growth and developmental activities to anticipate for Roland.

6. Roland's age puts him at risk for many potential problems. During the discussion, take care not to be judgmental with the parents, who probably already feel guilty about Roland's condition.

Evaluation (outcomes)

- Roland does not develop signs or symptoms of acetaminophen toxicity.
- Roland returns home free from injury.
- Mr. and Mrs. Petersen state four ways to prevent future injury to Roland.

Common poisonings in children

The substances listed here are the most common substances ingested by children. For more information specific to the substance ingested, call a poison control center.

SUBSTANCE	SIGNS AND SYMPTOMS	TREATMENT
Caustic agents (acids or alkalies)	• Oral burns • Inability to swallow • Seizures • Coma	• The child requires immediate emergency treatment. • If the child is awake, administer oral fluids to dilute the caustic agent, as ordered. • **Do not** induce vomiting because this would reexpose tissues to the caustic agent. • Tracheostomy may be necessary if airway edema is severe.
Drugs	• Vary with the substance ingested	• Administer ipecac, as ordered. • Make sure the child goes to the emergency department. • Administer oral charcoal, as ordered. • Monitor for signs and symptoms of drug toxicity. • If the serum drug level is toxic with the potential for severe injury, the child may need short-term hemodialysis.
Hydrocarbons	• Nausea • Vomiting • Confusion • Respiratory distress • Breath odor	• **Do not** induce vomiting because of the danger of aspiration and accompanying pneumonitis. • Arrange for a chest X-ray. • Monitor the child for at least 6 hours to evaluate response to treatment and identify late-appearing symptoms.

PRESCHOOLER (AGE 3 TO 6)

Acute lymphocytic leukemia

Overview

Leukemia, the most common form of childhood cancer, is characterized by abnormal proliferation and development of white blood cells (WBCs, or leukocytes) and their precursors in the blood and bone marrow. In acute lymphocytic leukemia (ALL), which accounts for roughly 80% of childhood leukemia cases, large numbers of immature cells resembling lymphocytes appear in the bloodstream, lymph nodes, liver, spleen, and other organs. Called leukemic blast cells or stem cells, these immature cells function inappropriately. Because the bone marrow produces large amounts of leukemic blast cells, it cannot produce enough red blood cells (RBCs) and platelets.

Abnormal blood cell counts cause many of the signs and symptoms of ALL. For example, high levels of immature WBCs cause repeated infections; the decreased RBC count results in signs and symptoms of anemia; a low platelet count may lead to petechiae and purpura.

In some cases, the diagnosis of ALL is delayed because the physician may fail to draw blood for a CBC, instead treating the child for routine infections, bruising, or anemia. Then, when a CBC eventually is done and shows an abnormal blood profile, the child is referred to an oncologist or a hematologist for definitive testing.

Clinical situation

José Benavides, age 5, is admitted to the pediatric unit with a diagnosis of ALL. He has had frequent respiratory infections, for which he received antibiotics. He is pale and lethargic. Petechiae cover his trunk; purpura appear on his lower extremities where he fell last week. Mr. and Mrs. Benavides seem anxious as they accompany José to the hospital.

Assessment

Nursing behaviors	Nursing rationales
1. Obtain a detailed history from Mr. and Mrs. Benavides, including the onset of José's symptoms.	**1.** A detailed history helps confirm the diagnosis. Keep in mind that the parents may still be in shock over José's diagnosis and that the history may seem confused because José has had signs and symptoms for several months.
2. Measure José's baseline vital signs.	**2.** José's temperature may be elevated on admission, indicating an infection. Along with anemia, an elevated temperature may lead to tachycardia. José's respiratory rate also may be increased. On the other hand, his blood pressure may be normal (from vascular compensation) or slightly elevated from fear.
3. Weigh José.	**3.** José's weight serves as the basis for determining medication dosages; measurement will help detect any weight loss from induction chemotherapy.
4. Assess and document the appearance of José's skin.	**4.** A low platelet count may cause petechiae and purpura. (A normal platelet count is 150,000 to 450,000/mm³.) Such evidence of bleeding must be documented on admission because chemotherapy may reduce his platelet count further.

PEDIATRIC NURSING

5. Assess José's mouth and perianal region for ulcers.

5. Because the oral cavity and anus are covered with mucous membranes, they are especially vulnerable to ulcers, which may become infected and bleed.

6. Assess Mr. and Mrs. Benavides to determine the stage of grief they are in.

6. Grief typically occurs in stages. If the Benavides are in the denial stage, they may have trouble understanding José's medical treatment. If they are in the anger stage, they may be hostile to the staff.

7. Assess José's reactions to the hospital environment.

7. Nursing care should take into account José's level of fear. Because he is only 5, he will need simple explanations immediately before treatments and comfort measures after painful procedures.

Nursing diagnoses
- Potential for infection related to immature WBCs
- Potential for injury related to hemorrhage

Planning and goals
- José's vital signs will return to within normal limits.
- José's RBC and platelet counts will stabilize.
- José will remain free from signs and symptoms of infection.
- Mr. and Mrs. Benavides will express an understanding of the purpose of José's treatments.
- José will enter remission with induction chemotherapy.

Implementation

Nursing behaviors

1. Protect José from infection by placing him in a private room on a clean hospital unit. Make sure all staff and visitors wash their hands thoroughly before entering José's room and having contact with him.

Nursing rationales

1. ALL reduces the ability to fight infection. Once José begins chemotherapy, he will become immunosuppressed, further increasing his infection risk. Staff members with infections should not care for José. Family members with infections should wear a mask when visiting José and should minimize the time they spend with him. José probably will receive co-trimoxazole (Bactrim) prophylactically to prevent *Pneumocystis carinii* pneumonia—an infection that may be fatal to an immunosuppressed patient.

2. Protect José from trauma by keeping the bed side rails up, using a sponge toothbrush (Toothette) rather than a toothbrush for oral care, using medicated (Tucks) pads to clean the perineal area after bowel movements, and administering stool softeners, as ordered.

2. Chemotherapy will reduce José's low platelet count even further because it decreases the number of platelets produced by the bone marrow. Keeping the side rails up helps prevent trauma from a fall, which could cause local bleeding. Using a sponge toothbrush and medicated pads helps avoid trauma and bleeding of fragile mucous membranes. Administering stool softeners helps reduce straining at stool resulting from immobility and medications that cause constipation. In a patient with a low platelet count, straining at stool could cause increased intracranial pressure leading to intracranial bleeding, as well as rectal or anal bleeding.

PEDIATRIC NURSING

3. Perform guaiac tests on all urine, stools, and emesis.

3. A guaiac test detects blood. A positive test should be reported to the team leader.

4. Measure and record José's vital signs frequently. Report any deviations to the team leader.

4. Once chemotherapy begins, even a slight temperature elevation could indicate infection. José also will receive blood products, which may cause a transfusion reaction that alters vital signs. Chemotherapy itself also can cause vital sign changes.

5. Check the I.V. site frequently; report any redness or irritation to the team leader immediately.

5. In an immunocompromised patient, such as José, any skin break can bleed or become infected. Infiltration of I.V. chemotherapy drugs can damage subcutaneous tissue.

6. Keep accurate fluid intake and output records. Encourage oral fluids, if José can tolerate them.

6. Leukemia causes rapid cell turnover; induction chemotherapy rapidly destroys large numbers of aberrant cells. The resulting cellular debris (including large amounts of uric acid) must be processed through the kidneys. To avoid renal toxicity, José must be well hydrated.

7. Administer allopurinol (Lopurin) orally, as ordered.

7. Allopurinol blocks uric acid formation, decreasing hyperuricemia and the risk of uric acid renal stones.

8. Administer prednisone (Deltasone), as ordered.

8. Prednisone is administered to patients with ALL because it suppresses WBC production.

9. Prepare José and his family for any invasive or anxiety-provoking procedures. Provide simple explanations for José.

9. José will undergo many painful and distressing procedures during hospitalization, including finger sticks, venipunctures, and bone marrow aspiration. At his age, he needs simple explanations immediately beforehand. Mr. and Mrs. Benavides also need explanations at an appropriate level so they can provide emotional support for José.

10. Assist with lumbar puncture, as necessary.

10. With leukemia, the first metastatic site typically is the central nervous system. At the time of diagnosis, lumbar puncture is performed to check for leukemic cells in cerebrospinal fluid. If none are present, methotrexate (Folex) is administered intrathecally for prophylaxis. If leukemic cells are present, intrathecal methotrexate is given to treat the metastasis.

Evaluation (outcomes)
- José's vital signs remain within normal limits.
- José's RBC and platelet counts stabilize at low-normal levels.
- José remains free from signs and symptoms of infection.
- Mr. and Mrs. Benavides express an understanding of the purpose of Jose's treatments without undue anxiety.
- José enters remission.

SCHOOL-AGE CHILD (AGE 6 TO 12)

Nephrosis

Overview

In nephrosis (nephrotic syndrome), the nephron's capillary permeability increases markedly, causing significant protein loss in the urine. The cause of nephrosis is unknown; the disorder may be associated with an allergic reaction or previous infection. Urinary protein loss causes severe hypoalbuminemia and osmotic pressure changes, with fluid leaving the vascular system and entering the interstitial spaces. These changes lead to severe generalized edema, particularly in dependent areas, along with anorexia and fatigue.

Clinical situation

Phillip Sullivan, age 7, is admitted to the hospital with significant edema that has developed over the last 2 weeks. He is irritable and slightly dyspneic. His rectal temperature measures 99° F (37.2° C); pulse rate, 100 beats/minute; and respiratory rate, 26 breaths/minute. He weighs 58 lb (26.3 kg) — 6 lb (2.7 kg) more than on his last visit to the physician 1 week ago. He has had no prior illnesses.

Assessment

Nursing behaviors

1. Take Phillip's baseline vital signs.

Nursing rationales

1. Nephrosis and urinary protein loss impair immunologic function, increasing the infection risk. Also, Phillip's edematous skin is at risk for splitting and could become a source of infection. Once Phillip begins treatment (steroid therapy), the medication will increase his risk for infection.

2. Weigh Phillip, and compare the measurement with the previous weight his mother reported during the history interview. Measure Phillip's weight daily.

2. Severe edema from nephrosis causes significant weight gain. Once Phillip begins therapy, he should lose weight daily until edema resolves. Daily measurement helps monitor the effectiveness of therapy.

3. Measure Phillip's baseline abdominal girth; continue to measure abdominal girth daily.

3. Nephrosis commonly causes ascites. Daily weight and abdominal girth measurement provide data that help gauge Phillip's response to therapy.

4. Assess Phillip's psychological status.

4. Phillip may become depressed during the acute stage of nephrosis because of the severity of the illness. If his abdomen distends so much that he no longer can see his penis, this may cause marked anxiety or contribute to depression. Also, steroid therapy may cause mood swings.

Nursing diagnoses

- Potential for infection related to steroid therapy
- Potential for impaired skin integrity related to edema

Planning and goals

- Phillip's weight will return to normal.
- Phillip's fluid intake and output will be equal.
- Phillip's edema will resolve, with no skin breakdown noted.
- Philip will remain free from infection.
- Phillip will remain free from depression.

PEDIATRIC NURSING

Implementation

Nursing behaviors	Nursing rationales
1. Measure and record vital signs frequently. Report any abnormalities, no matter how slight, to the team leader.	**1.** Throughout Phillip's treatment, vital signs provide important data on his progress. Because he has a high risk for infection, he must be protected from exposure to anyone with an infection. Edema may cause tachypnea from pleural effusions or abdominal pressure on the diaphragm. After steroid therapy starts and fluid begins to return from the interstitium to the vascular system, Phillip may experience tachycardia and hypertension.
2. With each urine specimen, perform ordered diagnostic tests and document the results.	**2.** A dipstick is used to test each urine sample for protein, blood, and specific gravity. Normally, urine should contain no red blood cells or protein. Specific gravity in a patient with nephrosis typically is high because of the heavy protein molecules and decreased urine volume. When Phillip starts to respond to therapy, his specific gravity should return to normal (1.010 to 1.025).
3. Provide meticulous skin care and turn Phillip frequently. As necessary, provide scrotal support.	**3.** Edema makes the skin taut, placing Phillip at high risk for skin breakdown. Skin creases (such as in the neck, groin, and other moist areas) should be checked frequently for signs of breakdown. Phillip may need scrotal support during ambulation because of the heavy edematous scrotal sac. Cotton clothing helps protect skin surfaces.
4. Maintain accurate fluid intake and output records.	**4.** Maintaining accurate intake and output records is a key nursing responsibility. Because of the fluid shift into the interstitium, Phillip's urine output may be below normal or low-normal. If his edema increases, he may need fluid restrictions until steroid therapy takes effect.
5. Provide a high-protein diet with adequate carbohydrates and fats.	**5.** Nephrosis usually reduces the appetite; Phillip may need much encouragement to eat. Dietary protein must be replaced because nephrosis causes protein loss. Without adequate carbohydrates and fats, the body breaks down fats for energy; urea, the end product of protein breakdown may tax the already stressed kidneys.
6. Administer oral prednisone, as ordered. Monitor Phillip for signs of infection, mood swings, and return of appetite.	**6.** Prednisone, the preferred drug for treatment of nephrosis, stabilizes capillary membranes in the nephron, reducing urinary protein loss. However, like other steroids, it also suppresses the immune system, increasing the risk for infection, and may cause mood swings. Prednisone also stimulates the appetite.

7. Prepare Phillip and his family for his discharge.

7. Phillip will be discharged when his urine is free of protein and his weight returns to normal. Teach him and his family about the need to continue oral prednisone for at least 1 month and to check his urine for protein at home. Instruct them to call the physician if his urine contains protein or his edema returns. Also instruct them not to discontinue prednisone unless the physician approves.

Evaluation (outcomes)

- Phillip returns to his preillness weight of 52 lb (23.6 kg).
- Phillip's fluid intake and output remain equal for 72 hours.
- Phillip is free from edema.
- Phillip has no signs or symptoms of infection.
- Phillip has no signs or symptoms of depression.

Rheumatic fever

Overview

A multisystem inflammatory disease, rheumatic fever is an antigen-antibody reaction to a previous streptococcal infection. It arises roughly 6 weeks after an inadequately treated Group A beta-hemolytic streptococcal infection of the upper respiratory tract (such as strep throat or scarlet fever). Most common in school-aged children, rheumatic fever causes such early signs and symptoms as joint pain, fever, abdominal pain, and vomiting. Carditis also may occur, manifesting as chest pain, tachycardia, palpitations, or even congestive heart failure (CHF). The diagnosis of acute rheumatic fever is on the basis of the modified Jones criteria (see *Modified Jones criteria,* page 172).

Clinical situation

Samantha Perry, age 10, is admitted to the pediatric unit with arthralgia, fever, tachycardia, and a history of strep throat 3 weeks earlier. The physician suspects rheumatic fever.

PEDIATRIC NURSING

Assessment

Nursing behaviors

1. Take Samantha's baseline vital signs.

Nursing rationales

1. A child with rheumatic fever usually has tachycardia (from carditis) and may have afternoon fevers. Vital signs taken on admission provide baseline data for later comparison.

2. Weigh Samantha.

2. Because a child with rheumatic fever may develop CHF, Samantha's weight must be established at admission for comparison with later measurements.

3. Assess Samantha's perception of the pain she is experiencing.

3. Migratory arthritis accompanies rheumatic fever. The joints may appear red and feel warm to the touch. Samantha's complaints of pain may seem disproportionate to objective data.

Modified Jones criteria

This table lists the criteria that serve as the basis for diagnosing rhuematic fever. The presence of two major criteria or one major criterion plus two minor criteria establish the diagnosis.

MAJOR CRITERIA	MINOR CRITERIA
Arthritis	Arthralgia
Carditis	Elevated antistreptolysin O titer
Erythema marginatum	Elevated erythrocyte sedimentation rate
Subcutaneous nodules	Fever
Sydenham's chorea	History of rheumatic fever
	Leukocytosis
	Positive C reactive protein
	Rheumatic heart disease
	Previous streptococcal infection
	Prolonged PR interval on electrocardiogram

---

4. Assess Samantha frequently for signs and symptoms of CHF, such as tachycardia, edema, increasing fatigue, and congested breathing.

4. CHF calls for aggressive treatment. If Samantha develops CHF signs and symptoms, the physician may order corticosteroids, digoxin (Lanoxin), and furosemide (Lasix).

Nursing diagnoses
- Activity intolerance related to bed rest
- Pain related to arthritis

Planning and goals
- Samantha's vital signs will return to normal.
- Samantha's weight will remain stable.
- Samantha will be discharged without permanent heart damage.

Implementation

Nursing behaviors	Nursing rationales
1. Assist with diagnostic tests, as ordered and necessary.	**1.** The physician will order blood samples, an electrocardiogram, and a chest X-ray to gather data that will confirm the diagnosis. Because of Samantha's history of strep infection, a throat culture also may be done.
2. Organize nursing care so that Samantha can rest frequently.	**2.** A child with acute rheumatic fever requires several weeks of bed rest to allow the inflammatory response to subside. If Samantha also is anemic, she will need even more rest.
3. Provide comfort measures for Samantha. Turn her every 2 hours if she cannot do so herself.	**3.** Warmth or cold application may provide some relief for painful joints. A bed cradle can be used to keep the weight of the bedclothes off Samantha's knees and ankles. She may need help to turn because of the pain.
4. Administer prescribed anti-inflammatory medications (such as aspirin), as ordered. Observe Samantha carefully for signs of aspirin toxicity.	**4.** Aspirin, the drug of choice for rheumatic fever, reduces the inflammatory response and acts as an antipyretic and analgesic.

5. Administer prescribed antibiotics, such as penicillin, as ordered. (A child who is penicillin-sensitive will receive erythromycin [Ilotycin] or sulfonamides.)

5. Even if Samantha's throat culture is negative, she must receive penicillin or a substitute to ensure complete eradication of the causative organism and prevent future streptococcal infections. After rheumatic fever resolves, prophylactic antibiotic therapy continues indefinitely to prevent potential heart damage.

6. Implement safety measures to prevent injury, especially if Samantha develops Sydenham's chorea (a complication of the strep infection that causes rheumatic heart disease).

6. Sydenham's chorea causes random purposeless movements, muscle twitching, weakness, and difficulty concentrating and performing fine motor skills (important developmental tasks for the school-aged child). The disorder also may cause anxiety and anger, which may exhaust Samantha.

7. Maintain Samantha on bed rest if she develops signs of CHF.

7. Bed rest decreases the work load of the heart and may prevent heart valve damage caused by inflammation. Such valvular damage causes the permanent heart damage that sometimes follows rheumatic fever.

Evaluation (outcomes)

- Samantha's vital signs return to normal.
- Samantha's weight remains stable.
- Samantha avoids permanent heart damage.

Type I diabetes mellitus

Overview

Diabetes mellitus is a chronic disease of disturbed carbohydrate metabolism resulting from insulin deficiency or target-tissue insulin resistance. Type I (insulin-dependent) diabetes mellitus (IDDM, formerly called juvenile or brittle diabetes) stems from lack of insulin production by the pancreatic beta cells. It may stem from exposure to a virus that stimulates the immune system to destroy beta cells. Type I diabetes has been diagnosed in children as young as age 1.

Classic signs and symptoms of Type I diabetes include polyphagia, polyuria, and polydipsia. Other manifestations may include weight loss, fatigue, irritability, and dry skin. Diabetes may lead to diabetic ketoacidosis (DKA), a life-threatening condition caused by buildup of fat metabolites that lower the serum pH.

Clinical situation

Katy King, age 12, has had Type I diabetes since age 2. She has been performing her own glucose checks and self-administering insulin since age 10 (with help from her mother when necessary). Two days ago, she was admitted to the pediatric intensive care unit to receive treatment for DKA. Today, she is transferred to the pediatric unit. Her insulin has been switched from I.V. to subcutaneous administration.

Assessment

Nursing behaviors
1. Assess Katy's knowledge level regarding her diabetes.

Nursing rationales
1. At age 12, Katy probably has only a basic understanding of her disease. As she approaches adolescence, she may need clarification or elaboration of some points.

2. Assess Katy's attitude toward having a chronic disease that sets her apart from her peers.

2. The fear of being different may reduce Katy's compliance with treatment. She may be tempted to test whether she still has diabetes by neglecting treatment.

3. Measure Katy's weight.

3. Katy may have had a growth spurt, calling for a change in her insulin requirements.

Nursing diagnoses
- Altered nutrition (less than body requirements) related to disturbed carbohydrate metabolism
- Potential for injury related to hyperglycemia and hypoglycemia

Planning and goals
- Katy's serum glucose level will stabilize.
- Katy will demonstrate the correct method for checking her glucose levels.
- Katy will demonstrate the correct technique to self-administer insulin.
- Katy will state two positive facts about herself.

Implementation

Nursing behaviors

1. Observe Katy as she performs glucose checks. Compare the serum glucose level recorded by the hospital monitor with the level recorded by Katy's home monitor.

Nursing rationales

1. By observing Katy, the nurse can determine whether she performs her glucose checks correctly. Comparing the results recorded by the two monitors can determine whether Katy's home monitor functions correctly.

2. Observe Katy as she draws up and self-administers her insulin.

2. A 12-year-old child may require help with psychomotor skills, such as drawing up and self-injecting insulin. Watching her perform these skills provides an opportunity for positive reinforcement or tactful correction of her technique.

3. Review with Katy the signs and symptoms of hyperglycemia and hypoglycemia as well as the measures she should take in response to either disorder.

3. Hypoglycemia causes irritability, shakiness, and pale, wet skin. If Katy has these symptoms, she should eat food containing simple sugar to elevate her glucose level quickly. (For severe hypoglycemia, her parents should administer glucagon.) Hyperglycemia causes lethargy, confusion, thirst, nausea, vomiting, and dry skin. Katy should check her urine for ketones and serum glucose level for hyperglycemia. She and her parents should notify the physician if her blood glucose level rises dramatically.

4. Reinforce the need for regular exercise.

4. Regular exercise helps regulate carbohydrate metabolism and insulin needs and improves glucose utilization. Lack of exercise may raise Katy's glucose level, increasing her insulin requirements.

5. Provide positive reinforcement when Katy follows the diabetes care protocol.

5. Adolescents need approval from caregivers. (Also, by showing other adolescents how she uses her glucose monitor, Katy can receive peer approval for her knowledge and discipline, increasing her self-esteem.)

PEDIATRIC NURSING

| **Evaluation (outcomes)** | • Katy's glucose level remains consistent and within normal limits.
• Katy demonstrates the correct method for checking her glucose level.
• Katy demonstrates the correct method for self-administering insulin.
• Katy has a positive self-concept. |

ADOLESCENT (AGE 12 TO 19)

Scoliosis

| **Overview** | A lateral curvature of the spine, scoliosis may result from a congenital defect, muscle weakening caused by myelomeningocele, or unknown factors (idiopathic scoliosis). If the condition progresses without treatment, it can lead to respiratory and cardiac compromise. In idiopathic scoliosis, the curvature occurs gradually and may go unnoticed until a school nurse identifies it in an adolescent and refers the child to a physician. Scoliosis incidence is highest among adolescent females.

Scoliosis can be treated conservatively with exercises, braces, and traction. Treatment equipment may include a Milwaukee brace, an orthoplast jacket, a Risser localizing cast, and a body jacket with halo apparatus. (For an illustration of the Milwaukee brace, see *Milwaukee brace,* page 176.) If the curvature advances to more than 40 degrees, the child will require surgical intervention, such as Harrington, Dwyer, or Lugue instrumentation. |
| **Clinical situation** | Melinda Fiddler, age 14, has worsening scoliosis and must make periodic visits to the orthopedic clinic. Initially, she will be treated with a Milwaukee brace. |

Assessment

Nursing behaviors	**Nursing rationales**
1. Assess Melinda for signs of scoliosis.	**1.** Signs of scoliosis include asymmetry, such as one shoulder higher, one hip more protruding, or one scapula more prominent than the other. Also, Melinda may have had trouble finding clothes that fit her.
2. Assess Melinda's psychosocial status.	**2.** Adolescents typically are sensitive to being different from their peers. Anticipation of a medical problem requiring long-term treatment may cause Melinda to suffer depression, which could reduce her compliance with treatment.

| **Nursing diagnoses** | • Body image disturbance related to biophysical changes
• Potential for noncompliance, related to denial of being different |
| **Planning and goals** | • Melinda will cooperate with the treatment regimen.
• Melinda will continue her normal school activities as allowed.
• Melinda will maintain friendships with her peers. |

PEDIATRIC NURSING

Milwaukee brace

The Milwaukee brace, used to control scoliosis, extends from the chin to the hip region, maintaining an upright stretched posture.

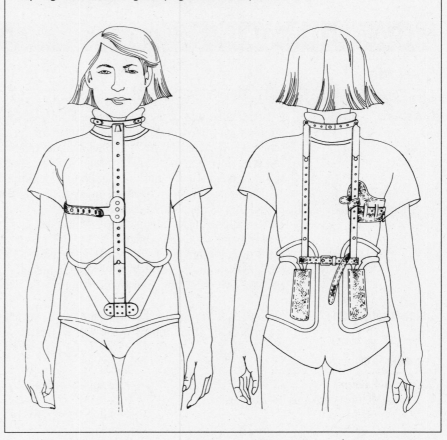

Implementation

Nursing behaviors	Nursing rationales
1. Teach Melinda how to use the Milwaukee brace.	**1.** Melinda will have to wear the brace 23 hours daily. She must understand that if she refuses to wear it as prescribed, she may need surgery.
2. Show Melinda how to inspect her skin.	**2.** The Milwaukee brace, made of leather and metal, is heavy and hot. Melinda should wear a T-shirt under the brace to decrease irritation. She must check her skin each day after removing the brace to bathe.
3. Assist Melinda to walk while she wears the brace.	**3.** The brace is heavy and forces Melinda's body into an unfamiliar position. Therefore, she may feel awkward and fear that she will fall when walking. Assisting her to walk will help her overcome this fear.
4. Discuss with Melinda how to choose clothes that cover the brace and conform to her adolescent tastes.	**4.** If Melinda feels attractive and likes her clothing, she is more likely to comply with treatment. (She may need to wear the brace for up to 2 years.)

5. Teach Melinda about the importance of returning for visits to the orthopedic physician.

5. Melinda will need to see the orthopedic physician regularly for an extended period for X-rays and physical examinations to determine her progress. If conservative treatment fails to correct scoliosis, she will need surgery.

Evaluation (outcomes)

- Melinda performs her exercises and wears her brace.
- Melinda maintains her normal school activities as allowed.
- Melinda maintains friendships with her peers.

SELECTED NURSING PROCEDURES

The nursing procedures described below commonly are used when caring for pediatric patients. (Procedure steps preceded by an asterisk are especially important.)

Caring for a child in a Croupette

Introduction

A Croupette is a plastic tent that provides large amounts of humidified oxygen to liquefy secretions. Young children are more tolerant of oxygen administered by this method because they feel less restrained than with a face mask or cannula.

Steps

*1. Take the child's temperature every 2 hours.

2. Change the child's clothing every 2 hours if wet. Change the bedding if wet.

*3. Keep the child's head elevated, if possible.

4. Keep the edges of the Croupette tucked securely under the mattress. Place several folded sheets over the end of the Croupette.

*5. If the child becomes frantic and refuses to remain in the Croupette, allow the parent's head inside the tent to distract and help calm the child. To prevent oxygen loss, tuck the edges of the Croupette securely around the parent's waist.

Rationales

*1. Humidity in a Croupette dampens clothing, causing cooling by evaporation and possible hypothermia.

2. Humidity dampens all fabric items in the Croupette.

*3. Elevating a child's head reduces respiratory distress. (However, an infant may benefit from lying prone with a diaper roll under the abdomen to promote expiration. Alternatively, an infant may sit in an infant seat; in this case, monitor the infant to prevent a sideways fall, which could compromise diaphragmatic movement.)

4. Because oxygen is heavy, it drops to the bottom of the Croupette, where it can escape if the tent edges are not secured.

*5. Toddlers particularly are fearful of being separated from their parents. A toddler who becomes frantic and starts to scream cannot benefit from Croupette therapy. The parent's presence at the bedside comforts the child, promoting cooperation. Tucking the edges of the Croupette around the parent's waist prevents oxygen loss.

PEDIATRIC NURSING

6. Allow only soft toys with no moving metal parts inside the Croupette.

6. Because the Croupette provides oxygen, toys with moving metal parts are a fire hazard.

7. After the child is removed from the Croupette, assess frequently for signs of recurrent respiratory distress.

7. The child may be removed from the Croupette briefly, such as for bathing or feeding. If respiratory and pulse rates change, the child may need to return to the Croupette.

8. Document the child's response to being in a Croupette.

8. Documentation proves that the procedure was done, assures high-quality care, and provides legal protection. It also provides data for evaluating the effectiveness of oxygen administration via the Croupette.

Assisting with bone marrow aspiration or biopsy

Introduction

To examine the bone marrow for blast cells, marrow may be removed from the bone marrow cavity by aspiration via a special needle. Typically, 1 to 2 ml are removed. If the bone marrow is too congested to allow aspiration, a specimen is removed via biopsy. In a child, the site of the aspiration or biopsy usually is the anterior or posterior iliac crest. More than 5% blast cells indicates leukemia.

Steps

1. Administer a sedative before the procedure, as ordered.

Rationales

1. A sedative (usually administered I.M.) reduces the child's anxiety, promoting cooperation.

*2. Position the child prone and place a towel under the hips to elevate them. (Allow the child to practice lying in this position before the procedure.)

*2. This position most effectively exposes the posterior iliac crest.

*3. Clean the hip area with povidone-iodine (Betadine) solution.

*3. Povidone-iodine solution has antibacterial properties.

4. Help restrain the child during administration of a local anesthetic. (The child may feel a stinging sensation.)

4. A local anesthetic is given to decrease pain caused by passage of the aspiration needle through the skin.

5. Continue restraining the child while the aspiration needle is inserted through the iliac crest and into the bone marrow cavity. The child may feel a popping sensation.

5. To pass the bone marrow needle through the bone, the physician must push it with pressure. A popping sensation occurs when the needle enters the bone marrow cavity.

6. The physician will aspirate the bone marrow by suction with a syringe attached to the needle (causing a deep or sharp pain), then place the aspirate on a slide and examine it for bone marrow spicules. If spicules are present, tell the child that the procedure will be over soon.

6. Pain arises as suction is applied to the bone marrow needle, which creates a negative pressure within the marrow cavity. If bone marrow spicules are present, the specimen is adequate. Telling the child that the procedure is almost over helps relieve anxiety.

*7. After the physician withdraws the needle, a pressure dressing is placed over the puncture site. Check the dressing every 15 minutes for signs of bleeding.

*7. Because the child may have a low platelet count, the aspiration site may bleed.

8. After the procedure, encourage the child to sleep or play quietly if the effects of the sedative have decreased.

8. The child probably will be tired from adrenalin expenditure and anxiety, and will sleep without difficulty. Quiet play helps prevent bleeding from the aspiration site.

9. Document the procedure.

9. Documentation proves that the procedure was done, assures high-quality care, and provides legal protection.

Teaching insulin self-administration

Introduction

In this procedure, the nurse teaches the patient with Type I diabetes mellitus how to self-administer insulin to ensure adequate carbohydrate metabolism. Such teaching helps to avoid adverse reactions from incorrect insulin administration. Children are more prone to adverse insulin reactions because of their unpredictable food intake, growth pattern changes, and inconsistent exercise. Many children receive a combination of short-acting regular insulin and intermediate-acting NPH insulin. Regular insulin is clear; NPH insulin is cloudy. To prevent contamination of regular fast-acting insulin by intermediate-acting NPH insulin, the child must draw up regular insulin into the syringe before NPH insulin (in other words, clear before cloudy).

Steps

1. Wash your hands thoroughly.

2. Gather needed supplies: both types of insulin, a syringe, and alcohol.

*3. Clean the tops of both insulin vials with alcohol.

*4. Inject an amount of air equal to the insulin dosage into the NPH insulin vial, then into the regular insulin vial.

5. Without removing the needle from the regular insulin vial, draw out the amount of insulin needed.

6. Without injecting more air into the NPH insulin vial, carefully withdraw the prescribed amount of NPH insulin.

*7. Select an injection site that is at least 1″ (2.5 cm) from a previous site.

8. Document patient teaching.

Rationales

1. This removes dirt and bacteria that could cause infection.

2. Gathering supplies in advance eliminates the need to interrupt the procedure to obtain a missing supply.

*3. This prevents introduction of bacteria into the vials.

*4. Injecting air before removing insulin prevents a vacuum from forming within the vial.

5. This puts the regular insulin dose into the syringe.

6. The total combined dosage of regular and NPH insulin now is ready for injection.

*7. Rotating injection sites prevents lipoatrophy and ensures adequate insulin absorption. Using one part of the body for 1 week is an easy guideline for a child to remember.

8. This proves that the patient has received teaching, assures high-quality care, and provides legal protection.

PEDIATRIC NURSING

Adult medical-surgical nursing

Introduction 186

Cardiovascular system

Anatomy and physiology 186

Congestive heart failure 191

Myocardial infarction 192

Hypertension 194

Arteriosclerosis 195

Applying and monitoring rotating tourniquets 198

Assisting with an electrocardiogram 199

Performing basic cardiopulmonary resuscitation 200

Applying elastic stockings 202

Respiratory system

Anatomy and physiology 208

Lobar pneumonia 210

Pulmonary edema 212

Lung cancer 213

Chronic obstructive pulmonary disease 216

Pulmonary tuberculosis 217

Caring for the patient with a chest tube 222

Teaching deep-breathing and coughing exercises 224

Performing postural drainage 225

Administering intermittent positive-pressure breathing treatments 227

Assisting with incentive spirometry 228

Administering oxygen 228

Assisting with thoracentesis 229

Performing tracheal suctioning 230

Providing tracheostomy care 232

Caring for a patient requiring mechanical ventilation 233

Musculoskeletal system

Anatomy and physiology 238

Patient in a cast (fracture of the tibia and fibula) 241

Patient in traction (fracture of the femur) 244

Fracture of the femoral neck 247

Osteoarthritis 253

Rheumatoid arthritis 256

Performing neurovascular checks 263

Assisting with cast application 264

Assisting with cast removal 267

Teaching about skin care after cast removal 268

Applying a sling 268

Assisting with application of balanced-suspension skeletal traction for a
fractured femur 269

Teaching a patient to use crutches, a cane, or a walker 272

Adult medical-surgical nursing *(continued)*

Gastrointestinal system

Anatomy and physiology 282

Gastrointestinal ulcer 288

Obstruction of the small intestine 292

Colon cancer 296

Inserting a nasogastric tube 300

Inserting a Miller-Abbott intestinal tube 302

Inserting a Cantor intestinal tube 303

Maintaining a gastrointestinal tube 305

Removing a nasogastric, Miller-Abbott, or Cantor tube 306

Providing tube feedings 307

Providing gastrostomy or jejunostomy tube feedings 310

Providing jejunal tube feedings 311

Assisting with paracentesis 312

Providing ileostomy care 314

Providing colostomy care 317

Administering a cleansing enema 321

Applying an abdominal binder 323

Inserting a rectal tube 325

Removing a rectal tube 326

Listening for bowel sounds 327

Assisting with proctoscopy 328

Neurologic system

Anatomy and physiology 333

Head injury and increased intracranial pressure 338

Cerebrovascular accident 341

Epilepsy 346

Brain tumor 350

Parkinson's disease 352

Performing neurologic checks 357

Placing a patient on a CircOlectric bed 360

Turning a patient on a CircOlectric bed 361

Turning a patient on a Stryker Wedge Frame bed 363

Positioning a patient in bed 365

Assisting with lumbar puncture 368

Genitourinary system

Anatomy and physiology 373

Glomerulonephritis 375

Benign prostatic hyperplasia 377

Kidney or bladder tumor 380

Dialysis 383

Inserting a urinary catheter 387

Caring for an indwelling urinary catheter 388

ADULT
NURSING

Adult medical-surgical nursing (continued)

Removing an indwelling urinary catheter 389

Caring for a nephrostomy tube 390

Applying a condom catheter 390

Caring for an arteriovenous shunt 391

Measuring fluid intake and output 393

Measuring urine specific gravity 394

Applying a T-binder 395

Endocrine system

Anatomy and physiology 397

Hyperthyroidism 399

Hypothyroidism 401

Cushing's syndrome 403

Addison's disease 405

Type II diabetes mellitus 407

Teaching blood glucose self-monitoring 412

Assisting with the glucose tolerance test 413

Assisting with the radioactive iodine uptake test 414

Collecting 24-hour urine specimens 415

Part IV

Integumentary system

Anatomy and physiology 420

Third-degree burn 421

Caring for pressure ulcers 429

Immune system

Anatomy and physiology 432

Acquired immunodeficiency syndrome 435

Oncology nursing

Malignant cell development 439

Ovarian cancer and chemotherapy 441

Lung cancer and radiation therapy 445

Breast cancer and mastectomy 449

Starting an I.V. line 455

Caring for a peripheral venous catheter 458

Providing oral hygiene 459

Changing a central line dressing 461

ADULT
NURSING

Introduction

This section contains a wealth of information about many common adult medical-surgical conditions and clinical situations likely to be tested on NCLEX-PN. Like the rest of this book, it presents a selective review of the nursing care you need to know to succeed on this examination; it is not meant to be comprehensive. The disorders, drugs, and procedures described are those encountered frequently by the practical nurse.

Organized by body system, this section presents clinical situations in the nursing process framework. For each body system, it provides a review of anatomy and physiology, anatomical illustrations, a glossary for easy review and enhanced understanding, case studies demonstrating common disorders, and step-by-step descriptions of selected nursing procedures. Information on complications associated with each body system and commonly used drugs appears in charts. To avoid redundancy, the text refers the reader to other parts of this book for details on general nursing concepts, growth and development, nutritional aspects of medical and nursing care, history taking and physical examination, and certain commonly encountered conditions (such as shock and inflammation).

Be aware that because this section takes a national rather than regional perspective, it presents certain nursing activities as required for a given patient condition and related nursing care. However, these activities are not practiced uniformly by all licensed practical nurses. (As the nursing profession continues to evolve, the activities of licensed practical nurses will become defined more clearly and performed more universally.) The text provides rationales for specific nursing activities to help clarify the roles of nursing and other health care personnel.

ADULT NURSING

CARDIOVASCULAR SYSTEM

Anatomy and physiology

I. **Anatomy**
    A. Heart
       1. The heart is a muscular organ containing four chambers—two atria and two ventricles (see *Reviewing the heart*)
       2. The heart pumps blood through an elaborate network of vessels
    B. Blood vessels
       1. Arteries carry oxygenated blood from the heart to body tissues
          a. Arteries are elastic and contractile; the latter quality causes the pulsations felt when assessing an artery or seen when observing an arterial hemorrhage
          b. Arteries constrict and dilate in response to certain medications and changes in surrounding muscles
       2. Veins carry deoxygenated blood from body tissues to the heart
          a. They have lower internal pressure than arteries
          b. They lack contractility
       3. Capillaries are microscopic vessels through which carbon dioxide, oxygen, nutrients, and waste products are exchanged between blood and body tissues.

Reviewing heart structures

The cardiovascular system transports oxygen from the lungs to body cells and transports carbon dioxide from body cells to the lungs. It also carries nutrients for cell metabolism. This illustration shows the heart as viewed from the front. The superior and inferior venae cavae supply blood to the right atrium; the pulmonary veins supply blood to the left atrium. The right ventricle, located just beneath the sternum, is the heart's most anterior structure. It obtains venous blood from the right atrium during ventricular diastole, then pumps this blood through the pulmonary valve into the pulmonary artery. The left ventricle gets blood from the left atrium during ventricular diastole, then ejects it through the aortic valve into the systemic arterial circulation during ventricular systole. Thick muscle tissue surrounding the left ventricle increases the expulsive force that delivers blood to peripheral tissues.

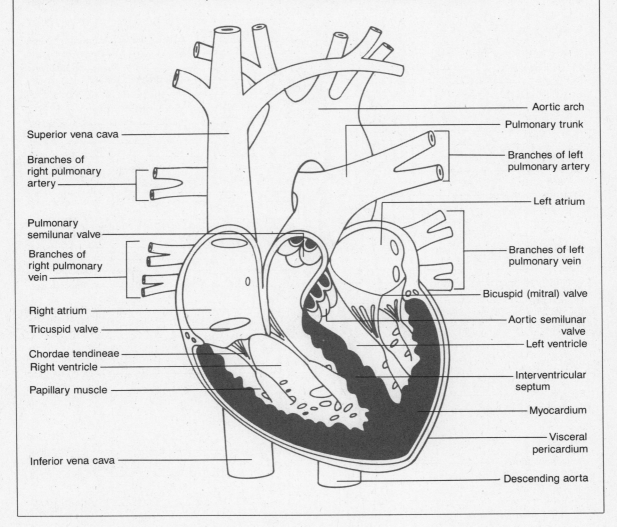

Superior vena cava

Branches of right pulmonary artery

Pulmonary semilunar valve

Branches of right pulmonary vein

Right atrium

Tricuspid valve

Chordae tendineae

Right ventricle

Papillary muscle

Inferior vena cava

Aortic arch

Pulmonary trunk

Branches of left pulmonary artery

Left atrium

Branches of left pulmonary vein

Bicuspid (mitral) valve

Aortic semilunar valve

Left ventricle

Interventricular septum

Myocardium

Visceral pericardium

Descending aorta

II. Physiology
A. Functions
1. The cardiovascular system transports oxygen from the lungs to body cells and transports carbon dioxide from body cells to the lungs
2. It also carries nutrients for cell metabolism
B. Blood circulation
1. The complete cycle (the time it takes blood to circulate throughout the body) occurs roughly every 1.5 seconds

Circulatory system

The anterior view shows the major arteries and veins. The venous system is in dark gray; the arterial system is light gray.

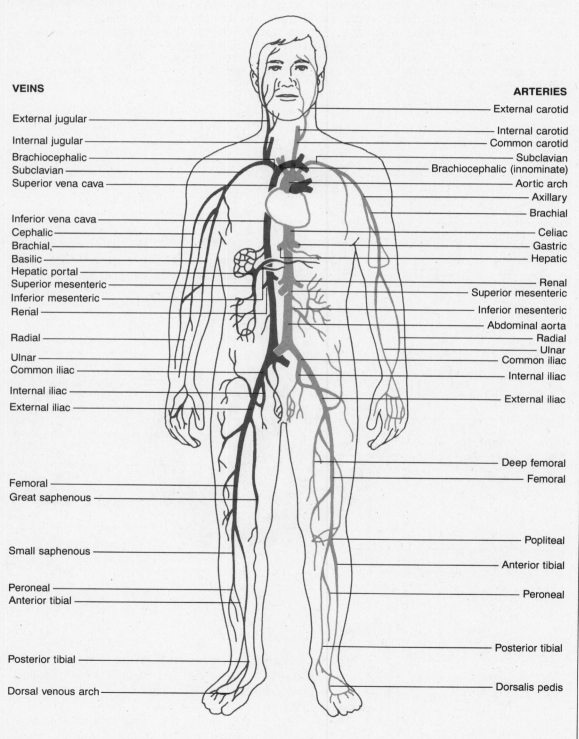

VEINS

External jugular

Internal jugular

Brachiocephalic
Subclavian
Superior vena cava

Inferior vena cava
Cephalic
Brachial
Basilic
Hepatic portal
Superior mesenteric
Inferior mesenteric
Renal

Radial

Ulnar
Common iliac

Internal iliac

External iliac

Femoral
Great saphenous

Small saphenous

Peroneal
Anterior tibial

Posterior tibial

Dorsal venous arch

ARTERIES

External carotid

Internal carotid
Common carotid
Subclavian
Brachiocephalic (innominate)
Aortic arch
Axillary
Brachial

Celiac
Gastric
Hepatic

Renal
Superior mesenteric
Inferior mesenteric
Abdominal aorta
Radial
Ulnar
Common iliac

Internal iliac

External iliac

Deep femoral
Femoral

Popliteal

Anterior tibial

Peroneal

Posterior tibial

Dorsalis pedis

2. Within the general circulation, arteries carry oxygenated blood and veins carry unoxygenated blood
3. Within the pulmonary circulation, the situation is reversed (see *Circulatory system*)

C. Cardiac conduction

1. The heart contains specialized structures that generate and conduct electrical impulses (see *Cardiac conduction system*)

   a. The sinoatrial (SA) node initiates impulses that spread in a wavelike fashion through the right and left atria, causing atrial contractions

   b. The atrioventricular (AV) node receives the impulse from the SA node when atrial contraction ends

   c. The impulse continues to the atrioventricular bundle (bundle of His), then travels to the Purkinje fibers, which trigger ventricular contraction

Cardiac conduction system

This illustration shows the heart structures that initiate and conduct electrical impulses causing the heart to beat.

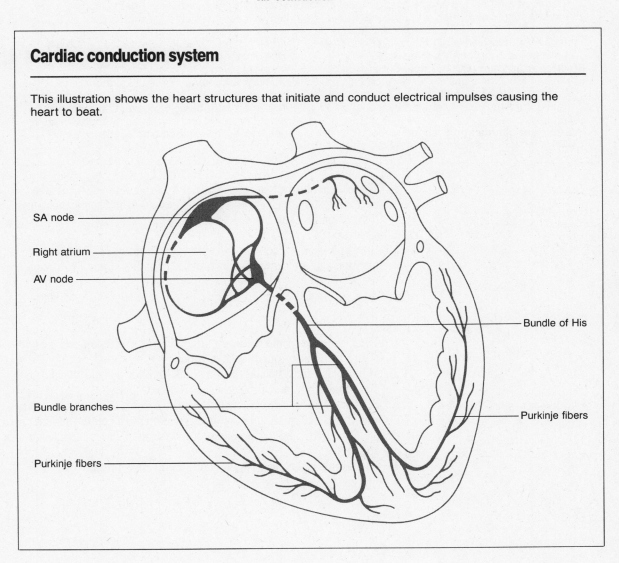

Glossary

Angina pectoris: recurrent chest pain and choking sensation caused by insufficient oxygen supply to the heart

Cardiac output: volume of blood expelled by either ventricle each minute

Cerebrovascular accident (CVA): abnormal condition of the vessels of the brain characterized by occlusion resulting from cerebrovascular hemorrhage or an embolus; leads to ischemia of brain tissues normally perfused by the damaged vessels. CVA may alter neurologic function.

Coronary artery disease (CAD): collective term for a group of abnormal conditions involving the arteries of the heart, characterized by a decreased supply of oxygen and nutrients to the myocardium. The most common CAD form is coronary atherosclerosis, in which lipid plaques accumulate in the inner layers of the vessel walls.

Electrocardiogram (ECG): paper or oscilloscope tracing of electrical activity within the heart produced by an electrocardiograph; used to evaluate the cardiac rate, rhythm, and conduction pattern

Intermittent claudication: abnormal condition characterized by severe pain in a limb after physical activity, followed by reduction or absence of pain at rest. The condition results from insufficient arterial blood supply to the involved limb.

Ischemia: reduced blood supply to an organ or other part of the body

Myocardium: contractile middle layer of muscle cells that forms the bulk of the heart wall

Necrosis: localized death of tissue in groups of cells resulting from prolonged lack of blood supply

Shock: a state of acute circulatory failure characterized by inadequate cellular perfusion and decreased oxygenation; may lead to cellular death

Transient ischemic attack: brief episode of cerebrovascular insufficiency typically caused by partial occlusion of an artery by an embolus or atherosclerotic plaque; may cause temporary loss of consciousness, vision, or sensory or motor function

Valsalva's maneuver: forced expiratory effort against a closed airway (as in straining at stool) that alters intrathoracic pressure; in response, the pulse slows and blood supply to the heart decreases, reducing cardiac output

2. The conduction system is specialized to respond to cues from the nervous system, changes in vascular pressure, and chemical changes (oxygen and carbon dioxide levels)

D. Blood pressure

1. Blood pressure reflects the strength and adequacy of heart muscle function and arterial pressure (resistance) as blood pumps through the arteries

2. Average normal blood pressure is 120/80 mm Hg for an average-size adult

E. Pulse

1. The pulse is palpable where an artery lies near the skin surface and over a firm background (such as a bone)

2. Major pulse sites include the temporal, carotid, apical, brachial, radial, femoral, popliteal, and pedal arteries

3. Peripheral pulses are assessed bilaterally for presence, rhythm, rate, amplitude, and quality. If asymmetry is noted, the pulse proximal to the asymmetrical pulse is assessed to determine where the change occurred

4. The normal pulse (heart) rate is 60 to 100 beats/minute

Congestive heart failure

Overview

In congestive heart failure (CHF), the myocardium cannot pump enough blood to meet the body's needs, compromising ventricular performance. CHF may follow injury to the myocardium (such as from myocardial infarction) or it may develop gradually in response to hypertension. CHF is characterized by signs and symptoms of general systemic debilitation, pulmonary congestion, and systemic congestion.

Three main causes of CHF include:
- conditions resulting in indirect heart damage, such as myocardial infarction (MI)
- conditions resulting in ventricular overload, such as I.V. fluid overload and hypertension
- conditions resulting in ventricular constriction, such as pericarditis.

Clinical situation

Nelson Bricker, age 60, is admitted to the medical-surgical unit after an acute MI. Since his admission, he has complained of worsening fatigue and seems increasingly anxious about his condition. At night, he complains of orthopnea and has a hacking cough. The physician suspects CHF.

Assessment

Nursing behaviors

1. Assess Mr. Bricker for respiratory distress by evaluating his respiratory rate and depth, observing skin and nail color, auscultating the lungs for crackles (rales), and observing sputum for the presence and amount of blood and froth.

2. Assess for other signs of CHF: increased apical pulse rate; abnormal apical pulse rhythm; increased blood pressure; decreased urine output (oliguria): decreased bowel sounds; cool, pale skin; and changes in orientation or level of consciousness.

3. Assess for early signs and symptoms of right ventricular failure: edema of the periorbital area, hands, feet, or dependent areas; distended neck veins; increased central venous pressure; and ascites.

4. Assess for signs and symptoms of pulmonary edema, such as restlessness, pallor, tachycardia, blood-tinged or frothy productive cough, and wheezing.

Nursing rationales

1. Respiratory distress is an early sign of CHF, which commonly complicates MI.

2. Inadequate pump function causes decreased cardiac output, which affects all body systems.

3. Right ventricular failure commonly follows left ventricular failure.

4. Pulmonary edema is a complication of CHF.

Nursing diagnoses

- Activity intolerance related to fatigue and orthopnea
- Ineffective breathing pattern related to pulmonary congestion

ADULT NURSING

Planning and goals

• Mr. Bricker's breathing pattern will remain within normal limits.
• Mr. Bricker will get enough physical and emotional rest to decrease his oxygen requirements.
• Mr. Bricker and his family will demonstrate knowledge of and compliance with his prescribed treatment regimen.

Implementation

Nursing behaviors	**Nursing rationales**
1. Encourage activity limitations (such as bed rest) and advance Mr. Bricker's activities progressively according to the physician's orders.	**1.** Rest decreases oxygen requirements.
2. Administer oxygen, as ordered.	**2.** Supplemental oxygen increases oxygen supply to body cells.
3. Place Mr. Bricker in a semi- to high-Fowler's position.	**3.** A semisitting position promotes lung expansion.
4. Institute strict fluid intake and output limitations. Weigh Mr. Bricker daily, and assist with assessment for tissue edema.	**4.** These assessments help detect fluid retention from CHF.
5. Administer prescribed diuretics, digitalis preparations, and vasodilators.	**5.** Diuretics increase the urine flow and reduce circulating volume, thereby decreasing the cardiac work load. Digitalis preparations increase myocardial contraction strength and improve cardiac output. Vasodilators decrease the cardiac work load by reducing systemic vascular resistance.
6. Encourage sodium restriction, according to the diet prescription.	**6.** Sodium restriction helps control edema.
7. Assist with teaching Mr. Bricker and his family about the need for rest, oxygen therapy, dietary restrictions, and drug therapy.	**7.** Explanation and reinforcement enhance Mr. Bricker's understanding and compliance.

Evaluation (outcomes)

• Mr. Bricker demonstrates effortless breathing patterns.
• Mr. Bricker alternates activity with rest.
• Mr. Bricker understands the purpose of his medication regimen and dietary restrictions and demonstrates compliance.
• Mr. Bricker remains free from CHF complications.

Myocardial infarction

Overview

Myocardial infarction (MI) occurs when blood flow through one or more major coronary arteries is blocked. The blockage reduces oxygenation of myocardial tissue (ischemia), leading to cellular death (necrosis) and impairing the heart's pumping ability. This, in turn, reduces blood supply to all body systems, possibly leading to shock. A common cause of MI is narrowing of the coronary vessels, which may stem from plaque formation (atherosclerosis) or vessel occlusion by an embolus (clot).

Clinical situation   Nora Popowitz, age 63, is admitted to the hospital complaining of crushing chest pain. She reports that the pain persists even though she has taken several nitroglycerin tablets and rested. She states that the pain began when she was working in the yard in the retirement community where she lives.

Assessment

Nursing behaviors

1. Assist with assessing the nature of Mrs. Popowitz's pain, such as a viselike or crushing (substernal) chest pain and referred pain to other body areas (including the epigastrium, jaw, neck, or arm).

2. Assess Mrs. Popowitz for other associated signs and symptoms of MI: nausea, dyspnea, apprehension, diaphoresis, and weakness.

3. Assess Mrs. Popowitz for signs of shock: pallor, increased pulse rate, and decreased blood pressure.

4. Note any electrocardiographic (ECG) changes.

5. Review laboratory results of creatine phosphokinase (CPK-MB), aspartate aminotransferase (AST; formerly known as serum glutamic-oxaloacetic transaminase), lactic dehydrogenase (LDH), white blood cell (WBC) count, and erythrocyte sedimentation rate (ESR) tests.

Nursing rationales

1. These pain characteristics are common with an MI.

2. These signs and symptoms result from changes in cardiac output stemming from MI.

3. Shock may result from a severe drop in cardiac output. It warrants immediate intervention.

4. MI may cause cardiac arrhythmias. (However, the extent of heart damage from an MI may not appear on ECG for several days.)

5. Levels of the enzymes CPK, AST, and LDH (released by damaged cardiac tissue) typically rise after MI. The WBC count increases up to $15,000/mm^3$ within a few hours of pain onset. ESR rises within 1 week of MI.

Nursing diagnoses
- Pain related to decreased myocardial blood supply
- Altered tissue perfusion related to diminished cardiac output

Planning and goals
- Mrs. Popowitz will obtain pain relief.
- Mrs. Popowitz will maintain adequate function of other body systems.
- Mrs. Popowitz will comply with a teaching plan to decrease cardiac stress.

Implementation

Nursing behaviors

1. Monitor Mrs. Popowitz's vital signs.

2. Maintain oxygen administration, as ordered.

3. Elevate the head of Mrs. Popowitz's bed.

4. Encourage bed rest and a quiet environment.

5. Assist Mrs. Popowitz with hygiene.

Nursing rationales

1. Changes in vital signs may reflect changes in cardiac status.

2. Supplemental oxygen increases tissue oxygenation.

3. A raised position improves lung expansion.

4. Bed rest and quiet decrease tissue oxygen needs.

5. Assistance helps reduce physical exertion, thereby decreasing tissue oxygen needs.

6. Record Mrs. Popowitz's fluid intake and output during each shift.

6. Fluid balance must be monitored and maintained to prevent fluid excess and cardiac overload.

7. Report any complaints of pain to the nurse-manager or team leader immediately.

7. This helps ensure prompt treatment of pain.

8. Instruct Mrs. Popowitz not to strain at stool.

8. Straining at stool induces the Valsalva maneuver, which slows the pulse rate (causing bradycardia) and decreases blood return to the heart.

9. Reinforce patient and family teaching about medications, adequate rest, caffeine and fluid restrictions, reduction of dietary cholesterol and sodium intake, and signs and symptoms to report to the physician.

9. Reinforcing teaching promotes learning. Mrs. Popowitz must understand the treatment regimen to comply with it.

Evaluation (outcomes)

• Mrs. Popowitz expresses pain relief.
• Mrs. Popowitz maintains adequate tissue oxygenation, as reflected by normal vital signs.
• Mrs. Popowitz complies with a schedule allowing progressive return to activities of daily living.
• Mrs. Popowitz expresses an understanding of her medication regimen and the measures she should take if she experiences chest pain again.

Hypertension

Overview

Hypertension is defined as a consistent systolic blood pressure above 140 mm Hg and a diastolic pressure above 90 mm Hg. It occurs when vascular resistance to blood flow is impeded, such as from changes in blood vessel diameter (related to atherosclerosis), increased blood viscosity, or fluid overload. Hypertension is extremely dangerous because it may be silent (asymptomatic) and result in cardiac failure and cerebrovascular accident (CVA). Risk factors for hypertension include a positive family history (especially among American blacks), obesity, smoking, excessive alcohol intake, sodium and water retention, renal disease, and emotional stress. In the United States, the incidence of hypertension increases with age.

Clinical situation

Ormond King, age 53, is admitted to the hospital with a diagnosis of hypertension and poor blood pressure control. The president of a large electronics company, Mr. King is married and black, with two children in college. He smokes one pack of cigarettes daily and is 25 lb (11.3 kg) overweight.

Assessment

Nursing behaviors

1. Measure blood pressure in both arms frequently, with Mr. King sitting, standing, and supine.

Nursing rationales

1. This will reveal any rise or fall in blood pressure associated with postural changes.

2. Assess Mr. King's apical and peripheral pulses.

2. This reveals any circulatory changes related to hypertension.

3. Measure blood pressure before and after administration of antihypertensive drugs.

3. This helps evaluate the effectiveness of antihypertensive drug therapy.

4. Evaluate Mr. King for headaches, vertigo, visual disturbances, and nosebleeds (epistaxis).

4. These signs and symptoms may stem from multi-system changes caused by uncontrolled hypertension.

Nursing diagnoses
• Knowledge deficit related to control of hypertension risk factors
• Altered tissue perfusion related to atherosclerosis

Planning and goals
• Mr. King will express an understanding of the disease and the need to control his blood pressure.
• Mr. King will remain free from hypertensive crisis.

Implementation

Nursing behaviors

1. Monitor Mr. King's blood pressure, using proper cuff size and placement, at least 30 minutes after he smokes or exercises. Keep the manometer at eye level, and compare the measurement obtained with his baseline blood pressure.

Nursing rationales

1. Following these guidelines will help ensure consistent, accurate blood pressure measurement.

2. Teach Mr. King about the prescribed antihypertensive drug regimen, including the need for strict compliance, follow-up blood pressure monitoring, and side effects.

2. Mr. King's full understanding of drug therapy will aid compliance.

3. Teach Mr. King about required dietary modifications (sodium and fat restriction), weight control (through decreased calorie intake and increased exercise), and life-style changes (stress reduction and smoking cessation).

3. Reducing or eliminating risk factors for hypertension is crucial to the success of treatment.

4. Refer Mr. King to appropriate community support groups for help with stress reduction, weight control, and smoking cessation.

4. Support group involvement promotes health-habit changes.

Evaluation (outcomes)
• Mr. King complies with his prescribed drug regimen.
• Mr. King expresses an understanding of controllable risk factors to prevent hypertensive crisis.
• Mr. King demonstrates weight loss and stops smoking.
• Mr. King complies with follow-up medical evaluation.

Arteriosclerosis

Overview

Arteriosclerosis is an abnormal condition in which the arterial walls thicken, harden, calcify, and become less elastic. These changes result from lipid plaque accumulation in the inner layers of the vessel wall. Arteriosclerosis reduces blood supply to body tissues and eventually may cause cellular death (necrosis). The condition commonly is associated with aging and has a higher incidence in males. Other risk factors for arteriosclerosis include high serum cholesterol levels, obesity, hypertension, cigarette smoking, diabetes mellitus, lack of exercise, and genetic predisposition.

ADULT NURSING

Clinical situation   Richard Collins, age 73, is admitted to the medical unit after his daughter, who cares for him in her home, brings him to the hospital. She explains that her father has memory lapses and episodes of dizziness, which have become more frequent over the past month. Mr. Collins weighs 20% more than the standard for his height and age. His brother died last year after a cardiovascular accident.

Assessment

Nursing behaviors	Nursing rationales
1. Assess Mr. Collins for orientation to time, place, and person.	**1.** This determines Mr. Collins's mental function.
2. Assess Mr. Collins for signs and symptoms of arteriosclerosis: headache, intermittent claudication, angina, changes in skin temperature (coolness) and color (pallor), and transient ischemic attacks.	**2.** This helps determine the body regions where arteriosclerosis is most pronouced.
3. Assess Mr. Collins's vital signs, paying special attention to intensity of pulses.	**3.** This reveals whether tissue perfusion is adequate.

Nursing diagnoses
- Potential for injury related to dizziness
- Altered tissue perfusion related to arterial circulatory changes

Planning and goals
- Mr. Collins will remain free from injury.
- Mr. Collins will modify risk factors for further arterial changes.

Implementation

Nursing behaviors	Nursing rationales
1. Institute safety measures, such as placing the call device within easy reach, putting the side rails up, placing the bed in the lowest position, clearing a path for ambulation, and ensuring safe patient transfer.	**1.** Like any elderly patient with arteriosclerosis, Mr. Collins is at risk for falls.
2. Avoid exposing Mr. Collins to cold environmental temperatures.	**2.** This helps prevent further vasoconstriction caused by cold exposure.
3. Provide for safe, supervised activities and frequent rest periods.	**3.** This helps avoid further complications and mental depression.
4. Teach Mr. Collins to eliminate smoking, lose weight, and reduce his saturated fat intake.	**4.** These measures help prevent complications associated with arteriosclerosis.
5. Provide adequate sensory stimulation and check his reality orientation.	**5.** These measures improve cognitive functioning.

Evaluation (outcomes)
- Mr. Collins remains free from accidental injury.
- Mr. Collins complies with dietary restrictions and eliminates or reduces modifiable risk factors for arteriosclerosis.
- Mr. Collins remains oriented to time, place, and person and shows an improved memory.

Complications of cardiovascular disorders

Cardiovascular disorders cause more deaths than all other disorders combined; any cardiovascular disorder can cause complications. This chart presents the most serious or life-threatening complications of cardiovascular disorders, along with interventions that are crucial to patient safety and comfort.

COMPLICATION	CAUSE	NURSING INTERVENTIONS
Cerebrovascular accident Brain function alteration caused by decreased blood supply to one or more brain regions	• Cerebral ischemia • Embolus of a blood vessel in the brain or neck • Embolus that travels to the brain from outside the cardiovascular system • Rupture of a cerebral vessel, causing bleeding into brain tissue	• Monitor for neurologic changes. • Position the patient to maintain cardiopulmonary and musculoskeletal function. • Ensure patient safety in and out of bed. • Take steps to prevent complications of immobility, such as pneumonia, decreased gastrointestinal motility, skin breakdown, muscle contractions, and urinary stasis. • Provide a way for the patient to communicate needs. • Help the patient attain maximum function to perform activities of daily living. • Reduce joint pain (resulting from disuse) through range-of-motion exercises and positioning.
Cardiac arrest Sudden cessation of myocardial contraction	• Myocardial changes, such as myocardial infarction (MI), myocardial rupture, ventricular arrhythmias, or complete heart block • Shock • Pulmonary arrest	• Rapidly assess for absent carotid pulse and pupil dilation. • Begin cardiopulmonary resuscitation (CPR) immediately. • Ensure emergency medical treatment.
Ventricular rupture Rupture of the ventricle, causing blood loss into the pericardial sac (cardiac tamponade) and inefficient myocardial pumping	• Weakness of the ventricular wall caused by infection, MI, pericardial disease, or trauma	• Prepare the patient for pericardiocentesis (drainage of blood from the pericardial sac). • Prepare the patient for surgery to repair the myocardium.
Cardiac arrhythmias Abnormal cardiac rate or rhythm (for example, bradycardia, tachycardia, atrial or ventricular flutter or fibrillation, premature beats, or heart block). Arrhythmias range in severity from benign to fatal.	• Increased myocardial irritability • Alteration in the cardiac conduction system • Myocardial tissue damage • Emotional disturbances • Hypoxia • Electrolyte changes • Drug toxicity • Electrical shock	• Rapidly assess the apical pulse and electrocardiographic status. • Position the patient at rest. • Administer appropriate drugs, as ordered. • Administer CPR, if necessary. • Prepare the patient for defibrillation or cardioversion. • Prepare the patient for pacemaker implantation.
Gangrene Tissue death (necrosis) caused by inadequate blood supply; most commonly affects the toes. Gangrene may be a complication of peripheral vascular disease or diabetes mellitus.	• Trauma or infection	To prevent gangrene: • Assess circulation to the patient's hands and feet by checking their color, temperature, mobility, pulses, and capillary refill. • Assess the patient's skin and nails to evaluate peripheral circulatory status. • Keep the patient's nails trimmed properly. • Gently clean the patient's feet with warm water and mild soap and dry them thoroughly. • Instruct the patient to avoid constricting hose or shoes, which may cause friction. • Teach the patient to avoid walking barefoot. • Warn the patient never to cut calluses. • Advise the patient to seek medical attention for cuts or wounds of the feet.

ADULT NURSING

Applying and monitoring rotating tourniquets

Introduction

Rotating tourniquets may be used in conjunction with drug therapy to treat pulmonary edema. The tourniquets are applied to three extremities at a time to trap venous blood, thereby reducing blood return to the right ventricle and preventing fluid overload in the pulmonary capillaries. Because stagnant blood leads to clot formation, this technique is reserved for patients with severe pulmonary edema.

Steps

1. Explain the procedure to the patient.

2. Assess the patient's vital signs.

3. Assess and mark the distal pulses.

4. Apply tourniquets to the upper parts of three extremities—for example, both arms and one leg. Make sure the arterial pulses remain palpable.

5. Rotate the tourniquets every 15 minutes by moving them from one extremity to another in a clockwise direction.

6. Monitor the patient's blood pressure every 15 minutes.

7. When ordered to discontinue the procedure, remove one tourniquet every 15 minutes until all extremities are free.

8. Assess each extremity for temperature, color, pulse, and mobility.

9. Document the procedure, the patient's vital signs, circulatory assessment findings, and how well the patient tolerated the procedure.

Rationales

1. Explanations help calm the patient, who already is anxious because of the life-threatening nature of the disease.

2. This provides a baseline for later comparison.

3. This aids pulse monitoring during treatment.

4. Blood flow must be maintained to ensure tissue oxygenation.

5. This method prevents confusion and ensures that each extremity is occluded for a maximum of 45 minutes and unoccluded for 15 minutes every hour.

6. This helps detect hypotension caused by decreased circulating volume.

7. This removal schedule prevents a sudden increase in circulating volume, which can cause recurrent pulmonary edema.

8. This helps determine whether all extremities have sufficient arterial blood supply.

9. Documentation proves that the procedure was done, assures high-quality care, and provides legal protection.

ADULT NURSING

Assisting with an electrocardiogram

Introduction

An electrocardiogram (ECG) is a graphic record produced by an electrocardiograph that shows the heart's electrical activity on a paper tracing or an oscilloscope. The 12-lead ECG demonstrates the electrical activity of the heart in twelve anatomic positions, using externally placed electrodes. (Although the procedure below specifies an ECG tracing, the same steps apply when an oscilloscope is used—except that no paper tracing is produced.) An ECG is used to assess cardiac abnormalities caused by abnormal cardiac impulse transmission, detect cardiac arrhythmias and myocardial damage or enlargement, and help gauge the effectiveness of medical treatment.

Steps

1. Properly identify the patient.

2. Teach the patient about the procedure.

3. Remove the patient's clothing from the waist up and provide for privacy.

4. Help the patient to a comfortable supine position.

5. Clean the skin surfaces where electrodes will be placed, then apply electrode paste and saline pads to these sites.

6. Assist the technician in placing one electrode at each of these sites:
• on each limb
• at V_1 (fourth intercostal space at the right sternal border)
• at V_2 (fourth intercostal space at the left sternal border)
• at V_3 (between V_2 and V_4)
• at V_4 (fifth intercostal space at the midclavicular line)
• at V_5 (fifth intercostal space at the anterior axillary line)
• at V_6 (fifth intercostal space at the midaxillary line).

7. After the technician has completed the ECG, remove the electrodes, wipe off the paste, and help the patient dress.

8. Label the ECG tracing with the patient's name and other appropriate information, as instructed.

9. Deliver the ECG tracing to the physician for interpretation.

Rationales

1. This helps prevent errors.

2. Teaching decreases patient anxiety.

3. ECG electrodes must be placed on bare skin.

4. A supine position promotes proper electrode placement and helps prevent movement, which could reduce recording clarity.

5. These measures ensure proper recording of electrical activity.

6. Placing the electrodes on these sites ensures proper recording from all anatomic areas.

7. These measures increase patient comfort.

8. This helps prevent errors.

9. This helps ensure review of the ECG tracing.

ADULT
NURSING

10. Document the procedure in the patient's chart.

10. Documentation proves that the procedure was done, assures high-quality care, and provides legal protection.

Performing basic cardiopulmonary resuscitation

Introduction

Cardiopulmonary resuscitation (CPR) is a basic emergency life-support procedure involving external manual chest compression and rescue breathing. It maintains blood circulation and oxygenation in a patient lacking a pulse and respiration, thereby preventing biologic death (permanent brain cell death from lack of oxygen). CPR must proceed according to the standardized steps of the American Heart Association.

Steps

1. Assess the patient's responsiveness by shouting, "Are you OK?"

2. If the patient does not respond, start CPR immediately by positioning the patient supine on a firm surface.

3. Open the airway by using the head-tilt-chin-lift method.

4. Assess the patient for spontaneous respirations. If none are present, give two mouth-to-mouth breaths, each lasting 1 to 1½ seconds.

5. Assess the patient's carotid pulse. If absent, begin external cardiac compressions.
• If one rescuer is present, use 15 compressions and 2 ventilations.
• If two rescuers are present, one rescuer ventilates the patient once for every five compressions done by the second rescuer.

6. Continue to perform CPR until one of these criteria is met:
• The patient resumes pulse and respirations spontaneously.
• You are relieved by another certified rescuer.
• You are physically unable to continue.
• You are instructed to discontinue CPR by a physician.

Rationales

1. Trying to elicit a response can determine if the patient is asleep, semicomatose, or intoxicated rather than suffering grave cardiac or respiratory dysfunction. If done unnecessarily, CPR can cause damage to the rib cage, lungs, and heart.

2. CPR must begin immediately because brain damage starts 4 minutes after perfusion stops. For CPR to be effective, the patient's head must be at heart level.

3. The head-tilt-chin-lift method clears the airway of obstruction by the tongue.

4. The patient requiring CPR has a dire need for oxygen. Giving breaths of this duration fills the lungs with air.

5. Cardiac compressions circulate blood by squeezing the heart.

6. Once CPR is initiated, you are bound legally to continue until one of these criteria is met.

ADULT NURSING

Proper positioning for CPR

The top illustration shows the proper position of the rescuer during CPR, with the body positioned over the victim's midline and the arms held straight. The bottom illustration shows proper hand placement on the sternum to ensure maximal heart compression.

BODY POSITION

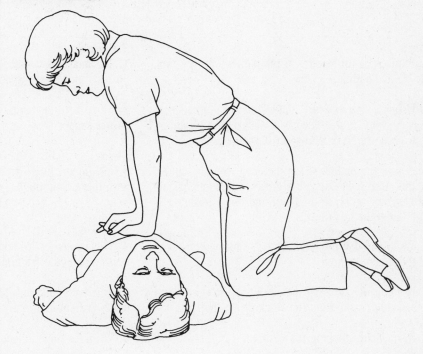

HAND POSITION

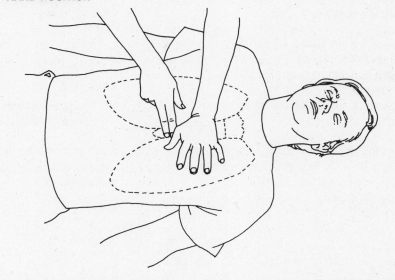

Applying elastic stockings

Introduction

Elastic stockings may be applied to the legs of an immobilized patient to reduce the risk of orthostatic hypotension and clot formation. These stockings decrease blood stasis in the legs by improving muscle tone and compressing superficial blood vessels to force blood into deeper vessels. This, in turn, enhances blood return to the central circulation.

Steps	Rationales
1. Explain the procedure to the patient and position the patient supine.	1. Explanations decrease patient anxiety. A supine position aids stocking application.
2. Using a tape measure, determine what size stockings the patient will need by measuring thigh and calf circumferences and foot-to-knee length.	2. Manufacturers specify stocking measurements to ensure proper fit.
3. Assess the patient's skin for open wounds, cold temperature, cyanosis, skin grafts, and signs of pulmonary edema (such as pallor and diaphoresis or right-sided heart failure).	3. Elastic stockings are contraindicated in patients with these conditions.
4. Wash and dry the patient's legs thoroughly, then apply talcum powder.	4. This promotes hygiene and aids stocking application by reducing friction.
5. Holding the stocking inside out, place the patient's foot inside it and glide the stocking up the leg.	5. This technique aids stocking application and promotes patient comfort.
6. Inspect the stocking for wrinkles.	6. Wrinkles impede leg circulation.
7. Warn the patient not to remove or roll the stocking down without help.	7. Removing or rolling the stocking down may constrict the veins, impairing circulation.
8. Assess leg circulation 1 hour after applying the stockings by checking leg color, temperature, pulses, mobility, and capillary refill.	8. This helps detect impaired circulation.
9. Assess leg circulation during every shift.	9. Regular assessment helps ensure prompt detection of inadequate circulation.
10. Document the date and time of stocking application, type of stocking applied, circulatory assessment findings, skin condition, and the patient's response to stocking application.	10. Documentation proves that the procedure was done, assures high-quality care, and provides legal protection.

ADULT
NURSING

Drugs used to treat cardiovascular disorders

This chart presents information about drugs commonly prescribed for cardiovascular disorders, including the drug action, dosage, and common side effects. Nursing considerations focus on patient comfort and teaching.

DRUG	ACTION	USUAL ADULT DOSAGE	COMMON SIDE EFFECTS	NURSING CONSIDERATIONS
Antiarrhythmics				
Quinidine sulfate (Quinidex)	• Inhibits impulse generation from areas other than the sinoatrial (SA) node • Slows impulse conduction throughout the myocardium	200 to 600 mg P.O. q 6 hours	• Slow pulse rate • Hypotension • Nausea and vomiting • Diarrhea • Worsening of arrhythmias	• Administer with meals. • Assess vital signs. • Stress the importance of follow-up blood tests to monitor therapeutic and toxic effects.
Procainamide (Pronestyl)	• Slows impulse conduction through the heart • Decreases abnormal cardiac impulses	Loading dose: 1 g P.O. Maintenance dose: 250 to 500 mg P.O. q 3 to 4 hours	• Lupus erythematosus syndrome (LES) with chronic use • Worsening of arrhythmias	• Give at evenly spaced intervals. • Monitor the pulse. • Assess for signs and symptoms of LES (joint pain, sore throat, fever, and bradycardia). • Stress the importance of follow-up blood tests to monitor therapeutic and toxic effects.
Disopyramide (Norpace)	• Slows impulse conduction through the heart • Inhibits abnormal cardiac impulses	Loading dose: 200 to 300 mg P.O. Maintenance dose: 100 to 200 mg P.O.	• Hypotension • Bradycardia • Dry mouth • Blurred vision • Urine retention • Worsening of arrhythmias	• Monitor vital signs. • Avoid administering to patients with congestive heart failure (CHF). • Stress the importance of follow-up blood tests to monitor therapeutic and toxic effects. • This drug is available in both immediate-release and sustained-release capsules. Be sure to give the right one.
Lidocaine (Xylocaine)	• Prevents ventricular arrhythmias	Loading dose: 50 to 100 mg I.V. Maintenance dose: 1 to 4 mg/minute I.V.	• Drowsiness • Confusion • Seizures • Respiratory arrest	• Never give P.O. • Administer with an I.V. pump, as ordered. • Monitor vital signs. • Monitor level of consciousness. • Monitor the electrocardiogram (ECG).
Bretylium (Bretylol)	• Controls ventricular arrhythmias	I.V. bolus: 5 mg/kg I.V. infusion: 5 to 10 mg/kg q 6 hours I.M.: 5 to 10 mg/kg q 6 to 8 hours	• Hypotension	• Monitor vital signs. • Monitor the ECG.
Antihypertensives				
Diuretics Hydrochlorothiazide (HydroDIURIL)	• Decreases blood volume • Promotes vasodilation	25 to 100 mg P.O., once or twice daily	• Hypokalemia • Dehydration • Nausea and vomiting	• Give early in the day. • Monitor vital signs. • Monitor fluid intake and output. • Monitor serum electrolyte, blood urea nitrogen, and creatinine levels. • Observe for signs and symptoms of dehydration. • Instruct the patient to take this drug with meals. • Stress the importance of a potassium-rich diet.

(continued)

Drugs used to treat cardiovascular disorders *(continued)*

DRUG	ACTION	USUAL ADULT DOSAGE	COMMON SIDE EFFECTS	NURSING CONSIDERATIONS
Antihypertensives *(continued)*				
Diuretics *(continued)*				
Furosemide (Lasix)	• Decreases blood volume • Inhibits sodium and chloride reabsorption	40 mg P.O. or I.V. b.i.d. (may increase dosage gradually)	• Dehydration • Hypokalemia • Hyponatremia	• Give early in the day. • Monitor fluid intake and output. • Monitor vital signs. • Monitor for dizziness and weakness. • Weigh the patient daily. • Monitor serum electrolyte levels. • Teach the patient to eat potassium-rich foods.
Beta blockers				
Atenolol (Tenormin)	• Decreases cardiac output • Reduces the heart rate • Decreases renin output, suppressing angiotensin II and decreasing blood pressure • Decreases myocardial oxygen needs • Decreases arrhythmias	50 to 100 mg P.O. daily	• Bradycardia • Bronchoconstriction • Insomnia • Sexual dysfunction	• Do not administer to patients with asthma or second- or third-degree heart block. • Assess the pulse before administering. • Monitor blood pressure. • Atenolol may mask some signs of hypoglycemia, such as tachycardia or sweating. • Use cautiously in a diabetic patient.
Propranolol (Inderal)	• Reduces the heart rate • Decreases ventricular contraction force • Decreases renin output, causing decreased blood pressure • Reduces arrhythmias	40 mg P.O. b.i.d. (up to 240 mg daily)	• Bradycardia • Bronchoconstriction • Depression • Nightmares • Heart block • CHF	• This drug is contraindicated in patients with CHF, sinus bradycardia, atrioventricular (AV) heart block, and asthma. • Measure blood pressure and pulse before administering. • Discontinue gradually. • Carefully monitor blood glucose levels. • Propranolol may mask signs of hypoglycemia.
Antiadrenergic agents				
Clonidine (Catapres)	• Decreases sympathetic nervous system action • Promotes vasodilation • Decreases blood pressure	0.2 to 0.8 mg P.O. b.i.d. (may increase dosage gradually to 2.4 mg daily)	• Dry mouth • Drowsiness • Impotence • Anxiety • Depression	• Monitor blood pressure with the patient standing and supine. • Monitor for changes in mental function. • Advise the patient to chew gum or suck on hard candy to reduce dry mouth. • Warn the patient to avoid operating hazardous machinery if drowsiness occurs. • Discontinue gradually. • Rebound hypertension may occur with sudden withdrawal.
Methyldopa (Aldomet)	• Acts within the central nervous system (CNS) to promote vasodilation, causing decreased blood pressure	250 mg P.O. b.i.d. or t.i.d. (to a maximum of 3 g daily)	• Hemolytic anemia • Dry mouth • Sexual dysfunction • Liver toxicity • Orthostatic hypotension	• This drug is contraindicated in patients with a history of liver dysfunction. • Monitor blood pressure with the patient standing and supine. • Teach the patient to move slowly when rising to a standing position. • Instruct the patient to avoid hot showers and baths.

Drugs used to treat cardiovascular disorders *(continued)*

DRUG	ACTION	USUAL ADULT DOSAGE	COMMON SIDE EFFECTS	NURSING CONSIDERATIONS
Antiadrenergic agents *(continued)*				
Reserpine (Serpasil)	• Acts within the CNS to decrease cardiac output • Promotes vasodilation	Initial dose: 0.25 to 0.5 mg P.O. daily; reduce gradually to 0.1 to 0.25 daily	• Depression • Bradycardia • Orthostatic hypotension • Nasal congestion • Peptic ulcers • Abdominal cramps • Diarrhea	• Administer with food. • Monitor blood pressure with the patient standing and supine. • Observe for mental changes. • Side effects may persist for several weeks after the drug is discontinued.
Guanethidine (Ismelin)	• Decreases cardiac output • Decreases smooth muscle tone	Initial dose: 10 mg P.O. daily (may increase dosage by 10 mg weekly until maintenance is established) Maintenance dose: 25 to 50 mg P.O. daily (to a maximum of 300 mg daily)	• Orthostatic hypotension • Bradycardia • Diarrhea • Severe hypertension (in patients with pheochromocytoma)	• This drug is contraindicated in patients with adrenal tumors. • Instruct the patient to avoid standing up abruptly. • Warn the patient to avoid using alcohol while taking this drug. • Teach the patient to avoid hot showers or baths. • Tricyclic antidepressants reduce the effects of guanethidine when taken concomitantly.
Angiotensin-converting enzyme inhibitors				
Captopril (Capoten)	• Inhibits conversion of angiotensin I to angiotensin II • Promotes vasodilation • Increases cardiac output • Promotes sodium and water excretion	Initial dose: 25 mg P.O. b.i.d. or t.i.d; increase gradually to a maximum of 450 mg daily	• Rashes • Impaired taste • Severe hypotension (during initial therapy) • Reduced neutrophil count • Nausea and vomiting • Diarrhea • Headache • Fatigue • Dizziness • Persistent cough	• Administer 1 hour before a meal. • Monitor blood pressure, especially 2 hours after the initial dose. • Monitor serum electrolyte levels. • Monitor fluid intake and output. • Report signs and symptoms of infection. • Do not give with diuretics during initial therapy. • Instruct the patient not to take excessive amounts of potassium and not to use a salt substitute.
Enalapril (Vasotec)	• Promotes vasodilation • Increases cardiac output • Promotes sodium and water excretion	10 to 40 mg P.O. daily in a single or divided dose	• Headache • Dizziness • Fatigue • Neutropenia • Proteinuria • Hypotension (after the initial dose) • Persistent cough	• This drug can be given with meals. • Monitor blood pressure, especially 2 hours after the initial dose. • Monitor serum electrolyte levels. • Monitor fluid intake and output. • Report signs and symptoms of infection. • Use cautiously in patients with renal disease. • Instruct the patient not to take excessive amounts of potassium and not to use a salt substitute.
Lisinopril (Zestril)	• Inhibits conversion of angiotensin I to angiotensin II • Promotes sodium and water excretion	Initial dose: 10 mg P.O. daily Maintenance dose: 20 to 40 mg P.O. daily in a single dose	• Dizziness • Fatigue • Headache • Persistent cough • Nasal congestion • Diarrhea	• Discontinue diuretics before starting this drug. • Instruct the patient to not change positions abruptly. • Warn the patient not to discontinue the drug abruptly. • Food does not affect drug absorption. • Instruct the patient not to take excessive amounts of potassium and not to use a salt substitute.

(continued)

ADULT NURSING

Drugs used to treat cardiovascular disorders *(continued)*

DRUG	ACTION	USUAL ADULT DOSAGE	COMMON SIDE EFFECTS	NURSING CONSIDERATIONS
Calcium-channel blockers				
Verapamil (Isoptin)	• Blocks entry of calcium into cardiac and smooth muscle cells • Dilates arteries, causing decreased blood pressure • Increases blood flow to the myocardium • Reduces the heart rate • Increases myocardial contraction force	40 to 120 mg P.O. q 6 to 8 hours	• Hypotension • Peripheral edema • Bradycardia • Nausea • Constipation • Dizziness • Fatigue • Headache • Ventricular tachyarrhythmias	• Monitor blood pressure and pulse before administering. • Use cautiously when giving concomitantly with digoxin or beta blockers because heart failure may occur. • Assess for edema. • Instruct the patient to move slowly when rising to a standing position.
Nifedipine (Procardia)	• Blocks entry of calcium into cardiac and smooth muscle cells • Promotes vasodilation • Decreases blood pressure • Relieves angina pectoris	10 to 20 mg P.O. t.i.d.	• Hypotension • Headache • Edema • Tachycardia	• Measure blood pressure and pulse before administering. • Assess for edema. • Nifedipine may be prescribed in combination with beta blockers to prevent tachycardia. • Store capsules in a dark, dry place.
Diltiazem (Cardizem)	• Blocks entry of calcium into cardiac and smooth muscle cells • Reduces blood pressure • Relieves angina pectoris	30 to 60 mg P.O. q.i.d.	• Hypotension • Headache • Peripheral edema • Arrhythmias	• Measure blood pressure and pulse before administering. • Assess for edema. • Instruct the patient to move slowly when rising to a standing position.
Digoxin (Lanoxin)	• Increases myocardial contraction force • Decreases SA node activity and impulse conduction through the AV node, reducing the heart rate	Loading dose: 0.75 to 1.25 mg I.V. or P.O. in divided doses given 6 to 8 hours apart Maintenance dose: 0.125 to 0.25 mg I.V. or P.O. daily	• Arrhythmias • Hypokalemia • Vomiting • Diarrhea • Headache • Blurred or yellow halo vision	• Measure the pulse before administering. If it is below 60 beats/minute, withhold the dose and call the nurse-manager or physician. • Monitor serum digoxin levels. • Monitor serum potassium levels. • Teach the patient to take digoxin only as directed. • Concomitant quinidine (Quinidex) therapy increases serum digoxin levels. • Anorexia may be an early sign of toxicity, especially in elderly patients.
Organic nitrate				
Nitroglycerin (Nitro-Bid)	• Dilates vessels • Reduces myocardial oxygen demands • Relieves anginal pain	P.O.: 2.5 to 9 mg given 2 to 3 times daily Sublingual: 0.15 to 0.6 mg p.r.n. Topical disc: Apply once daily • I.V.: 5 mg/minute	• Headache • Orthostatic hypotension • Tachycardia	• Measure blood pressure and pulse before administering. • Use cautiously if the patient is receiving other drugs that reduce blood pressure, such as beta blockers, calcium-channel blockers, or diuretics. • Warn the patient to avoid alcohol. • Rotate application sites when using the topical disc. • Store in a cool, dark place.

Drugs used to treat cardiovascular disorders *(continued)*

DRUG	ACTION	USUAL ADULT DOSAGE	COMMON SIDE EFFECTS	NURSING CONSIDERATIONS
Anticoagulants				
Heparin sodium (Hep Lock)	• Inactivates thrombin, preventing fibrin formation	I.V.: 5,000 to 10,000 units q 4 to 6 hours S.C.: 10,000 to 12,000 units q 8 to 12 hours Prophylactic S.C.: 5,000 units q 12 hours	• Hemorrhage • Decreased platelet count • Chills • Fever • Urticaria • Hematomas	• Do not give I.M. • Avoid administering to patients at risk for spontaneous hemorrhage (such as those with aneurysms, spinal or brain trauma, ulcers, or hemophilia). • Monitor activated partial thromboplastin time (APTT) to help determine therapeutic drug level (not to exceed 1½ to 2 times the normal APTT). • Assess for bleeding from the mouth, rectum, and injection sites. • Assess for hematomas. • Monitor vital signs. • Do not administer with aspirin. • Teach the patient to use a soft toothbrush and an electric razor. • Discontinue heparin before surgery. • Protamine sulfate is an antidote to heparin. • Heparin has a rapid action (20 to 30 minutes) and a short duration.
Warfarin sodium (Coumadin)	• Prevents vitamin K-dependent activation of clotting factors • Antagonizes clotting factors II, VII, IX, X, and prothrombin	Loading dose: 10 to 15 mg P.O. Maintenance dose: 2 to 10 mg P.O. daily	• Hemorrhage	• Monitor prothrombin time (not to exceed 1½ to 2 times the normal value). • Assess for bleeding from the mouth, rectum, and injection sites. • Assess for hematomas. • Monitor vital signs. • Do not give with aspirin. • Avoid administering to patients at risk for spontaneous hemorrhage (such as those with aneurysm, spinal or brain trauma, ulcers, or hemophilia). • Instruct the patient to use a soft toothbrush and an electric razor. • Discontinue warfarin before surgery. • Vitamin K_1 (phytonadione) is an antidote to warfarin. Vitamin K_3 (menadione) is not effective.

ADULT NURSING

RESPIRATORY SYSTEM

Anatomy and physiology

I.   **Anatomy**
A. Upper respiratory tree: nose; pharynx; larynx; trachea; left main bronchus; right main bronchus
B. Thoracic cavity
1. This is the portion of the body cavity between the neck and the respiratory diaphragm
2. It contains the two lungs, two pleural sacs, heart, pericardial sac, and mediastinum (the space between the pleurae)
C. Lungs
1. The lungs are composed of millions of alveoli (air sacs), the sites of oxygen and carbon dioxide exchange
2. The right lung has three lobes
3. The left lung has two lobes
4. The lungs are surrounded by a pleural sac, which reduces friction as the lungs move during respiration

II.   **Physiology**
A. Ventilation
1. Ventilation supplies oxygen to and removes carbon dioxide from the blood, maintains the normal pH of the blood, helps maintain normal body temperature, and helps eliminate water by way of the upper airway structures
2. During ventilation, gases move in and out of the lungs in two phases — inspiration and expiration
3. About 500 ml of gas are exchanged with each ventilation
4. Ventilatory control centers in the medulla and pons of the brain regulate respiratory rate, depth, and rhythm by sending impulses through the cervical and thoracic spine to stimulate movement of the intercostal, abdominal, and diaphragmatic muscles
B. Air passage into the lungs
1. Air enters the respiratory system via the nose or mouth
a. The nose or mouth warms and humidifies air
b. The nose also filters air
2. The pharynx (throat), serves as the first internal passageway for air
a. It provides resonance for vocal sounds
b. It also helps prevent dust particles from entering the lungs
3. The larynx (voice box), which links the pharynx with the trachea, contains structures that help convert vibrations into speech sounds
4. The trachea (windpipe) serves as a passageway for air; its mucous membrane protects against dust particles
5. The bronchi are passageways through which air enters either the right or left lung; these structures decrease progressively in size (becoming bronchioles) until air reaches the alveoli of the lungs
6. Factors that influence air passage into the lungs include the radius of the passage, lung tissue elasticity, surface tension created by the pleural sac, and changes in atmospheric pressure

Reviewing the respiratory system

The illustrations show an anterior view of the anatomy of the major structures of the respiratory system and a schematic of the basic respiratory unit.

RESPIRATORY SYSTEM

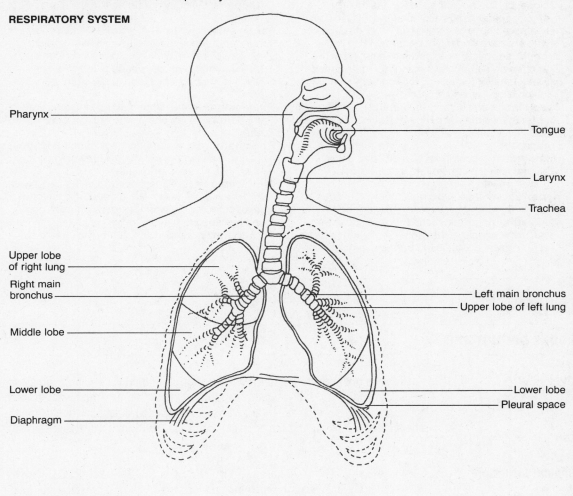

Pharynx

Tongue

Larynx

Trachea

Upper lobe of right lung

Right main bronchus

Left main bronchus

Upper lobe of left lung

Middle lobe

Lower lobe

Lower lobe

Pleural space

Diaphragm

RESPIRATORY UNIT

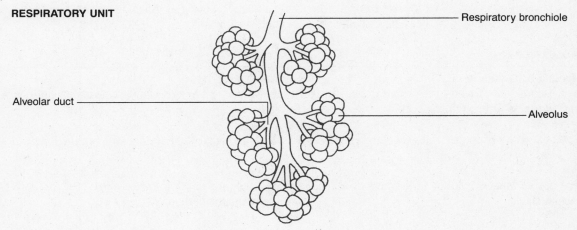

Respiratory bronchiole

Alveolar duct

Alveolus

Glossary

Arterial blood gases: oxygen, carbon dioxide, pH, bicarbonate, and other components of arterial blood; can be measured to assess the adequacy of oxygenation and ventilation (such as in patients who have respiratory or other diseases or who are receiving oxygen therapy)

Bronchoscopy: endoscopic examination of the trachea and bronchial passages with a lighted tube; used for diagnosis, foreign body removal, lesion excision, and biopsy

Dyspnea: difficult or labored breathing, as from interference with air entering or leaving the air passages or insufficient blood oxygen-carrying capacity

Hemothorax: accumulation of blood and fluid in the pleural cavity as the result of trauma, infection, or tumor growth

Hypoxia: decrease in oxygen supply to tissues; can be life-threatening if severe or prolonged

Mediastinum: portion of the thoracic cavity that lies in the middle of the thorax, between the pleural sacs; contains the trachea, heart, major cardiopulmonary vessels, esophagus, thymus, and lymph nodes

Orthopnea: difficulty breathing except in an upright position

Paroxysmal nocturnal dyspnea: difficult or labored breathing that occurs suddenly at night; caused by return of fluid from the legs to the central circulation, which overloads the heart and leads to fluid accumulation in the pulmonary system

Pneumonia: acute inflammation of the lungs resulting from infection, chemical irritation, or fluid aspiration

Pneumothorax: accumulation of air in the pleural cavity; results from trauma or chest surgery, or may have no apparent cause

Thoracentesis: surgical puncture of the chest wall into the pleural cavity with a needle to aspirate fluid for therapeutic or diagnostic purposes or to remove specimens for biopsy

Thoracotomy: surgical incision of the chest wall

Lobar pneumonia

Overview

Lobar pneumonia is a bacterial infection and inflammation of one or more lung lobes. Typically, it results from alveolar infection by a microorganism, such as *Streptococcus pneumoniae*. Inflamed tissue, fluid, and mucus become trapped. This clogs the alveoli and impedes gas exchange, resulting in decreased ventilation.

Clinical situation

Glenda Arnold, age 80, is hospitalized with a fever of 104° F (40° C), which arose suddenly 2 days ago. She complains of fatigue, pain on inspiration, and a productive cough. On examination, she appears flushed and diaphoretic; her nail beds are cyanotic. Mrs. Arnold has a history of cigarette smoking.

Assessment

Nursing behaviors

1. Observe Mrs. Arnold for tachypnea, tachycardia, and shortness of breath (dyspnea).

2. Assist with respiratory assessment, staying alert for rales (crackles) on auscultation.

3. Observe Mrs. Arnold for restlessness or change in mental status.

Nursing rationales

1. These are common signs and symptoms of pneumonia.

2. Rales signal fluid accumulation in the lungs.

3. These are signs of decreased oxygenation, especially in an elderly patient.

ADULT NURSING

Nursing diagnoses	• Ineffective airway clearance related to excessive mucus production • Activity intolerance related to decreased oxygenation
Planning and goals	• Mrs. Arnold will demonstrate improved airway clearance. • Mrs. Arnold will conserve energy needed for recovery. • Mrs. Arnold will maintain adequate hydration. • Mrs. Arnold will demonstrate understanding of and compliance with her treatment regimen.

Implementation

Nursing behaviors	**Nursing rationales**
1. Encourage Mrs. Arnold to consume fluids frequently.	**1.** Adequate hydration helps thin pulmonary secretions, improving expectoration.
2. Administer humidified oxygen, as ordered.	**2.** Humidified oxygen helps thin secretions while increasing oxygen supply, thereby improving gas exchange.
3. Assist Mrs. Arnold with pulmonary hygiene and frequent repositioning.	**3.** These measures mobilize secretions and ease expectoration.
4. Teach Mrs. Arnold how to splint the chest when coughing, and help her to do this.	**4.** Splinting decreases pain.
5. Elevate the head of Mrs. Arnold's bed.	**5.** Head elevation improves lung expansion.
6. Provide frequent rest periods and assist Mrs. Arnold with activities of daily living (ADLs), as needed.	**6.** Rest and assistance with ADLs will help Mrs. Arnold to conserve energy.
7. Teach Mrs. Arnold about proper antibiotic use, deep-breathing techniques, and smoking cessation.	**7.** Patient teaching increases therapeutic effectiveness and promotes compliance. Teaching Mrs. Arnold about antibiotics helps ensure their effective use. Teaching her about deep-breathing techniques promotes mucus removal. Instructions on smoking cessation help prevent further destruction of the lungs' natural defenses.

Evaluation (outcomes)	• Mrs. Arnold is afebrile. • Mrs. Arnold's sputum has a normal consistency and color. • Mrs. Arnold's mucous membranes and skin are free from signs of dehydration. • Mrs. Arnold rests when appropriate, especially during the acute phase of illness. • Mrs. Arnold demonstrates that she understands and complies with patient teaching by the time of discharge.

ADULT
NURSING

Pulmonary edema

Overview

Pulmonary edema occurs when the left ventricle of the heart cannot pump efficiently (such as after myocardial infarction). Reduced cardiac pumping causes blood to accumulate in the pulmonary capillary bed, increasing pressure within the capillaries. As a result, capillary fluid and blood leak into the lungs and alveoli. Other causes of pulmonary edema include excess I.V. fluid administration and severe burn injury (in the latter, pulmonary edema arises from fluid overload caused by fluid shift from the interstitial tissues into the plasma).

Clinical situation

Alfred Robinson, age 63, is hospitalized after a myocardial infarction. His recovery has progressed well, although he often stays out of bed for longer periods than prescribed. At 2 A.M., he rings his call light to complain of restlessness and inability to sleep.

Assessment

Nursing behaviors

1. Assist in assessing Mr. Robinson for signs and symptoms of left ventricular failure:
- dyspnea
- increased respiratory rate
- orthopnea
- paroxysmal nocturnal dyspnea
- frothy, blood-tinged mucus
- distended neck veins.

2. Assist in assessing Mr. Robinson for restlessness and other signs of decreased oxygenation: rapid, weak pulse; cyanotic nail beds; cool, moist skin; and pale to gray skin color.

Nursing rationales

1. These cardiopulmonary signs result from lung and alveolar congestion.

2. Restlessness may accompany pulmonary edema because the central nervous system is sensitive to decreased oxygenation. In response to decreased oxygenation, the pulse accelerates (in an attempt to improve circulating volume); nail beds become cyanotic; and the skin becomes cool and moist, taking on a pale or gray appearance (this reflects the body's attempt to redirect blood from the periphery to vital organs).

Nursing diagnoses
- Ineffective airway clearance related to inability to clear lung secretions
- Anxiety related to inadequate oxygenation

Planning and goals
- Mr. Robinson will regain normal tissue perfusion.
- Mr. Robinson will show decreased anxiety.
- Mr. Robinson will repair normal respirations.

Implementation

Nursing behaviors

1. Institute measures to prevent pulmonary edema from worsening:
- Monitor I.V. fluids closely.
- Encourage frequent rest.
- Restrict dietary sodium intake.

Nursing rationales

1. Preventing a disease from worsening is easier than treating a disease that has progressed.

ADULT NURSING

2. Elevate Mr. Robinson's head and thorax and place his legs in a dependent position.

2. Such positioning reduces circulating volume by increasing blood volume in the legs.

3. Administer oxygen, as ordered.

3. Supplemental oxygen increases the amount of oxygen available for gas exchange.

4. Monitor vital signs and central venous pressure frequently.

4. This helps detect any changes and gauge the effectiveness of therapy.

5. Administer prescribed drugs, such as diuretics, digitalis, morphine, and bronchodilators, as ordered.

5. Drug therapy is a major treatment modality for pulmonary edema. Diuretics promote fluid excretion. Digitalis improves ventricular contraction force and cardiac output. Morphine decreases pulmonary vascular pressure and relieves apprehension. Bronchodilators improve airway patency.

6. Assist in applying and monitoring rotating tourniquets.

6. Rotating tourniquets decrease circulating blood volume by trapping venous blood in the extremities.

7. Assist with phlebotomy.

7. This procedure helps relieve pulmonary congestion by removing blood from a peripheral vein. (Some authorities consider this a radical procedure.)

8. Provide emotional support.

8. This helps reduce fear and anxiety, which could increase Mr. Robinson's oxygen needs and elevate his pulse rate and arterial pressure.

Evaluation (outcomes)

- Mr. Robinson's respiratory rate returns to within normal limits.
- Mr. Robinson's lung congestion subsides (as heard on auscultation).
- Mr. Robinson's tissue perfusion improves (as shown by improved arterial blood gas findings and normal skin and nail-bed color).
- Mr. Robinson is less anxious.

Lung cancer

Overview

Cancer is characterized by uncontrolled growth of abnormal cells. Lung cancer (also called bronchogenic carcinoma) frequently is associated with cigarette smoking and environmental or occupational exposure to airborne carcinogens, such as asbestos dust. Although the success of lung cancer treatment continues to improve, the disease still carries a high mortality because of the late onset of recognizable signs and symptoms. Primary lung cancer may spread (metastasize) to the brain, bones, liver, lymphatic system, and adrenal glands.

Clinical situation

Thomas Wright, age 50, is admitted to the hospital for a diagnostic workup to investigate complaints of a productive, purulent, occasionally blood-tinged cough; increasing upper back pain; and appetite loss. He has worked in a plastics processing plant for 25 years. The suspected diagnosis is lung cancer.

ADULT NURSING

Assessment

Nursing behaviors	**Nursing rationales**
1. Assess Mr. Wright's respiratory status, including respiratory rate, depth, and rhythm, and auscultate his lungs for abnormal sounds.	**1.** A cancerous lung tumor causes lung tissue changes that alter airway patency and gas exchange.
2. Assess Mr. Wright for signs and symptoms of infection, such as an elevated temperature, abnormal culture and sensitivity test results, and changes in respiratory and urinary status.	**2.** Infection is common in patients with depressed immune responses.
3. Assess for blood in the sputum and other secretions.	**3.** Bleeding is a common sign of lung cancer.
4. Assess Mr. Wright's pain level and response to pain-relief interventions.	**4.** Pain increases as lung cancer progresses.
5. Assess Mr. Wright for changes in nutritional status.	**5.** Lung cancer can cause loss of appetite (from pain, fatigue, and anxiety).

Nursing diagnoses
- Ineffective airway clearance related to pain and thick, purulent sputum
- Altered nutrition (less than body requirements) related to anorexia

Planning and goals
- Mr. Wright's airway will remain patent and his respiratory rate will stay within normal limits.
- Mr. Wright will remain free from nosocomial (hospital-acquired) infection.
- Mr. Wright will remain free from injury and hemorrhage.
- Mr. Wright's pain will decrease.
- Mr. Wright's nutritional status will improve, as shown by weight maintenance.

Implementation

Nursing behaviors	**Nursing rationales**
1. Elevate the head of Mr. Wright's bed.	**1.** Head elevation increases lung expansion.
2. Administer humidified oxygen, as ordered.	**2.** This increases the amount of oxygen available for gas exchange.
3. Encourage Mr. Wright to perform deep-breathing and coughing exercises.	**3.** These techniques help eliminate secretions.
4. Minimize multiple venipunctures and invasive procedures.	**4.** This reduces the risk of infection and hemorrhage.
5. Monitor wounds and I.V. sites for signs of inflammation or infection.	**5.** Any skin break could serve as an entry point for infectious organisms.
6. Provide a soft diet, an electric razor, stool softeners, and a soft toothbrush. Take appropriate safety measures to prevent falls. Apply direct pressure over venipuncture sites; try to avoid multiple injections.	**6.** Preventing or minimizing trauma to the skin, mucous membranes, and musculoskeletal system reduces the risk of hemorrhage.

ADULT NURSING

Surgical lung resection

Total or partial lung resection is the most common type of thoracic surgery. To enter the pleural space, the surgeon must use a chest tube and water-seal drainage to restore negative pressure. This chart compares surgical lung resection procedures.

PROCEDURE	DESCRIPTION	INDICATIONS	TYPE OF POSTOPERATIVE CHEST-TUBE DRAINAGE
Segmental resection	Removal of one or more lung segments (not performed on the right middle lobe)	• Lung cancer	Closed
Wedge resection	Removal of a pie-shaped lung section without regard for segmental lines	• Lung cancer • Well-defined benign lung tumor • Lung biopsy • Tuberculosis	Closed
Lobectomy	Removal of an entire lung lobe	• Lung cancer • Bronchiectasis • Fungal infection • Emphysematous bleb	Closed (two tubes: upper tube for air, lower tube for fluid)
Pneumonectomy	Removal of an entire lung; performed only when lesser resections will not remove all diseased tissue	• Widespread cancer • Abscess • Tuberculosis • Bronchiectasis	None (lung tissue does not need to be reexpanded)

7. Assist with pain-control measures, such as:
• positioning Mr. Wright for comfort
• providing a quiet environment
• using appropriate distraction techniques
• encouraging Mr. Wright to report pain early
• administering analgesics promptly and regularly.

7. Pain-control measures improve patient comfort and reduce tissue oxygen demands. A comfortable position and quiet environment help decrease pain. Distractions can reduce Mr. Wright's perception of pain. Early reporting of pain ensures prompt intervention, which can prevent prolonged excessive pain. Analgesics also help prevent prolonged excessive pain.

8. Take measures to improve Mr. Wright's nutritional intake, such as:
• determining which foods he prefers
• providing small, frequent meals
• limiting fluids given with meals
• serving food in an attractive manner
• avoiding environmental odors
• administering an antiemetic agent before meals, as needed
• offering nutritional supplements between meals
• increasing Mr. Wright's intake of calories, protein, and vitamins
• avoiding serving foods that are very hot or very cold.

8. Serving preferred foods may help stimulate Mr. Wright's appetite. Small, frequent meals can help motivate him to eat; large meals, on the other hand, may discourage him from even attempting. Limiting fluids helps prevent a feeling of fullness and leaves more room for solid foods. Attractive food presentation may help stimulate Mr. Wright's appetite. Antiemetics help prevent nausea and vomiting. Nutritional supplements increase calorie and nutrient intake. Increased intake of calories, protein, and vitamins helps meet metabolic needs of cell repair and growth. Extreme food temperatures may cause oral and esophageal discomfort.

Evaluation (outcomes)

• Mr. Wright's respirations remain within normal limits.
• Mr. Wright shows no signs or symptoms of infection.
• Mr. Wright remains free from trauma and bleeding.
• Mr. Wright obtains pain relief.
• Mr. Wright eats six small meals daily and maintains his current weight.
• Mr. Wright is discharged for follow-up care.

ADULT NURSING

Chronic obstructive pulmonary disease

Overview

Chronic obstructive pulmonary disease (COPD) refers to a group of progressive, irreversible conditions characterized by airway obstruction. Such obstruction may lead to mucus accumulation (chronic bronchitis); loss of elasticity and increased resistance to air flow (emphysema); or inflamed, narrowed airways (chronic irreversible asthma). COPD is linked with environmental factors (such as air pollution), genetic factors, and cigarette smoking.

Clinical situation

Howard Gonzales, age 62, is admitted to the hospital complaining of shortness of breath on exertion, a productive cough, and frequent respiratory infections. He reports that he has smoked cigarettes since age 15. He is married, with three children and seven grandchildren.

Assessment

Nursing behaviors	Nursing rationales
1. Assess Mr. Gonzales's vital signs, especially noting his respiratory rate, rhythm, and depth.	1. Vital signs reflect the severity of respiratory dysfunction.
2. Observe Mr. Gonzales for use of accessory chest muscles to breathe.	2. This helps determine the extent of his respiratory distress.
3. Observe Mr. Gonzales's sputum for color, consistency, and amount.	3. This helps detect any infection.
4. Observe Mr. Gonzales's skin and nail-bed color.	4. Changes in skin and nail-bed color signal altered gas exchange.
5. Assess Mr. Gonzales's level of consciousness.	5. Decreased oxygenation can affect the central nervous system, leading to a change in level of consciousness.
6. Assess Mr. Gonzales's sleeping and eating patterns.	6. Changes in respiratory function can affect sleeping and eating patterns.

Nursing diagnoses

• Ineffective airway clearance related to excessive mucus production
• Impaired gas exchange related to chronic respiratory disease

Planning and goals

• Mr. Gonzales will demonstrate improved airway clearance.
• Mr. Gonzales will perform basic activities of daily living independently.
• Mr. Gonzales will understand and comply with measures to improve his respiratory function.

Implementation

Nursing behaviors	Nursing rationales
1. Place Mr. Gonzales in Fowler's position, or have him fold and rest his arms on a padded pillow on the overbed table.	1. These positions increase lung expansion.

ADULT NURSING

2. Maintain oxygen therapy (not to exceed 2 liters/minute), and monitor Mr. Gonzales frequently.

2. Oxygen therapy helps correct hypoxemia. Mr. Gonzales needs to be monitored because too much oxygen can depress the breathing stimulus of a patient with COPD, which hinges on a high partial pressure of arterial carbon dioxide ($PaCO_2$).

3. Assist with nebulizer and aerosol treatments.

3. These treatments are used to administer medications (such as bronchodilators), liquefy secretions, and stimulate effective coughing.

4. Encourage Mr. Gonzales to maintain a high fluid intake.

4. Good hydration helps liquefy secretions.

5. Teach Mr. Gonzales how to perform pursed-lip and diaphragmatic breathing.

5. These breathing techniques improve respiratory rate and depth.

6. Assist with chest and respiratory therapy.

6. Postural drainage, clapping, and aerosol therapy aid bronchial secretion removal.

7. Instruct Mr. Gonzales to limit his activities and rest frequently.

7. Activity limitations and frequent rest will help Mr. Gonzales avoid dyspnea and fatigue.

8. Teach Mr. Gonzales how to decrease his exposure to respiratory infection and recognize early signs and symptoms of infection.

8. Like any patient with COPD, Mr. Gonzales is susceptible to respiratory infection. Patient participation in treatment helps maintain an optimal functioning level.

9. Inform Mr. Gonzales about smoking cessation programs and related support groups.

9. Smoking cessation is important because smoking causes severe respiratory irritation, hypoxia, and depressed respiratory function.

10. Teach Mr. Gonzales about measures to reduce his exposure to respiratory irritants (such as air pollution, hair sprays, and paint fumes) and temperature extremes.

10. Exposure to respiratory irritants and temperature extremes can cause bronchospasm.

Evaluation (outcomes)

- Mr. Gonzales demonstrates reduced dyspnea and improved skin color.
- Mr. Gonzales has fewer coughing episodes.
- Mr. Gonzales participates in basic self-care and alternates physical activity with rest.
- Mr. Gonzales uses proper positioning and breathing techniques to enhance respiration.
- Mr. Gonzales avoids smoking cigarettes and avoids exposure to other respiratory irritants.

Pulmonary tuberculosis

Overview

Pulmonary tuberculosis is a chronic infection caused by *Mycobacterium tuberculosis*, an airborne organism usually transmitted by inhalation or ingestion of infected drops. The organism enters the pulmonary system and remains in the alveoli, where it multiplies and inflames tissues. Unless the disease is treated,

ADULT NURSING

tubercules (small nodules) form, walling off the fibrotic tissue from healthy tissue. These tubercles enlarge and coalesce to form larger tubercles that become necrotic; the organism is swept into the surrounding tissue and lymphatic system. Tubercles can become dormant or inactive; an inactive tubercle can become activated at any time, especially after physical or emotional stress. Tuberculosis is associated with crowded living conditions, poor sanitation, and immunosuppression.

Clinical situation   Aida Lee, age 43, visits the health clinic after coughing up blood. She reports that she has lost weight recently, frequently coughs up thick mucus, and wakes up in the middle of the night covered with sweat. Ms. Lee immigrated to the United States from Asia 1 year ago. She works 16 hours a day in a local restaurant and lives with her sister's family of six in a two-bedroom apartment.

Assessment

Nursing behaviors

1. Assess Ms. Lee for risk factors for tuberculosis:
• exposure to an infected person
• a history of cancer, acquired immunodeficiency syndrome (AIDS), or steroid therapy
• alcohol abuse
• malnutrition
• scarred lung tissue
• recent visit to an underdeveloped country.

2. Evaluate the site of the tuberculin skin test (Mantoux test) in 48 hours and 72 hours. An induration (red, hardened area) measuring 5 mm to 9 mm or more indicates a positive result.

3. Assess Ms. Lee for signs and symptoms of active tuberculosis, such as weight loss, fever, night sweats, mucopurulent cough, hemoptysis (bloody sputum), and anemia.

Nursing rationales

1. Early recognition and proper treatment of tuberculosis help prevent disease transmission.

2. The tuberculin skin test is used to diagnose and identify patients infected with tuberculosis.

3. These are common signs and symptoms of active tuberculosis.

Nursing diagnoses   • Knowledge deficit related to the disease and its transmission
• Ineffective airway clearance related to productive cough and hemoptysis

Planning and goals   • Ms. Lee will express an understanding of the disease, including its transmission and medications used to treat it.
• Ms. Lee will comply with her treatment regimen and keep follow-up medical visits until cleared by the physician.
• Ms. Lee will take prescribed cough medication and demonstrate proper coughing technique.

Implementation

Nursing behaviors

1. Take universal precautions when handling Ms. Lee's respiratory secretions. Provide her with tissues and show her how to dispose of them properly. Use a mask when caring for her, if necessary.

Nursing rationales

1. These measures help prevent the spread of tuberculosis through mucus secretions.

2. Teach Ms. Lee how to create positive environmental conditions, including adequate sunlight and fresh air.

3. Encourage Ms. Lee to take cough medications and use proper positioning.

4. Take measures to improve Ms. Lee's appetite and calorie intake, such as teaching her how to perform good oral hygiene and providing favorite foods in small, frequent meals.

5. Teach Ms. Lee how to prevent tuberculosis transmission, such as by washing her hands frequently, covering her mouth when coughing or sneezing, and disposing of tissues properly.

6. Teach Ms. Lee how to take prescribed medications, stressing that she must take them consistently on a long-term basis. Inform her that members of her household should take prophylactic medications.

7. Teach Ms. Lee to avoid respiratory irritants, such as dust, smoke, and chemicals.

8. Refer Ms. Lee to a community health service nurse for follow-up medical care and family evaluation for tuberculosis.

2. Ultraviolet light from sunlight destroys the tuberculosis-causing organism. Fresh air dilutes the concentration of airborne organisms.

3. Cough suppressants and a semi-Fowler's position enhance comfort and promote rest.

4. These measures stimulate the appetite and increase calorie intake.

5. These measures help prevent the spread of mucus and droplets containing the tuberculosis organism.

6. This helps ensure the success of treatment. Noncompliance with drug therapy by an infected patient and household members is the most common cause of treatment failure.

7. This helps prevent further lung damage.

8. This helps remove sources of tuberculosis transmission and determines if family members are infected.

Evaluation (outcomes)

• Ms. Lee takes her medications as prescribed and complies with follow-up medical appointments.
• Ms. Lee expresses an understanding of disease transmission and encourages household members and others with whom she has had contact to seek medical attention.

Ensuring medical asepsis

Medical asepsis refers to the removal or destruction of disease organisms or infected material to limit or interrupt the chain of events leading to infection spread.

By following these measures, you can help maintain medical asepsis:
● Wash your hands before and after providing treatment, serving a meal, or having other patient contact.
● Keep patient areas well ventilated.

● Dispose of contaminated materials properly (in closed containers).
● Avoid shaking bed linens.
● Clean all bedside equipment before using it with another patient.
● Do not let your nurse's uniform touch bed linens.
● Dispose of soiled bed linens in a closed container.
● Use gloves when directly handling body secretions or materials contaminated with secretions.

ADULT NURSING

Complications of respiratory disorders

This chart presents the most serious or life-threatening complications of respiratory disorders, along with interventions that are crucial to patient safety and comfort.

COMPLICATION	CAUSE	NURSING INTERVENTIONS
Atelectasis Abnormal condition characterized by alveolar collapse. The condition impedes gas exchange, causing dyspnea, cyanosis, chest pain, tachycardia, and a sense of doom.	• Airway obstruction by a foreign body or mucus secretions • Shallow breathing, such as from immobility, pain, or drugs that depress respirations • Chest wall injury • Increased thoracic cavity pressure • Pneumothorax • Tumor • Heart enlargement • Diaphragm displacement • Hemothorax	• Assess respiratory rate, depth, and rhythm. • Auscultate the lungs. • Encourage deep-breathing and coughing exercises. • Encourage early ambulation. • Perform chest physiotherapy.
Lung abscess Formation of a lung cavity containing pus (dead leukocytes and fluid) where lung tissue has become necrotic and collapsed. Signs and symptoms include a productive cough, chills, fever, painful respirations, and decreased breath sounds.	• Infection secondary to tumor growth • Pneumonia • Aspiration of infected mucus secretions • Chest trauma	• Assess respirations for rate and depth. • Auscultate the lungs for abnormal sounds. • Administer antibiotics, as ordered. • Encourage adequate fluid intake. • Monitor fluid intake and output. • Encourage deep-breathing and coughing exercises. • Perform chest physiotherapy.
Mediastinal shift Abnormal condition in which air leaks into the intrapleural space and cannot escape. The resulting increase in thoracic pressure causes compression of the heart and great vessels on the side opposite the pressure increase, severely reducing cardiac output and possibly causing shock and death. Signs and symptoms include dyspnea, shock, and a displaced apical beat.	Tension pneumothorax (air in the intrapleural space) caused by spontaneous lung rupture, lung puncture (as from rib fracture), blunt chest trauma, an open chest wound, or interruption of a closed-chest tube drainage system	• Notify the physician immediately. • Assess for deviation of the trachea from its normal midline position. • Assess the patient's respirations and auscultate the chest. • Monitor the vital signs and electrocardiogram. • Enforce complete bed rest. • Place the patient in semi-Fowler's position. • Prepare for chest tube insertion.
Pleural effusion Abnormal fluid accumulation in the pleural space. Signs and symptoms include painful respirations, decreased breath sounds, dyspnea, fever, and chills (if pleural effusion stems from pneumonia).	• Movement of plasma into the pleural space, as from heart failure, infection, trauma, or tumor • Inflammation that causes fluid accumulation in the pleural sac, such as from lung infection or tumor	• Assess vital signs and breath sounds. • Elevate the head of the bed and place the patient in semi-Fowler's position. • Position the patient for comfort. • Administer pain medication, as ordered and needed. • Prepare the patient for a thoracotomy.

Complications of respiratory disorders *(continued)*

COMPLICATION	CAUSE	NURSING INTERVENTIONS
Pneumothorax Accumulation of air in the thoracic cavity, causing increased pressure and lung collapse (atelectasis). Signs and symptoms include sudden chest pain, tachypnea, and decreased breath sounds in the affected area.	• Open chest wound that creates positive pressure in the thoracic cavity • Closed chest injury causing laceration of lung tissue and escape of air from alveoli into the pleural cavity	• Assess respirations for rate and depth. • Auscultate the lungs for abnormal sounds. • Elevate the head of the bed and place the patient in semi-Fowler's position. • Administer oxygen therapy, as ordered. • Restrict the patient's activity. • Teach the patient how to perform deep-breathing and coughing exercises. • Prepare the patient for a thoracotomy.
Pulmonary embolism Obstruction of a pulmonary artery by an embolus (such as a thrombus, foreign matter, air, or tumor tissue). Commonly, the embolus originates in the deep veins of the legs and becomes dislodged, moving through the circulatory system to a pulmonary artery. Pulmonary embolism decreases circulation to the affected lung tissue, causing tissue death (necrosis) and preventing gas exchange in the affected area. The heart tries to compensate by pumping harder, until it fails; shock ensues. Signs and symptoms of pulmonary embolism include dyspnea, sudden chest pain, anxiety, tachycardia, and syncope. Symptom severity depends on the size of the embolus and the occluded pulmonary artery.	Conditions that decrease blood flow, including immobility, crossing the legs when sitting or lying in bed, constrictive clothing (especially of the legs), dehydration, and abnormal blood coagulation	• Place the patient in semi-Fowler's position. • Administer oxygen therapy, as ordered. • Monitor vital signs. • Administer narcotics for pain relief, as ordered. • Provide emotional support. • Administer anticoagulant therapy, as ordered. • Enforce bed rest. • Instruct the patient to wear elastic stockings, if ordered. • Prepare the patient for an embolectomy. • To help *prevent* pulmonary embolism, encourage proper fluid intake and early ambulation; perform range-of-motion exercises (for the immobilized patient); and instruct the patient not to cross the legs while lying in bed or sitting and not to dangle the legs over the side of bed.
Respiratory failure Failure of the respiratory system to meet the body's oxygen needs	• Chronic conditions that cause gradual structural changes leading to decreased PaO_2 and increased $PaCO_2$ (such as emphysema and bronchitis) • Acute conditions that cause a sudden change in thoracic structure or depress the central nervous system (such as drug overdose, head or spinal cord injury, anesthesia, upper airway obstruction, or chest trauma)	• Assess for presence of respirations. • Elevate the head of the bed. • Administer oxygen therapy, as ordered. • Restrict the patient's activity to conserve oxygen. • Encourage fluids (if not contraindicated) to prevent fluid imbalance. • Perform chest physiotherapy.

ADULT NURSING

Caring for the patient with a chest tube

Introduction

A chest tube is a firm rubber or plastic tube that is inserted through the chest wall into the thoracic cavity to remove air and fluid. It helps prevent lung tissue from collapsing and creates negative thoracic pressure (needed for normal respiration) after pneumothorax, hemothorax, or thoracic surgery. The chest tube is attached to one or more collection bottles or to a disposable commercial chest drainage system, such as a Pleurovac unit. The drainage receptacle is sealed tightly to prevent air and fluid from reentering the thoracic cavity. Gravity or suction is used to promote drainage. (Procedure steps preceded by an asterisk are especially important.)

Steps	**Rationales**
1. Before chest tube insertion, assess the patient's baseline vital signs.	**1.** Changes in vital signs may signal cardiopulmonary changes, such as tension pneumothorax or mediastinal shift.
*2. Explain the procedure to the patient and make sure a signed informed consent has been obtained.	***2.** Explanations reduce patient anxiety; informed consent is needed because chest tube insertion is an invasive procedure.
3. After chest tube insertion, mark the drainage level in the receptacle with tape, including the date and time of the marking.	**3.** This helps determine how much chest tube drainage is collected during each shift.
*4. Keep the drainage receptacle below the patient's chest level.	***4.** This enhances drainage flow by gravity.
5. Loop the tubing on the bed and fasten it to keep it free from kinks.	**5.** This helps prevent dependent loops, which decrease the system's effectiveness.
6. Ensure that the water-seal tube is below water level.	**6.** This prevents air from reentering the thoracic cavity.
7. Check for fluctuation of the fluid level of the water-seal bottle or chamber when the patient breathes or coughs.	**7.** Fluctuation means that the chest tube system is functioning properly.
8. Place the patient in a semi-high Fowler's position.	**8.** This position promotes drainage.
*9. Check for gentle continuous bubbling in the suction-control bottle or chamber.	***9.** Bubbling ensures that the suction device is working properly. The correct amount of suction is maintained when the long tube is under 4″ to 8″ (10.2 to 20.3 cm) of water.
10. Keep two hemostats at the patient's bedside.	**10.** Hemostats are used when changing drainage collection bottles or the commercial drainage system. (However, do not clamp tubes when the system malfunctions because this may cause a tension pneumothorax, lung collapse, or mediastinal shift.)

ADULT NURSING

Closed chest drainage systems

The illustrations show underwater seal drainage systems from the simplest (one-bottle) to the more complex (three-bottle). Each system is designed to keep air from entering the chest by providing a water seal.

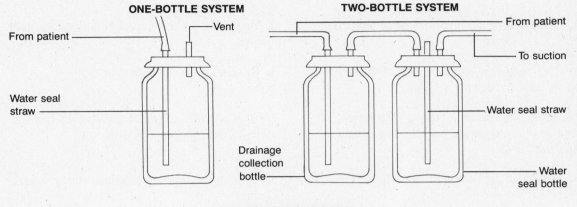

ONE-BOTTLE SYSTEM

From patient

Vent

Water seal straw

Drainage collection bottle

TWO-BOTTLE SYSTEM

From patient

To suction

Water seal straw

Water seal bottle

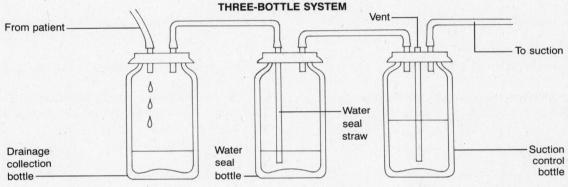

THREE-BOTTLE SYSTEM

From patient

Vent

To suction

Drainage collection bottle

Water seal bottle

Water seal straw

Suction control bottle

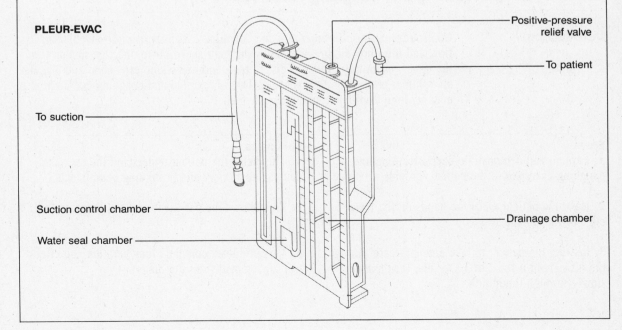

PLEUR-EVAC

To suction

Suction control chamber

Water seal chamber

Positive-pressure relief valve

To patient

Drainage chamber

11. Encourage frequent turning and deep-breathing exercises.

11. These measures promote lung expansion.

12. Assess the patient's lung sounds.

12. This helps evaluate lung reexpansion.

During chest tube removal

1. Explain the removal procedure to the patient.

1. Explanations decrease patient anxiety.

2. Administer medication (such as an antianxiety agent), as ordered.

2. Medication promotes comfort during chest tube removal.

3. Have the patient sit on the side of the bed or lie on the unaffected side.

3. These positions aid chest tube removal.

*4. Instruct the patient to take a deep breath and hold it, or to exhale and hold the breath until the tube is removed.

*4. This prevents air from reentering the thoracic cavity through the chest wound.

5. Assist with application of an occlusive dressing.

5. An occlusive dressing promotes aseptic wound closure.

6. Assess the patient's vital signs.

6. Vital signs may reflect changes in the patient's status.

7. Assess the dressing for drainage.

7. This helps determine the status of the wound site.

8. Document the procedure and the patient's response.

8. Documentation proves that the procedure was done, assures high-quality care, and provides legal protection.

Teaching deep-breathing and coughing exercises

Introduction

Controlled, purposeful breathing and coughing exercises increase alveolar air flow and intrathoracic pressure, allowing high-speed air to dislodge mucus from the upper respiratory airway. This, in turn, improves lung expansion and alveolar air volume, promoting gas exchange. Deep-breathing and coughing exercises also may be done to promote pulmonary hygiene.

Steps

1. Explain and demonstrate deep-breathing and coughing exercises to the patient; provide a rationale.

Rationales

1. This helps the patient understand the exercises, decreasing anxiety and promoting compliance.

2. Have the patient place the hands on the lower edge of the rib cage.

2. This allows the patient to feel the lungs expand.

3. Instruct the patient to take a deep breath through the nose, hold it for 2 to 3 seconds, then exhale slowly through the mouth.

3. This promotes complete lung aeration and effective air removal from the lungs.

4. Have the patient take several deep breaths, then another deep breath. Instruct the patient to hold this second breath for 2 to 3 seconds, then cough forcefully once or twice using chest and abdominal muscles.

4. This promotes airway clearance by increasing airway diameter and forces a large volume of air beneath the mucus to push it outward with each cough.

5. If the patient has a chest or abdominal incision, demonstrate how to splint the incision site with the hands or a pillow.

5. Splinting supports the incision site during coughing, reducing pain and promoting more effective coughing.

6. Place an appropriate receptacle at the bedside for sputum collection or tissue disposal.

6. This ensures hygienic handling of sputum and tissues.

7. Provide oral hygiene after coughing exercises.

7. Oral hygiene promotes patient comfort.

8. Document the procedure and the patient's response.

8. Documentation proves that the procedure was done, assures high-quality care, and provides legal protection.

Performing postural drainage

Introduction

Postural drainage, a technique involving special patient positioning and the use of gravity, helps drain secretions from various segments of the bronchi and lungs into the trachea. This allows easier removal of thick secretions by coughing and suctioning, maintains open airways, and decreases mucus accumulation, reducing the risk of respiratory infection. (Procedure steps preceded by an asterisk are especially important.)

Steps

1. Assemble needed supplies: tissues, sputum collection container, pillows, adjustable bed.

Rationales

1. Assembling supplies beforehand promotes proper handling of secretions and helps the patient assume the required positions.

2. Assess the patient's lung sounds for crackles, wheezes, and gurgling.

2. These sounds help identify which lung and bronchial segments need to be drained.

3. Assess the patient for contraindications to postural drainage: recent myocardial infarction, heart failure, head trauma, thoracic hemorrhage, or pulmonary distress.

3. Postural drainage can cause cardiovascular, pulmonary, or neurologic trauma.

4. Explain the procedure to the patient.

4. Explanations reduce patient anxiety and promote compliance.

5. Drape the patient appropriately, using bed linens or pajamas.

5. This maintains patient privacy.

*6. Position the patient for appropriate lung segment drainage:
• semi-Fowler's position for the anterior upper lobes
• upright sitting position in bed or in a chair, leaning forward over pillows with the arms crossed, or lying on the side with a pillow under the chest, for the posterior upper lobes
• Trendelenburg's position (right or left side), with the chest supine and the knees flexed, for the anterior middle lobes
• prone, with pillows under the abdomen and hips, for the posterior middle lobes
• Trendelenburg's position and supine, for the anterior lower lobes
• right or left side-lying position and Trendelenburg's position, for the lateral segments of the right or left lower lobe
• prone position and Trendelenburg's position, for the posterior lower lobes.

*6. These positions promote the most effective use of gravity to drain secretions from the affected lung segment.

7. Have the patient remain in the appropriate position for 10 to 15 minutes.

7. This allows enough time for drainage.

8. Use the appropriate percussion and vibration techniques, as ordered.

8. These techniques loosen mucus from the airways to promote mucus removal.

9. Assist the patient with coughing techniques or suctioning.

9. This helps remove mucus.

10. Collect a sputum specimen and examine it.

10. This determines the need for increased fluids and may reveal signs of infection.

11. Provide the patient with mouthwash for oral hygiene.

11. This increases patient comfort.

12. Encourage the patient to rest.

12. Positional changes cause fatigue.

13. Schedule postural drainage two to four times times daily. Avoid performing it shortly after a meal.

13. Postural drainage can cause fatigue; treatments must be spaced to allow enough rest. When done immediately after a meal, postural drainage can cause vomiting.

14. Document the procedure and the patient's response.

14. Documentation proves that the procedure was done, assures high-quality care, and provides legal protection.

ADULT
NURSING

Administering intermittent positive-pressure breathing treatments

Introduction

Intermittent positive-pressure breathing (IPPB) is a technique in which the lungs are inflated periodically with compressed air or oxygen under pressure and allowed to empty through a valve by passive exhalation. The cycle recurs as inhalation triggers the flow of gas. IPPB delivers more air to the alveoli for gas exchange, thereby improving lung expansion, preventing atelectasis, and increasing oxygenation. *Note:* In most institutions, portable incentive spirometry has replaced IPPB. However, IPPB treatment commonly is used to deliver medications that dilate the bronchi and remove mucus. (Procedure steps preceded by an asterisk are especially important.)

Steps

1. Assess the patient's lungs by auscultation.

2. Explain the procedure to the patient.

3. Place the patient in semi-Fowler's position.

4. Add ordered medication to the medication chamber (which is part of the IPPB machine).

*5. Instruct the patient to close the lips around the IPPB mouthpiece and start inhaling. Then allow the machine to complete the inspiratory cycle.

6. Instruct the patient to exhale passively and maintain a slow respiratory rate.

7. Encourage productive coughing during and after the procedure.

8. Observe sputum characteristics.

9. Document the procedure, the patient's response to treatment, coughing results, and post-treatment lung sounds.

Rationales

1. This helps determine the need for IPPB treatment and establishes a baseline for later comparison.

2. Explanations decrease patient anxiety and promote compliance.

3. This position promotes maximum lung expansion.

4. This allows proper dispersion of medication.

*5. This allows the IPPB machine to deliver the accurate air volume.

6. This prevents hyperventilation.

7. Productive coughing helps remove pulmonary secretions.

8. This helps determine the patient's hydration status (for example, thick, tenacious sputum may mean poor hydration). It also helps detect signs of infection (such as an abnormal color).

9. Documentation proves that the procedure was done, assures high-quality care, and provides legal protection.

ADULT NURSING

Assisting with incentive spirometry

Introduction

An incentive spirometer is a hand-held, patient-operated device that promotes voluntary deep breathing. By providing visual feedback, the spirometer allows the patient to see the results of increased inspiratory effort. Incentive spirometry is used to increase lung expansion, prevent atelectasis, improve oxygenation, and measure the effort needed to sustain maximal inspiration. (Procedure steps preceded by an asterisk are especially important.)

Steps	**Rationales**
1. Assess the patient's respiratory status.	**1.** This provides baseline data used to evaluate therapeutic effectiveness.
2. Explain the procedure to the patient.	**2.** Explanations decrease anxiety and promote compliance.
3. Place the patient in semi-Fowler's position.	**3.** This position promotes lung expansion.
***4.** Instruct the patient to close the lips tightly around the spirometer's mouthpiece, then inhale slowly through the mouthpiece while watching the device to achieve the desired inspiratory volume.	***4.** Closing the lips tightly around the mouthpiece ensures the tight seal needed for proper spirometer use. A lighted display or floating balls provide visual feedback.
5. Instruct the patient to inhale as deeply as possible, hold the breath for 2 to 3 seconds, then exhale slowly.	**5.** This permits enough time for alveolar expansion.
6. Instruct the patient to take several normal breaths intermittently between uses of the spirometer.	**6.** This prevents hyperventilation.
7. After the patient completes the procedure, clean the mouthpiece and store the spirometer in a clean place.	**7.** This prevents contamination of the device.
8. Document the procedure and the patient's response.	**8.** Documentation proves that the procedure was done, assures high-quality care, and provides legal protection.

Administering oxygen

Introduction

Supplemental air with a greater oxygen concentration than normal atmospheric air is administered to prevent or treat hypoxia. Oxygen can be delivered by such devices as a nasal catheter, cannula, and face mask. (Procedure steps preceded by an asterisk are especially important.)

Steps

1. Assess the patient for respiratory distress or hypoxia.

2. Explain the procedure to the patient.

3. Assemble needed supplies and post "No smoking" signs outside the room.

4. Apply the appropriate oxygen administration device, as ordered. If using a nasal cannula or catheter, place the tips of the device in the nostrils and adjust the plastic slide comfortably around the patient's head. If using a face mask, select the appropriate type and proper size. Securely cover the patient's nose and mouth with the mask, then secure the mask in place with an elastic strap.

*5. Attach the oxygen tubing to a humidifying unit filled with distilled sterile water.

6. Drain excess water from the humidifier tubing, as needed.

*7. Check the water level of the humidifying unit every 4 hours, and refill as needed.

*8. Evaluate the patient's response to oxygen therapy, for example, by assessing skin color, vital signs, and arterial blood gas findings.

9. Document the procedure and the patient's response to supplemental oxygen.

Rationales

1. Hypoxia must be prevented or treated early to avoid permanent organ damage.

2. Explanations decrease anxiety and promote compliance.

3. Having needed supplies on hand ensures efficient and rapid completion of the procedure. Posting "No smoking" signs helps prevent fire (oxygen supports combustion and fuels fire).

4. Proper placement and good fit of the administration device help ensure delivery of the prescribed oxygen concentration.

*5. Providing humidified oxygen prevents drying of the oral and nasal mucosa.

6. This prevents bacterial growth within the oxygen administration system.

*7. This promotes adequate oxygen humidification.

*8. This helps determine the effectiveness of oxygen therapy.

9. Documentation proves that the procedure was done, assures high-quality care, and provides legal protection.

ADULT NURSING

Assisting with thoracentesis

Introduction

Thoracentesis is a medical procedure in which the physician perforates the chest wall and pleural space with a needle. It is done to remove air or fluid from the pleural cavity, thereby reducing friction and promoting lung expansion; instill antibiotics or chemotherapeutic drugs into the pleural cavity; or diagnose a respiratory disorder (for instance, by evaluating fluid characteristics or obtaining a biopsy specimen). (Procedure steps preceded by an asterisk are especially important.)

Steps	Rationales
1. Assemble needed supplies.	**1.** This promotes patient safety and comfort.
2. Explain the procedure to the patient.	**2.** Explanations decrease anxiety and promote cooperation and informed consent.
*3. Make sure the patient has signed an informed consent form.	***3.** Thoracentesis is an invasive procedure and requires signed informed consent.
*4. Maintain sterile technique and asepsis.	***4.** This helps prevent infection.
5. Before the procedure, assess the patient's vital signs and respiratory status.	**5.** This provides baseline data for later comparison.
6. Position the patient upright with the arms supported by an overbed table padded with pillows, or in a side-lying position with the head of the bed elevated and the arm on the involved side raised.	**6.** Either position promotes patient comfort and safe needle insertion between the ribs.
7. Warn the patient to avoid sudden movements, such as coughing, during the procedure.	**7.** This helps prevent trauma while the needle is inserted into the pleural cavity.
8. Provide emotional support during the procedure.	**8.** This decreases patient anxiety and promotes comfort.
*9. After the procedure, assess the patient's respiratory status, vital signs, and skin color. Evaluate the dressing for drainage.	***9.** This helps detect hemorrhage caused by an abnormal fluid shift or by liver, spleen, or lung injury resulting from the procedure.
10. Document the procedure and the patient's response.	**10.** Documentation proves that the procedure was done, assures high-quality care, and provides legal protection.

ADULT NURSING

Performing tracheal suctioning

Introduction   To suction the trachea, the nurse inserts a flexible sterile plastic tube into the trachea and uses suction to remove excess secretions. Tracheal suctioning maintains a patent airway, promoting optimal oxygenation; reduces the risk of infection from secretions harboring microorganisms; and helps stimulate coughing, enhancing the effectiveness of pulmonary hygiene. (Procedure steps preceded by an asterisk are especially important.)

Steps	Rationales
1. Near a wall suction source, gather needed supplies: sterile kit containing gloves, catheter, and rinse cup; and connecting tubing.	**1.** Gathering supplies in advance promotes a smooth work flow and aids patient comfort.
2. Explain the procedure to the patient.	**2.** Explanations reduce anxiety and promote cooperation.

3. Assess the patient's vital signs and auscultate the lungs.

3. This provides baseline data for later comparison.

4. Place the patient in semi-Fowler's position.

4. This position promotes lung expansion and prevents aspiration of gastric contents.

5. Open the sterile supply tray and fill the receptacle with sterile saline solution or water.

5. This helps maintain aseptic technique.

6. Turn on the suction machine and set it at 80 to 120 mm Hg of pressure for a child or 120 to 150 mm Hg for an adult.

6. This negative pressure level prevents irritation of tracheal tissue.

*7. Have the patient hyperinflate the lungs by taking several deep breaths. (If the patient is unconscious, use a manual resuscitation bag to hyperinflate the lungs.)

*7. Suctioning reduces breathing ability; hyperinflation ensures adequate oxygenation during suctioning.

8. Put on sterile gloves and attach a sterile catheter to the suction tubing.

8. This helps maintain aseptic technique.

*9. With the suction turned off, insert the catheter about 4″ to 5″ (10.2 to 12.7 cm) into the trachea.

*9. This ensures proper catheter placement within the trachea.

Placement of a suction catheter

The illustration shows the proper placement of a suction catheter using a Y-connector that prevents tissue injury.

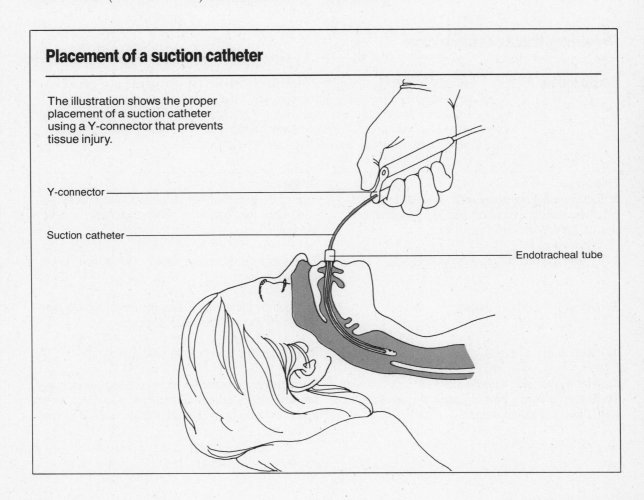

Y-connector

Suction catheter

Endotracheal tube

ADULT NURSING

10. Turn on the suction machine and apply intermittent suction for 5 to 10 seconds while gently rotating, then removing, the catheter.

11. Rinse the catheter with sterile saline solution or water.

12. Repeat suctioning only if necessary.

13. Properly dispose of used supplies.

*14. Have the patient hyperinflate the lungs (as described in step 7).

15. Auscultate the patient's lungs.

16. Document the procedure, its results, and the patient's response.

10. This prevents severe oxygen depletion and tissue irritation.

11. This clears the suction catheter.

12. Repeating suctioning only when necessary helps prevent oxygen depletion and tissue damage from excessive suctioning.

13. This helps prevent the spread of microorganisms.

*14. This replaces oxygen lost during suctioning.

15. This helps evaluate the effectiveness of suctioning.

16. Documentation proves that the procedure was done, assures high-quality care, and provides legal protection.

Providing tracheostomy care

Introduction

In this procedure, the nurse systematically cleans the inner and outer cannulas and the skin surrounding a tracheostomy. Tracheostomy care promotes airway clearance and cleanliness, improving oxygenation; it also maintains the integrity of skin surrounding the tracheostomy, reducing the risk of infection. (Procedure steps preceded by an asterisk are especially important.)

Steps

1. Prepare a tracheostomy care kit. Pour hydrogen peroxide into one receptacle and sterile saline solution or sterile water into the other.

2. Explain the procedure to the patient.

3. Suction the patient's trachea.

4. Put on sterile gloves.

5. Remove the inner cannula and soak it in peroxide. Then scrub it with a pipe cleaner and rinse it with sterile water or saline solution.

Rationales

1. Preparing needed supplies in advance promotes a good work flow and helps prevent contamination of the field.

2. Explanations decrease anxiety and promote cooperation.

3. Tracheal suctioning before the inner cannula is removed removes excess mucus secretions.

4. This helps prevent stoma contamination.

5. Hydrogen peroxide loosens dried secretions; rinsing with sterile saline solution or sterile water prevents peroxide from entering the trachea and causing irritation.

6. Dry the cannula with sterile cotton.

6. This prevents liquid from entering the trachea.

*7. Reinsert the clean inner cannula and lock it in place.

*7. This maintains airway patency.

*8. Using a cotton-tipped applicator, clean the periostomal tissue with peroxide and rinse with sterile water or saline solution.

*8. Peroxide loosens dried secretions; rinsing with sterile water or saline solution removes peroxide, which can irritate the skin.

9. Apply antibiotic ointment (if ordered) and a dry sterile tracheostomy dressing.

9. This helps maintain a clean environment and minimizes the risk of infection.

*10. Change the tracheostomy ties and make sure they are securely in place before leaving the patient's bedside.

*10. This helps prevent extubation of the tracheostomy cannula.

11. Properly dispose of all contaminated dressings and cleaning materials.

11. This helps prevent the spread of microorganisms.

12. Position the patient comfortably.

12. This promotes rest.

13. Document the procedure and the patient's response.

13. Documentation proves that the procedure was done, assures high-quality care, and provides legal protection.

Caring for a patient requiring mechanical ventilation

Introduction

A mechanical ventilator is a machine that assists or controls ventilation. It is used to prevent irreversible tissue damage or death in a patient with decreased partial pressure of arterial oxygen (PaO_2) and elevated partial pressure of arterial carbon dioxide ($PaCO_2$). Mechanical ventilation is used for patients who are apneic (lacking spontaneous respirations) or who cannot breathe adequately to meet tissue oxygenation needs. Such patients typically include those recovering from thoracic surgery and those with advanced COPD, multisystem trauma, or central nervous system or spinal cord injury. Several types of mechanical ventilators are available; all operate on the same basic principle. Nursing care aims to maintain airway patency, prevent infection, avoid problems of immobility, and meet the emotional needs of the patient and family.

ADULT NURSING

Steps
1. Assess the patient's vital signs and respiratory function.

Rationales
1. Vital signs may reflect changes in respiratory and cardiovascular function. Assessing respiratory function is important in case the ventilator malfunctions or becomes disconnected.

2. Using a checklist, assess the mechanical ventilator for proper function and settings.

2. Although the respiratory therapist usually is responsible for ensuring proper ventilator function, the nurse is responsible for the patient's safety.

3. Assess for proper endotracheal or tracheostomy tube alignment and cuff inflation.

3. This helps ensure proper oxygen delivery to the lungs without oxygen leakage.

4. Auscultate the patient's lungs at least every 2 hours during mechanical ventilation.

4. This helps verify proper ventilator function.

5. Maintain proper positioning, depending on the patient's condition. Reposition the patient every 2 hours.

5. This helps maintain a patent airway and prevent fluid accumulation with consequent atelectasis.

6. Maintain the proper level of sterile distilled water in the humidifier unit.

6. This prevents drying of the mucous membranes and helps liquefy and remove secretions.

7. Provide endotracheal tracheostomy tube care and oral hygiene at least every 8 hours.

7. This helps prevent infection.

8. Assess the patient's abdomen for distention and bowel sounds.

8. This helps determine gastrointestinal (GI) function, which typically decreases from prolonged immobility.

9. Perform range-of-motion exercises on all extremities every 4 hours.

9. This helps prevent contractures and stimulates circulatory, respiratory, and GI function.

10. Ensure an alternative communication method for the patient (if conscious), such as by having the patient blink the eyes to indicate a certain response or use a letter board, pencil and pad, or gestures.

10. Mechanical ventilation impairs the patient's oral communication. An alternative communication method ensures that the patient can communicate needs.

11. Explain all procedures to the patient and family. Use stress-reduction techniques, such as music, massage, and diversion.

11. Explanations and stress-reduction techniques decrease anxiety and help the patient cope.

12. Document the procedure and the patient's response.

12. Documentation proves that the procedure was done, assures high-quality care, and provides legal protection.

ADULT
NURSING

Drugs used for respiratory disorders

This chart presents information about drugs commonly prescribed for respiratory disorders, including the drug action, dosage, and common side effects. Nursing considerations focus on patient comfort and teaching.

DRUG	ACTION	USUAL ADULT DOSAGE	COMMON SIDE EFFECTS	NURSING CONSIDERATIONS
Bronchodilators				
Aminophylline (Aminophyllin)	• Relieves bronchospasm by relaxing bronchial smooth muscle	P.O.: 600 to 1,600 mg daily in 3 or 4 divided doses I.V.: loading dose of 6 mg/kg followed by maintenance infusion adult nonsmokers: 0.7 mg/kg/hour for 12 hours, then 0.5 mg/kg/hour; adult smokers: 1 mg/kg/hour for 12 hours, then 0.8 mg/kg/hour	• Nausea, vomiting • Epigastric pain • Diarrhea • Palpitations, tachycardia • Flushing • Dizziness, vertigo • Headache • Insomnia • Agitation	• This drug is converted to theophylline, the active form. Monitor theophylline blood levels for effectiveness (usual therapeutic range is 10 to 20 mcg/ml; a level above 20 mcg/ml may produce toxic effects. • Warn the patient to avoid caffeine because it may increase the incidence or severity of side effects. • Warn the patient that smoking may worsen the disease • Patients with liver or heart disease, older patients, and patients with cor pulmonale require dosage adjustment.
Epinephrine (Adrenalin)	• Stimulates bronchodilation, relieves bronchospasm and nasal congestion • Promotes vasoconstriction and relieves nasal congestion, counters anaphylactic shock	S.C.: 0.2 to 0.5 ml of 1:1,000 solution; may be repeated after 20 minutes Inhalation: 1% dilution; 1 to 2 puffs four to six times daily	• Elevated blood pressure • Increased pulse rate • Angina • Increased blood glucose level • Nervousness • Tachycardia	• Monitor vital signs. • Encourage rest to decrease oxygen requirements. • Instruct the patient to reduce intake of caffeine-containing foods and beverages. • When administering by inhalation, teach the patient how to use the inhaler. • Epinephrine's effects may be increased and prolonged when given concomitantly with monoamine oxidase (MAO) inhibitors and tricyclic antidepressants. • Warn the patient that smoking may worsen the disease.
Isoetharine (Bronkosol)	• Relieves bronchospasms by relaxing smooth bronchial muscles, promoting bronchodilation	1 to 2 puffs by inhalation q.i.d.	• Tachycardia • Nervousness • Nausea	• Wait about 1 minute before giving the second puff. • Caution the patient against excessive use. • Monitor the pulse and blood pressure. • Warn the patient that smoking may worsen the disease.
Metaproterenol sulfate (Alupent)	• Provides long-acting bronchodilation to relieve bronchospasms	P.O.: 10 to 20 mg q 6 to 8 hours Inhalation: 1 to 3 puffs q.i.d. (up to 12 puffs daily)	• Tachycardia • Tremors • Nausea	• Wait 1 minute before giving the second puff. • Give P.O. dose with meals. • Caution the patient against excessive use. • Monitor pulse and blood pressure. • Warn the patient that smoking may worsen the disease.
Terbutaline (Brethine)	Provides long-acting bronchodilation	P.O.: 2.5 to 5 mg q 6 to 8 hours S.C.: 0.25 mg; repeat in 15 to 30 minutes, if needed	• Tachycardia • Tremors • Palpitations • Dizziness	• Give P.O. dose with meals. • Monitor the pulse rate. • Warn the patient that smoking may worsen the disease.

(continued)

ADULT NURSING

Drugs used for respiratory disorders *(continued)*

DRUG	ACTION	USUAL ADULT DOSAGE	COMMON SIDE EFFECTS	NURSING CONSIDERATIONS
Bronchodilators *(continued)*				
Theophylline (immediate release: Elix-ophyllin) (sustained release: Aerolate, Theo-dur)	• Relieves bronchospasm by relaxing smooth muscle	P.O.: 6 mg/kg followed by 2 to 3 mg for 2 doses, then 1 to 3 mg/kg every 8 to 12 hours. Or give sustained-release tablet or capsule every 12 or 24 hours.	• Nausea, vomiting • Epigastric pain • Diarrhea • Palpitations, tachycardia • Flushing • Dizziness, vertigo • Headache • Insomnia • Agitation	• Monitor theophylline blood levels for effectiveness (usual therapeutic range is 10 to 20 mcg/ml; levels above 20 mcg/ml may produce toxic effects). • Warn the patient to avoid caffeine because it may increase the incidence or severity of side effects. • Warn the patient that smoking may worsen the disease. • Patients with liver or heart disease, older patients, and patients with cor pulmonale require dosage adjustment.
Antihistamines				
Diphenhydramine hydrochloride (Benadryl)	• Blocks histamine action, helping to control the allergic response • Provides sedation	P.O.: 25 to 50 mg three to four times daily I.V.: 10 to 50 mg	• Drowsiness • Blood pressure changes • Dry mouth	• Monitor blood pressure. • Warn the patient not to drink alcohol or operate dangerous machinery when taking this drug. • Concomitant use of a CNS depressant increases this drug's sedative effects.
Hydroxyzine hydrochloride, hydroxyzine pamoate (Vistaril)	• Blocks histamine action, helping to control the allergic response • Antiemetic (controls nausea and vomiting) • Provides sedation	P.O.: 75 to 100 mg three to four times daily I.M.: 25 to 100 mg	• Dry mouth • Drowsiness	• Monitor the patient closely when administering with other central nervous system (CNS) depressants. • Carry out safety measures, such as use of side rails. • Caution the patient not to operate dangerous machinery when taking this drug.
Tripelennamine citrate, tripelennamine hydrochloride (PBZ)	• Blocks histamine action, helping to control the allergic response • Depresses or stimulates the CNS • Promotes mucous membrane drying	P.O.: 5 mg/kg/day in four to six divided doses	• GI distress • Drowsiness	• Administer with meals. • Warn the patient not to operate dangerous machinery or take this drug with other CNS depressants, such as alcohol, hypnotics, or sedatives.
Promethazine hydrochloride (Phenergan)	• Blocks histamine action, helping to control the allergic response • Relieves motion sickness • Antiemetic (controls nausea and vomiting)	P.O.: 12.5 mg q 12 hours Rectal suppository: 25 mg I.M. or I.V.: 12.5 mg q 12 hours	• Pulse and blood pressure changes • Drowsiness • Nervousness • Tremors • Light sensitivity	• Carefully monitor pulse and blood pressure. • Monitor the patient during ambulation. • Sensitivity to light signals a toxic reaction; notify the physician immediately.

ADULT NURSING

Drugs used for respiratory disorders *(continued)*

DRUG	ACTION	USUAL ADULT DOSAGE	COMMON SIDE EFFECTS	NURSING CONSIDERATIONS
Antituberculars				
Isoniazid (INH) (Laniazid)	• Bactericidal to tubercle bacilli	P.O.: 300 mg daily for 9 months	• Tingling • Numbness • Burning sensation of the hands and feet • Anorexia • Dizziness • GI distress • Muscle aches • Jaundice	• Administer 1 hour before or 2 hours after a meal • Teach the patient about the need for long-term therapy. • Warn the patient not to drink alcohol when taking this drug. • Concomitant use of pyridoxine (Hexacrest; 25 to 50 mg P.O. daily) is recommended to prevent neuropathy. • Concomitant use of phenytoin (Dilantin) may cause phenytoin toxicity. • Monitor serum aspartate aminotransferase (AST) and alanine aminotransferase (ALT) levels.
Rifampin (Rifadin)	• Bactericidal to tubercle bacilli	P.O.: 600 mg daily for 9 months	• Red-orange discoloration of urine, sweat, and tears • Anorexia • Nausea • Vomiting • Jaundice • Flulike syndrome	• Drug absorption increases when taken on an empty stomach. Instruct the patient to take the drug 1 hour before or 2 hours after a meal. • Monitor AST and ALT levels. • Inform the patient that discoloration of urine, sweat, and tears is harmless. • Teach the patient to report flulike syndrome or jaundice • Advise the patient to avoid wearing soft contact lenses because this drug may discolor lenses. • Instruct the patient about the need for long-term therapy. • This drug reduces the effectiveness of oral contraceptives, methadone, (Dolophine) glucocorticoids, and digitoxin (Crystodigin).
Ethambutol (Myambutol)	• Bacteriostatic against tubercle bacilli	P.O.: 800 to 1,600 mg daily for 60 days	• Blurred vision • Gastric upset	• This drug is absorbed well even when taken with food. • Instruct the patient to report any vision changes. • Teach the patient about the need for long-term therapy. • Not recommended for children under age 13.
Mucolytic agent				
Acetylcysteine (Mucomyst)	• Dilutes mucus • Improves cough productivity	Nebulizer: 20% solution 3 to 5 ml three or four times daily Tracheal instillation: 1 to 2 ml q 4 hours	• GI distress • Drowsiness	• Do not give immediately before or after a meal. • Inform the patient that the drug smells like rotten eggs. • Do not heat the solution.

ADULT NURSING

MUSCULOSKELETAL SYSTEM

Anatomy and physiology

I. **Anatomy**
   A. Bones
      1. These are dense, hard tissue structures containing calcium for strength
      2. Types of bones include long bones (such as the femur), short bones (such as the carpals), flat bones (such as the sternum), and irregular bones (such as the skull bones)
   B. Muscles
      1. These are bands of fibers held together in bundles
      2. Muscle fibers are classified as striated or smooth
         a. Striated muscle consists of cells arranged in striations, or stripes, which help the muscle contract for movement
            (1) This type of muscle is found in all skeletal muscles

Reviewing the musculoskeletal system

**ANTERIOR VIEW OF
SUPERFICIAL MUSCLES**

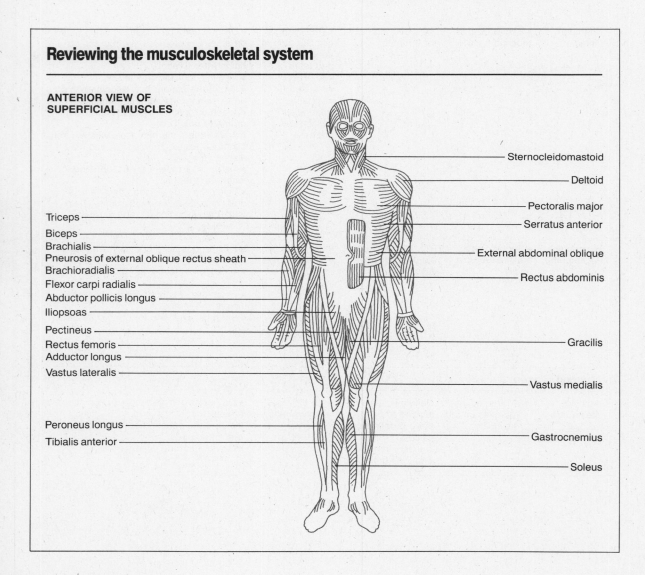

Sternocleidomastoid

Deltoid

Pectoralis major

Serratus anterior

External abdominal oblique

Rectus abdominis

Gracilis

Vastus medialis

Gastrocnemius

Soleus

Triceps

Biceps

Brachialis

Pneurosis of external oblique rectus sheath

Brachioradialis

Flexor carpi radialis

Abductor pollicis longus

Iliopsoas

Pectineus

Rectus femoris

Adductor longus

Vastus lateralis

Peroneus longus

Tibialis anterior

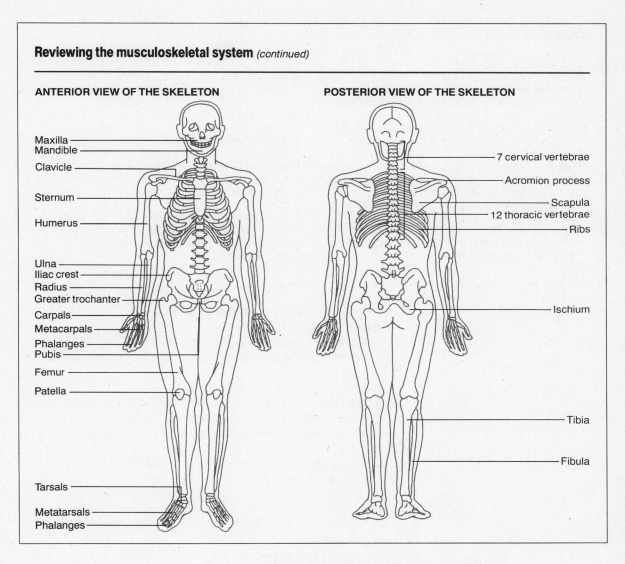

Reviewing the musculoskeletal system *(continued)*

ANTERIOR VIEW OF THE SKELETON

- Maxilla
- Mandible
- Clavicle
- Sternum
- Humerus
- Ulna
- Iliac crest
- Radius
- Greater trochanter
- Carpals
- Metacarpals
- Phalanges
- Pubis
- Femur
- Patella
- Tarsals
- Metatarsals
- Phalanges

POSTERIOR VIEW OF THE SKELETON

- 7 cervical vertebrae
- Acromion process
- Scapula
- 12 thoracic vertebrae
- Ribs
- Ischium
- Tibia
- Fibula

        (2) It is responsible for voluntary movement

    b. Smooth muscle, which comprises all visceral muscles, is responsible for involuntary movement (controlled by the autonomic nervous system)

C. Ligaments
    1. These are strong, short, flexible bands of fibrous tissue
    2. They bind joints together and connect various bones and cartilages

D. Tendons
    1. These are white, fibrous bands of tissue found at the ends of muscles
    2. They attach the muscle to bone

E. Joints
    1. These are connections between bones covered by ligaments, tendons, synovium, and synovial fluid
    2. Joints are classified as freely movable, partially movable, or immovable (such as skull bones)

F. Synovium
    1. This membrane, or thin tissue layer, covers the inside of moveable joints

---

Glossary

Arthritis: inflammation of one or more joints

Autoimmune disease: group of disorders in which the body fails to recognize its own tissues and the immune system is directed against itself

Callus: bony deposit that develops between and around the broken ends of a fractured bone during healing

Cast: firm, solid dressing made of plaster of Paris or other material that is wrapped around a body part to keep it from moving during healing

Fracture: injury in which the continuity of bone tissue is broken

Neurovascular check: series of eight assessments used to evaluate circulatory and nerve function in an injured body part

Osteoarthritis: degenerative joint condition affecting mainly large, weight-bearing joints; associated with "wear and tear" and aging

Osteomyelitis: infection of bone or the bone marrow

Osteoporosis: disorder marked by loss of bone density that increases the risk of fracture

Rheumatoid arthritis: chronic disease with an autoimmune component, characterized by synovial (joint) inflammation and increased synovial exudate

Traction: pulling force exerted on a body part through such devices as ropes, pulleys, and weights; used to immobilize, position, and align a fractured bone to aid healing

---

       2. It produces synovial fluid, which lubricates the joint and aids movement

       3. Synovium also helps remove wastes from joints, provides white blood cells for immune functions, and supplies oxygen and nutrients to joint cartilage

    G. Cartilage

       1. This fibrous connective tissue is found mainly in the joints, between vertebrae, and in rigid tubes, such as the trachea

       2. It permits pain-free weight bearing

    H. Bursae

       1. These are fibrous sacs situated between certain tendons and the bones beneath them

       2. They lubricate tendons and ligaments to aid movement

II. Physiology

    A. Gives the body shape and form

    B. Protects internal organs

    C. Serves as the site for blood cell production, producing red blood cells, white blood cells, and the megakaryocyte — the "mother cell" of platelets

    D. Makes movement possible

       1. Skeletal muscles produce movement by pulling on bones

          a. One muscle in a pair of opposing muscles pulls on the bone to which it is attached (flexes)

          b. The opposing muscle relaxes (extends)

       2. Joints permit movement between bones

          a. Flexion refers to shortening of the joint angle

          b. Extension denotes lengthening of the joint angle

          c. Abduction is movement away from the body's midline

          d. Adduction is movement toward the body's midline

          e. Rotation refers to pivoting of a bone on its axis

          f. Circumduction denotes turning in a circular motion (flexion, abduction, extension, and adduction in succession)

Patient in a cast (fracture of the tibia and fibula)

Overview

A cast may be used to immobilize a fractured (broken) bone until it heals or to move a bone into a more desirable position, such as in talipes (clubfoot). The cast promotes healing by helping to overcome muscle tension and rotational forces. A cast made from plaster of Paris hardens to form a rigid wrap; a fiberglass cast also becomes rigid after hardening but is lighter than a plaster cast. A plaster cast typically is used for a leg fracture because it is stronger than fiberglass; also, it can withstand the weight borne on a walking heel (which may be applied if X-rays of a transverse fracture show some callus formation). Casts must be applied carefully.

Clinical situation

Arlene Archer, age 20, a college sophomore, is taken to the emergency department of a nearby hospital after slipping and falling on icy pavement while walking to a class. She states that she felt pain immediately in the lower part of her right leg and could not put her weight on the leg when she stood up and tried to walk. X-rays reveal transverse fractures of the tibia and fibula (the bones of the lower leg). The physician recommends application of a plaster cast. Ms. Archer and her parents consent to this, and a short leg cast is applied from the knee to the base of the toes. After waiting 30 minutes for the plaster to become firm, another X-ray is taken to confirm that the reduction (alignment) of the fractured bones is satisfactory.

Assessment

Nursing behaviors	**Nursing rationales**
1. Assess the size, shape, and condition of Ms. Archer's cast.	**1.** This determines the dampness and integrity of the cast. A plaster cast takes 2 to 3 days to dry completely. A transverse fracture may be less stable than other fractures because of the muscle-pulling forces involved in the injury.
2. Assess the condition of the skin around the edges of the cast.	**2.** Rough plaster can cause skin breaks leading to inflammation or infection. To prevent this, the edges of the cast should be covered with pieces of turned-down stockinette to make them smooth.
3. Assess the casted toes for color, temperature, and capillary refill. Compare them with the opposite toes. (For details on this assessment, see "Performing neurovascular checks," pages 263 and 264.)	**3.** Comparing injured and uninjured tissues helps establish normal findings.
4. Assess Ms. Archer's reaction to having the cast.	**4.** Patients who must wear a cast may become anxious, angry, and claustrophobic. However, these reactions do not necessarily stem directly from the cast but may result from the injury, loss of a sense of control, or other factors.

ADULT
NURSING

5. Assess Ms. Archer for complaints of pain or a too-tight cast.

5. Pain, which reflects pressure on nerve endings, may be minimal or severe depending on the injury and the patient's usual response to pain. Pain usually subsides after cast application because the cast prevents movement of the fractured bones. Tightness may signify edema in the injured tissues.

6. Assess Ms. Archer's ability to move all of her toes. Count the toes to make sure they are all visible.

6. All toes should move freely and be fully visible to prevent pressure.

7. Assess Ms. Archer for complaints of numbness or tingling in the affected foot and toes.

7. Numbness and tingling signal pressure on nerve endings. If these sensations persist, the cast may need to be cut in half (bivalved) to relieve the pressure.

8. Assess Ms. Archer's understanding of home care instructions, including cast drying techniques, use of pain medications, and using crutches.

8. Ms. Archer should receive written instructions and be able to repeat them in her own words. To ensure that she knows how to use the crutches safely, she should practice using them with a nurse or a technician present.

Nursing diagnoses

- Altered peripheral tissue perfusion related to fractures
- Impaired physical mobility related to the cast and fractures

Planning and goals

- Ms. Archer will achieve bone union over time.
- Ms. Archer will use crutches to move about with weight-bearing restrictions, as ordered.
- Ms. Archer will maintain the cast in the proper position until it dries completely.
- Ms. Archer will regain pain-free mobility over time.
- Ms. Archer will participate in self-care and her usual activities, as her condition allows.

Implementation

Nursing behaviors

1. Elevate Ms. Archer's cast and right leg on a pillow covered with plastic. Place a cotton blanket between the pillow and cast, and keep the cast uncovered until it dries.

Nursing rationales

1. Elevation helps prevent edema and increases venous return. The pillow provides a firm surface, yet will not deform the cast while it is damp. The plastic covering protects the pillow; however, it also prevents the plaster from drying. Therefore, a blanket should be placed between the cover and cast to aid drying.

2. Explain the need for Ms. Archer to turn to her side and change position every 2 to 4 hours while the cast is damp.

2. Plaster must dry thoroughly in all areas. Turning and changing position help the cast dry as well as help maintain muscle and joint strength and function.

3. When lifting or moving the casted extremity, support the cast by placing the palms of your hands under the joints above and below the injured area (in this case, the knee and ankle). Avoid pressing your fingertips into the damp plaster.

3. Supporting the joints above and below the injured area prevents bone dislocation and lessens pain. Using the palms avoids undue pressure on damp areas, which could cause indentations in the cast and exert pressure on the skin (indentations remain after the cast dries).

ADULT
NURSING

4. Keep the cast uncovered while it is damp. To aid drying, use a fan or a hair dryer set on low temperature.

4. Covering the cast reduces evaporation and delays drying. A fan or hair dryer increases air circulation and enhances drying. (However, do not use these drying aids if the patient has an open area or an incision inside the cast because this could blow microorganisms into the cast, where they can grow in the warm, dark environment.) A low temperature prevents skin burns.

5. Perform all eight neurovascular checks every hour until Ms. Archer is discharged (see "Performing neurovascular checks," pages 263 and 264).

5. Hourly neurovascular checks help detect early signs of complications.

6. Apply ice bags to the cast at the injury site.

6. Ice relieves pain by constricting vessels, decreasing bleeding, and reducing edema.

7. Note any patient complaints of pain.

7. Initially, Ms. Archer may have minimal pain because of numbness or pressure on nerve endings. However, as nerve functions return, pain typically increases. Later, bruises and pain (caused by the fall) may arise in other body areas.

8. Administer pain medications every 4 hours, as ordered and needed, until Ms. Archer is discharged.

8. Initially, the physician typically orders narcotic analgesics for pain relief. Administering these medications every 4 hours maintains a therapeutic blood level that enhances pain relief. Later, pain relief typically involves only nonnarcotic analgesics.

9. Before Ms. Archer is discharged, review and clarify home-care instructions. Teach her how to walk with crutches, and assist her as she practices. Teach her about side effects of medications and tell her which signs and symptoms to report to the physician. Have her repeat the instructions in her own words. Schedule a return appointment to the physician.

9. Ms. Archer may not comprehend initial explanations about her injury and self-care regimen because of anxiety, pain, or lack of understanding about the injury severity and required treatments. Therefore, you may need to reinforce the physician's explanations and instructions. Having her repeat these in her own words helps assess her level of understanding. A return appointment ensures patient well-being.

10. Document all findings in Ms. Archer's chart.

10. Timely documentation helps ensure safe care, aids later comparison, and ensures continuity of care.

Clinical situation
(continued)

The nurse reviews the physician's instructions to Ms. Archer on self-care, cast care, and use of crutches. After receiving prescriptions for pain medication and making an appointment for a return visit to the physician, Ms. Archer is discharged and goes home with her parents.

Six weeks later, Ms. Archer returns to the physician's office. The physician orders an X-ray to check for bone alignment and sufficient callus (bony deposits between and around the broken ends of the fractured bones). The X-ray shows good alignment of both fractured bones, with significant callus formation. The physician then removes the cast and instructs Ms. Archer to reduce use of the crutches gradually by progressively increasing weight-bearing on her right leg and asks the nurse to give Ms. Archer a pamphlet on skin care and review it with her.

ADULT NURSING

**Evaluation
(outcomes)**

• Ms. Archer can perform her own self-care, resumed her college activities on the second day after cast application, and continues with these activities throughout the fracture-healing period.
• Ms. Archer regains bone union with good alignment.
• Ms. Archer walks safely with crutches, following weight-bearing restrictions, until permitted to begin full weight-bearing.
• Ms. Archer maintains an intact cast for the full 6 weeks that she needs the cast.
• Ms. Archer gradually regains pain-free mobility approximately 6 weeks after cast removal.

Patient in traction (fracture of the femur)

Overview

Traction, a pulling force exerted on a body part, is used to immobilize, position, and align a fractured bone before cast application or surgery or during healing. Traction also may be used to relieve muscle spasms or tightness or to relieve pain in the neck, back, or other areas.

Traction may involve skin traction or skeletal traction. In skin traction, pull is applied to an affected body part by straps attached to the surrounding skin. Skin traction is used for less serious injuries and shorter periods than skeletal traction. It is intermittent (can be removed for brief periods) and requires relatively little weight (usually only 2 to 8 lb [0.9 to 3.6 kg]) to prevent epidermal dislodgment from underlying tissues. Types of skin traction include Buck's extension, Russell's traction, Dunlop's traction, pelvic belt traction, head halter traction, Bryant's traction, and Cotrel's traction.

Skeletal traction refers to traction applied directly to the bone by a firm wire, thick pin, or metal pin attached to weights. Types of skeletal traction include skull tongs for cervical traction, balanced-suspension skeletal traction to the femur and 90-degree-to-90-degree skeletal traction to the femur. Skeletal traction is used for more serious injuries in which muscle spasms cause overriding bone ends. It helps overcome muscle spasms by pulling fractured bones apart. Once applied, skeletal traction is used continuously. Maintained for long periods (at least 6 to 8 weeks), it requires more weight than skin traction (at least 10 to 30 lb [4.5 to 13.6 kg]). (For details on skeletal traction, see *Types of skeletal traction* and *Special nursing assessments for a patient in skeletal traction,* page 246.)

Clinical situation

Brian Cook, age 25, is hit by a car while riding his motorcycle. The impact throws him from the motorcycle, and his left thigh strikes a sharp rock. Because he is wearing a helmet, he does not lose consciousness or suffer a head injury. A medical emergency squad ambulance takes him to the emergency department of a nearby hospital. There, Mr. Cook reports that he heard a sharp crack and felt immediate pain in his thigh. X-rays show an oblique fracture of the left femur, with shortening and overriding of the distal fractured bone on the proximal fragment. He is transferred to the orthopedic nursing unit, where he will be placed in balanced-suspension skeletal traction.

ADULT
NURSING

Types of skeletal traction

Skeletal traction may involve balanced-suspension traction (described in "Fracture of the femur"), Dunlop's traction to the humerus, or skeletal tongs. Dunlop's traction is used to reduce, align, and treat fractures of the shaft or distal humerus. A Kirschner wire or Steinmann pin is inserted through the distal humerus and connected to a spreader, ropes, and weights. The forearm is held at a right angle to the humerus by Buck's extension traction (a type of skin traction). The nurse removes and rewraps the skin traction to the forearm daily; however, skeletal traction is maintained continuously until discontinued by the physician.

Skeletal tongs (such as Barton, Crutchfield, Gardner-Wells, and Vinke tongs) are used to immobilize fractures of the cervical vertebrae. The tongs are inserted into the skull bones, then connected to ropes and weights. Usually, the patient with a cervical vertebral fracture is paralyzed and may be maintained on a special bed, such as a CircOlectric bed or Stryker Wedge Frame bed.

Assessment

Nursing behaviors

1. Assess the whole patient, including Mr. Cook's personal and family concerns as well as his general physical condition (such as bruises, open wounds, and injury site) and his orientation to time, place, and person.

2. Assess Mr. Cook's vital signs.

3. Assess the neurovascular status of the affected leg (see "Performing neurovascular checks," pages 263 and 264).

4. Assess Mr. Cook for complaints of pain, including its type, duration, and character. Note his description of pain intensity.

5. Assess the time of Mr. Cook's last food and fluid intake. Determine whether he is thirsty, feels nauseated, or is vomiting.

6. Assess Mr. Cook's understanding of upcoming events (such as placement in traction, immobility problems, and anticipated nursing care) by asking pertinent questions.

Nursing rationales

1. Incorporating personal and family concerns into the assessment helps determine Mr. Cook's strengths and health needs, aiding planning of care.

2. This determines his present condition and helps detect any signs of shock.

3. This determines the leg's circulatory status and neurologic function.

4. This helps determine the pattern of pain and Mr. Cook's response to it, aiding planning of care.

5. Recent food and fluid intake may necessitate a delay in anesthetic administration. Thirst may indicate bleeding or dehydration. Nausea or vomiting may indicate head injury.

6. This determines whether Mr. Cook heard and understood the initial explanation fully (patients who are injured or in shock commonly need a repeat explanation).

Nursing diagnoses
- Pain related to the injury
- Impaired physical mobility related to bed rest, skeletal traction, and fracture of the femur

ADULT NURSING

Special nursing assessments for a patient in skeletal traction

When caring for a patient in skeletal traction, follow these guidelines:
● Perform all eight neurovascular checks every 1 to 2 hours initially.
● Assess all bony prominences, such as the elbows, styloid process (bulge at the outer wrist), greater trochanter (at the hip), malleoli (bones on the inside and outside of the ankle),

heels, back of the head, and ears. Check for excoriation, redness, and tenderness.
● Evaluate all parts of the traction apparatus — ropes (for fraying and for proper position in pulleys), pulleys, knots (for intactness), weights (for free hanging) — and the patient (for proper position).

Planning and goals

• Mr. Cook will achieve bone union after appropriate treatment.
• Mr. Cook will remain free from complications, such as fat embolism.
• Mr. Cook will regain mobility through the use of crutches and partial weight-bearing.
• Mr. Cook will resume his usual roles and responsibilities.

Implementation

Nursing behaviors

1. Orient Mr. Cook to the nursing unit, his room, and roommate (if present).

2. Monitor Mr. Cook's vital signs closely and compare them with previous findings.

3. Perform all neurovascular checks.

4. Apply ice bags to the injured thigh area, as ordered.

5. Note any patient complaints of pain, including the description of pain characteristics, duration, and intensity.

6. Assemble all equipment for traction application; order a sterile Steinmann pin tray.

7. Administer narcotic analgesics and muscle relaxants at the specified times, as ordered.

8. Explain the traction application procedure to Mr. Cook. Then assist with the procedure, such as by holding the affected limb as requested for Steinmann pin insertion, suspending the thigh and leg, and applying weights (see "Assisting with application of balanced-suspension skeletal traction to treat a fractured femur," pages 269 to 271).

Nursing rationales

1. This promotes patient comfort in unfamiliar surroundings.

2. Mr. Cook's temperature may be subnormal if he is in shock. His blood pressure may be low-normal if bleeding is minor. Pulse and respirations may be elevated slightly from pain, anxiety, fear, or the extent of trauma.

3. This provides baseline data for later comparison.

4. Ice causes vasoconstriction and decreases bleeding into the injury site.

5. Pain, a response to injury, is individualized in experience, expression, and tolerance.

6. Assembling all supplies in advance eases traction application and minimizes patient trauma.

7. Analgesics and muscle relaxants increase patient comfort during traction application.

8. Explanations promote patient comfort. Assistance makes traction application more efficient and minimizes patient discomfort.

ADULT
NURSING

9. After traction is established, check all traction parts for proper function and amount of weight; document your findings.

9. This ensures that traction is working properly and that the amount of weight is recorded, helping to ensure continuity of care.

10. Monitor Mr. Cook's vital signs and perform neurovascular checks periodically.

10. This provides data on Mr. Cook's tolerance for traction and helps detect any new trauma or bleeding.

Clinical situation
(continued)

Mr. Cook remains in balanced-suspension skeletal traction for 2 weeks. X-rays taken at that time show reduced overriding and good alignment of bone fragments. Mr. Cook undergoes surgery for intramedullary nail insertion in closed fashion (using minimal incisions) under fluoroscopic guidance. After an uneventful postoperative recovery, he is discharged to his home using crutches with touch-down weight-bearing.

Evaluation (outcomes)

• Mr. Cook achieves bone union over time (6 to 9 months). The intramedullary nail holds the fractured bones in approximation (with ends touching).
• Mr. Cook remains free from fat embolism and other fracture complications.
• Mr. Cook walks with crutches, then progresses to full weight-bearing, as permitted by X-ray evidence of healing.
• Mr. Cook returns to his family and resumes his normal roles and responsibilities.

Fracture of the femoral neck

Overview

Fracture of the femoral neck (a part of the hip joint) typically results from a fall or a fairly minor injury, such as a sudden twist or turn with the foot held stationary. This type of fracture poses a major problem for older patients with reduced bone density (such as from osteoporosis). It affects more women than men.

A fracture of the femoral neck or head is called an intracapsular fracture because it is located inside the hip capsule, which surrounds the head and neck of the femur and encloses the acetabulum (see *Types of hip fractures*, page 248). Blood enters the capsule from arteries and the ligamentum teres, a ligament in the center of the femoral head that extends to the middle of the acetabulum. A fracture of the femoral neck may disrupt blood supply to the femoral head, possibly causing avascular necrosis. To prevent this complication, the femoral head is removed and replaced by a metallic prosthesis.

Clinical situation

Sally Kircher, age 69, a widow who lives alone in a small apartment, falls over a small stool while watering her plants. She immediately feels pain in her left hip and cannot rise to stand or walk. She slowly drags herself to the phone and calls 911. The emergency squad arrives quickly and gets a key to her apartment from her building superintendent. After checking Mrs. Kircher's orientation and vital signs, the paramedics notice that her left leg is lying in an externally rotated and shortened position. They lift her to the stretcher gently, secure her with straps (holding her left leg in the externally rotated position), and take her to the emergency department. There, physicians determine that she has a fracture of the femoral neck. X-rays also show moderate osteoporosis of the hip and femoral areas. Mrs. Kircher is transferred to the orthopedic nursing unit and scheduled for surgical implantation of a femoral prosthesis.

ADULT NURSING

Types of hip fractures

The illustrations below show the most commonly occuring fractures of the hip.

SUBCAPITAL FRACTURE

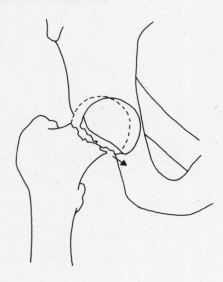

FEMORAL NECK FRACTURE

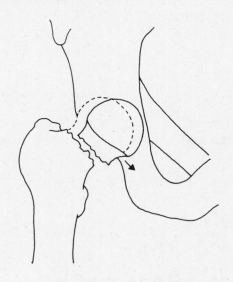

**IMPACTED FRACTURE
OF FEMORAL NECK**

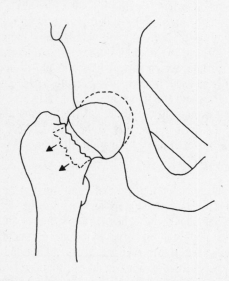

**INTERTROCHANTERIC
FRACTURE**

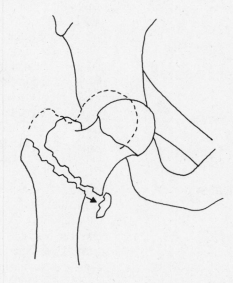

Assessment

Nursing behaviors	Nursing rationales
1. Assess the "whole" patient, including Mrs. Kircher's family characteristics, nutritional status, and mental orientation.	**1.** Incorporating personal and family concerns into the assessment helps determine Mrs. Kircher's strengths and health needs, aiding planning of care.
2. Assess the affected leg for position and signs of bleeding (bruises or ecchymoses), edema, and skin breaks.	**2.** Bruising and edema signal bleeding into interstitial tissues and venous stasis. Shortening and external rotation of the leg result from the fracture and muscle spasms. Skin breaks may indicate lacerations or abrasions, which require treatment.
3. Assess Mrs. Kircher's vital signs and temperature.	**3.** This provides baseline data. Mrs. Kircher's temperature may be decreased and her pulse and respirations increased slightly if she is in shock. Shock and bleeding also may cause a subnormal blood pressure.
4. Assess Mrs. Kircher's appetite and determine the time of her last food and fluid intake.	**4.** Mrs. Kircher may require emergency surgery. However, if she has consumed food or fluids within the last 4 hours, she risks nausea, vomiting, and aspiration from anesthesia.
5. Assess Mrs. Kircher for complaints of pain, including its nature and severity.	**5.** Pain, which results from pressure on nerve endings, may be acute and sharp and will increase when the affected parts are moved.
6. Assess Mrs. Kircher for urine output and a sensation of bladder fullness or pressure.	**6.** Pain may cause urine retention, leading to bladder fullness and pressure.
7. Perform all neurovascular checks (see "Performing neurovascular checks," pages 263 and 264).	**7.** Neurovascular checks provide data about circulatory and neurologic status.

Nursing diagnoses	• Impaired physical mobility related to fracture of the femoral neck • Self-care deficit related to trauma and surgery
Planning and goals	• Mrs. Kircher will regain limited mobility after surgical repair and wound healing. • Mrs. Kircher will remain free from additional injuries related to osteoporosis or wound infection. • Mrs. Kircher will be able to perform activities of daily living (ADLs) independently by the time of discharge. • Mrs. Kircher will return to her family and social roles after an interim period in an extended-care facility.

Implementation

Nursing behaviors	Nursing rationales
1. Orient Mrs. Kircher to the nursing unit and roommate (if present).	**1.** This will increase Mrs. Kircher's comfort and understanding of routines.
2. Position Mrs. Kircher as comfortably as possible, using pillows if necessary.	**2.** Because of her upcoming surgery, Mrs. Kircher will not be placed in skin traction to increase her comfort or relieve muscle spasms. Therefore, she will need other comfort measures.

3. Assist with additional diagnostic studies, such as an electrocardiogram, blood samples, and chest X-ray, as needed.

4. Assist with insertion of an indwelling urinary (Foley) catheter if Mrs. Kircher cannot void (if ordered). Connect the catheter to a sterile drainage system.

5. Withhold all oral intake for the period ordered.

6. Assist with insertion of an I.V. line and solution; adjust the I.V. flow rate, as needed.

7. Prepare Mrs. Kircher for surgery physically and emotionally (as described in the "Perioperative nursing" section).

8. Administer preoperative medications, if permitted and ordered, or confirm that these have been administered.

9. Make sure that required laboratory data and results of special examinations are recorded on Mrs. Kircher's chart.

10. Send Mrs. Kircher's X-rays and an abduction pillow to surgery with her.

11. Assist with transfer of Mrs. Kircher to a gurney or to the surgical suite.

12. Complete all required documentation on the nursing notes, and send Mrs. Kircher's chart to surgery with her.

3. Because of Mrs. Kircher's age and possible medical problems, her cardiopulmonary status and blood chemistry must be evaluated.

4. Because Mrs. Kircher cannot bend her knee and plant her left foot, the urethral orifice cannot be visualized optimally. Therefore, assistance is needed during catheter insertion.

5. This reduces the risk of nausea, vomiting, and aspiration from anesthesia.

6. I.V. fluids help maintain blood volume.

7. Preoperative implementations help ensure Mrs. Kircher's safety before, during, and after surgery.

8. Preoperative medications are given to reduce muscle tension, lessen secretions, prevent aspiration, and delay the memory of perioperative events.

9. Laboratory results must be obtained before anesthesia is administered to determine if Mrs. Kircher has any abnormalities requiring correction.

10. X-rays show the extent and nature of the injury; an abduction pillow is used postoperatively.

11. To reduce trauma resulting from transfer to a gurney, Mrs. Kircher may be taken in her own bed to the surgical suite.

12. Documentation helps ensure safety and continuity of care.

Clinical situation
(continued)

After 2 hours in the postanesthesia care unit following surgery, Mrs. Kircher returns to the nursing unit. An I.V. line is in place, and the abduction pillow is positioned between her legs. Mrs. Kircher appears drowsy and responds to questions slowly.

Assessment

Nursing behaviors

1. Assess Mrs. Kircher's orientation to time, place, and person.

2. Assess the wound site, including the wound drainage system and amount of drainage.

Nursing rationales

1. This helps determine how well she tolerated anesthesia and surgery and may reveal any neurologic complication, such as cerebrovascular accident.

2. Drainage should be bright to dark red. If a drainage system is not in use, the dressing may show a slight to moderate amount of red drainage (unless the dressing was reinforced in the recovery room).

3. Assess Mrs. Kircher's vital signs.

3. The stress of surgery and anesthesia may cause a slight decrease in blood pressure and temperature and a slight increase in respirations (compared with preoperative findings).

4. Assess Mrs. Kircher for complaints of pain, noting the pain location.

4. Mrs. Kircher may have received narcotic analgesics in the recovery room. Sites other than the hip area may be sore or bruised from her fall.

5. Assess and count the I.V. drip rate.

5. The actual drip rate may vary from the ordered rate because of Mrs. Kircher's transfer and movements.

6. Assess urine output from the catheter, if it is still in place.

6. This helps determine the adequacy of fluid replacement.

Implementation

Nursing behaviors

1. Assist Mrs. Kircher to bathe, or bathe her, as needed. Assist with or provide oral hygiene.

Nursing rationales

1. Mrs. Kircher will need help with daily care for 24 hours postoperatively because of the effects of anesthesia and surgical trauma.

2. Continue to monitor Mrs. Kircher's vital signs.

2. Mrs. Kircher's temperature may be slightly elevated (to 100° F [37.8° C]) from the inflammatory response to surgical trauma.

3. Encourage Mrs. Kircher to breathe deeply and cough every 2 hours. If her cough is productive, assess sputum amount and color. Help her use an incentive spirometer every 2 hours.

3. Deep breathing helps oxygenate all lung areas to maintain respiratory function; coughing clears respiratory secretions. A productive cough may result from the respiratory effects of anesthesia or from infection (as shown by yellow or green sputum). Slightly bloody sputum may stem from endotracheal intubation during surgery. Use of an incentive spirometer keeps the lungs and alveoli expanded, aiding gas exchange.

4. Monitor breath sounds in all lung lobes every 4 hours.

4. Breath sounds should be audible in all lobes. Absent breath sounds may signal developing atelectasis.

5. Turn or reposition Mrs. Kircher onto the nonoperative side every 4 hours; make sure the operative leg is well supported on an abduction pillow. Place a pillow against her back and keep the side rails up.

5. Turning Mrs. Kircher to the nonoperative side helps maintain abduction. A patient with a prosthetic replacement of the femoral head should keep the legs abducted to maintain the prosthesis in the acetabulum. Pillows help Mrs. Kircher maintain a side-lying position. Side rails provide safety and security.

6. Give Mrs. Kircher clear liquids when ordered and when bowel sounds return. Monitor bowel sounds every 4 hours. Remove the I.V. line when oral intake is adequate, as ordered.

6. Return of bowel sounds (reflecting peristalsis) signals resumption of normal bowel function. Giving food or fluids before bowel function returns may cause paralytic ileus. The I.V. line is discontinued when oral intake is adequate.

ADULT NURSING

7. Assist Mrs. Kircher to sit on the bedside and pivot to a chair when this is permitted. Make sure she bears only the permitted amount of weight on the operative leg.

7. Usually, the patient is allowed to sit up on the first or second postoperative day, depending on general condition and the prosthetic fit. Permitted weight-bearing may vary from no weight to touch-down weight, or as tolerated.

8. Teach Mrs. Kircher how to use a walker (see "Teaching a patient to use crutches, a cane, or a walker," pages 272 and 273). Help her ambulate with the walker every 4 hours.

8. Typically, the patient uses a walker initially because it provides greater stability than crutches. As Mrs. Kircher's strength increases, she will use crutches for 2 to 3 months until X-rays show sound healing.

9. Change wound dressings, as required. Assess wound healing by checking for the presence and amount of redness, edema, drainage, or pain. Replace the dressing if drainage is present; otherwise, the incision may be left uncovered.

9. Initially, the wound site may be moderately red, edematous, and painful, with slight to moderate drainage. If a drainage system is in place, drainage may measure 200 ml or more. As inflammation subsides during the first 5 postoperative days, redness and edema decrease, pain subsides to tenderness, and drainage stops. Leaving the incision uncovered exposes it to air and light, promoting epithelial healing.

10. Encourage Mrs. Kircher to do range-of-motion (ROM) exercises of the ankles, arms, and shoulders every 4 hours.

10. ROM exercises help maintain strength and circulation of joints, muscles, and other tissues, and may prevent further osteoporosis by keeping calcium in the bones.

11. Perform neurovascular checks every 4 hours, as ordered.

11. Neurovascular checks may reveal a complication, such as thrombophlebitis, venous stasis, or delayed wound healing. (See *Complications of musculoskeletal disorders*, pages 261 and 262.)

12. Administer narcotic analgesics every 4 hours, as needed and ordered. If Mrs. Kircher is using a patient-controlled analgesia (PCA) pump, monitor the amount of medication used and pain relief obtained. Note any complaints of nausea, vomiting, diarrhea or constipation, and headache.

12. Narcotic analgesics relieve pain when given at regular intervals that maintain therapeutic (desired) blood levels. A PCA pump can help Mrs. Kircher control pain independently. Nausea, vomiting, diarrhea or constipation, and headache are potential side effects of narcotics.

13. Monitor urine output after the indwelling catheter is removed. Note any complaints of urinary urgency, frequency, or burning as well as decreased urine output or inability to void.

13. An indwelling catheter may cause urinary tract infection, which may manifest as urinary burning, frequency, urgency, and decreased output. Inability to void, signalled by urine retention, may reflect sphincter constriction caused by narcotics.

14. Obtain a social service consultation for home care or discharge planning, or discuss the need for social services with Mrs. Kircher's primary care nurse.

14. Because Mrs. Kircher is a widow, she may need assistance after discharge. If such assistance is not available, she may be discharged to an extended-care facility.

15. Assist with removal of skin clips or sutures, when ordered (usually on the fifth or sixth postoperative day). Apply adhesive skin closures (Steri-strips) to wound edges.

15. Skin clips or sutures are removed when wound edges are well approximated and no signs of wound infection appear. Adhesive skin closures support the wound until the skin can maintain closure.

16. Prepare Mrs. Kircher for discharge or transfer to an extended-care facility, when appropriate.

16. Adherence to proper procedures helps ensure thorough and safe discharge or transfer.

17. Discuss special dietary considerations (such as calcium supplementation) with Mrs. Kircher to help her overcome the effects of surgical trauma and osteoporosis progression.

17. Mrs. Kircher must increase her intake of proteins, carbohydrates, and minerals to meet surgical and wound-healing demands. Increased calcium and vitamin D intake may help keep calcium in the bones, slowing osteoporosis progression.

18. Schedule a return appointment with the physician. Review the actions and side effects of discharge medications with Mrs. Kircher.

18. Return visits to the physician ensure proper follow-up and continuity of care. Helping Mrs. Kircher understand the expected actions and side effects of medications promotes her compliance.

19. Assist with Mrs. Kircher's transfer to an extended-care facility, when ordered. Transfer all supplies or equipment that Mrs. Kircher already has used (such as a walker, incentive spirometer, and personal supplies).

19. Sending Mrs. Kircher's personal items and required supplies eases her transfer.

20. Complete all information required on the continuity-of-care form. Notify the extended-care facility and discuss Mrs. Kircher's care needs. (In some cases, this may be done by the primary care nurse.)

20. This promotes continuity of care.

21. Complete all required documentation on Mrs. Kircher's chart. Record the time of discharge, Mrs. Kircher's present condition and special needs, and items sent to the extended-care facility.

21. Thorough documentation is crucial to fulfill safety and legal requirements.

Evaluation (outcomes)

• Mrs. Kircher regains limited mobility with use of a walker after surgery (weight-bearing on the left side will be limited for 3 months).
• Mrs. Kircher remains free from complications of surgery and osteoporosis.
• Mrs. Kircher performs her own activities of daily living with some assistance by the time of discharge.
• Mrs. Kircher will be able to return to her own apartment and usual roles after a 2- to 3-month stay at an extended-care facility.

ADULT NURSING

Osteoarthritis

Overview

Osteoarthritis is a degenerative condition of the joints characterized by loss of articular cartilage. It primarily affects the large, weight-bearing joints, such as the hip and knee. Osteoarthritis may arise after an injury or other overt cause (secondary osteoarthritis); or it may have no known cause (primary or idiopathic osteoarthritis). Contributing factors include obesity and abnormal bone alignment within joints or relative to one another (for example, knock-knees or bowlegs). Such abnormal positions cause excessive pressure and uneven wear on cartilage during weight-bearing activities. Also, researchers have discovered a defective cartilage gene that may be linked with the degenerative changes of primary osteoarthritis.

Osteoarthritis is a disease of aging, most common after age 50. It affects more than 50 million Americans; the incidence among males and females is nearly equal.

Surgical procedures used to treat osteoarthritis include replacement of the femoral head with a metallic prosthesis, osteotomy of the femur to change the weight-bearing surface of the femoral head in the acetabulum, and total joint replacement. More than one joint may need to be replaced or corrected. Surgery is performed only when medical treatments no longer relieve symptoms.

Clinical situation

Polly Hart, age 68, a widow, visits the physician complaining of a recurring dull ache in her right hip. She enters the examining room slowly, with a marked limp, and holds onto the door and furniture for support. She is accompanied by her daughter, who is quite protective toward her. Mrs. Hart states that the ache spreads to her thigh and knee and often awakens her at night.

Assessment

Nursing behaviors	Nursing rationales
1. Assess Mrs. Hart's height, posture, and gait.	**1.** Changes in height, posture, and gait may result from age-related muscle or joint changes (such as loss of muscle mass and strength) rather than disease. In an elderly patient, a gait change commonly stems from a change in the angle of the femoral head within the acetabulum.
2. Assess Mrs. Hart for pain, including its nature, intensity, site, and duration.	**2.** Patients with osteoarthritis commonly describe the pain as a dull, deep ache in a joint, which may spread to surrounding tissues. Typically, the pain awakens the patient at night, recurs during weight-bearing, and subsides with rest.
3. Assess Mrs. Hart's vital signs and temperature.	**3.** Mrs. Hart's vital signs may increase from pain and fear of the unknown (such as the course of the disease). Her temperature should be normal, however, because osteoarthritis does not involve systemic inflammation.
4. Assess or assist with assessment of Mrs. Hart's joint range of motion (ROM).	**4.** Joints affected by osteoarthritis have decreased ROM; movements stop as pain occurs. Other joints may have normal or only slightly decreased ROM.
5. Assist with assessment of Mrs. Hart's muscle strength and reflexes.	**5.** Mrs. Hart will have reduced muscle strength, although this may stem solely from age. Her reflexes may be within the normal range.
6. Assess Mrs. Hart for other medical conditions.	**6.** Many patients over age 65 have one or more chronic illnesses.

Nursing diagnoses

• Impaired physical mobility related to decreased ROM in the affected joint or joints
• Knowledge deficit related to required life-style adjustments and the treatment regimen

Planning and goals
- Mrs. Hart will regain pain-free mobility.
- Mrs. Hart will comply with the prescribed treatment regimen.
- Mrs. Hart will regain joint congruity within normal limits with treatment.

Implementation

Nursing behaviors	Nursing rationales
1. Explain upcoming events to Mrs. Hart, such as the health history interview, physical examination, X-rays, and laboratory studies (blood studies, urinalysis, and possibly an electrocardiogram).	**1.** Explanations reduce anxiety and promote cooperation.
2. Assist with diagnostic studies, as needed.	**2.** Assistance improves the quality of care and shows attentiveness to Mrs. Hart's needs.
3. Gather laboratory and X-ray data, when available.	**3.** This promotes diagnosis and treatment.
4. Clarify the physician's explanations of Mrs. Hart's condition, proposed treatment regimen, and possible outcomes. As appropriate, use pictures, posters, or charts.	**4.** Mrs. Hart may need repeated explanations because she is anxious or unfamiliar with medical terms. Visual aids enhance comprehension of verbal explanations.
5. Teach Mrs. Hart how to use a cane; explain that when stepping forward with her *right* foot, she must have the cane in the *left* hand and move it forward.	**5.** Placing the cane in the opposite hand and moving it forward while moving the affected foot forward simulates normal walking. If Mrs. Hart carries the cane in her right hand instead, she will limp rather than walk normally.
6. Watch Mrs. Hart practice walking with the cane.	**6.** This eases patient concerns and may reveal the need for additional explanations or practice.
7. Teach Mrs. Hart and her daughter about the prescribed medication regimen. For example, the physician may prescribe buffered aspirin (600 to 1,000 mg) every 4 hours, taken alone or with another anti-inflammatory medication, such as ibuprofen (Motrin, 400 mg taken four times daily) or piroxicam (Feldene, 20 mg taken once daily).	**7.** Mrs. Hart and her significant other must understand the medication regimen and schedule needed to maintain a therapeutic blood drug level.
8. Teach Mrs. Hart about potential side effects of prescribed medications, such as gastric irritation, ulcers, and gastrointestinal (GI) bleeding. Instruct her to take medications with food and check the color of the stool and water in the toilet for signs of bleeding. Instruct her to to stop taking the medications and to call the physician if side effects occur.	**8.** Anti-inflammatory medications are known GI irritants and may cause GI ulcers and bleeding. To counteract these problems, the physician also may prescribe cimetidine (Tagamet) or famotidine (Pepcid).
9. Arrange for an appointment for physical therapy, if this service is not available in the physician's office.	**9.** Exercises, gait training, and diathermy may relieve Mrs. Hart's symptoms, helping her regain greater mobility.
10. Make a follow-up medical appointment for Mrs. Hart.	**10.** Mrs. Hart will require extended follow-up care because joint cartilage does not regenerate on its own.

ADULT NURSING

11. Stress the need for Mrs. Hart to comply with the treatment regimen.

11. Patient compliance may help delay the need for surgery for many years—or avoid it entirely.

Evaluation (outcomes)

• Mrs. Hart eventually regains nearly pain-free mobility after using a cane, taking prescribed medications, and undergoing physical therapy.
• Mrs. Hart complies with the treatment regimen over an extended period (2 years).
• Mrs. Hart regains joint congruity with treatment.

Rheumatoid arthritis

Overview

Rheumatoid arthritis, a chronic inflammatory disease with an autoimmune component, causes joint inflammation and increased synovial exudate. It may involve the heart, lungs, kidneys, and skin. In early disease stages, joints of the fingers, hands, and wrists are affected more frequently than major weight-bearing joints. Typically, symptoms are more pronounced in winter.

Rheumatoid arthritis sometimes arises during childhood (juvenile rheumatoid arthritis, such as Still's disease). However, onset most commonly occurs between ages 30 and 50. It affects three times as many females as males. The disease has a familial basis, typically occurring in more than one family member.

Signs and symptoms of rheumatoid arthritis include:
• swelling in one or more joints (swelling commonly is symmetrical, affecting corresponding joints on opposite sides of the body)
• pain in one or more joints
• edema in one or more joints
• joint stiffness on awakening that lessens gradually throughout the day
• Raynaud's phenomenon (white to bluish or red color change of the fingers or toes)
• joint deformities of the hands and wrists
• changes in hand or foot sensations
• joint stiffening or fusing
• pneumonitis
• carditis
• dryness of the mouth and conjunctivae
• anemia
• involvement of the cells lining the renal glomeruli
• partial joint dislocation (subluxation)
• subcutaneous nodules.

Clinical situation

Sarah Frankford, age 45, is admitted to the nursing unit to undergo surgical bilateral synovectomies (synovial membrane excision) of joints affected by rheumatoid arthritis. An executive secretary, she is accompanied by her husband, an airline pilot.

Assessment

Nursing behaviors
1. Assess Mrs. Frankford's health history and physical condition.

Nursing rationales
1. This helps determine Mrs. Frankford's current condition, past or present treatments, and understanding of the disease.

2. Measure Mrs. Frankford's weight and height and assess her vital signs.

3. Assess the condition of joints throughout the body. Determine Mrs. Frankford's range of motion (ROM), muscle strength, and reflexes.

4. Assess Mrs. Frankford's ability to perform activities of daily living (ADLs) independently.

5. Assess Mrs. Frankford's current medication regimen.

6. Assess Mrs. Frankford for adverse effects of medications.

7. Assess Mrs. Frankford's rest and exercise habits, physical therapy regimen, and use of heat or cold application and orthoses (such as splints, inserts, and braces).

2. This helps assess the effects of rheumatoid arthritis on the entire body. For instance, Mrs. Frankford may have an elevated temperature because rheumatoid arthritis is an inflammatory disease.

3. Involved joints will appear edematous and deformed, with partial dislocations and tendon shortening. They also will feel hot and show reduced ROM. Near involved joints, muscle strength will be decreased and reflex reactions altered slightly.

4. Mrs. Frankford may require assistance with some ADLs.

5. Prescribed medications vary with the stage of the disease or therapy (see *Treatments for rheumatoid arthritis*).

6. Anti-inflammatory agents, steroids, and other medications may cause multiple adverse effects.

7. Physical therapy regimens for rheumatoid arthritis vary with the patient's condition.

Treatments for rheumatoid arthritis

Treatments for rheumatoid arthritis are multiple and typically proceed in levels, or steps, according to the patient's response. However, some treatments in higher levels may be prescribed before all treatments in a lower level have been attempted.

Level 1
- Patient teaching
- Physical and occupational therapy
- Rest and exercise
- Orthotic devices
- Heat or cold applications
- Nonnarcotic analgesic medications and nonsteroidal anti-inflammatory drugs (NSAIDS)

Level 2
- Salicylates (such as aspirin)
- Joint injection with corticosteroids
- NSAIDS
- Gold therapy
- Antimalarial medications
- Low-dose oral corticosteroids

Level 3
- Surgical correction
- Plasmapheresis
- Penicillamine

Level 4
- Cytotoxic medications (such as methotrexate)
- Immunosuppressive medications

ADULT NURSING

8. Assess results of Mrs. Frankford's laboratory tests and synovial fluid analysis.

8. In 95% of patients with rheumatoid arthritis, blood studies indicate anemia (a low hemoglobin level), and positive rheumatoid factor, which is a specific immunoglobulin. Synovial fluid analysis may reveal yellow fluid with a white blood cell (WBC) count above 200/mm³, a positive culture indicating infection, and higher-than-normal volume (over 3.5 ml). Normally, synovial fluid is clear and colorless or straw-colored, with less than 200 WBCs/mm³, and negative for culture.

Nursing diagnoses

- Impaired physical mobility related to joint changes
- Knowledge deficit related to the disease process and treatment plan

Planning and goals

- Mrs. Frankford will regain satisfactory joint movement in her fingers after the synovectomies.
- Mrs. Frankford will gradually regain the ability to perform ADLs.
- Mrs. Frankford will continue her usual medical treatments for rheumatoid arthritis.
- Mrs. Frankford will return to her job after an uncomplicated recovery.

Implementation

Nursing behaviors

1. Orient Mrs. Frankford to the nursing unit and personnel.

2. Explain the procedures and purposes of scheduled diagnostic studies, such as an electrocardiogram, I.V. pyelogram, repeated serum studies, X-rays, and urinalysis.

3. Administer medication for rheumatoid arthritis, as ordered.

4. Prepare Mrs. Frankford for scheduled treatments or diagnostic tests.

5. Teach Mrs. Frankford about required skin preparation or cleaning before her surgery.

6. Perform preoperative preparations and provide care the evening before and morning of surgery (for details, see the section on "Perioperative nursing").

7. Complete required nursing documentation before transferring Mrs. Frankford to the surgical suite.

Nursing rationales

1. Orientation eases patient anxiety and concern in the unfamiliar environment.

2. Explanations promote compliance and understanding. Thorough data help determine Mrs. Frankford's present status and predict her ability to tolerate surgery and anesthesia.

3. Mrs. Frankford must continue taking medications to maintain control of the disease.

4. Preparation reduces stress on all involved parties.

5. Mrs. Frankford may be required only to shower daily, or she may need to use special cleaning solutions, as ordered. Skin preparation may be done in the preoperative preparation area in the surgical suite.

6. Thorough preparation helps ensure that Mrs. Frankford will be in optimal condition for surgery.

7. This helps ensure the safety and continuity of care.

ADULT NURSING

Clinical situation
(continued)

Mrs. Frankford is taken to surgery, where she undergoes bilateral synovectomies of the proximal interphalangeal joints of all fingers and both thumbs with silicone spacers. (Spacers help maintain the joint space; silicone is almost inert and reduces the reaction.) Then she is transferred to the postanesthesia recovery room.

Implementation

Nursing behaviors

1. Assist in transferring Mrs. Frankford to her bed when she returns to the nursing unit from the recovery room.

2. Elevate Mrs. Frankford's hands and forearms on pillows or place them in vertical cotton restraints attached to I.V. poles.

3. Apply ice bags to the operative areas.

4. Perform neurovascular checks STAT and as ordered, such as every 30 minutes to 1 hour for the first 24 hours, then every 2 to 4 hours (see "Performing neurovascular checks," pages 263 and 264).

5. Monitor Mrs. Frankford's vital signs, as ordered.

6. Monitor I.V. fluid administration while oral fluids are withheld.

7. Administer narcotic analgesics, as needed and ordered. (Although these drugs frequently are given via a patient-controlled analgesia pump, Mrs. Frankford would not be able to activate the pump because both of her hands are bandaged.)

8. Check the elastic wraps around Mrs. Frankford's hands for tightness and capillary refill changes, and note any complaints of throbbing.

9. When Mrs. Frankford can resume oral intake, administer medications for rheumatoid arthritis, as ordered.

10. Teach Mrs. Frankford about iron-rich foods to consume to help overcome anemia.

Nursing rationales

1. Mrs. Frankford will need help during transfer because she cannot use her fingers or hands.

2. This increases venous return by reducing edema.

3. Ice causes vasoconstriction, reducing edema.

4. Neurovascular checks provide information about the circulation and motor and sensory functions of involved tissue.

5. Vital signs provide data about Mrs. Frankford's recovery from anesthesia and surgery, and may signal complications.

6. Oral fluids are withheld, as ordered, until Mrs. Frankford is alert and has regained a gag reflex. In the meantime, she needs I.V. fluids to maintain hydration.

7. Mrs. Frankford may need narcotics for several days or longer because of her multiple incisions and significant soft-tissue involvement.

8. Elastic wraps may become too tight because of edema. They usually can be loosened or unwrapped by the RN. Sluggish capillary refill may indicate arterial compromise and a too-tight bandage. Throbbing signals excessive pressure on arteries.

9. Continued medications are required to treat rheumatoid arthritis.

10. Nonsteroidal anti-inflammatory drugs, given to treat rheumatoid arthritis, may cause anemia. To counter this effect, Mrs. Frankford should consume such iron-rich foods as raisins and other dried fruit, spinach, red meats, liver, and tuna.

ADULT NURSING

11. Change Mrs. Frankford's dressings, as needed but at least every 24 hours.

11. Dressings must be changed every 24 to 48 hours to permit increased joint movement.

12. Schedule physical therapy, as ordered.

12. Exercises typically can begin as early as the first or second postoperative day.

13. Monitor breath sounds in all lung lobes. Encourage Mrs. Frankford to use a respiratory aid every 2 hours.

13. Inhalation anesthetics and rheumatoid arthritis affect the lungs, necessitating frequent pulmonary monitoring. Use of a respiratory aid improves the quality of respirations and helps prevent respiratory complications.

14. Monitor Mrs. Frankford's vital signs every 1 to 4 hours. Check the apical pulse every 4 hours.

14. Rheumatoid arthritis may cause inflammatory cardiac changes. The apical pulse is a good index of cardiac function.

15. Monitor Mrs. Frankford's fluid intake and output every 8 hours.

15. Rheumatoid arthritis affects renal function, calling for careful monitoring of fluid intake and output.

16. Monitor Mrs. Frankford's bowel sounds every 4 hours. Check for daily bowel movements.

16. Narcotics, bedrest, and lack of oral intake may alter bowel function.

17. Arrange for a consultation with an occupational therapist to determine which modifications are needed for Mrs. Frankford's self-care and home management.

17. Mrs. Frankford probably will need modifications for self-care and home management to help conserve muscle and joint strength. For instance, she may need modified utensils or appliances to prevent injury and use musculoskeletal tissues most efficiently.

18. Observe Mrs. Frankford's ability to perform ADLs; provide assistance, as needed.

18. Mrs. Frankford will need assistance with ADLs in the early postoperative period because of her surgery.

19. Use aseptic technique and gentle movements when performing dressing changes and wound care.

19. This helps prevent infection of Mrs. Frankford's multiple incisions.

20. Provide a back massage and encourage Mrs. Frankford to change her position every 2 to 4 hours.

20. Massage increases circulation and promotes waste removal. Changing position reduces pressure on all tissues.

21. Review with Mrs. Frankford the actions and adverse effects of any newly prescribed medications.

21. This ensures that Mrs. Frankford has current, correct information.

22. Encourage Mrs. Frankford to express her concerns and feelings about the disease and its effect on her role performance.

22. Expression helps clarify Mrs. Frankford's feelings and concerns.

23. Consult with the social worker for discharge planning assistance.

23. Social workers have special expertise for meeting patient needs after discharge.

24. Complete a continuity-of-care referral for a community nurse to visit Mrs. Frankford at home after discharge.

24. Because of Mrs. Frankford's chronic disease, she will need long-term follow-up care.

25. Complete nursing documentation appropriately.

25. Proper documentation provides a complete record of Mrs. Frankford's care and progress.

Evaluation (outcomes)

• Mrs. Frankford regains satisfactory joint movements in her fingers after recovering from the synovectomies and insertion of silicone spacers.
• Mrs. Frankford regains the ability to perform some ADLs by the time of discharge.
• Mrs. Frankford continues her ongoing medical treatments.
• Mrs. Frankford should be able to resume employment after a 3- to 6-month recovery.

Complications of musculoskeletal disorders

This chart presents the most serious or life-threatening complications of musculoskeletal disorders, along with interventions that are crucial to patient safety and comfort.

COMPLICATION	CAUSE	NURSING INTERVENTIONS
Bone union problems		
Nonunion Failure of bone ends to join firmly because of lack of calcification at the fracture site. Signs and symptoms include persistent pain and inability to use or bear weight on the involved body part.	• Lack of approximation of bone segments • Inadequate reduction • Insufficient nutrients	• Encourage the patient to increase dietary calcium intake. • Instruct the patient to seek continuing medical care. • Advise the patient to use an ambulatory aid, sling, or splint, as appropriate.
Malunion Healing of a fracture in a less-than-optimal position. Signs and symptoms include unusual or abnormal position of the distal fracture fragment and inability to use normally or bear full weight on the involved body part.	• Inadequate reduction • Excessive or premature weight-bearing	• Encourage the patient to discuss concerns related to malunion. • Instruct the patient to return to the physician if dissatisfied with the function or shape of the involved body part. (The physician may need to refracture and reset the bone.)
Delayed union Prolonged healing of a fracture (usually longer than 9 months). Signs and symptoms include inability to regain full use and strength in the involved area for a prolonged period.		• Encourage the patient to seek continuing medical care. • Advise the patient to continue using an ambulatory aid, splint, or brace, as needed. • Encourage the patient to maintain an adequate intake of vitamins A, B, C, and D and zinc and calcium to aid bone healing.
Wound or joint infection Infection of a wound or joint tissues. Signs and symptoms of wound infection include fever, soreness, pain, swelling, abscess, and purulent drainage at the wound site. Signs and symptoms of joint infection include inability to use the involved joint normally, marked soreness or pain, swelling, redness, and an enlarging mass in the joint area. With an infected joint, purulent drainage may appear within a fistula that develops to the skin.	• Bacterial contamination of the wound or joint	• Monitor vital signs closely. • Assess the wound or joint area frequently for an increase in inflammation or infection. • Administer antibiotics, if ordered. • Assist with wound opening to permit drainage. • Apply moist soaks and perform irrigation, as ordered. • Use strict aseptic technique when performing wound care. • If joint infection follows total joint replacement, the joint area may need to be opened and the prosthesis removed. Irrigating tubes may be inserted into the joint; the prosthesis may be replaced later or bone grafts may be inserted to increase joint stability. The patient will receive long-term I.V. antibiotics, followed by oral antibiotics. • Wound or joint infections in orthopedic patients are serious complications that should be prevented, if possible.

(continued)

ADULT NURSING

Complications of musculoskeletal disorders *(continued)*

COMPLICATION	CAUSE	NURSING INTERVENTIONS
Nerve palsy Weakness or paralysis of one or more nerves. Signs and symptoms include inability to move or feel a muscle, joint, or body part after injury or treatment.	• Nerve damage caused by injury or treatments	• Help the patient perform passive range-of-motion exercises to reduce muscle atrophy. • Conduct careful neurovascular checks. • Avoid using a hot water bottle or heating pad because the patient cannot sense high temperatures. • Use a sling, brace, or splint to hold the affected part in a functional position. • Encourage the patient to seek continuing medical care.
Unequal leg length Inequality of leg length after treatment, joint replacement, or tumor removal. Signs include a discrepancy in the measured lengths of the right and left legs.	• Operative repair	• Orthotic devices, lifts, shoe alterations, and other treatments may reduce the discrepancy. • Encourage the patient to seek continuing medical care.
Fat embolism Obstruction of one or more areas of the lung, skin, or other organs by fat molecules released after fracture of a long bone. This complication most commonly arises within 1 to 3 days after a fracture. Signs and symptoms include: • changes in vital signs, such as increased pulse and respiratory rates and reduced blood pressure (shock is common) • a fine petechial rash over the chest, neck, and conjunctivae • subjective feeling that something is wrong • chest pain • confusion or disorientation.	• Mobilization (freeing) of fat molecules into the bloodstream from a long-bone fracture	• Arrange for immediate medical attention. • The patient may require I.V. line insertion, supplemental oxygen, steroids, antibiotics, and other treatments (such as dextran or other volume expanders). • Monitor the patient continuously to prevent death.
Compartment syndrome Condition in which increased tissue pressure in a confined area leads to reduced blood flow, resulting in ischemia and nerve and muscle dysfunction in the affected area. Signs and symptoms include marked edema of the involved area; increasing pain (especially on passive movement, such as when joints near the involved area are moved); and weak or absent peripheral pulses distal to the injury site.	• Marked increase in venous pressure at the injury site that leads to decreased arterial inflow, causing ischemia	• Maintain a high index of suspicion for patients at risk for this complication, such as those with a fracture of one or more extremities. • Elevate the affected limb to heart level. • Apply ice bags to the affected area to decrease edema. • Perform careful neurovascular checks. • Report increased pain or edema or changes in peripheral pulses to the team leader. • This is a serious complication that must be corrected within 6 to 12 hours to prevent permanent damage to the affected area.

Performing neurovascular checks

Introduction

To evaluate peripheral circulation and nerve function, the nurse performs a series of eight assessments focusing on peripheral neurologic and vascular tissues. (Procedure steps preceded by an asterisk are especially important.)

Steps

*1. Check the color of injured tissues, which may be pink, pale, bluish, or red. Compare with corresponding tissues on the opposite side of the body.

*2. Check the temperature of injured tissues, which may feel warmer than, cooler than, or the same as corresponding tissues on the opposite side.

*3. Check for edema (swelling) distal to (farther from) injured tissues, and compare with corresponding tissues on the opposite side.

*4. Assess the patient's ability to move joints distal to the injury. Compare these movements with those of corresponding joints on the opposite side.

*5. Assess the patient for complaints of numbness, tingling, or a "pins and needles" or "asleep" sensation in injured tissues or tissues distal to the injury.

*6. Check capillary refill by compressing the middle nail on the patient's injured limb (use moderate pressure when doing this). Continue compressing the nail for as long as it takes to say "refill" (about 1 second). Then release, and assess how long the nail takes to regain its normal pink color. To validate refill times, repeat this step.

Rationales

*1. Skin color reflects circulatory adequacy. Injured tissues usually are slightly paler than normal tissues. Pink skin reflects adequate arterial flow. Pallor may indicate decreased arterial flow; bluish skin, venous stasis causing tissue deoxygenation (bluish blood is deoxygenated). Reddened skin may signal inflammation, infection, or vasodilation caused by an allergic response.

*2. Like skin color, skin temperature reflects arterial circulatory adequacy. Injured tissues usually are cooler than normal tissues. Coolness indicates reduced circulation; coldness, absent or inadequate arterial circulation. Abnormal warmth signals localized tissue inflammation or infection.

*3. Edema signals venous stasis or decreased venous return to the heart. Injured tissues usually are edematous for several days or more.

*4. The patient should be able to move tissues distal to the injury site (although such movement may be slower than that of healthy tissues). *Sudden inability to move joints actively should be reported immediately.*

*5. These sensations reflect pressure on nerves. If they arise suddenly, report them immediately because they may signal an abnormal rise in venous pressure.

*6. Pink nail color indicates that capillary refill has occurred. Refill within 2 to 4 seconds indicates adequate arterial blood flow. Refill in 4 to 6 seconds is considered prolonged or sluggish, which may signal arterial compromise. Refill that takes more than 6 seconds may signal inadequate arterial blood flow or increased venous pressure; *report this finding immediately.*

ADULT NURSING

*7. Check for patient complaints of pain, noting severity, type, duration, and site. Record specific descriptions, such as "a sharp pain that feels like a bad toothache."

*7. Pain is a response to noxious (harmful) stimuli; it also may result from pressure on nerve endings. Responses to pain are highly individualized. Some patients can tolerate significant pain without complaining; other patients may complain of pain repeatedly. Keep in mind that *pain is as severe as the patient says it is* and must be dealt with, not ignored. Report any increasing pain not relieved by prescribed medications.

8. As you complete each neurovascular check, compare findings from injured tissues with those from corresponding tissues on the opposite side.

8. Comparison provides a basis for evaluating normal or abnormal findings.

9. Document all findings.

9. Documentation proves that the procedure was done, assures high-quality care, and provides legal protection. (Flow sheets may be available for recording results of neurovascular checks, or you may document the results on nursing sheets.)

Assisting with cast application

Introduction

To provide the safest and most effective care enviornment, the nurse assists with cast application and provides appropriate care before, during, and afterward. (Procedure steps preceded by an asterisk are especially important.)

Steps

1. Assess the patient's understanding of cast application (if the patient is a young child, assess the parent's understanding).

Rationales

1. This helps correct any misunderstandings or knowledge deficit, eases anxieties, and increases patient comfort.

*2. Assess the skin areas over which the cast will be placed for cleanliness, open areas (such as skin breaks), rashes, bruises, and blisters.

*2. Skin should be clean and free of bruises, blisters, rashes, and open areas before the cast is applied. Blisters may result from altered circulation caused by the injury, especially if a bone has been fractured.

*3. Assemble needed supplies (these may be stored on a cast cart or in the cast room). These include:
• plaster rolls in various sizes (2″, 3″, 4″, or 6″ [5.1, 7.6, 10.2, or 15.2 cm]), or fiberglass packages if a fiberglass cast will be applied
• pail filled with warm water (to dampen the plaster rolls or fiberglass)
• materials used to cover or pad the skin (such as a stockinette or felt, webril, or sheet wadding)
• gloves and apron
• scissors
• paper or plaster sheets
• cast saw.

*3. Assembling supplies in advance eases cast application and reduces patient discomfort. Plaster, which is stronger and heavier than fiberglass, is used if weight-bearing will be permitted. Warm water triggers the chemical actions that set plaster or fiberglass. Skin coverings or padding prevent pressure over bony prominences (more padding may be needed for an older patient, who has less subcutaneous fat than a younger patient). Gloves and an apron protect the nurse's skin and clothing. Scissors are used to cut materials to size and shape to fit various areas. Paper or plaster sheets protect the table or floor surfaces. A cast saw is used to trim the plaster or fiberglass to the desired shape and size.

4. Place the patient in the most comfortable position possible. Depending on the type of cast to be applied, the best position may be sitting, standing, or lying. If needed, support the affected body part, and keep it exposed.

4. These measures aid cast application.

5. Assist with applying and shaping the padding.

5. Padding should be smooth, wrinkle-free, and dry, with no lumpy areas.

6. Assist with cast application by performing one of the following steps, as appropriate:
• Dampen the plaster rolls or fiberglass in the warm water for several seconds, then squeeze gently to remove excess water.
• Support the involved body part while the plaster rolls are unrolled.
• Hold the involved body part while the fiberglass or cast tape is wrapped around the body part, then smooth the tape edges.

6. Plaster or fiberglass must be dampened so that it can be applied and molded to the body part. Supporting the body part maintains the part in the proper position. Fiberglass or cast tape must be dampened to activate adhesive on the strips (which dries within 3 to 5 minutes of application). Smoothing the tape edges prevents roughness.

7. Turn down the ends of the stockinette over the damp plaster or fiberglass, then cover the ends of the stockinette with the plaster or fiberglass.

7. This creates a smooth surface that helps prevent skin injury from rough plaster or fiberglass.

*8. Hold the body part firmly while the plaster or fiberglass is molded around it for final shaping of the cast.

*8. Sufficient plaster is needed to make the cast strong; fiberglass is lightweight but strong and only a few rolls are needed.

9. Assist with trimming the plaster or fiberglass, if needed.

9. The cast should fit snugly without restricting finger or toe movement.

10. Help apply a stabilizing bar, brace, or walking heel (if used).

10. A bar is used to stabilize the legs of a spica cast. A knee brace may be used with a brace (called a cast brace). A walking heel aids full or partial weight-bearing.

ADULT NURSING

*11. If a plaster cast was applied, rest the affected limb on one or more pillows to let the plaster set. (Cast tapes dry in 3 to 5 minutes.) Keep the cast uncovered.

12. Discard unused supplies, empty water from the pail, return supplies to the appropriate places, and clean the area.

13. Assist with patient transfer to the nursing unit or to the home after discharge. While the cast is damp, provide the following patient teaching:
• Keep the cast uncovered until it dries, which may take 2 to 5 days depending on cast size and the materials used.
• Keep the casted part elevated on a pillow for 2 to 3 days.
• Lift the cast from beneath, supporting the casted part at two joints (one above and one below the injury site).
• Use the palms, not fingers, to hold or lift the casted part while the cast is damp.
• Continue to use an ice bag for 24 hours, or as ordered.
• Continue to take prescribed analgesics every 4 to 6 hours.
• Keep follow-up medical appointments.
• Notify the physician if any of the following signs or symptoms arise: numbness, tingling, marked swelling, increased pain, inability to move the fingers or toes, or prolonged capillary refill (longer than 6 seconds).

*14. If the cast is on an upper extremity, apply a sling, as ordered (see "Applying a sling," pages 268 and 269). If the cast is on a lower extremity, teach the patient how to use crutches, as appropriate (see "Teaching a patient to use crutches, a cane, or a walker," pages 272 and 273).

15. After the cast has set, perform neurovascular checks on the affected body part.

16. Document cast application, the patient's response, patient teaching, and results of neurovascular checks. Also document the time of discharge and the patient's condition at discharge.

*11. Pillows provide a firm but soft surface to prevent deformity of the cast while it is damp. Keeping the cast uncovered promotes drying.

12. This readies the area and equipment for use by other patients and personnel.

13. The patient may be an inpatient or outpatient. Patient teaching helps ensure safe care. Exposing the cast to air allows it to dry thoroughly, both inside and outside. Elevation minimizes edema. Supporting the casted part at these joints prevents pain and additional injury. Using the palms distributes pressure over a wider area than the fingertips. Ice causes vasoconstriction, which decreases bleeding and edema. Therapeutic blood drug levels help maintain pain relief. Follow-up care is vital to maintaining continuity of care, assessing the patient's recovery, and detecting abnormalities. The signs and symptoms listed may signal complications.

*14. Suspension in a sling helps support the joints of the affected extremity. Crutches permit ambulation during bone healing.

15. This determines if the patient has adequate circulation without pressure on nerve points.

16. Documentation proves that the procedure was done, assures high-quality care, and provides legal protection.

Assisting with cast removal

Introduction   To make cast removal as trauma-free as possible, the nurse helps remove a cast from the patient's body part.

Steps	**Rationales**
1. Place the patient in a comfortable position, with the cast exposed completely.	**1.** This aids cast removal.
2. Obtain large blunt-ended scissors and a cast saw. Plug the saw into an electrical outlet.	**2.** Gathering the proper equipment makes cast removal easier.
3. Reassure the patient that the saw will not cut through the skin surface.	**3.** This eases patient anxiety.
4. Hold the affected body part or cast while the physician or orthopedic technician cuts through the cast on two sides.	**4.** This increases patient comfort and reduces the risk of injury.
5. Assist with (or perform) cutting of the padding or stockinette with the scissors.	**5.** Scissors must be used to remove the padding or stockinette (the saw cuts only plaster or fiberglass).
6. Carefully slide the affected body part out of the cast, or gently lift the cast from the body part.	**6.** Careful cast removal reduces the risk of injury to tissues that have been weakened by enclosure in the cast.
7. After the cast and padding have been removed, gently wash the skin with mild soap and water.	**7.** Gentle handling helps prevent injury to weakened skin tissues.
8. If a new cast will not be applied, teach the patient about skin care (as described in "Teaching about skin care after cast removal," page 268).	**8.** A new cast may be applied if healing is incomplete. Skin care promotes healing.
9. Assist with discharge care. Remind the patient of the need for follow-up X-rays or medical appointments, if ordered.	**9.** This promotes safety and continuity of care.
10. Document cast removal, the condition of the involved tissues, and the patient's response to the procedure.	**10.** Documentation proves that the procedure was done, assures high-quality care, and provides legal protection.

ADULT NURSING

Teaching about skin care after cast removal

Introduction
After cast removal, the nurse teaches the patient how to care for injured skin and tissues. Skin care promotes continued healing and helps prevent injury to weakened tissues. (Procedure steps preceded by an asterisk are especially important.)

Steps

1. Teach the patient how to remove dead skin cells and debris by applying a liquid enzyme-containing, cold-water washing solution (such as Woolite or Delicare) on the affected skin and leaving it there for at least 20 minutes. Then instruct the patient to immerse the body part in warm water gently, wash it with a soft cloth, flush it with clear warm water, and gently pat the skin dry without rubbing or scratching. Teach the patient to cover the skin with a moisturizing lotion, then repeat the wash in 24 hours.

*2. Inform the patient that the affected part may become mildly to moderately swollen (edematous) for several days. If this occurs, the patient should elevate the limb on a pillow until the swelling recedes.

*3. Inform the patient that the limb may feel sore and painful with increased weight-bearing. To relieve discomfort, advise the patient to take a nonnarcotic analgesic (usually aspirin) every 4 hours for 24 to 48 hours.

4. Instruct the patient to notify the physician if edema or soreness persists more than 2 to 4 weeks.

5. Document teaching and the patient's response.

Rationales

1. Enzymes in cold-water washing solution emulsify fats, aiding removal of dead cells and debris. Applying a moisturizer and avoiding skin breaks help reduce trauma to skin cells that have become dry and delicate from enclosure in the cast. After the second washing and lotion application, skin cells usually regain normal health and require no further special care.

*2. Edema develops because the restrictive cast has been removed. Elevation increases venous return and reduces edema.

*3. Pain and soreness arise as previously disused muscles and joints suddenly must resume normal function. Aspirin is an effective anti-inflammatory analgesic that relieves mild to moderate pain.

4. Relief of discomfort and return of full function depend on the specific injury, individual response, and treatment.

5. Documentation proves that the procedure was done, assures high-quality care, and provides legal protection.

Applying a sling

Introduction
A sling is used to provide support to an injured upper extremity.

Steps

1. Obtain a triangle muslin sling or manufactured sling, if available.

Rationales

1. A sling may be made from muslin or strong cotton material in a formed shape.

2. Place the patient in a comfortable sitting or standing position.

3. With the patient's elbow bent, slide the corner of the triangle muslin sling under the patient's arm. Place the end of the triangle near the elbow and the under-arm end of the sling on the opposite shoulder. Bring the last end of the triangle over the cast and forearm to the shoulder on the casted side. Adjust the sling to fit snugly under the cast, with the elbow slightly lower than the wrist. Secure the ends of the sling around the patient's neck with pins, or tie a knot to the side of the nape (bony area) of the neck.

4. If applying a manufactured sling, slide it under and over the patient's forearm and arm with the elbow bent. Close and adjust the pressure-sensitive (Velcro) straps for comfort.

5. Teach the patient to relax ("drop") the shoulder in the sling so that the muscles will be relaxed and comfortable.

6. If needed, adjust the sling several minutes after applying it. Remind the patient to relax the shoulder when adjusting the sling.

7. If ordered, apply an arm swath over the sling by closing the pressure-sensitive strap. Make sure the swath is snug.

8. Document the sling application and the patient's response.

2. Proper positioning aids sling application.

3. Applying the sling in this method provides a snug, comfortable resting area for the arm and forearm.

4. Various sizes of manufactured slings are available to provide safety and comfort.

5. Muscle tenseness or contraction may cause pain or soreness, counteracting the benefits of the sling.

6. The patient may need several minutes to adjust to or become comfortable in the sling.

7. An arm swath helps keep the arm close to the body for additional support.

8. Documentation proves that the procedure was done, assures high-quality care, and provides legal protection.

ADULT NURSING

Assisting with application of balanced-suspension skeletal traction for a fractured femur

Introduction

In this procedure, the nurse helps place a patient in balanced-suspension skeletal traction—a system of pins, pulleys, ropes, weights, and suspension supports. Such traction helps align or immobilize a fractured femur, permitting healing and reducing or eliminating muscle spasms. (Procedure steps preceded by an asterisk are especially important.)

Steps

*1. Gather all needed supplies on a cart, and take the cart to the cast room or the patient's room where traction will be applied. (If the patient is on an orthopedic nursing unit, a bed frame and trapeze should be on the patient's bed. If they are not, obtain these items in advance.) Supplies to gather include a sterile Steinmann pin tray (obtained from the operating room or central supply); local anesthetic (usually 1% to 2% lidocaine); antiseptic solution for skin cleaning; sterile gloves; Harris or Thomas splint; Pearson attachment; towels; felt strip and stockinette; drill; extension cord; nylon rope on a roll; 1-, 5-, and 10-lb (0.5-, 2.3-, and 4.5-kg) weights; weight holders; foot support; adhesive tape or small corks; and a wastebasket with plastic liner.

2. Reinforce or clarify the physician's explanation of the purpose of traction.

3. Position the patient properly in bed—usually in a recumbent position.

4. Place the Steinmann pin tray on the overbed table. Open the sterile drapes using surgical aseptic technique, touching only the outer covers of the tray and opening the flaps away from you. Move the overbed table close to the bed and patient area.

5. Assist the physician as requested by holding the affected extremity still. Be sure to handle only *nonsterile* equipment, such as the extension cord, splint, and foot support.

6. Unless the physician does so, explain that the skin will be prepared with an antiseptic and that a local anesthetic will be injected into the pin entry and exit sites (usually the upper tibia).

7. Continue to support the affected extremity as the physician drills through bone with the Steinmann pin. Explain that drilling will be brief—usually 1 to 2 minutes—and may cause a sensation of pressure or heat but not frank pain, because bones do not feel pain. Reassure the patient that the pin entry and exit sites have been numbed with local anesthetic.

Rationales

*1. Gathering supplies in advance makes the procedure smoother and helps ensure optimal nursing care.

2. This increases patient understanding and eases anxiety.

3. This helps the patient remain in the desired position for traction application.

4. Having supplies within easy reach promotes traction application. Using aseptic technique prevents introduction of pathogens to a sterile area.

5. Providing assistance allows the physician to maintain glove sterility and ensures that the patient is supported properly.

6. Explanations ease patient anxiety. An antiseptic reduces the risk of skin contamination; a local anesthetic deadens nerve endings to prevent pain.

7. Drilling is noisy and may upset the patient. Explanations help reduce patient anxiety.

ADULT NURSING

*8. After the pin has been placed properly, assist with completing the traction application. For instance, you may need to hold the patient's leg while the physician places a Harris or Thomas splint under the thigh and a Pearson attachment under the leg, with foot support placed on the Pearson attachment at the heel or sole area. When lifting the leg, support it at the joints above and below the injury site. Avoid moving tissues unnecessarily.

*8. Supporting the leg at the joints above and below the injury site stabilizes the bone to prevent additional injury or pain.

9. Apply ropes, weights, and weight holders to spreaders and pulleys for traction, suspension, and countertraction (or assist the physician in doing this).

9. Traction is created by the use of weights that pull tissues apart. Suspension elevates the body parts in traction. Countertraction pulls in the opposite direction.

*10. Ask the physician which positions the patient can assume during traction.

*10. Usually, the patient in balanced-suspension skeletal traction must lie on the back (dorsal recumbent position) and may lift the body, but should not turn to the side.

11. Monitor the patient's response to skeletal traction, once established. Clarify patient concerns, as needed.

11. Initial patient responses may include fear, anxiety, and claustrophobia.

*12. Check all parts of the traction apparatus, including ropes, pulleys, knots, corks on pin ends, weights, weight holders, suspension, and countertraction.

*12. Weights must hang freely from the rope with no restrictions on movement. *Never lift weights once skeletal traction is established.* Lifting can cause sudden muscle contraction, resulting in pain and disruption of alignment or other injury.

*13. Teach the patient how to lift the body, using a trapeze and the uninjured foot and leg, by providing these instructions: Bend the knee, place the foot flat on the bed, then put weight on the bent leg and foot and pull the body up with the hands on trapeze. Keep the back straight.
   When instructing the patient, avoid calling the uninjured leg the "good leg" and the injured leg the "bad leg." Instead, refer to them simply as the left leg and right leg.

*13. Teaching the patient how to lift the body properly during traction helps the patient adjust body position and achieve some independence; it also promotes care. Using such terms as "good leg" and "bad leg" may foster negative feelings toward the injured leg. By avoiding such judgments, the nurse helps the patient cope with the injury and view it less negatively.

14. Monitor the patient's vital signs and complaints of pain, as appropriate. Perform neurovascular checks until the patient's condition is stable.

14. This provides data needed for ongoing care.

15. Remove the used Steinmann pin tray and remaining supplies. Restore furniture to the normal position and replace supplies as needed.

15. This provides a safe, clean environment.

*16. Document the time of traction application, name of the physician who applied it, traction type and site, amount of weight applied, and the patient's response (including vital signs and results of neurovascular checks).

*16. Documentation proves that the procedure was done, assures high-quality care, and provides legal protection.

ADULT
NURSING

Teaching a patient to use crutches, a cane, or a walker

Introduction To increase the patient's mobility, the nurse teaches the patient how to move about using a special ambulatory aid. (Procedure steps preceded by an asterisk are especially important.)

Steps

1. Check the patient's chart for the medical order specifying crutches, a cane, or a walker.

2. Obtain the ordered ambulatory aid, along with needed pads or tips.

3. Clarify with the patient the purpose and use of the ambulatory aid (such as to permit mobility with limited or no weight-bearing, thereby reducing pain or permitting a tender, surgically repaired fractured bone or joint to heal).

*4. If the physician has ordered crutches, explain and demonstrate how to use them, as follows:
   Depending on the physician's order, use one of these gaits (walking methods).
• Four-point gait: Each crutch and each foot are considered a point. First, move one crutch forward, then the opposite foot. Next, move the second crutch forward, then move the second foot forward.
• Three-point gait: Each crutch is considered one point; one foot is the third point. (The second foot does not touch the ground.) Move both crutches forward together with the injured foot or leg (to avoid putting weight on the injured limb), then step with the uninjured leg.
• Two-point gait: One crutch and one foot (opposite the injured limb) move forward as one point, then the other crutch and foot move forward together. (A paraplegic patient who can ambulate may use a two-point gait in which both crutches are considered one point and both feet the second point. To move forward, the patient puts all the weight on the wrists, raises or hunches the shoulders to lift the body, propels the body and legs forward ahead of the crutches, balances the body, then brings the crutches forward together ahead of the body.)

*5. If the physician has ordered a cane, explain and demonstrate how to use it, as follows:
   Place the cane in the hand opposite the injured limb and move it forward with the injured limb.

Rationales

1. Special ambulatory aids require a written physician's order.

2. Rubber or foam pads or tips on an ambulatory aid increase patient comfort and safety.

3. This promotes patient understanding.

*4. Demonstrating various gaits and explaining the purpose of each aids patient understanding and promotes treatment. The four-point gait simulates normal walking and is used when weight-bearing is permitted. The three-point gait is used when the patient is not allowed to bear weight on the foot of the injured leg. The three-point gait, used when one foot or leg is injured, initially calls for the patient to put all the weight on one foot. (The two-point gait used by the paraplegic patient is extremely tiring; until stamina increases, the patient can walk only a short distance.)

*5. This technique simulates a normal gait.

*6. If the physician has ordered a walker, shorten or lengthen it to conform to the patient's height by pressing the button on each side until it pops out of the hole above or below its original position. If the patient is not permitted to bear weight on one limb, have the patient stand upright with the walker in front of the body. Next, explain and demonstrate how to use the walker, as follows:

Lift and move the walker forward 8″ to 10″ (20.3 to 25.4 cm) while bearing all weight on the uninjured limb. The injured limb can be placed on the floor without bearing weight on the foot. Place all weight on the wrists, with elbows straight, and step up to the walker with the uninjured limb. While moving the uninjured limb, do not put any weight on the injured limb. Bend the knee of the injured limb and move it forward so that it is just even with the opposite foot. Pause to rest and breathe deeply, then repeat these steps to move from place to place. (If no weight-bearing is permitted, remember not to bear weight on the injured limb.)

*7. For the patient using crutches, explain and demonstrate how to climb and descend stairs, as follows:

To climb stairs, step up to the stairs and place both crutches in one hand. Place the other hand on the bannister or railing, and put all the weight on the hands. Step up to the first stair with the uninjured limb, then bring the crutches and injured limb up to the first stair. Rest, then repeat this procedure for each stair.

To descend the stairs, step close to the edge of the top stair. Place both crutches in one hand and grasp the railing with the other hand. Move the injured limb and crutches down to the next step, then bring the uninjured limb down to the same step with the weight on both wrists and crutches. Rest, then repeat the procedure for each stair.

8. Have the patient practice climbing and descending stairs. (A patient who is weak or tires easily should walk up or down only two to three stairs to practice.) For support and stability, hold the patient at the waist.

*9. Document the patient's use of an ambulatory aid, noting the type of gait used and the patient's strength and skill at using the aid.

*6. The walker must be adjusted to a height that allows the patient to stand upright with elbows straight and feel comfortable without leaning or bending over. Most patients using a walker can put touch-down weight (up to 25 lb [11.3 kg]) on the injured limb. The injured limb should not precede the uninjured limb; otherwise, some weight might be placed on the injured limb inadvertently with the next step. If touch-down weight is permitted, test the amount of weight the patient is applying by putting your hand under the foot periodically.

*7. This method increases patient comfort because it allows the patient to move the injured limb last when climbing stairs and first when descending stairs, preventing weight-bearing on the injured limb.

8. Practice increases patient confidence and skill and promotes safe care.

*9. Documentation proves that the procedure was done, assures high-quality care, and provides legal protection.

ADULT NURSING

Drugs used to treat musculoskeletal disorders

This chart presents information about drugs commonly prescribed for musculoskeletal disorders, including the drug action, dosage, and common side effects. Nursing considerations focus on patient comfort and teaching.

DRUG	ACTION	USUAL ADULT DOSAGE	COMMON SIDE EFFECTS	NURSING CONSIDERATIONS
Salicylates				
Aspirin (acetyl-salicylic acid), plain or buffered	• Inhibits prosta-glandin synthe-sis, which blocks pain impulse generation	325 to 4,000 mg/day P.O.	• Anorexia • Nausea • Vomiting • Gastric upset • Gastrointestinal (GI) bleeding • Tinnitus (ringing in the ears) • Increased bleeding time	• Monitor for excessive bleeding. • Teach the patient to take the drug with food or an antacid or to use a buffered product, if ordered. • Instruct the patient to take the drug as ordered to maintain proper blood drug levels.
Choline magne-sium trisalicylate (Trilisate)	• Inhibits prosta-glandin synthe-sis, which blocks pain impulse generation	500 to 1,000 mg P.O. b.i.d. or t.i.d.	• Anorexia • Nausea • Gastric upset • Headache	• Monitor for magnesium toxicity when giving high doses. • Instruct the patient to take the drug as ordered to maintain proper blood drug levels. • Teach the patient to take the drug with food or an antacid.
Choline salicy-late (Arthropan)	• Inhibits prosta-glandin synthe-sis, which blocks pain impulse generation	1,000 to 3,000 mg P.O. t.i.d.	• Anorexia • Nausea • Gastric upset • Headache	• Monitor the patient's response to the drug. • Teach the patient to take the drug with food or an antacid or to use a buffered product, if ordered. • Instruct the patient to take the drug as ordered to maintain proper blood drug levels.
Salsalate (Disalcid)	• Inhibits prosta-glandin synthe-sis, which blocks pain impulse generation	2,000 to 3,000 mg/day P.O.	• Anorexia • Nausea • Gastric upset • Headache	• Monitor the patient's response to the drug. • Teach the patient to take the drug with food, an antacid, or 8 oz of milk or water. • Instruct the patient to take the drug as ordered to maintain proper blood drug levels.

Drugs used to treat musculoskeletal disorders *(continued)*

DRUG	ACTION	USUAL ADULT DOSAGE	COMMON SIDE EFFECTS	NURSING CONSIDERATIONS
Nonsteroidal anti-inflammatory agents				
Diclofenac (Voltaren)	• Inhibits prostaglandin synthesis, which blocks pain and reduces fever	25 mg P.O. q.i.d to 100 mg P.O. b.i.d.	• Peptic ulcers • GI bleeding • Nausea • Abdominal cramps • Diarrhea or constipation • Headache • Tinnitus • Rash • Edema	• Monitor the patient's response to the drug. • Weigh the patient and assess vital signs regularly. • Teach the patient the signs and symptoms of GI bleeding (such as black, tarry stools), and stress the need to report these to the physician immediately. However, be aware that serious GI toxicity can occur at any time without warning; elderly or debilitated patients and those on high-dose, long-term therapy may be at increased risk. • Instruct the patient to take with food if GI upset occurs • Stress the need to take the drug as prescribed to maintain proper blood drug levels.
diflunisal (Dolobid)	• Inhibits prostaglandin synthesis, which blocks pain and reduces fever	250 to 500 mg P.O. b.i.d., to a maximum daily dosage of 1.5 g	• Peptic ulcers • GI bleeding • Nausea • Abdominal cramps • Diarrhea or constipation • Headache • Tinnitus • Rash • Edema	• See "Nursing Considerations" for diclofenac.
fenoprofen (Nalfon)	• Inhibits prostaglandin synthesis, which blocks pain and reduces fever	300 to 600 mg P.O. q.i.d., to a maximum daily dosage of 3.2 g	• Peptic ulcers • GI bleeding • Nausea • Abdominal cramps • Diarrhea or constipation • Headache • Tinnitus • Rash • Edema	• See "Nursing Considerations" for diclofenac.
flurbiprofen (Ansaid)	• Inhibits prostaglandin synthesis, which blocks pain and reduces fever	200 to 300 mg P.O. in divided doses b.i.d. to q.i.d.	• Peptic ulcers • GI bleeding • Nausea • Abdominal cramps • Diarrhea or constipation • Headache • Tinnitus • Rash • Edema	• See "Nursing Considerations" for diclofenac.

(continued)

ADULT NURSING

Drugs used to treat musculoskeletal disorders *(continued)*

DRUG	ACTION	USUAL ADULT DOSAGE	COMMON SIDE EFFECTS	NURSING CONSIDERATIONS
Nonsteroidal anti-inflammatory agents *(continued)*				
ibuprofen (Advil, Medipren, Motrin, Rufen, Trendar)	• Inhibits prostaglandin synthesis, which blocks pain and reduces fever	400 to 800 mg P.O. q.i.d.; not to exceed 3.2 g daily	• Peptic ulcers • GI bleeding • Nausea • Abdominal cramps • Diarrhea or constipation • Headache • Tinnitus • Rash • Edema	• Tell the patient not to self-administer more than 1.6 g daily without the advice of a physician. • See "Nursing Considerations" for diclofenac.
indomethacin (Indocin)	• Inhibits prostaglandin synthesis, which blocks pain and reduces fever	25 to 50 mg P.O. b.i.d.	• Peptic ulcers • GI bleeding • Nausea • Abdominal cramps • Diarrhea or constipation • Headache • Tinnitus • Rash • Edema	• See "Nursing Considerations" for diclofenac.
ketoprofen (Orudis)	• Inhibits prostaglandin synthesis, which blocks pain and reduces fever	25 to 75 mg P.O. q.i.d., to a maximum daily dosage of 300 mg	• Peptic ulcers • GI bleeding • Nausea • Abdominal cramps • Diarrhea or constipation • Headache • Tinnitus • Rash • Edema	• See "Nursing Considerations" for diclofenac.
meclofenamate (Meclomen)	• Inhibits prostaglandin synthesis, which blocks pain and reduces fever	50 to 100 mg P.O. b.i.d. to q.i.d., to a maximum daily dosage of 400 mg	• Peptic ulcers • GI bleeding • Nausea • Abdominal cramps • Diarrhea or constipation • Headache • Tinnitus • Rash • Edema	• See "Nursing Considerations" for diclofenac.
naproxen (Naprosyn)	• Inhibits prostaglandin synthesis, which blocks pain and reduces fever	250 to 500 mg P.O. b.i.d.	Peptic ulcers • GI bleeding • Nausea • Abdominal cramps • Diarrhea or constipation • Headache • Tinnitus • Rash • Edema	• See "Nursing Considerations" for diclofenac.

Drugs used to treat musculoskeletal disorders *(continued)*

DRUG	ACTION	USUAL ADULT DOSAGE	COMMON SIDE EFFECTS	NURSING CONSIDERATIONS
Nonsteroidal anti-inflammatory agents *(continued)*				
naproxen sodium (Anaprox)	● Inhibits prostaglandin synthesis, which blocks pain and reduces fever	275 mg P.O. every 6 to 8 hours	● Peptic ulcers ● GI bleeding ● Nausea ● Abdominal cramps ● Diarrhea or constipation ● Headache ● Tinnitus ● Rash ● Edema	● See "Nursing Considerations" for diclofenac.
piroxicam (Feldene)	● Inhibits prostaglandin synthesis, which blocks pain and reduces fever	10 mg P.O. b.i.d. or 20 mg P.O. daily	● Peptic ulcers ● GI bleeding ● Nausea ● Abdominal cramps ● Headache ● Diarrhea or constipation ● Headache ● Tinnitus ● Rash ● Edema	● See "Nursing Considerations" for diclofenac.
sulindac (Clinoril)	● Inhibits prostaglandin synthesis, which blocks pain and reduces fever	150 to 200 mg P.O. b.i.d.	● Peptic ulcers ● GI bleeding ● Nausea ● Abdominal cramps ● Diarrhea or constipation ● Headache ● Tinnitus ● Rash ● Edema	● See "Nursing Considerations" for diclofenac.
tolmetin sodium (Tolectin)	● Inhibits prostaglandin synthesis, which blocks pain and reduces fever	400 mg P.O. t.i.d. or q.i.d., to a maximum daily dosage of 2 g	● Peptic ulcers ● GI bleeding ● Nausea ● Abdominal cramps ● Diarrhea or constipation ● Headache ● Tinnitus ● Rash ● Edema	● See "Nursing Considerations" for diclofenac.
Muscle relaxants				
Baclofen (Lioresal)	● Reduces nerve impulses from the spinal cord to the muscles	10 to 20 mg P.O. q.i.d.	● Drowsiness ● Dizziness ● Weakness ● Fatigue ● Headache ● Dry mouth ● Depression ● Insomnia ● Blurred vision ● Tremors ● Muscle pain ● Nausea ● Constipation ● Bloody stools ● Rash	● Warn the patient to avoid abrupt drug withdrawal because this could cause seizures or hallucinations. ● Monitor stools for blood. ● Warn the patient to avoid driving or operating dangerous machinery while taking this drug.

(continued)

ADULT NURSING

Drugs used to treat musculoskeletal disorders *(continued)*

DRUG	ACTION	USUAL ADULT DOSAGE	COMMON SIDE EFFECTS	NURSING CONSIDERATIONS
Muscle relaxants *(continued)*				
Carisoprodol (Soma)	• Reduces nerve impulses from the spinal cord to the muscles	350 mg P.O. t.i.d. and at bedtime	• Drowsiness • Dizziness • Ataxia • Depressive reaction • Rash • Hives • Nausea • Vomiting	• After one to four doses, some patients have an unusual reaction characterized by extreme weakness, dizziness, temporary vision loss, and disorientation. This reaction may necessitate hospitalization. • Warn the patient to avoid driving or operating dangerous machinery while taking this drug.
Chlorzoxazone (Paraflex, Parafon Forte DSC)	• Reduces nerve impulses from the spinal cord to the muscles	250 mg P.O. t.i.d.	• GI upset • Drowsiness • Dizziness • Rash • Dry mouth	• Monitor for side effects. • Warn the patient to avoid driving or operating dangerous machinery while taking this drug.
Cyclobenzaprine (Flexeril)	• Reduces nerve impulses from the spinal cord to the muscles	10 mg P.O. t.i.d.	• Drowsiness • Dizziness • Dry mouth • Fatigue • Nausea • Constipation • Rash • Tinnitus	• Do not administer if the patient has cardiac arrhythmias, is receiving mono-amine oxidase (MAO) inhibitors, or is recovering from a myocardial infarction. • Warn the patient to avoid driving or operating dangerous machinery while taking this drug.
Dantrolene (Dantrium)	• Reduces nerve impulses from the spinal cord to the muscles	25 to 100 mg P.O. b.i.d., t.i.d., or q.i.d.	• Drowsiness • Dizziness • Constipation • Nausea • GI bleeding • Headache • Seizures • Elevated liver function test results	• Stay alert for side effects. • Monitor results of liver function tests. • Warn the patient to avoid driving or operating dangerous machinery while taking this drug.
Diazepam (Valium)	• Reduces nerve impulses from the spinal cord to the muscles	2 to 20 mg P.O. q.i.d.	• Drowsiness • Dizziness • Fatigue • Ataxia • Confusion • Disorientation • Headache • Constipation • Changes in libido • Blurred vision	• Monitor for desired drug effects and side effects. • Warn the patient to avoid driving or operating dangerous machinery while taking this drug.
Methocarbamol (Robaxin)	• Reduces nerve impulses from the spinal cord to the muscles	500 mg P.O. q.i.d.	• Dizziness • Lightheadedness • Drowsiness • Nausea • Rash • Blurred vision • Headache • Fever	• Instruct the patient not to consume alcohol while taking this medication. • Monitor for side effects. • Warn the patient to avoid driving or operating dangerous machinery while taking this drug.

Drugs used to treat musculoskeletal disorders *(continued)*

DRUG	ACTION	USUAL ADULT DOSAGE	COMMON SIDE EFFECTS	NURSING CONSIDERATIONS
Muscle relaxants *(continued)*				
Orphenadrine (Norflex)	• Reduces nerve impulses from the spinal cord to the muscles	100 to 200 mg P.O. b.i.d.	• Dry mouth • Confusion • Urine retention • Tachycardia • Blurred vision • Increased intraocular pressure • Nausea • Vomiting • Headache • Gastric irritation	• Do not administer if the patient has glaucoma, an enlarged prostate, or bladder neck obstruction. • Monitor for side effects. • Warn the patient to avoid driving or operating dangerous machinery while taking this drug.
Narcotics				
Opiate analgesics				
Codeine sulfate	• Acts on opiate receptors in the brain and spinal cord to reduce the perception of pain	30 to 60 mg P.O. q 4 to 6 hours	• Nausea • Vomiting • Constipation • Respiratory depression • Restlessness • Depressed cough reflex	• Observe for side effects. • Force fluids and increase dietary fiber intake to aid bowel elimination. • Warn the patient to avoid driving and operating dangerous machinery.
Hydromorphone hydrochloride (Dilaudid)	• Acts on opiate receptors in the brain and spinal cord to reduce the perception of pain	P.O.: 2 to 4 mg q 4 to 6 hours Rectal suppository: 3 mg q 6 to 8 hours	• Nausea • Vomiting • Respiratory depression • Constipation	• Observe for side effects. • Force fluids and increase dietary fiber intake to aid bowel elimination. • Warn the patient to avoid driving and operating dangerous machinery.
Levorphanol (Levo-Dromoran)	• Acts on opiate receptors in the brain and spinal cord to reduce the perception of pain	2 mg P.O. or S.C. q 4 to 6 hours	• Nausea • Vomiting • Headache • Dizziness • Respiratory depression • Urine retention • Decreased blood pressure	• Monitor vital signs frequently. • Observe or assist with ambulation • Assess for constipation • Warn the patient to avoid driving and operating dangerous machinery.
Meperidine hydrochloride (Demerol)	• Acts on opiate receptors in the brain and spinal cord to reduce the perception of pain	25 to 150 mg I.M. q 3 hours	• Respiratory depression • Nausea • Vomiting • Constipation • Dry mouth • Headache • Dizziness • Disorientation • Tremors	• Monitor vital signs frequently. • Observe or assist with ambulation. • Assess for constipation; provide increased fluids and dietary fiber, if needed. • Warn the patient to avoid driving and operating dangerous machinery.

(continued)

ADULT NURSING

Drugs used to treat musculoskeletal disorders *(continued)*

DRUG	ACTION	USUAL ADULT DOSAGE	COMMON SIDE EFFECTS	NURSING CONSIDERATIONS
Narcotics *(continued)*				
Morphine sulfate	• Acts on opiate receptors in the brain and spinal cord to reduce the perception of pain	S.C.: 4 to 5 mg q 4 hours Patient-controlled analgesia pump: 3 to 4 mg/ml q 3 to 4 hours (20-minute lockout)	• Respiratory depression • Euphoria • Disorientation • Nausea • Vomiting • Constipation • Headache	• Monitor vital signs frequently. • Observe or assist with ambulation. • Assess for constipation; provide increased fluid and dietary fiber, if needed. • Warn the patient to avoid driving and operating dangerous machinery.
Oxycodone hydrochloride (Roxicodone), oxycodone terephthalate (Percodan), oxycodone 5 mg with acetaminophen 325 mg (Percocet-5), oxycodone 5 mg with acetaminophen 500 mg (Tylox)	• Acts on opiate receptors in the brain and spinal cord to reduce the perception of pain	Oxycodone hydrochloride: 1 to 1.5 mg I.M. or I.V. q 4 hours Oxycodone terephthalate: 5 mg P.O. q 6 hours Oxycodone 5 mg with acetaminophen 325 mg: 1 tablet P.O. q 6 hours Oxycodone 5 mg with acetaminophen 500 mg: 1 tablet P.O. 1 6 hours	• Constipation • Sedation • Headache • Nausea • Vomiting • Dizziness	• Monitor vital signs frequently. • Observe or assist with ambulation. • Assess for constipation; provide increased fluids and dietary fiber, if needed. • Warn the patient to avoid driving and operating dangerous machinery.
Propoxyphene (Darvon), propoxyphene with aspirin (Darvon N with ASA), propoxyphene with acetaminophen (Darvocet N-50 or 100)	• Acts on opiate receptors in the brain and spinal cord to reduce the perception of pain	1 capsule P.O. q 4 hours	• Nausea • Vomiting • Dizziness • Headache • Constipation • Rash • Sedation	• Monitor vital signs frequently. • Observe or assist with ambulation • Assess for constipation • Warn the patient to avoid driving and operating dangerous machinery.

Drugs used to treat musculoskeletal disorders *(continued)*

DRUG	ACTION	USUAL ADULT DOSAGE	COMMON SIDE EFFECTS	NURSING CONSIDERATIONS
Mixed agonists-antagonists				
Buprenorphine (Buprenex)	• Acts on opiate receptors in the brain and spinal cord to reduce the perception of pain	1 ml by I.M. injection or slow I.V. push (1 ml contains 0.324 mg buprenorphine)	• Sedation • Nausea • Dizziness • Vertigo • Hypotension • Vomiting • Headache • Hypoventilation	• Monitor vital signs frequently. • Observe or assist with ambulation. • Assess for constipation; provide increased fluids and dietary fiber, if needed. • Warn the patient to avoid driving and operating dangerous machinery.
Butorphanol (Stadol)	• Acts on opiate receptors in the brain and spinal cord to reduce the perception of pain	I.M.: 2 mg q 3 to 4 hours I.V.: 1 mg q 3 to 4 hours	• Respiratory depression • Sedation • Nausea • Vomiting • Headache • Dizziness • Confusion • Flushing • Dry mouth • Blood pressure changes	• Observe for respiratory or cardiovascular changes.
Pentazocine (Talwin), pentazocine with acetaminophen 650 mg (Talacen)	• Acts on opiate receptors in the brain and spinal cord to reduce the perception of pain	P.O.: 2 caplets t.i.d. or q.i.d. I.M. (Talwin only): 30 to 60 mg q 3 to 4 hours (also may be given I.V. or S.C.)	• Nausea • Dizziness • Vomiting • Respiratory depression • Sedation • Headache • Dry mouth	• Give I.M. preferably; rotate injection sites. • S.C. administration may cause tissue damage. • This drug can be habit-forming.
Nonnarcotic analgesic				
Acetaminophen (Anacin-3, Datril, Excedrin, Panadol, Tylenol)	• Blocks pain impulse generation	Varies with the specific medication; usually 1 to 2 tablets or capsules P.O. q 4 hours	• Nausea • Vomiting • Hepatic or renal toxicity in sensitive patients	• Assess for symptomatic relief. • For short-term therapy, do not exceed 4 g daily; for long-term therapy, 2.4 g daily. • Overdose can be fatal and must be treated immediately.
Corticosteroid				
Prednisone (Deltasone)	• Stabilizes lysosomal membranes; prevents inflammatory response to injury by cellular mediators	Varies with patient status and indications; typically 2 to 20 mg or more P.O. daily	When given for prolonged periods, this drug may cause multiple side effects, including increased blood pressure; acne; edema; changes in carbohydrate, protein and fat metabolism; potassium excretion; sodium retention; weight gain; skin striae; subcapsular cataracts; and easy bruising.	• For weaning, decrease dosage over several days; never discontinue this drug suddenly.

ADULT
NURSING

GASTROINTESTINAL SYSTEM

Anatomy and physiology

I. **Anatomy**
A. The mouth (oral or buccal cavity) includes the lips surrounding the orifice, the cheeks that give it shape, the hard palate making up the front (anterior) portion, the soft palate making up the back (posterior) portion, and the tongue
B. The esophagus extends from the back of the throat (pharynx) to the stomach
   1. It is a hollow tube
   2. It contains muscles to help move food and fluids along its length to the stomach
C. The stomach is located just below the diaphragm
   1. It consists of three sections
      a. The fundus, the upper portion, is located above and left of the esophageal opening into the stomach
      b. The body is the stomach's central portion
      c. The antrum (pylorus) is the stomach's lowest portion
   2. The stomach contains several sphincters
      a. The cardiac sphincter, located at the esophageal opening into the stomach, controls the entry of food and fluids into the stomach
      b. The pyloric sphincter, located at the opening of the pylorus into the first section of the small intestine, allows chyme (food mass) to leave the stomach
D. The small intestine is a hollow tube measuring 22' to 25' (6.7 to 7.6 m) long, with a diameter of approximately 1" (2.5 cm)
   1. It has three sections
      a. The duodenum, the uppermost section, starts at the pyloric sphincter and extends about 10" (25.4 cm)
      b. The jejunum, the middle section, is approximately 8' (2.4 m) long
      c. The ileum, the lowest section, is approximately 12' (3.7 m) long and is separated from the first section of the large intestine by the ileocecal valve or sphincter
   2. The small intestine has four layers, or coats
      a. The tunica serosa is the outer layer
      b. The tunica muscularis is the muscular layer
      c. The submucosa tela is the submucous layer
      d. The tunica mucosa is the inner mucous layer
E. The large intestine is approximately 5' to 6' (1.5 to 1.8 m) long and about 2" (5.1 cm) in diameter
   1. It consists of three sections
      a. The cecum extends about 2" to 3" (5.1 to 7.6 cm) from the ileocecal valve
      b. The colon extends from the ileocecal valve to the rectum; its four subdivisions are the ascending colon, transverse colon, descending colon, and sigmoid colon
      c. The rectum extends from the sigmoid colon to the anal opening

Reviewing the gastrointestinal system

As this illustration shows, the gastrointestinal system includes the:
- mouth
- esophagus
- stomach
- small intestine, with its three main sections — duodenum, jejunum, and ileum
- large intestine, with its five main sections —

cecum, ascending colon, transverse colon, descending colon, and sigmoid colon
- rectum.

Sphincter muscles are located at the opening of the esophagus into the stomach (cardiac sphincter), opening from the pyloric portion of the stomach into the duodenum (pyloric sphincter), opening of the cecum (ileocecal sphincter), and the anus (anal sphincter).

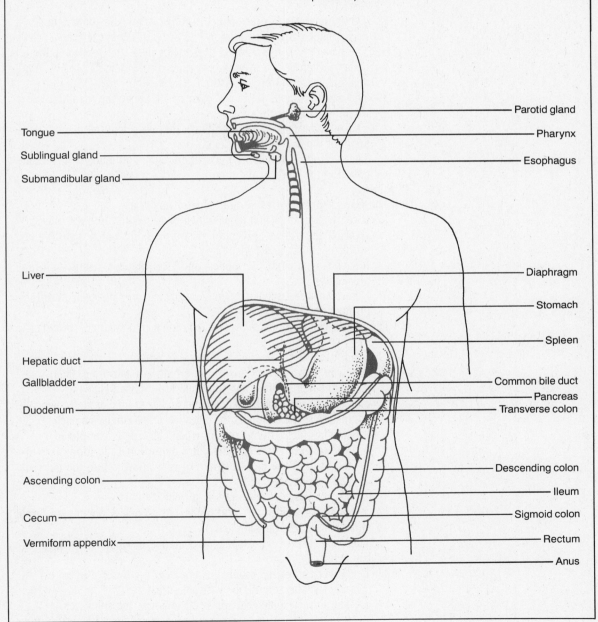

Tongue

Sublingual gland

Submandibular gland

Liver

Hepatic duct

Gallbladder

Duodenum

Ascending colon

Cecum

Vermiform appendix

Parotid gland

Pharynx

Esophagus

Diaphragm

Stomach

Spleen

Common bile duct

Pancreas

Transverse colon

Descending colon

Ileum

Sigmoid colon

Rectum

Anus

ADULT NURSING

2. The four coats of the large intestine are the same as those of the small intestine
   a. The outer layer of the tunica muscularis has strips called taenia coli, which extend along the length of the intestine
   b. Haustra, or sacs, give the large intestine a puckered appearance
   c. Internal and external muscles form the muscle coat of the anus and control anal opening and closing
F. Three organs attached to the GI tract facilitate and influence its functions
   1. The liver, the largest internal organ in the body, lies in the right upper abdominal quadrant just below the diaphragm; it has two lobes
   2. The gallbladder, a pear-shaped, saclike organ, lies under the liver; it is connected to the common bile duct by the cystic duct
   3. The pancreas, a many-lobed organ, lies in the left upper abdominal quadrant behind the greater curvature of the stomach
G. Various glands also are part of the GI tract
   1. The parotid glands lie inside each cheek above the mandible, next to and in front of the ears
   2. The submandibular salivary glands lie just below the mandibular angle of the jaw
   3. The sublingual glands lie under the tongue and mucous membrane covering the floor of the mouth

II. Physiology

A. The GI system performs several general functions
   1. It carries out digestion (breakdown of foodstuffs into simpler substances) and allows absorption (the process by which digestive endproducts enter the bloodstream)
   2. It secretes enzymes, hormones, and electrolytes to assist with food breakdown
   3. It performs peristalsis (the movement that propels foods and fluids through the GI tract)
B. The mouth chews foods to break them down into smaller, smoother pieces
   1. Food mixes with the digestive enzyme ptyalin, or amylase, contained in saliva (secretions of the mouth and parotid glands)
      a. Saliva helps soften and lubricate food during chewing
      b. Ptyalin begins the breakdown of starches to smaller molecules called maltoses, and continues the digestive actions in the stomach
   2. Swallowing (deglutition) occurs when chewing is completed
      a. The tongue, cheeks, and palates help propel the food mass to the back of the mouth, where it is swallowed into the pharynx and esophagus
      b. The swallowed food mass is termed a bolus
C. The esophagus receives the food bolus and propels it downward through its entire length into the stomach
   1. The upper end of the esophagus contains the upper esophageal sphincter
   2. The lower end of the esophagus contains the lower esophageal sphincter in the ampulla or vestibule area
      a. The lower esophageal sphincter is not a true sphincter
      b. It is an area of greater pressure that provides a barrier to prevent reflux (backward flow) of stomach fluids and acids into the esophagus

Glossary

Cholecystitis: inflammation of the gallbladder

Choledocholithiasis: calculi (biliary gallstones) in the common bile duct

Cirrhosis: chronic degenerative liver disease characterized by hepatic fibrosis, parenchymal degeneration, and fat infiltration of the lobules; although associated with chronic alcoholism, the condition may arise secondary to biliary disease or hepatitis

Enzyme: protein substance that catalyzes (facilitates) chemical reactions inside the cells or, in the case of digestive enzymes, outside the cells in the lumen of the digestive tube

Flatulence: large amounts of air or gas in the stomach or intestine

Hepatitis: liver inflammation characterized by liver enlargement, jaundice, and abnormal liver function; may result from bacterial or viral infection, drugs, toxins, or incompatible blood transfusions

Intrinsic factor: substance secreted in the gastric mucosa that is crucial to intestinal vitamin B_{12} absorption; combines with extrinsic factor (cyanocobalamin)

Pancreatitis: acute or chronic inflammation of the pancreas; typically results from alcohol, drugs, trauma, or infection

Peritonitis: inflammation of the peritoneum (abdominal cavity lining) caused by bacteria or irritants (such as toxins) released from an inflamed appendix, gallbladder, liver, or intestine

Tenesmus: persistent ineffective rectal or bladder spasms accompanied by the urge to empty the bowel or bladder

D. The stomach stores, mixes, liquefies, and continues the breakdown of foodstuffs
1. Gastric (stomach) glands secrete 1,500 to 3,000 ml/day of gastric juice, which consists mainly of hydrochloric acid, pepsin, mucus, intrinsic factor, and gastrin
   a. Intrinsic factor is needed for vitamin B_{12} absorption
   b. Gastrin stimulates hydrochloric acid secretion, promotes digestion, and relaxes the ileocecal sphincter
   c. Mucus helps liquefy the bolus
2. Initial protein breakdown begins with hydrochloric acid and the enzyme pepsin, which breaks proteins into smaller molecules called proteases, peptones, and polypeptides
3. Starch breakdown continues in the fundus of the stomach with ptyalin
4. Limited fat breakdown takes place in the stomach through the effects of the enzyme lipase
5. Foods may stay in the stomach for varying times as digestion goes through three phases
   a. The cephalic phase is triggered by hunger and the odor or sight of food
   b. The gastric or hormonal phase occurs as the bolus reaches the lower portion of the stomach (antrum)
   c. The intestinal phase starts when food enters the duodenum
      (1) The small intestine secretes enterogastrone, an enzyme similar to gastrin, which stimulates the stomach to secrete gastrin and mucus
      (2) It also secretes a hormone called secretin, which slows gastric secretion and emptying (stimulation of the vagus nerve also slows gastric secretion and emptying)

ADULT NURSING

E. The small intestine has several major functions
   1. It secretes hormones to control pancreatic juice, bile, and intestinal secretions
   2. It completes food digestion
      a. The action of enzymes, intestinal secretions, bile, and pancreatic juices cause the breakdown of chyme into carbohydrates, proteins, fats, and end products
      b. The duodenum accepts the food bolus (chyme) and fluids from the stomach, then continues digestion by secreting secretin and cholecystokinin in response to the presence of fats and sugars
      c. Chyme digestion and absorption may take 3 to 10 hours, depending on chyme content, intestinal motility (movement), and intestinal flora
      d. Secretin decreases gastric acid secretion and helps boost production of pancreatic juices by the pancreas and bile by the liver
         (1) Pancreatic juices enter the duodenum through the sphincter of Oddi in the ampulla of Vater
         (2) The alkalinity of pancreatic juices protects the duodenal mucosa
      e. Cholecystokinin induces secretion of pancreatic juices, triggers the gallbladder to empty its bile, slows gastric emptying, and increases small intestinal motility
      f. The duodenum also secretes gastric inhibitory peptide (GIP) and somatostatin
         (1) GIP slows gastric motility and stimulates secretion of insulin and intestinal juice
         (2) Somatostatin slows secretion of gastrin, secretin, and GIP
            (a) Gastrin, secretin, and GIP reduce duodenal and gallbladder motility
            (b) They also decrease intestinal sodium and chloride absorption
      g. The jejunum (along with the duodenum) secretes 2 to 3 liters/day of succus entericus, a yellowish fluid that is acidic in the duodenum and jejunum but neutral in the ileum (from the alkaline effects of pancreatic juices)
         (1) Enzymes in the succus entericus continue digestion through the actions of enterokinase, which increases trypsin to break down polypeptides and peptones to amino acids; maltase, sucrase, and lactase, which break down carbohydrates; and nuclease, which helps break down some proteins and nucleic acids
         (2) Succus entericus and pancreatic juices continue the breakdown of carbohydrates, proteins, and fats in the duodenum and jejunum
   3. The small intestine also absorbs digested end products and fluids
      a. All three portions of the small intestine absorb approximately 1.8 to 2.1 gallons (7 to 8 liters) of fluids (including water, gastric juices, intestinal juices, pancreatic juices, and bile)
      b. Consequently, only about 17 to 34 oz (500 to 1,000 ml) of fluid enters the large intestine
      c. In the jejunum (the site of most carbohydrate digestion), carbohydrates are absorbed as glucose molecules

(1) Absorption of water-soluble vitamins, some fats, and proteins also takes place in the jejunum

(2) Iron may be absorbed in the jejunum and duodenum

d. The ileum absorbs vitamin B_{12} (if calcium ions are present in the ileum and intrinsic factor in the stomach) and, along with the duodenum, also promotes sodium transport

e. Carbohydrates are absorbed through the intestinal villi as monosaccharides (simple sugars) and a few disaccharides

f. Proteins are broken down mainly into amino acids, with a few dipeptides

g. Fats are broken down into fatty acids, monoglycerides, diglycerides, and a few triglycerides

h. Carbohydrates and proteins are absorbed along with sodium (neither can be absorbed without the other)

i. Fatty acids and water are absorbed by diffusion into the intestinal villi

j. Electrolytes are absorbed by active transport through the intestinal villi

F. The large intestine has three major functions

1. It manufactures vitamin K and some B vitamins

2. It absorbs water, sodium, and chloride, thereby reducing the volume of chyme into a mass called feces

3. It stores and expels feces from the anus and rectum

   a. Peristaltic movements, or waves, propel the fecal mass through the large intestine to the rectum for storage

   b. The colon secretes mucus (to ease movement of the fecal mass), water, potassium, and bicarbonate (to make the feces alkaline)

   (1) This allows colonic bacteria to reproduce

   (2) In turn, the remaining proteins and indigestible residue are broken down

      (a) The large intestine primarily contains lactobacillus, staphylococcus, streptococcus, *Escherichia coli, Proteus, Pseudomonas, Streptococcus faecalis, Candida albicans, Aerobacter aerogenes,* and *Bacteroides* organisms

      (b) Intestinal bacteria convert urea to ammonium salts and ammonia and produce intestinal gases to provide more fecal bulk and dead bacterial bodies; this helps to propel the fecal mass into the rectum

   c. Absorption of water, sodium, and chloride in the large intestine reduces the fecal liquid content to about 34 oz (100 ml)

   (1) Approximately 90% of the sodium and chloride entering the large intestine is absorbed

   (2) Consequently, little sodium and chloride remain in the fecal mass

   d. The fecal mass is expelled from the rectum through defecation

   (1) Defecation is stimulated by rectal distention

   (2) Rectal distention increases rectal pressures and relaxes the internal and external sphincters, permitting rectal emptying

G. The liver has multiple functions

1. It produces bile to aid fat metabolism and digestion

2. It stores glycogen and releases glucoses (converted from glycogen) into the bloodstream as needed

ADULT NURSING

3. It converts or breaks down proteins into amino acids
4. It stores vitamins
5. It makes plasma proteins for clotting and immune defenses
6. It detoxifies (breaks down) hormones, drugs, and other chemicals

H. The gallbladder collects, stores, concentrates, and releases bile into the duodenum in the presence of fats in foodstuffs

I. The pancreas has both endocrine and exocrine functions
   1. As an endocrine gland, it secretes insulin and glucagon into the bloodstream for carbohydrate use
   2. As an exocrine gland, it secretes pancreatic juice (containing enzymes that aid fat and protein metabolism) into the duodenum through the ampulla of Vater and the sphincter of Oddi

J. The parotid, submandibular, and sublingual glands produce various substances to aid digestion
   1. The parotid gland produces saliva (containing amylase) to begin digestion of starches in the mouth
   2. The submandibular and sublingual glands produce saliva and mucus to aid digestion and lubrication of foodstuffs in the mouth

Gastrointestinal ulcer

Overview

A gastrointestinal ulcer is a common medical condition occurring between ages 30 and 60, with peak incidence from age 40 to 50. The condition is nearly twice as common in men as in women. The precise cause of GI ulcers is unknown; genetic and environmental factors may contribute to their development.

Types of ulcers include *peptic ulcers*, which may occur in the esophagus, stomach, or duodenum. Peptic ulcers include *gastric ulcers*, which develop in the stomach, and *duodenal ulcers*, which form in the duodenum. Ulcers arise when gastric cells lack resistance to gastric acid; duodenal ulcers result from increased gastric acid and rapid emptying of stomach contents. Duodenal ulcers account for about 80% of peptic ulcers; esophageal and gastric ulcers make up the remaining 20%. Another type of GI ulcer is a stress ulcer, usually caused by severe stress, such as from a severe burn, trauma, shock, or head injury.

GI ulcers initially are treated with medications, dietary changes, and reduced intake of stimulants (such as alcohol and caffeine) to reduce gastric acid production. Surgical correction may be needed to treat ulcer complications, such as perforation or hemorrhage.

Clinical situation

John Murphy, age 47, a stockbroker, is admitted to the hospital to investigate complaints of severe pain and occasional vomiting of blood and to review ulcer management. He has received treatment for recurrent duodenal ulcers for the past 3 years.

ADULT
NURSING

Surgical repair of ulcers

Because current medications heal ulcers so effectively, the need for surgical ulcer repair is rare. When it is necessary, one of the following procedures may be performed:
- Laser cauterization of the bleeding site. In this procedure, the source of bleeding is removed and small ulcer craters are eradicated.
- Partial gastrectomy with gastroduodenostomy. The antrum (the stomach's acid-producing area), pyloric sphincter, and part of the ulcerated duodenum are removed. (Removal of the pyloric sphincter speeds emptying of foods and fluids into the remaining duodenum. This may cause dumping syndrome, a disorder characterized by shifting fluid volume, electrolyte, and blood glucose levels.)
- Partial gastrectomy with gastrojejunostomy. In this procedure, the antrum and part of the duodenum are removed, the remaining portion of the stomach is sutured to the jejunum, and the remaining portion of the duodenum is sutured to the omentum. (This duodenal portion contains the sphincter of Oddi and the ampulla of Vater, where the common bile duct empties into the small intestine.)

Assessment

Nursing behaviors

1. Assess Mr. Murphy's pain for type, location, severity, time of occurrence, accompanying signs and symptoms (such as eructation, nausea, vomiting, or hunger), and relief measures and their results.

2. Assess Mr. Murphy's vital signs and temperature.

3. Assess Mr. Murphy for risk factors for GI ulcers, such as life-style, job, coping behaviors, frequent intake of spicy foods, alcohol and caffeine consumption, smoking, use of stimulants and medications, and family history of ulcers.

Nursing rationales

1. Ulcer pain may be described as burning, gnawing, aching, sharp, dull, intermittent, brief (lasting only minutes), or prolonged. Mr. Murphy may identify its location as a small area under the xiphoid process (lower end of the sternum) and around the umbilicus. A gastric ulcer may cause pain in the left upper epigastric area; a duodenal ulcer, in the right epigastric area. Some patients with ulcers also have feelings of hunger, nausea, or fullness. Vomiting is rare but may be associated with a bleeding ulcer in the antrum of the stomach. Pain frequently occurs between meals, when the stomach is empty, and at night, awakening the patient. Ulcers tend to recur after periods of remission. Typically, food and antacids temporarily relieve pain from a duodenal ulcer.

2. The blood pressure of a patient with an ulcer may be within the normal range for sex and age. Pulse and respiratory rates may be slightly elevated, especially when pain recurs or when a bleeding ulcer causes mild anemia. The temperature usually is normal.

3. Patients with gastric and duodenal ulcers typically internalize their anxieties and feel they have little control over their work activities. Stress increases adrenal hormone production, promoting mucus secretion and predisposing the mucosa to ulceration. Stress and nicotine from cigarettes cause duodenal blood vessel constriction; the lining then becomes more vulnerable to injury from gastric acid. Alcohol and caffeine consumption increase gastric acid production. Anti-inflammatory medications, such as ibuprofen (Motrin), indomethacin (Inderal), and aspirin, decrease mucosal cell resistance to gastric acid. Ulcers have a slight familial tendency.

4. Assess Mr. Murphy's bowel functions and inspect stools for color and consistency.

4. Mr. Murphy may have diarrhea (from antacids containing magnesium salts) or constipation (from antacids containing aluminum). Dark stool color may reflect oozing blood or frank bleeding.

5. Assess for a history of dizziness, faintness, and weight changes.

5. These signs and symptoms may reflect intermittent or gross bleeding, leading to a reduced red blood cell count and anemia; or they may result from blood pressure changes on rising (orthostatic hypotension). Bleeding may lower the blood volume.

Nursing diagnoses
• Pain (intractable or uncontrollable) related to duodenal ulcer
• Potential for injury related to ulcer hemorrhage or perforation

Planning and goals
• Mr. Murphy will express relief of ulcer signs and symptoms with treatment.
• Mr. Murphy's ulcer will heal.
• Mr. Murphy will learn stress-management techniques.
• Mr. Murphy will express an understanding of the expected effects and side effects of prescribed and over-the-counter medications.

Implementation

Nursing behaviors

Nursing rationales

1. Explain the diagnostic regimen (or clarify the physician's explanations) to Mr. Murphy, as needed.

1. Mr. Murphy may be scheduled for an upper and lower GI series, endoscopic examination of the stomach and duodenum, gastric analysis, and blood studies.

2. Monitor Mr. Murphy's food intake, menu selections, and the effects of food on ulcer signs and symptoms.

2. The few dietary restrictions imposed by an ulcer include avoiding hot or spicy foods and fruit with peels or seeds. Food intake typically relieves ulcer pain for several hours.

3. Encourage Mr. Murphy to maintain exercises (such as walking) and other activities appropriate for his age, ability, and treatment regimen.

3. Maintaining activities and physical strength helps reduce stress and promotes a positive outlook.

4. Explain the desired effects and side effects of medications. For instance, explain that an antacid's side effects depend on whether it is aluminum-hydroxide based, magnesium-hydroxide based, or calcium-carbonate based, and that antacids may interact with other medications.

4. Explanations reduce or eliminate knowledge deficits. Antacids buffer (reduce) gastric acids, decreasing acidic effects on the gastric mucosa. They should be given 1 hour after meals and at regular intervals (every 2 or 3 hours) during periods of higher acid production (such as fasting). Side effects of antacids include diarrhea (with magnesium-based antacids), constipation (with aluminum- or calcium-based antacids), and acid rebound (with calcium-based antacids). Antacid absorption may increase if it is given with diazepam (Valium), dicumerol, or aspirin; it may decrease if given with digoxin (Lanoxin) or phenothiazines. Antacids decrease absorption of tetracycline (Sumycin), propranolol (Inderal), and iron. To avoid drug interactions, give antacids 1 to 2 hours before or after these medications.

5. Administer fluids, up to a total of 100 oz (3,000 ml) a day (unless contraindicated). Record fluid intake and output.

5. Fluids aid digestion and elimination and help maintain renal function and fluid balance.

6. If the physician does not order antacids, administer prescribed acid-blocking agents, such as cimetidine (Tagamet), ranitidine (Zantac), famotidine (Pepcid), or nizatidine (Axid), as ordered.

6. These agents block production of hydrochloric acid, speeding ulcer healing. Side effects are rare but may include dizziness, insomnia, constipation or diarrhea, and rash.

7. If ordered, administer anticholinergic drugs, such as dycyclomine hydrochloride (Bentyl) or propantheline bromide (Pro-Banthine).

7. These drugs slow gastric motility (by decreasing vagal stimulation), decrease hydrochloric acid secretion, and reduce spasms in the stomach and small intestine.

8. Prepare Mr. Murphy for diagnostic procedures. Withhold oral intake, as ordered and needed. Administer a laxative or enema, as ordered. Have Mr. Murphy wear a long gown, if required.

8. Proper patient preparation helps ensure the best diagnostic results, prevent delays, and reduce costs.

9. Provide frequent periods for Mr. Murphy to rest and review teaching materials.

9. Rest reduces stress, enhances healing, and decreases gastric stimulation. Reviewing explanations helps determine Mr. Murphy's level of understanding.

10. Explain to Mr. Murphy the need to modify his life-style and diet and to reduce stressors.

10. Mr. Murphy's ulcer may not heal completely unless he makes life-style and dietary changes.

11. With the physician's order, arrange for Mr. Murphy to consult with stress-management personnel.

11. Mr. Murphy and general nursing staff may need guidance to help reduce his stress and improve his coping mechanisms.

12. Explain to Mr. Murphy that his ulcer may recur if he discontinues maintenance therapy.

12. The ulcer recurrence rate after maintenance therapy stops may exceed 50%.

13. Instruct Mr. Murphy to read the labels on all nonprescription medications to see if they contain aspirin or other salicylates, steroids, or phenylbutazone (Azolid).

13. Salicylates, steroids, and phenylbutazone irritate gastric and duodenal mucosal cells and disrupt ulcer healing. If Mr. Murphy must take them for other conditions, teach him to take antacids and eat snacks between meals.

14. Include Mr. Murphy's significant other and family members in patient teaching sessions.

14. Assistance and understanding by the significant other and family members will help Mr. Murphy to cope and also will reduce their stress.

Evaluation (outcomes)

• Mr. Murphy obtains relief from ulcer signs and symptoms with treatment.
• Mr. Murphy's ulcer eventually heals.
• Mr. Murphy participates in and learns how to perform stress-management techniques.
• Mr. Murphy, his significant other, and family learn and can recite the expected effects and common side effects of his prescribed and over-the-counter medications.

ADULT NURSING

Obstruction of the small intestine

Overview

Small intestine (bowel) obstruction is a common, painful, serious condition that quickly can become a surgical emergency. Typically, it results from inflammatory disease, such as Crohn's disease or regional enteritis. In some cases, the cause is abdominal adhesions that restrict or inhibit normal bowel activity, or paralytic ileus arising from hypokalemia. The portion of the small bowel most frequently obstructed is the ileum (the third segment) because it is the narrowest.

Small bowel obstruction leads to buildup of pressure in the intestinal lumen, which halts peristalsis. Fluid and gas absorption also ceases and the bowel distends, reducing normal blood flow. Large amounts of fluids and electrolytes are lost as fluid moves from the plasma and cellular spaces into the bowel. In advanced stages of small-bowel obstruction, gangrene—a surgical emergency—may develop.

Clinical situation

Jamie Karle, age 28, a construction worker, is admitted to the hospital with a diagnosis of possible small bowel obstruction. On admission, he has dyspnea and marked abdominal distention. Mr. Karle seems quite anxious and objects to anyone touching his abdomen. He was hospitalized previously for treatment of small bowel obstruction caused by adhesions from an earlier appendectomy.

Assessment

Nursing behaviors

1. Assess the whole patient, including his age, sex, height, weight, and current condition.

2. Assess Mr. Karle's vital signs.

3. Assess Mr. Karle's abdomen for bowel sounds (for details, see "Listening for bowel sounds," pages 327 and 328). Evaluate the degree of abdominal distention by measuring abdominal girth. Note any complaints of tenderness or pain.

4. Assess Mr. Karle's skin turgor to evaluate hydration status. Also assess for dry mucous membranes and dry, flaky skin.

Nursing rationales

1. This helps determine Mr. Karle's current health status and potential nursing care needs.

2. This determines if his vital signs have changed. Mr. Karle's blood pressure may be low and his pulse and respiratory rates elevated from fluid loss and possible shock. His temperature may be 100° F (37.8° C) or higher from bowel inflammation or obstruction. Abdominal distention may cause dyspnea.

3. Bowel sounds should be present unless Mr. Karle has extensive obstruction. If obstruction is developing, bowel sounds may be high-pitched, squeaky, and abnormally slow (normally, peristaltic rushes occur approximately every 30 seconds). His abdominal girth will be increased from gas and fluid accumulation and bowel inflammation. (Abdominal girth increases as bowel obstruction becomes more acute or complete.) He also may have severe, acute abdominal pain or steady, dull pain over the entire abdomen.

4. Skin turgor may decrease from hypovolemia caused by fluid movement into the bowel. With dehydration, the skin tents (stays elevated) when pinched lightly and appears dry and flaky.

5. Assess Mr. Karle for nausea and vomiting, check for blood in his vomitus, and evaluate for burping or eructation (belching) of gas.

5. Nausea, vomiting, burping, and belching are common signs of obstruction. They result from reverse peristalsis—the body's attempt to relieve pressure in the bowel lumen.

6. Assess Mr. Karle for constipation and obstipation.

6. Constipation (infrequent bowel movement) is a sign of reduced peristalsis. Obstipation (no bowel movement) results from complete obstruction and lack of peristalsis.

7. Assess Mr. Karle's perineal and anal areas for signs of skin irritation or excoriation (epithelial loss).

7. Anal and perineal areas may be red, painful, sore, edematous, and excoriated from initial diarrhea.

8. Assess Mr. Karle's fluid intake and output.

8. Accurate assessment of fluid intake and output is crucial to ensuring an adequate hydration status.

Nursing diagnoses
- Fluid volume deficit related to collection of plasma and interstitial fluid in the bowel lumen
- Pain related to abdominal distention and dyspnea

Planning and goals
- Mr. Karle will recover from small-bowel obstruction without the need for surgery.
- Mr. Karle's vital signs will return to within normal limits.
- Mr. Karle will regain normal intestinal function with medications, proper diet, and fluids.
- Mr. Karle will regain fluid and electrolyte balance.

Implementation

Nursing behaviors

1. Explain upcoming treatments, including pain medication, anticholinergic or antispasmodic medications, antibiotics, nasogastric (NG) tube insertion, I.V. fluids and electrolytes, withholding of oral intake, and frequent monitoring.

Nursing rationales

1. Anxiety may prevent Mr. Karle from fully absorbing or understanding initial explanations. Therefore, reinforcement may be necessary.

2. Assemble the equipment needed for I.V. therapy.

2. Mr. Karle will need fluid and electrolyte replacement to replace volume deficits caused by diarrhea and fluid shifts. (Fluids may accumulate within the bowel lumen above the obstructed area, causing loss of intravascular fluids and electrolytes.)

3. Assemble the equipment needed for NG tube insertion. Assist with tube insertion, as needed, and connect the tube to suction equipment. (For details, see "Inserting a nasogastric tube," pages 300 and 301.)

3. An NG tube drains fluids and stomach contents. (An intestinal tube, such as a Miller-Abbott or Cantor tube, may be needed if the NG tube does not relieve the obstruction.)

4. Monitor the type, color, and amount of drainage from the NG tube. Check for occult blood in the drainage.

4. Drainage from an NG tube usually is yellowish green, but may include some blood streaks. Signs of occult (hidden) blood may appear. Drainage varies in amount and may exceed 500 to 1,000 ml. (With small-bowel obstruction, drainage from an intestinal tube may exceed 3,000 to 5,000 ml a day.)

ADULT NURSING

5. Monitor Mr. Karle's vital signs every 1 to 2 hours, as ordered.

5. Pulse and respiratory rates and blood pressure should return to normal as Mr. Karle's fluid levels normalize. Temperature may remain elevated or even spike to higher levels if perforation, peritonitis, or another complication occurs.

6. Monitor I.V. therapy closely. Replace solutions and electrolytes as needed to maintain adequate intake.

6. When oral intake is withheld, I.V. fluids are the only source of fluids and nutrients. Lost electrolytes must be replaced to restore homeostasis.

7. Administer I.V. antibiotics, if ordered, every 4 to 6 hours.

7. Antibiotics help prevent or eliminate infection. A therapeutic blood antibiotic level depends on regular antibiotic administration at appropriate times.

8. Monitor Mr. Karle's abdominal girth every 1 to 2 hours. Monitor abdominal tenderness and bowel sounds every 1 to 2 hours.

8. As the bowel obstruction is relieved, abdominal girth, distention, and tenderness should subside and bowel sounds should be audible in all areas. If bowel sounds remain high-pitched, suspect increasing obstruction (bowel sounds normally are low-pitched).

9. Monitor for bowel output every 1 to 2 hours. Also monitor for blood in stools.

9. Complete obstruction may cause obstipation (lack of bowel movements). However, even with complete obstruction, diarrhea may occur for several hours as lower bowel contents empty. Blood may result from bleeding in ulcerated areas.

10. Monitor laboratory data, including electrolyte levels, complete blood counts, hemoglobin and hematocrit values, and blood nitrogen levels, as ordered.

10. Laboratory data should reflect results of treatments. However, Mr. Karle may need additional adjustments to treatments over time as his condition stabilizes or worsens. If Mr. Karle's condition resolves or the obstruction is relieved, laboratory data should be within normal limits.

11. Monitor Mr. Karle for relief of abdominal pain after administration of pain medication and anticholinergic or antispasmodic medications.

11. Pain medication increases tolerance of discomfort from obstruction and distention. Anticholinergic and antispasmodic medications relax the intestinal sphincters, allowing fluids and bowel contents to pass. Antibiotics eliminate infectious organisms to reduce inflammation and relieve the obstruction.

12. Help Mr. Karle into a chair or help him ambulate as tolerated, when ordered.

12. During acute bowel obstruction, the patient usually needs bed rest. As Mr. Karle's condition improves, he will be permitted to get up and to ambulate for progressively longer distances to regain his strength and stability.

Clinical situation *(continued)*

With treatment, Mr. Karle's small-bowel obstruction diminishes. The physician orders removal of the NG tube, a clear liquid diet, continuation of I.V. and antibiotic therapy, and daily laboratory studies.

Implementation

Nursing behaviors	**Nursing rationales**
13. Explain upcoming events to Mr. Karle. Then remove the NG tube (see "Removing a nasogastric, Miller-Abbott, or Cantor tube," page 306).	**13.** The NG tube must be removed before Mr. Karle can start a clear liquid diet. After it is removed, he will require oral hygiene.
14. After permitting Mr. Karle to rest, provide a clear liquid diet. Monitor his appetite, intake, and tolerance for liquids.	**14.** Clear liquids allow the GI tract to readjust to intake gradually. After oral intake resumes, Mr. Karle's appetite may be minimal from lack of oral intake or fear of a recurrence of bowel obstruction.
15. Continue to monitor bowel sounds and abdominal girth, distention, and tenderness.	**15.** With relief of obstruction, bowel sounds should be lower-pitched and audible in all quadrants. Abdominal girth, distention, and tenderness should subside gradually as inflammation diminishes. (However, abdominal girth may increase temporarily as fluids and foods are introduced.)
16. Continue I.V. therapy, as ordered.	**16.** I.V. therapy may continue until Mr. Karle can tolerate fluids and foods adequately.
17. Continue to help Mr. Karle ambulate, as tolerated.	**17.** Repetitive ambulation increases strength.
18. When ordered, provide soft foods. Monitor Mr. Karle's food intake and tolerance. Increase to a normal diet, as tolerated.	**18.** Monitoring food intake and diet helps ensure that Mr. Karle can tolerate food and is not experiencing another obstruction.
19. Clarify the cause of bowel obstruction with Mr. Karle and discuss the importance of early treatment of any recurrence.	**19.** Adhesions are a common cause of obstruction. Obstruction may cause perforation and ulceration of the intestinal wall with bleeding, leading to peritonitis and gangrene.
20. When ordered, remove the I.V. line and discard I.V. equipment. Record the amount of fluid remaining in I.V. bags and the condition of the I.V. site.	**20.** The I.V. needle or intracatheter insertion site may be edematous and red from foreign body invasion. A red streak running up the arm could signify phlebitis (venous inflammation).
21. Consult with the dietitian about Mr. Karle's dietary modifications, if needed.	**21.** Bowel obstruction and fluid loss reduce levels of iron, potassium, and other nutrients. Therefore, Mr. Karle temporarily may need to increase his intake of fluids, potassium- and iron-rich foods, carbohydrates, proteins, and soft foods. He should avoid spicy foods and those with skins, peels, and seeds because they are hard to digest.
22. Assist with discharge planning, as needed.	**22.** Discharge planning will help ensure that Mr. Karle's needs are anticipated and dealt with in care plans and nursing actions.
23. Document all observations, monitoring data, and Mr. Karle's response to therapy.	**23.** This helps ensure that Mr. Karle's record is complete and accurate.

ADULT NURSING

24. Explain or clarify the expected effects and side effects of discharge medications to Mr. Karle.

24. Bowel obstruction is a serious illness. Typically, the patient needs daily medication to avoid infection and regain normal bowel function.

Evaluation (outcomes)

• Mr. Karle recovers from small-bowel obstruction with medical treatments and does not require surgery.
• Mr. Karle's vital signs are within normal limits at the time of discharge.
• Mr. Karle's daily intake consists of four small meals with soft foods and a fluid intake of 85 oz (2,500 ml). His appetite improves and he has no side effects from medications. By the time of discharge, he has had several soft, formed bowel movements with no blood detected.
• Mr. Karle starts to regain lost weight; his skin turgor and laboratory data are within normal ranges at the time of discharge.
• Mr. Karle is free from abdominal tenderness and requires no analgesic medications at the time of discharge.

Colon cancer

Overview

Cancer of the colon is a leading cause of cancer morbidity (sickness) and is the second leading cause of cancer death (mortality) in men and women combined. The most common site of colon cancer is the ascending colon. (Formerly, the disease occurred more frequently in the sigmoid or descending colon. The cause of this change in disease site is unknown.) Colon cancer usually manifests as polyps, which eventually break through the wall of the colon. Cancer spreads by direct extension or through the lymphatic or circulatory system.

Clinical situation

Florence Morris, age 60, a restaurant owner, is admitted to the nursing unit to investigate complaints of recent weight loss, marked weakness, fatigue, and pain in her lower right side. Her admitting diagnosis is possible colon cancer. She appears pale and anxious and expresses concern about her condition, her restaurant, and upcoming events.

Assessment

Nursing behaviors

1. Assess the whole patient, including her age, sex, occupation, health history, height, and weight.

Nursing rationales

1. Cancer of the colon affects both men and women age 30 and over, although it is more common in women. (Rectal cancer is more common in men.) The disease has been linked with dietary carcinogens (such as nitrites and chemically treated foods and additives) and low fiber intake. Weight loss is a common finding.

2. Assess Mrs. Morris's vital signs.

2. Mrs. Morris's blood pressure may be decreased slightly and pulse and respiratory rates increased from anemia (caused by tumor ulceration and bleeding). Unless she has an infection or inflammation, her temperature may be normal.

3. Assess Mrs. Morris's abdomen for distention, masses, pain, tenderness, bowel sounds, and abdominal girth. (For details on assessing bowel sounds, see "Listening for bowel sounds," pages 327 and 328.)

3. A mass in the right lower abdomen may cause partial obstruction, distention, tenderness, pain, and changes in abdominal girth and bowel sounds. Bowel sounds should be audible in all abdominal quadrants, unless the bowel is totally obstructed.

4. Assess Mrs. Morris for nausea, vomiting, diarrhea, and constipation.

4. Nausea and vomiting may accompany a tumor in the right colon. Diarrhea may occur occasionally as foods and fluids pass the tumor. Constipation is unlikely because the colon distends easily and fecal contents in this area are semiliquid. However, as the tumor enlarges, obstruction may occur, causing constipation or obstipation.

5. Assess Mrs. Morris's laboratory data for evidence of anemia.

5. Anemia results from tumor ulceration and bleeding.

6. Assess Mrs. Morris for weakness and fatigue.

6. These are symptoms of anemia.

7. Periodically assess Mrs. Morris's stools for blood (serial stool checks).

7. Occult blood may go unnoticed because the bleeding site may be far from the rectum. Blood may appear sometimes, but not with each bowel movement.

8. Assess Mrs. Morris for weight changes.

8. Weight loss is common with cancer of the ascending colon.

Nursing diagnoses

• Fatigue related to anemia and weight loss
• Constipation related to an abdominal mass

Planning and goals

• Mrs. Morris will undergo an uncomplicated surgical resection of the tumor.
• Mrs. Morris will regain adequate health after an uncomplicated postoperative recovery.
• Mrs. Morris will resume regular bowel elimination without diarrhea or constipation.
• Mrs. Morris will remain free from cancer recurrences.

Implementation

Nursing behaviors

1. Clarify upcoming events and diagnostic procedures with Mrs. Morris and her family.

Nursing rationales

1. This will help ease anxieties and concerns and promote patient cooperation with diagnostic procedures. (Anxiety is common in patients who have an uncertain diagnosis.)

2. Assemble needed equipment, then assist with insertion of a nasogastric (NG) tube or an intestinal tube, if used. (See "Inserting a nasogastric tube," pages 300 and 301, "Inserting a Miller-Abbott intestinal tube," pages 302 and 303, or "Inserting a Cantor intestinal tube," pages 303 to 305.)

2. An NG tube or an intestinal tube may be inserted to remove intestinal secretions and contents.

3. Monitor Mrs. Morris for nausea, vomiting, diarrhea, and constipation.

3. Nausea, vomiting, and constipation may stem from partial or complete bowel obstruction. Diarrhea may occur as secretions bypass the obstructed area.

ADULT NURSING

4. Prepare Mrs. Morris for GI examinations. Make sure to obtain a written order for a laxative and enemas before beginning these preparations.

4. Upper and lower GI examinations or an abdominal X-ray (flat plate of the abdomen) may be needed to aid diagnosis. Laxatives or enemas may cause perforation or bleeding of the bowel or tumor. Colonoscopy must be performed when Mrs. Morris has an empty colon; a low enema may be given or a sodium biphosphate-sodium phosphate (Fleet) enema may be used to empty the lower colon and rectum.

5. Administer I.V. therapy, as ordered. Withhold all oral intake.

5. To keep the GI tract empty, I.V. therapy is used to administer fluids and nutrients.

6. Administer I.V. antibiotics every 4 or 6 hours, if ordered.

6. Antibiotics help eliminate intestinal flora (in preparation for surgery) and prevent infection, if bowel obstruction causes perforation. The physician may order sulfonamides and neomycin (Mycifradin).

7. Irrigate the NG tube or intestinal tube as required, using normal saline solution. Reposition Mrs. Morris every 2 hours to aid drainage.

7. Irrigation helps maintain tube patency; using normal saline solution helps prevent excessive electrolyte loss. Repositioning or turning Mrs. Morris from side to side helps the intestinal tube pass to the obstruction site.

8. Encourage Mrs. Morris to perform deep-breathing exercises every 2 hours. Use an incentive spirometer, if needed.

8. Deep breathing enhances cellular oxygenation and helps maintain respiratory functions. An incentive spirometer helps expand the alveoli to aid gas exchange—important for any patient undergoing surgery.

9. Encourage Mrs. Morris to perform leg and foot exercises every 3 to 4 hours.

9. These exercises help prevent circulatory stasis and maintain musculoskeletal strength.

10. Prepare Mrs. Morris physically and emotionally for surgery, when ordered. (For details on patient preparation, see the "Perioperative nursing" section.)

10. This eases Mrs. Morris's anxiety about upcoming events and helps prevent complications.

Clinical situation
(continued)

Mrs. Morris undergoes resection of the cecum and right ascending colon, with anastomosis of the ileum to the transverse colon (ileocolostomy anastomosis). No cancer spread (metastasis) is noted at the time of surgery. She makes an uneventful recovery and is scheduled to begin chemotherapy with fluorouracil (5-fluorouracil) and levamisole as soon as her strength permits. (For details on chemotherapy, see the "Oncology nursing" section.)

Evaluation
(outcomes)

• Mrs. Morris undergoes successful resection of cancer of the ascending colon.
• Mrs. Morris regains adequate health without complications, as shown by normal fluid, electrolyte, hematocrit, and hemoglobin levels.
• Mrs. Morris regains regular bowel elimination with formed brown stools.
• Mrs. Morris remains free from recurrence of colon cancer and will begin chemotherapy soon.

Complications of gastrointestinal disorders

This chart presents the most serious or life-threatening complications of gastrointestinal disorders, along with interventions that are crucial to patient safety and comfort.

COMPLICATION	CAUSE	NURSING INTERVENTIONS
Paralytic ileus Lack of movement in the GI tract. Signs and symptoms include abdominal pain, marked abdominal distention, and absence of peristalsis and bowel sounds.	● Excessive handling of the bowel during surgery ● Resumption of feeding too soon after surgery	● Measure abdominal girth frequently. ● If a nasogastric tube is used, observe for proper tube functioning and drainage. ● Keep I.V. fluids infusing properly. ● Withhold oral intake, as ordered. ● Listen for bowel sounds. ● Determine if the patient is passing flatus. ● Measure fluid intake and output. ● Assess the patient for pain; administer pain medications, if needed and ordered (some analgesics slow resumption of bowel function).
Bowel perforation Rupture of the bowel into the peritoneal cavity. Signs and symptoms include abdominal pain and distention, fever, rectal bleeding, and absent bowel sounds.	● Injury ● Puncture by a rectal tube or colonic instrument during examination ● Bowel obstruction	● Be aware that the disorder calls for surgical correction. ● Monitor I.V. therapy for proper fluid delivery. ● Check vital signs. ● Observe closely for signs and symptoms of shock. ● Measure abdominal girth frequently. ● Monitor for abdominal pain and bleeding, if present. ● Administer antibiotics, as ordered. ● Monitor nasogastric tube drainage (if used).
Hemorrhage Bleeding from the stomach, small or large intestine, esophagus, or hemorrhoids. Signs and symptoms include pallor, shock, abdominal pain or rigidity, and bloody stools or emesis.	● Bleeding into the GI tract from an ulcer, a tumor, cirrhosis with esophageal varices, or hemorrhoids	● The patient may require immediate surgery to locate the bleeding site. A Sengstaken-Blakemore tube may be inserted to treat bleeding esophageal varices. ● Monitor vital signs frequently. ● Measure intake and output. ● Maintain proper I.V. infusion. ● Replace lost blood, as ordered.
Bowel obstruction Partial or complete obliteration of the bowel lumen, preventing peristalsis and absorption of fluids and nutrients from the bowel. Signs and symptoms include absent bowel movements and bowel sounds, abdominal distention, pain, and shock.	● Inflammatory disease ● Tumor ● Occlusion of an intestinal blood vessel	● Monitor vital signs carefully. ● Measure abdominal girth frequently. ● Withhold oral intake, as ordered. ● Measure fluid intake and output. ● Prepare the patient for surgery to correct the obstruction. ● Monitor nasogastric tube drainage, if used. ● Observe for emesis or nausea. ● Monitor I.V. fluids. ● Check for bowel sounds.
Peritonitis Inflammation of the peritoneal lining. Signs and symptoms include localized or generalized abdominal pain, muscle tenseness and rigidity, absent bowel sounds, nausea, vomiting, and low-grade fever.	● Infection ● Bowel perforation ● Inflammation of an abdominal organ	● Measure abdominal girth. ● Withhold oral intake, as ordered. ● Monitor I.V. infusions. ● Observe for signs and symptoms of shock. ● Monitor nasogastric or intestinal tube function and drainage (if used). ● Administer antibiotics and pain medications, as ordered. ● Keep the patient in semi-Fowler's position.
Constipation Change in bowel elimination characterized by decreased frequency or passing of hard, dry stools. Signs and symptoms include straining at stool; a feeling of rectal fullness; passage of small, hard stools; lack of bowel movements for 1 to 3 days; anorexia; and abdominal pain.	● Decreased fiber and food intake ● Decreased fluid intake ● Bedrest ● Spinal or general anesthesia	● Offer high-fiber foods, if tolerated. ● Increase fluid intake, if tolerated. ● Insert a rectal suppository, if ordered. ● Increase ambulation and activity, as tolerated. ● Encourage regular toileting habits. ● Administer a laxative, if ordered.

Inserting a nasogastric tube

Introduction

Nasogastric (NG) and other gastrointestinal tubes are made of flexible plastic. GI tubes are used to empty the contents of the GI tract; provide a means to administer foods, fluids, or medications; or relieve abdominal distention. An NG tube is inserted through the nose into the stomach; other GI tubes are inserted into the mouth or rectum. *Note:* In some health care facilities, only physicians or registered nurses are permitted to insert GI tubes. (Procedure steps preceded by an asterisk are especially important.)

Steps

1. Check the physician's order for the type of tube to be inserted and whether suction is to be used.

*2. Gather all needed supplies and equipment: NG tube, hypoallergenic tape, emesis basin, water-soluble lubricant, 50-ml syringe, basin with warm water (or ice for a rubber tube), suction apparatus (if ordered), towel or linen-saver pad, clamp, safety pin, stethoscope, glass of water with a straw, and tissues.

3. Clarify previous explanations given to the patient about the purpose of the tube and the insertion procedure.

4. Place the patient in high Fowler's position. Remove the pillow, if permitted, so the patient can tilt the head backward more easily.

*5. With the patient's head tilted backward, check each nostril to assess its condition for tube passage. To determine which nostril to use, have the patient close each nostril in turn, then breathe through the open nostril.

*6. To determine how far to insert the tube, use the tube to measure from the bottom of the ear lobe to the nose to the lower end of the sternum (breastbone). If the tube does not have premarked circles, place a small piece of tape on it to mark the distance from its end to the sternum.

*7. Rub water-soluble lubricant on the tip of the tube, to a length of 5″ (12.7 cm).

Rationales

1. A written physician's order is required for NG tube insertion.

*2. Having all needed supplies on hand facilitates the procedure. Immersing a plastic tube in warm water makes it more flexible for insertion; immersing a rubber tube in ice stiffens it for easier insertion. Hypoallergenic tape minimizes irritation.

3. An anxious patient may not understand initial explanations.

4. High Fowler's position helps the patient swallow the tube. Tilting the head backward straightens the neck and throat (oropharynx) area. Gravity aids tube passage.

*5. Some patients have a deviated nasal septum, making tube insertion in the affected nostril difficult or impossible.

*6. This measurement approximates the depth of tube insertion.

*7. Water-soluble lubricant eases tube insertion and helps prevent respiratory infection in case the tube is inserted into the trachea inadvertently.

ADULT
NURSING

8. Ask the patient to breathe deeply several times, then hold the breath as you gently but firmly insert the tube into the selected nostril. As the tube reaches the oropharynx, ask the patient to tilt the head backward.

8. Holding the breath closes the epiglottis, reducing the risk of the tube entering the trachea. The tube is curved slightly, aiding insertion through the nostril.

*9. When the tube reaches the oropharynx, ask the patient to tilt the head forward and take a few sips of water as you advance the tube into the esophagus. If the patient gags, stop advancing the tube until the gagging stops, then proceed as the patient again sips water. If the patient's eyes tear (from gagging), offer tissues to dry them.

*9. Sipping water helps the tube pass from the throat to the esophagus and then to the stomach. Gagging is a response to the sensation of the tube in the back of the throat; tilting the head forward moves the tube away from the back of the throat to reduce the gag reflex. Tearing is a response to gagging.

10. As the patient swallows, continue to advance the tube to the premarked length while aspirating it occasionally.

10. Aspiration helps ensure that the tube is in the stomach.

11. After verifying that the tube is in the stomach, tape the tube to the nose by bringing tape under and around the tube and crossing the ends over the tube and then each other. Tape the ends to the nose.

11. Tape secures the tube so that it does not rub against the nostril.

12. If suction is ordered, connect the tube to suction and turn the suction on. If suction is not ordered, the tube may be clamped off and the end covered with a gauze square.

12. Suction helps remove gastric secretions.

*13. Secure the tube to the patient's gown by placing some tape around the tube, bringing the ends together, and pinning through the ends to the gown.

*13. Securing the tube to the gown prevents the tube from pulling against the nose and dangling loosely.

14. Collect the linen-saver pad, any unused supplies, and the empty water basin. Discard used disposable supplies. Place the patient in a comfortable position, and ask whether the tube is causing any discomfort.

14. Discarding and replenishing supplies promotes safe, thorough care and a clean environment.

15. Document tube placement, type of tube inserted, the person who inserted the tube, the patient's response, and type of drainage.

15. Documentation proves that the procedure was done, assures high-quality care, and provides legal protection.

16. Make a notation on the care plan to irrigate the NG tube routinely with normal saline solution.

16. Irrigation helps ensure tube patency.

ADULT NURSING

Inserting a Miller-Abbott intestinal tube

Introduction

The insertion procedure for a Miller-Abbott tube (now used rarely) resembles that for a nasogastric tube. However, the Miller-Abbott tube is harder to insert because it has a metallic end and a large bag (balloon) for mercury. In some cases, air or saline solution is used instead of mercury to eliminate the risk of mercury poisoning if the bag breaks. (Procedure steps preceded by an asterisk are especially important.)

Steps

1. Check the physician's order for the type of tube to be inserted and whether suction is to be used.

*2. Gather all needed supplies and equipment: Miller-Abbott intestinal tube, emesis basin, water-soluble lubricant, 50-ml syringe, basin with warm water (or ice for a rubber tube), suction apparatus (if ordered), towel or linen-saver pad, clamp, safety pin, stethoscope, glass of water with a straw, and tissues.

3. Clarify previous explanations given to the patient about the purpose of the tube and the insertion procedure.

4. Place the patient in high Fowler's position. Remove the pillow, if permitted, so the patient can tilt the head backward more easily.

*5. With the patient's head tilted backward, check each nostril to assess its condition for tube passage. To determine which nostril to use, have the patient close each nostril in turn, then breathe through the open nostril.

*6. To determine how far to insert the tube, use the tube to measure from the nose to the bottom of the ear lobe to the lower end of the sternum (breastbone). If the tube does not have premarked circles, place a small piece of tape on it to mark the distance from its end to the sternum.

*7. Liberally apply water-soluble lubricant to the tip of the tube, to a length of 5″ (12.7 cm). Make sure the nostril that will accept the tube is patent.

Rationales

1. A written physician's order is required for Miller-Abbott tube insertion.

*2. Having all needed supplies on hand facilitates the procedure. Immersing a plastic tube in warm water makes it more flexible for insertion; immersing a rubber tube in ice stiffens it for easier insertion.

3. An anxious patient may not understand initial explanations.

4. High Fowler's position helps the patient swallow the tube. Tilting the head backward straightens the neck and throat (oropharynx) area. Gravity aids tube passage.

*5. Some patients have a deviated nasal septum, making tube insertion in the affected nostril difficult or impossible.

*6. This measurement approximates the depth of tube insertion.

*7. The tip must be well lubricated for insertion. The nasal septum must be in the midline to ensure enough space for tube passage.

ADULT
NURSING

8. Insert the tube beyond the nasal passages to the oropharynx. Then ask the patient to open the mouth. Grasp the end of the tube and bring it to the mouth.

8. The end of the tube must be passed gently to reduce the risk of injuring the nasal mucosa. Bringing the tube to the mouth allows visualization for air or mercury instillation and permits extra lubrication to promote swallowing.

9. Insert premeasured air (or mercury, if used) into the self-sealing rubber balloon; the balloon should be filled only partially.

9. A bolus of air or mercury aids tube passage through the intestinal tract and sphincters.

10. Gently withdraw the tube from the nostril until the bag is in the oropharynx again.

10. This positions the tube properly for swallowing.

11. While inserting the tube into the esophagus, have the patient swallow water and the balloon or bag.

11. Water aids tube passage into the stomach.

12. After the tube has been inserted to the premeasured length, withdraw gastric secretions.

12. Gastric secretions (usually yellowish green) verify that the tube is in the stomach.

*13. Leave the tube *untaped* but connect it to a suction source, as ordered.

*13. The tube must move through the sphincters freely without hindrance.

*14. Begin the patient turning procedure, as ordered, to promote tube passage through the GI tract and sphincters. Turn the patient onto the right side for 30 minutes, then onto the left side for 1 to 2 hours, and back to the right side as ordered. (Specific times must be ordered.)

*14. Turning allows gravity to help the Miller-Abbott tube pass through the GI tract and sphincters.

15. Document insertion of the Miller-Abott tube, the person who inserted it, and the patient's response.

15. Documentation proves that the procedure was done, assures high-quality care, and provides legal protection.

Inserting a Cantor intestinal tube

Introduction   Like the Miller-Abbott tube, the Cantor intestinal tube is now used rarely. The insertion procedure resembles that for nasogastric tube insertion. (Procedure steps preceded by an asterisk are especially important.)

Steps
1. Check the physician's order for the type of tube to be inserted and whether suction is to be used.

Rationales
1. A written physician's order is required for Cantor tube insertion.

*2. Gather all needed supplies and equipment: Cantor tube, emesis basin, water-soluble lubricant, 50-ml syringe, basin with warm water (or ice for a rubber tube), suction apparatus (if ordered), towel or linen-saver pad, clamp, safety pin, stethoscope, glass of water with a straw, and tissues.

*2. Having all needed supplies on hand facilitates the procedure. Immersing a plastic tube in warm water makes it more flexible for insertion; immersing a rubber tube in ice stiffens it for easier insertion.

3. Clarify previous explanations given to the patient about the purpose of the tube and the insertion procedure.

3. An anxious patient may not understand initial explanations.

4. Place the patient in high Fowler's position. Remove the pillow, if permitted, so the patient can tilt the head backward more easily.

4. High Fowler's position helps the patient swallow the tube. Tilting the head backward straightens the neck and throat area (oropharynx). Gravity aids tube passage.

*5. With the patient's head tilted backward, check each nostril to assess its condition for tube passage. To determine which nostril to use, have the patient close each nostril in turn, then breathe through the open nostril.

*5. Some patients have a deviated nasal septum, making tube insertion in the affected nostril difficult or impossible.

*6. To determine how far to insert the tube, use the tube to measure from the nose to the bottom of the ear lobe to the lower end of the sternum (breastbone). If the tube does not have premarked circles, place a small piece of tape on it to mark the distance from its end to the sternum.

*6. This measurement approximates the depth of tube insertion.

*7. Rub water-soluble lubricant on the tip of the tube, to a length of 5″ (12.7 cm).

*7. Water-soluble lubricant eases tube insertion and helps prevent respiratory infection in case the tube inadvertently is inserted into the trachea.

8. Before inserting the tube, wrap the rubber balloon (bag) around the end of the tube to reduce its size. Lubricate the bag well, then insert it into the patient's nostril, gently turning the tube to keep the bag flat and rolled around the tube.

8. A bag or balloon made of soft rubber can be wrapped easily around the end of the tube for insertion.

9. When the tube reaches the oropharynx, have the patient open the mouth; then withdraw the bag. Insert premeasured air or mercury (if used) into the self-sealing rubber bag; fill the balloon only partially.

9. A bolus of air or mercury aids tube passage through the intestinal tract and sphincters.

10. Gently withdraw the tube from the nostril until the bag is in the oropharynx again.

10. This positions the tube properly for swallowing.

11. While inserting the tube into the esophagus, have the patient swallow water and the balloon or bag.

11. Water aids tube passage into the stomach.

12. After the tube has been inserted to the premeasured length, withdraw gastric secretions.

12. Gastric secretions (usually yellowish green) verify that the tube is in the stomach.

*13. Leave the tube *untaped* but connect it to a suction source, as ordered.

*13. The tube must move through the sphincters freely without hindrance.

ADULT
NURSING

*14. Begin the patient turning procedure, as ordered, to promote tube passage through the GI tract and sphincters. Turn the patient to the right side for 30 minutes, then to the left side for 1 to 2 hours, and back to the right side, as ordered. (Specific times must be ordered.)

*14. Turning allows gravity to help the Cantor tube pass through the GI tract and sphincters.

15. Document insertion of the Cantor tube, the person who inserted it, and the patient's response.

15. Documentation proves that the procedure was done, assures high-quality care, and provides legal protection.

Maintaining a gastrointestinal tube

Introduction

Nursing support for a patient with a gastrointestinal (GI) tube ensures optimal care and helps maintain proper tube function. (Procedure steps preceded by an asterisk are especially important.)

Steps

1. Provide oral hygiene at 1- to 2-hour intervals. Caution the patient not to swallow the solutions.

Rationales

1. Because the patient with a GI tube cannot receive oral intake, oral hygiene is needed to maintain healthy oral mucosal tissue, prevent bacterial overgrowth, and stimulate saliva flow.

*2. Before administering a feeding or irrigating the GI tube, check for proper tube placement by using one of these two methods.
(a) Place a stethoscope over the epigastric area (below and left of the ribs). While inserting 10 cc of air into the tube, listen for a rush of air.
(b) Attach a syringe to the end of the tube and withdraw it to obtain secretions. To prevent gastric mucosal injury, do not pull too firmly on the plunger.

*2. Proper placement ensures patient safety and comfort. In the first method described, a rush of air verifies proper tube placement in the stomach. In the second method, gastric secretions are minimal when the tube is draining stomach contents properly.

*3. Remove secretions by cleaning the area around the nostrils with a damp cotton-tipped applicator. Dry the area with a dry cotton-tipped applicator.

*3. If secretions accumulate, they could cause nasal irritation or inflammation.

4. If the nostrils become red or irritated, apply a small amount of antibacterial ointment.

4. Antibacterial ointment keeps the nasal area moist and healthy.

5. If the tube is taped, remove tape that is loose or covered with secretions. After cleaning the nasal area, apply new tape.

5. Once the tube reaches the obstruction site (or other desired site), it must be taped securely to maintain the proper position.

6. Document intake and output accurately, using a separate line for GI tube drainage.

6. Accurate documentation makes needed adjustments easier to note and provide. It also proves that the procedure was done, assures high-quality care, and provides legal protection.

ADULT NURSING

Removing a nasogastric, Miller-Abbott, or Cantor tube

Introduction

The removal procedures for nasogastric, Miller-Abbott, and Cantor tubes are similar. However, after removing a Miller-Abbott or Cantor tube, be sure to open the bag containing mercury, then measure and save the mercury for reuse (to conserve mercury and ensure safety). After the tube is cleaned and sterilized for reuse, a new bag (balloon) is applied in the service area, unless the tube is damaged. (Procedure steps preceded by an asterisk are especially important.)

Steps

1. Check the physician's order for tube removal.

2. Cover the patient's gown and chest area with a linen-saver pad.

*3. Turn off the suction source and disconnect the tube from the suction apparatus. Unpin the tube from the patient's gown.

4. Ask the patient to loosen the tape securing the tube to the nose. (If the patient cannot do this, loosen it yourself.)

5. Insert 30 ml of air into the tube.

*6. Ask the patient to take a deep breath, exhale, and hold the breath. Then pull out the tube, using a smooth, steady, unhurried motion. Kink or clamp the tube as you remove it.

7. Wrap the tube in a linen-saver pad and discard it in a trash can in the utility room.

8. Provide oral hygiene supplies, including mouthwash, for the patient's use.

9. Ask the patient to blow the nose gently.

*10. Empty and measure the contents of the suction drainage bottle.

11. Move the suction apparatus to the proper service area. Clean the suction apparatus and drainage bottle.

12. Document tube removal and the patient's response.

Rationales

1. Tube removal requires a written order.

2. This ensures a clean surface.

*3. Suction no longer is needed.

4. The patient, if able, may wish to do this.

5. This removes irritating gastric secretions from the tube.

*6. Having the patient hold the breath closes the epiglottis to prevent aspiration. Kinking or clamping the tube prevents aspiration or leakage of secretions into the esophagus. Smooth, steady, unhurried tube withdrawal is less frightening to the patient.

7. Proper tube disposal promotes a safe care environment.

8. Oral hygiene removes oral secretions and helps maintain healthy tissues.

9. This removes nasal secretions.

*10. Drainage must be measured to monitor output accurately.

11. This helps maintain a clean, safe care environment.

12. Documentation proves that the procedure was done, assures high-quality care, and provides legal protection.

Providing tube feedings

Introduction

Feedings instilled through a nasogastric (NG), gastrostomy, jejunostomy, or jejunal tube are used to provide nutrients to a patient who cannot take oral feedings (such as from unconsciousness or inability to swallow) or to administer medication. The procedures below describe NG tube feeding by various methods—syringe, measured plastic bag (burette), and prefilled bottle. (Procedure steps preceded by an asterisk are especially important.)

Syringe feeding through a previously placed NG tube

Steps

1. Check the physician's order for the type and amount of solution and administration times.

2. Gather needed supplies. The feeding solution may consist of commercially prepared solution in bulk or premeasured amounts in cans or bottles; in some cases, it is prepared by institutional dietary personnel. Supplies to gather include a 50-ml syringe, glass or measured container for water, linen-saver pad, and emesis basin. (A special pump may be used to provide continuous feedings at a prescribed rate through a prefilled bag. To prevent organism growth, keep the bag cool or filled only with small amounts.)

3. Place the linen-saver pad over the patient's gown.

4. Place the patient in Fowler's position or sitting up in a chair. Close the curtain or door.

*5. Attach the syringe to the NG tube and aspirate stomach contents, or listen over the epigastric area for a rush of air while inserting 30 cc of air into the tube. Measure the total amount of gastric contents removed (if ordered) to determine the amount remaining in the stomach. If the amount is large, you may need to notify the nurse-manager.

*6. Remove the plunger from the syringe and reattach the barrel or syringe to the NG tube. Kink the tube and pour the feeding into the syringe. Then unkink the tube and allow the feeding to flow into the tube by gravity.

Rationales

1. Tube feedings require a written order, which must specify the type and amount of solution and administration times (or total amount to administer over 24 hours).

2. Having all supplies on hand aids the procedure and promotes safe care.

3. This ensures a clean surface and catches any spills.

4. A Fowler's or sitting position aids the flow of the feeding by gravity. Closing the curtain or door promotes privacy, reducing patient embarrassment.

*5. Aspirating stomach contents or listening for a rush of air verifies correct placement of the NG tube in the stomach and determines whether the previous feeding has been absorbed. If gastric contents total more than 50 ml in an adult or 10 ml in an infant, check with the nurse-manager before administering the feeding.

*6. Kinking the tube while filling the syringe prevents excess air from entering the stomach. Feedings should be administered at room temperature; a cold feeding solution may cause cramps.

ADULT NURSING

7. Fill the syringe barrel before it empties totally.

7. This prevents excess air from entering the stomach.

***8.** After the entire feeding has flowed into the tube, insert 50 ml of water into the tube.

***8.** Water clears the tube of feeding solution, ensuring that the patient has received the full amount. If the patient has discomfort, you may need to raise or lower the barrel to aid gravity flow or stop the flow temporarily.

9. Before the water has passed through the tube completely, clamp the NG tube.

9. This prevents excess air from entering the stomach.

10. Document the amount of feeding and the patient's response to feedings.

10. Documentation proves that the procedure was done, assures high-quality care, and provides legal protection.

NG tube feeding by measured plastic bag (burette)

Steps

1. Check the physician's order for the type and amount of solution and administration times.

Rationales

1. Tube feedings require a written order, which must specify the type and amount of solution and administration times (or total amount to administer over 24 hours).

2. Gather needed supplies. The feeding solution may consist of commercially prepared solution in bulk or premeasured amounts in cans or bottles; in some cases, it is prepared by institutional dietary personnel. Supplies should include a calibrated bag (burette), glass or measured container for water, linen-saver pad, and emesis basin. (A special pump may be used to provide continuous feedings at a prescribed rate through a prefilled bag. To prevent organism growth, keep the bag cool or filled only with small amounts.)

2. Having all supplies on hand facilitates the procedure and promotes safe care.

3. Attach the plastic bag to the infusion pole so that the bottom of the bag is about 12″ (30.5 cm) above the point where the tube enters the patient.

3. Placing the bag at this height aids flow by gravity.

4. Clamp the tubing and pour the feeding solution into the bag.

4. Clamping the tube allows for accurate measurement of the feeding solution. Exact amounts can be noted on the bag.

***5.** Unclamp the tubing and allow the feeding solution to clear the burette tubing of air. Then reclamp the tubing.

***5.** Removing air helps prevent excess air from entering the stomach.

***6.** Check NG tube placement by either method described in step 5 of the syringe feeding method.

***6.** Proper tube placement is mandatory for safe care.

7. After verifying that the tube is placed properly in the stomach, attach the burette tubing to the NG tube. Open the clamp and regulate the drip rate by adjusting the clamp.

7. The feeding solution should flow slowly and steadily to prevent cramps or a feeling of excessive fullness.

*8. Just as the feeding ends, clean the NG tube with 50 ml of water.

*8. Water clears feeding solution from the tube.

9. Before all the water is infused, reclamp the NG tube.

9. This prevents excess air from entering the stomach.

10. Document the amount of feeding and the patient's response to feedings.

10. Documentation proves that the procedure was done, assures high-quality care, and provides legal protection.

NG tube feeding by prefilled bottle

Steps

1. Check the physician's order for the type and amount of solution and administration times.

Rationales

1. Tube feedings require a written order, which must specify the type and amount of solution and administration times (or total amount to administer over 24 hours).

2. Gather needed supplies. The feeding solution kit consists of commercially prepared solution in bottles with tubing supplied by the solution manufacturer. Supplies should include a 50-ml syringe, glass or measured container for water, linen-saver pad, and emesis basin. (A special pump may be used to provide continuous feedings at a prescribed rate. To prevent organism growth, keep the bottle cool or filled only with small amounts.)

2. Having all supplies on hand facilitates the procedure and promotes safe care.

3. Unscrew the cap from the bottle. Screw on a drip chamber and the attached tubing supplied by the manufacturer. Close the clamp on the tubing.

3. This creates a closed system.

4. Hang the bottle on the I.V. pole about 12″ (30.5 cm) above the point where the tube enters the patient.

4. This promotes gravity to ensure a safe flow rate.

*5. Squeeze the drip chamber so that it is filled about one-third to one-half.

*5. This prevents air from entering the stomach.

6. Open the clamp and allow the feeding formula to flow through the tubing. Reclamp the tubing.

6. This prevents air from entering the stomach.

*7. Check NG tube placement by either method described in step 5 of the syringe feeding method.

*7. This verifies that the tube is placed properly in the stomach.

8. Attach the formula tubing to the NG tube. Open the clamp and allow the feeding to flow into the NG tube.

8. Attaching the tubing completes the connection. Allowing the flow to continue delivers the prescribed amount of feeding solution.

ADULT
NURSING

9. Clamp the tubing and remove it from the NG tube. Kink the NG tube to prevent entry of air, then unkink it and instill 50 ml of water.

9. Water clears the rest of the feeding solution from the NG tube.

10. Document the amount of feeding and water instilled as well as the patient's response to the feeding.

10. Documentation proves that the procedure was done, assures high-quality care, and provides legal protection.

Providing gastrostomy or jejunostomy tube feedings

Introduction

A gastrostomy tube is a large catheter (usually #16 French) with an inflatable balloon at the end to secure it. The physician inserts it into the stomach surgically and sutures it in place.

A jejunostomy tube, made of plastic or rubber, is inserted into the jejunum surgically. It usually has a small diameter to help prevent formation of a fistula (a persistent opening from the bowel to the skin) after it is removed. (Procedure steps preceded by an asterisk are especially important.)

Steps

1. Check the physician's order for the type and amount of solution and administration times.

Rationales

1. Tube feedings require a written order, which must specify the type and amount of solution and administration times (or total amount to administer over 24 hours).

2. Gather a measured amount of feeding solution, syringe, container of water, gauze square, elastic band, and linen-saver pad.

2. Having needed supplies on hand facilitates the procedure and promotes safe care.

3. Provide privacy by closing the curtain or door.

3. This maintains patient privacy. The upper abdomen is exposed during gastrostomy or jejunostomy tube feeding.

4. Position the patient in Fowler's position or in a chair (if tolerated), or have the patient turn slightly to the right side.

4. These positions aid stomach emptying and reduce the risk of esophageal reflux.

5. Check the tube insertion site; clear any secretions from the skin.

5. The site should not be inflamed and should remain free from secretions.

6. Place a linen-saver pad over the bed and abdomen just below the tube.

6. This reduces soiling of the patient and promotes safe care.

7. Remove the gauze at the end of the tube and attach the barrel of the syringe to the tube. Kink and unclamp the tube.

7. Gauze keeps the end of the tube clean. Kinking the tube prevents air from entering the stomach.

*8. Pour 30 ml of water into the syringe. Unkink the tube and allow water to flow into the stomach.

*8. Water flow helps ensure tube patency. If water does not flow freely, notify the nurse-manager.

ADULT
NURSING

9. When the water is almost gone, kink the tube. Fill the syringe with feeding solution and allow the solution to flow into the stomach.

9. This permits the feeding to flow slowly by gravity.

*10. As the feeding nears completion, flush the tube with 50 ml of water.

*10. This clears the tube of feeding solution.

11. Reclamp the tube and remove the syringe. Cover the end of the tube with clean gauze and secure the gauze with an elastic band.

11. This provides a clean environment for safe care.

12. Remove the linen-saver pad, replace the patient's gown, and leave the patient on the side or in Fowler's position.

12. These measures promote patient comfort. Fowler's and the side-lying positions permit the feeding solution to enter the duodenum as digestion takes place.

13. Document the amount of feeding solution administered, the condition of the tube insertion site, and the patient's response to the feeding.

13. Documentation proves that the procedure was done, assures high-quality care, and provides legal protection.

Providing jejunal tube feedings

Introduction

A jejunal tube is a small polyethylene catheter through which feedings are given by continuous 24-hour infusion (intermittent bolus feedings may cause diarrhea). A pump (such as a Kangaroo pump) may be used to administer feedings. (Procedure steps preceded by an asterisk are especially important.)

Steps

1. Gather needed equipment: a 50-ml syringe, feeding formula, and a disposable bag for formula. The pump should be at the patient's bedside.

Rationales

1. Having needed supplies on hand promotes safe care.

*2. Connect the tubing to the bag and fill the bag with formula. The formula can be warmed in a basin of warm water or left out to reach proper temperature. *Do not store formula at room temperature for more than 4 hours.* To displace air, fill the tubing with formula.

*2. Formula must be at room temperature when administered to prevent cramps. However, if left at room temperature for more than 4 hours, bacteria may flourish.

3. Place the patient in high Fowler's position by raising the head of the bed 30 degrees.

3. Elevation aids gravity flow in the intestines.

4. Listen for bowel sounds in all abdominal quadrants.

4. Bowel sounds signal that the bowels are functioning well enough to absorb nutrients.

5. Allow the ordered amount of feeding solution to flow through the pump tubing at the ordered rate.

5. This permits administration of proper nutrients.

*6. Carefully wash the previously hung bag and tubing to remove all formula. (If the bag is disposable, discard in a plastic bag and place in a trash container in the service room.)

*6. Washing prevents bacterial growth.

*7. Carefully observe the pump for proper functioning.

*7. This helps ensure that the patient is receiving nutrients as ordered.

*8. Check the jejunal tube entry site for signs of inflammation. Change the dressing as needed.

*8. The entry site may become inflamed from leakage. The GI tract contains enzymes that can irritate the skin.

9. Document the amount of formula given, the patient's response to feedings, and the quality of bowel sounds.

9. Documentation proves that the procedure was done, assures high-quality care, and provides legal protection.

*10. Monitor the patient periodically for diarrhea, abdominal distention, and weight changes. Also monitor laboratory data.

*10. Diarrhea may signify overfeeding, bacterial overgrowth, or other complications. Abdominal distention may indicate putrefaction or obstruction. Tube feedings can cause electrolyte imbalance and hyperglycemia.

Assisting with paracentesis

Introduction

Paracentesis is a procedure in which fluid is removed from the abdominal cavity. It is done to remove ascites (abnormal fluid accumulation), thereby relieving pressure, or to obtain fluid for examination to rule out bleeding and allow fluid analysis. (Procedure steps preceded by an asterisk are especially important.)

Steps

*1. Prepare the patient for paracentesis, as described below in steps 2 through 7.

Rationales

*1. This facilitates the procedure.

2. Clarify the procedure to the patient, as needed.

2. Explanations ease patient anxiety and concerns.

3. Check the patient's vital signs.

3. With ascites, pulse and respiratory rates may be elevated from increased abdominal pressure. Temperature should be normal.

4. Measure abdominal girth.

4. Abdominal girth increases in a patient with ascites.

5. Have the patient void.

5. The bladder should be empty during paracentesis to prevent possible trauma or perforation.

6. Ask the patient about allergies, especially to local anesthetics.

6. A local anesthetic will be injected at the site of trocar insertion (the trocar is used to puncture the skin and enter the abdominal cavity). An antiseptic such as povidone-iodine (Betadine) solution, will be used to clean the puncture site.

7. Determine if informed consent is needed. If so, make sure the patient has signed the consent form. (Consult with the team leader or physician.)

7. Signed informed consent is required if the health care facility considers paracentesis an invasive procedure.

*8. Gather needed supplies:
• paracentesis tray (from the central service area), with sterile drapes, syringes, needles, trocar and cannula with drainage tubing or catheter, antiseptic solution (usually povidone-iodine) in packets, gauze sponges, knife with a blade or just a knife blade, and local anesthetic solution (usually 1% or 2% lidocaine [Xylocaine])
• sterile gloves (two or three pairs)
• sterile containers or tubes for specimens, with specimen labels
• masks and cover gowns for all assisting personnel
• large container or pail for removed fluid
• adhesive tape or Montgomery straps or ties
• I.V. fluid (2 to 3 liters) and tubing (if needed).

*8. All supplies in the paracentesis tray must be sterile to avoid entry of microorganisms into the abdominal cavity. Masks and gowns must be clean but need not be sterile. (Estimate the size of the fluid container based on the degree of abdominal distention). Adhesive tape or Montgomery straps or ties are used with the dressing applied after the procedure is completed, if drainage persists. I.V. fluid and tubing are used for peritoneal lavage (if that is the reason for paracentesis) to determine whether blood is present in the abdomen, or as peritoneal dialysis fluid.

9. Help the patient to the position requested by the physician, such as high Fowler's position.

9. Fowler's position aids gravity, promoting fluid collection in the lower abdominal cavity.

10. Arrange the equipment conveniently for the physician at the patient's bedside. Open the sterile tray.

10. The physician may sit at the patient's bedside.

*11. Assist as needed while the physician:
• cleans the abdomen with antiseptic swabs or sterile gauze squares
• puts on mask and gown
• applies sterile gloves
• injects local anesthetic
• makes a small incision with the knife in the midline of the lower abdomen
• inserts the trocar into the abdominal cavity
• removes the trocar
• attaches the tubing to collect specimens and drain fluid, if desired.

*11. The nurse can assist by providing explanations, holding the hand, or just staying close to the patient. The trocar has sharp points to aid insertion. Fluid is drained slowly to prevent vascular or pressure changes that could compromise cardiovascular function.

12. When requested, apply gentle pressure over the patient's abdomen with your hands to consolidate or collect fluid in the desired area.

12. External pressure helps localize fluid.

*13. Periodically check the patient's blood pressure, pulse, and respirations. Report the findings to the physician.

*13. Vital signs may change from fluid loss or vascular responses.

14. Periodically measure the amount of fluid removed.

14. Removal of large amounts of fluid (1,200 to 1,500 ml) may lead to tachycardia and hypovolemic shock.

ADULT NURSING

15. When fluid withdrawal is completed (or when the physician is ready to remove the trocar), the physician removes the trocar and applies a dry, sterile dressing. Cover the dressing with tape or Montgomery straps or ties to secure it.

15. Fluid withdrawal signals that the procedure has ended. The sterile dressing helps prevent infection. If continued drainage is anticipated, the physician may request Montgomery straps to prevent skin excoriation from repeated tape removal.

16. Help the patient to a comfortable position.

16. Because abdominal fluid has been removed, the patient may be able to tolerate a lower head position.

*17. Recheck the patient's vital signs.

*17. Recording and comparing vital signs with previous results helps determine any changes caused by fluid removal.

18. Clean and return reusable supplies to the central service area. Discard disposable items.

18. Proper cleaning or disposal prevents the spread of microorganisms.

*19. Apply labels to specimen containers and send the containers to the laboratory.

*19. Specimen analysis aids patient care.

20. Measure the total amount of ascitic fluid, then discard the remaining fluid. Document the amount on the patient's intake and output sheet.

20. Documentation proves that the procedure was done, assures high-quality care, and provides legal protection.

Providing ileostomy care

Introduction

An ileostomy is the surgical creation of an opening in the ileum for temporary or permanent passage of feces. The surgeon brings the terminal ileum to the abdominal surface to divert fecal drainage and prevent it from entering the colon. Drainage collects in a plastic disposable pouch or an internal, surgically created pouch (Kock pouch). Nursing support for a patient with an ileostomy focuses on caring for the stoma site and surrounding skin areas to prevent skin irritation, such as by removing drainage that has collected. (Procedure steps preceded by an asterisk are especially important.)

Steps
*1. Assess the ileostomy area for the type of pouch used, signs of loosening, and the type and amount of drainage. Note any patient complaints of itching, burning, or tenderness under the pouch.

Rationales
*1. An ileostomy produces frequent drainage through the stoma because ileal secretions are semiformed. To prevent digestion of skin tissues from proteolytic enzymes, secretions and drainage must be removed from the skin surface as soon as possible.

*2. If assessment shows that the ileostomy pouch must be changed, gather needed supplies (which should be stored in the patient's bedstand or in a cupboard in the patient's room): disposable plastic ileostomy pouch with a bottom opening and an adhesive surface around the stoma, karaya ring or paste (Stomadhesive), paper bag, skin cleaning solution, measuring container, tape (usually hypoallergenic paper tape), bandage scissors, fitted gloves, wash basin, soap, water, towels, and toilet tissues.

*2. Patients with a conventional ileostomy must wear a pouch to prevent drainage from flowing onto the skin. The pouch should be emptied frequently so it does not loosen from the weight of the drainage. (Patients with a Kock pouch need wear only a gauze square because they drain the internal pouch by inserting a catheter every 3 to 4 hours. This pouch has a one-way valve to control or prevent spillage.) Skin cleaning solution is used to clean the area around the stoma and prevent irritation from pouch changes. Karaya is a protective skin preparation that helps prevent skin irritation. Commercially prepared karaya pads or rings can be cut to size. Karaya paste or powder also may be used. A paper pouch is needed to collect used materials. A measuring container is used to measure drainage in the pouch (more than 2,400 ml of drainage a day can cause fluid and electrolyte imbalance). Tape is used to secure the edge of the pouch to the skin. Bandage scissors are used to enlarge the hole in the pouch so that it fits with ⅛" (0.3 cm) clearance around the stoma. A precut template should be available for each patient so that all future holes are cut to the same size. Fitted gloves are worn to prevent the spread of organisms. A wash basin, soap, water, towels, and toilet tissues are used to clean the patient and patient area.

3. Arrange the supplies for convenient use.

3. This facilitates care.

4. Close the curtain. Fill the wash basin with warm water.

4. Closing the curtain provides privacy for the patient, whose abdomen will be exposed.

*5. Remove the ileostomy pouch gently from around the stoma. Retain the clamp at the bottom of the pouch for possible future use, then place the pouch in the measuring container for later drainage measurement.

*5. Careful pouch removal helps prevent skin injury.

6. Wipe the drainage from the stoma site with toilet tissues.

6. This prevents skin irritation from enzymes in the drainage.

*7. Thoroughly wash the skin with soap and water, up to and around the stoma. Rinse well.

*7. Skin must be washed thoroughly to remove all irritating drainage. Rinsing well permits a better surface for pouch adhesion.

*8. Observe the skin and stoma for signs of irritation, breaks, and inflammation.

*8. Bacteria can cause infection; an allergic reaction to the ostomy pouch or equipment may cause blisters, redness, or itching.

9. Dry the skin gently but thoroughly.

9. The skin must be dried thoroughly so that the new pouch will adhere well.

*10. Check the stoma for color, mucus, edema, and other signs, such as blood or bloody seepage.

*10. The stoma should be pale pink and only slightly edematous. Mucus should appear on mucosal surfaces. Small amounts of bloody seepage—but not bleeding—may be normal.

*11. If the skin around the stoma is irritated, apply karaya paste or powder or use a commercially prepared pad (Stomadhesive).

*11. Karaya paste or powder or a commercially prepared pad helps heal irritated areas and prevents inflammation from worsening.

*12. Apply a skin prep or adhesive liquid to the skin that will be under the adhesive of the new pouch. Allow the skin to dry thoroughly.

*12. This helps the new pouch adhere properly.

13. Cut the hole in the new pouch to the proper size, using the premeasured circle as a guide.

13. To prevent drainage from contacting the skin, the hole should be only ⅛" larger than the stoma.

*14. Remove the adhesive cover from the adhesive area of the pouch. Center the pouch over the stoma and apply it to the skin around the stoma. Press carefully to eliminate creases, wrinkles, and air bubbles from the adhesive area.

*14. To ensure that the pouch adheres to the skin, the adhesive area should fit smoothly around the stoma without creases, wrinkles, or air bubbles (which could allow drainage to loosen the pouch).

15. Tape the tops and sides of the plastic pouch to the patient's skin.

15. This secures the pouch to skin surfaces, aiding adherence.

*16. Fold over the bottom edges of the pouch several times. Remove air from the pouch, then close the pouch with the clamp.

*16. This prevents leakage.

17. Replace the patient's gown, if needed, and position the patient comfortably.

17. A clean gown reduces the spread of microorganisms. Patient comfort aids recovery.

*18. Measure drainage and discard the used pouch and supplies in a trash container in the service area. Retain and clean reusable items for later use.

*18. Proper disposal or cleaning of used items prevents the spread of microorganisms and eliminates distressing odors in the patient area.

19. Wash your hands.

19. This reduces the spread of microorganisms.

*20. Document the change of ileostomy pouch, condition of the skin and stoma, and any patient reactions or concerns.

*20. Documentation proves that the procedure was done, assures high-quality care, and provides legal protection.

ADULT
NURSING

Providing colostomy care

Introduction

A colostomy is a surgically created opening in the colon for temporary or permanent passage of feces. The surgeon creates an artificial anus by bringing the colon to the surface of the abdominal wall to divert fecal drainage. Colostomy of the transverse colon usually has a double-barrelled opening (both the distal and proximal loops open onto the abdomen); colostomy of the sigmoid colon, a single-barreled opening. A loop colostomy—typically done in an emergency, then closed within a few days—usually involves the ascending or transverse bowel.

The procedure for changing the colostomy pouch is similar for both transverse and sigmoid colostomy. However, a sigmoid colostomy must be irrigated by instilling a solution into the bowel through the stoma to eliminate feces and to control or manage bowel elimination. (Irrigation also may be needed to empty the bowel before surgery or diagnostic examination.) Initially, the nurse performs irrigation; then, when the patient recovers strength and interest, the nurse teaches the patient the necessary skills.

Drainage from a sigmoid colostomy usually consists of semiformed feces, flatus, and fluid. Because such drainage does not irritate the skin, no special skin or stoma care is required. During the initial postoperative period, the patient must use a colostomy pouch. However, once the wound heals and the patient learns how to regulate bowel emptying through colostomy irrigation, the stoma need be covered only with a small gauze square or piece of toilet tissue. Typically, the colostomy pouch used initially has a closed end because so little drainage collects between irrigations and the total drainage measures much less than in ostomies located higher in the colon or the small bowel. Consequently, the patient may need to use only one pouch daily. (Procedure steps preceded by an asterisk are especially important.)

Transverse colostomy care

Steps

*1. Check the colostomy pouch for size and type. Gather needed supplies: a new pouch, tissues, hypoallergenic tape, basin, wash cloth, towel, soap, plastic disposal pouch, and clean colostomy belt (if used). Take the supplies to the patient's bedside.

2. Arrange the supplies on the overbed table or bedstand. Open the plastic bag and place it in an accessible area. Close the curtain or door.

*3. Carefully remove the present colostomy pouch, avoiding injury to the stoma. Do not pull on the skin or any glass rod under the bowel. Place the colostomy pouch in a container for later drainage measurement.

4. Using tissues, remove drainage from around the stomas.

Rationales

*1. This facilitates optimal care.

2. This facilitates care and reduces the spread of microorganisms. Closing the curtain or door provides privacy (the patient's abdomen will be exposed).

*3. A glass rod may be placed under the transverse colon to help secure it to the skin. The ends of the rod may be connected with rubber or plastic tubing to keep the rod from sliding out from under the bowel. Transverse colostomy stomas usually are side by side and connected only partially by a small portion of the colon that was left intact.

4. This provides a cleaner area around the stomas.

*5. Wash the skin under and around the stomas gently but thoroughly. Dry the skin thoroughly.

*5. Skin surfaces must be free of secretions to prevent skin irritation and sores caused by enzymes in the secretions.

*6. Examine the stomas and skin surface for color, swelling, mucus, blood, open sores, and signs of irritation.

*6. Stomas usually appear slightly swollen and pink with mucus drainage, along with liquid or semisolid fecal drainage and gas (flatus). The skin surface may appear slightly red, with minimal swelling. No open sores should appear.

7. Cut an opening in the new colostomy pouch to fit around the stoma, using the precut circle as a guide.

7. The opening should be only ⅛" (0.3 cm) larger than the stoma to protect the skin from irritating drainage.

*8. Remove the backing from the adhesive surface. Carefully place the pouch around the stomas and glass rod. (The rod slides freely under the stomas and can be moved to one side while the pouch is placed around the stomas and rod.) Work slowly to prevent creases, wrinkles, or air bubbles in the adhesive backing. Press the adhesive firmly onto the patient's skin.

*8. The pouch must be centered around the stomas with the rod inside the pouch. Eliminating wrinkles, creases, and air bubbles in the adhesive ensures adherence and prevents drainage from contacting the skin.

9. Fold over the bottom end of the pouch several times, then close the pouch with the clamp.

9. Multiple folds help prevent the pouch from leaking.

10. Apply a belt (if used) around the patient's abdomen and attach it to the appropriate areas of the pouch.

10. Some patients use a belt for added security in holding the pouch snugly. Others find that the belt pulls on the pouch, loosening it.

11. Clean the care area and discard used items in a trash container.

11. This helps prevent the spread of microorganisms.

*12. Measure the drainage in the colostomy pouch, and record the amount on the patient's intake and output sheet.

*12. Accurate drainage measurement helps to guide fluid replacement and prevent fluid imbalance.

13. Wash your hands.

13. This helps prevent the spread of microorganisms.

14. Place the patient in a comfortable position.

14. This aids patient comfort and recovery.

*15. Document the change of colostomy pouch, amount of drainage, and condition of the skin and stomas.

*15. Documentation proves that the procedure was done, assures high-quality care, and provides legal protection.

Sigmoid colostomy irrigation

Steps

*1. Before surgery, ask the patient about the usual bowel movement time so that irrigation can be scheduled near this time.

Rationales

*1. Irrigation near the patient's usual bowel movement time promotes bowel regularity.

*2. Check the physician's order for the type and amount of irrigating solution to use (usually, irrigation begins with 500 ml of normal saline solution or soap suds). Also determine which stoma is to be irrigated; with a transverse colostomy, irrigation of the proximal or distal loop may be done before surgery to reconnect the bowel.

3. Assess the patient's condition and willingness to learn how to perform the procedure.

*4. Gather needed supplies:
• enema bag for the irrigating solution
• irrigating solution
• soap suds packet or salt (1 tsp [5 ml] for a 500-ml solution)
• irrigating tube with cone
• plastic irrigation sleeve
• belt to hold the sleeve to the abdomen
• water-soluble lubricant
• toilet tissue
• two clamps
• wash basin, washcloth, and towel
• bedpan (if the patient cannot sit on the toilet)
• gauze squares or a new colostomy pouch
• plastic bag for waste materials
• two linen-saver pads.

5. Explain the procedure to the patient, showing the patient each piece of equipment while discussing its purpose and use. Have the patient handle the equipment, if able.

6. Help the patient sit up in bed, sit in a chair by the toilet, or sit on a toilet facing the toilet flush tank.

7. Fill the solution bag with the ordered type and amount of solution, warmed to 105° F (40.6° C).

8. Remove (or have the patient remove) the present colostomy pouch. If the stoma site is very soiled, clean it. Place the colostomy pouch in the plastic trash bag for later disposal.

*9. Apply the sleeve around the stoma, placing the lower end in the toilet bowl or bedpan covered loosely with the linen-saver pad.

*2. The amount of irrigating solution varies with the amount of bowel remaining and the purpose of irrigation. Up to 1,000 ml may be needed to help empty the remaining bowel and regulate emptying.

3. To irrigate a colostomy, the patient must be willing and able to learn and perform a new task and focus on the procedure.

*4. Having needed supplies on hand facilitates care.

5. Explanations ease patient concerns and anxiety. Handling familiarizes the patient with the equipment.

6. These positions allow the patient to observe, participate if able, and empty the bowel. If the patient sits close to or on the toilet, the irrigating sleeve can empty into the toilet.

7. Warming the solution reduces the risk of bowel injury and minimizes cramping.

8. Having the patient remove the colostomy pouch (if able) promotes patient participation and encourages the patient's efforts.

*9. The sleeve should be snug enough to keep bowel drainage from irritating the skin. Covering the toilet bowl or bedpan with the linen-saver pad diverts odors away from the patient.

ADULT NURSING

*10. Explain each step to the patient while performing it. Lubricate the irrigator tip or cone, and allow the solution to fill the tubing before insertion to remove any air.

*11. Insert the tubing tip or cone into the stoma, using gentle but firm pressure, and direct the tip or cone upward.

*12. Allow the solution to flow into the bowel. If the patient complains of cramping, pinch the tubing for 2 to 3 seconds.

*13. After the solution has flowed into the bowel, clamp the tubing and remove the cone carefully, holding the sleeve closely to catch any solution that spurts out of the stoma as the cone or tip is removed.

14. Fold down the top of the sleeve and clamp each side.

15. Observe the solution for color, fecal amount and character, and gas.

*16. If the patient's condition permits and abdominal wounds have healed, show the patient how to massage the abdomen gently, using circular movements over the ascending, transverse, and descending colon. Begin at the right lower side, move upward and across the abdomen, then move down the left side to the stoma.

*17. After the solution and fecal matter stop discharging through the stoma, pour water through the sleeve to remove any adherent particles. Then remove the sleeve and wash it well with soap and water. Rinse it and hang to dry.

*18. Help the patient clean and wash the area around the stoma, as needed.

19. Apply a new colostomy pouch (if the patient still uses one), or cover the stoma with gauze pads.

20. Remove and clean reusable equipment and discard disposable materials.

*10. Lubrication eases insertion of the irrigator tip into the stoma. Removing air from the tubing with the solution minimizes entry of excess air into the bowel and subsequent cramping.

*11. The open top of the irrigating sleeve allows easy insertion of the cone or tip into the stoma.

*12. To maintain flow and prevent bowel injury, the solution bag should be hung or held so that the bottom of the pouch is about 18″ (46 cm) above the stoma. Cramping (caused by compression of gases in the bowel) can be reduced by stopping the solution flow temporarily.

*13. The solution will return in small or large quantities. It will be accompanied by feces and gas.

14. This helps control odors from return of the solution and feces.

15. The returning solution may be dark or light brown, with partially formed or well-formed feces. Gas may be expelled in small or large amounts.

*16. Gentle circular massage aids the flow of solution and gas through the bowel to the stoma.

*17. Return of the solution and feces may take 20 to 30 minutes or more. Allow enough time for the solution to return so that the patient need not worry about discharges throughout the day.

*18. The patient will need progressively less help as normal strength returns.

19. Initially, the patient will feel more comfortable wearing a colostomy pouch until bowel output becomes better regulated. Later, the patient may need only cover the stoma with gauze pads between irrigations.

20. Cleaning reduces the spread of microorganisms. Disposal helps maintain a clean care environment.

ADULT
NURSING

21. Wash your hands. Help the patient to a comfortable position.

21. Handwashing reduces the spread of microorganisms. A comfortable position aids patient recovery.

*22. Document irrigation time, type of irrigating solution used, results of irrigation, patient participation and response, stoma condition, and any unexpected occurrences (such as failure to expel the solution or retain it in the bowel, bleeding at the stoma site, or complaints of pain during inflow, with abdominal tightness and marked distention).

*22. Documentation provides evidence of patient learning and participation (or lack of participation). It also proves that the procedure was done, assures high-quality care, and provides legal protection. Bleeding may signal that the stoma or bowel is fragile. Severe pain with abdominal distention and tightness may indicate bowel perforation. The stoma should appear pink and slightly edematous, with no bleeding.

Administering a cleansing enema

Introduction

Fluid is instilled into the rectum and sigmoid colon to empty the colon of feces, gas, and bacteria and to promote defecation. (Procedure steps preceded by an asterisk are especially important.)

Steps

*1. Determine the patient's need for an enema by:
• checking the time of the last bowel movement
• evaluating the patient for stool hardness, straining, diarrhea, anal sphincter control, and hemorrhoids
• checking the diagnostic procedure that necessitates the enema.

Rationales

*1. This assessment may reveal that the patient needs an oil-retention or medicated enema rather than a cleansing enema.

2. Check the physician's order for the enema.

2. Enema administration requires a written order.

3. Explain to the patient the need for and purpose of the enema.

3. An enema may be needed before a diagnostic procedure or surgery. Explanations reassure and comfort the patient.

*4. Gather needed supplies:
• enema bag and tubing
• water-soluble lubricant
• rectal tube of the appropriate size
• bath thermometer
• linen-saver pad
• ordered solution (usually 500 to 1,000 ml of soap suds or normal saline solution [1 tsp salt to 500 ml water])
• bath blanket
• clean disposable gloves
• bedpan, bedside commode, or bathroom facilities
• toilet tissue
• sink or wash basin, soap, and towels for handwashing.

*4. Having all needed supplies on hand promotes safe, efficient care. (Supplies may be prepackaged.) The patient's size and age help determine the rectal tube size. A bath thermometer is used to check the temperature of the solution, which should range from 104° to 108° F (40° C to 42.2° C). Cold solution may cause cramping; hot solution may injure the rectal mucosa. The linen-saver pad protects bed linens. The amount of solution ordered depends on the patient's age and size (from 150 ml for a child to 1,000 ml for adult). A bath blanket provides privacy. Clean disposable gloves prevent contamination. The patient's condition determines whether the enema solution will be expelled in a bedpan, bedside commode, or bathroom. Toilet tissue is used to clean the anal and perineal areas after the enema solution is expelled. The patient probably will want to wash the hands at the end of the procedure.

ADULT NURSING

5. Clamp the enema tubing and fill the bag with the proper solution, after checking its temperature carefully. Expel air from the tubing and reclamp.

5. Using solution of the correct amount and temperature prevents patient injury. Removing air from the tubing reduces cramping.

6. Hang the bag on an I.V. pole so that the bottom of the bag is about 12″ (30.5 cm) above the rectal area.

6. This height allows fluid to flow into the rectum and sigmoid colon without excessive pressure.

*7. Close the curtain and turn the patient to a left side-lying position.

*7. Closing the curtain provides privacy; a left side-lying position aids the flow of solution by following the sigmoid colon curvature.

8. Place the linen-saver pad under the patient's hips.

8. This protects bed linens.

9. Place the bedpan on the bed, or bring the bedside commode next to the bed.

9. The patient may feel the urge to defecate as soon as the solution is inserted.

10. Put on clean disposable gloves. Lubricate the tip of the rectal tube liberally.

10. Gloves prevent the spread of microorganisms. Lubricating the tube prevents injury to the rectal mucosa.

*11. Ask the patient to breathe slowly through the mouth.

*11. This diverts the patient's attention and promotes anal sphincter relaxation.

12. Raise the patient's upper buttock and locate the anus.

12. This helps locate and visualize the anus.

*13. Gently insert the tip of the rectal tube into the anus, then into the rectum—about 3″ to 4″ (7.6 to 10.2 cm) for an adult or 2″ to 3″ (5.1 to 7.6 cm) for a child. With one hand, hold the tube in place; with the other, open the clamp on the tubing to allow the solution to enter the rectum and sigmoid colon.

*13. Gentle movements help prevent injury to the anus and the rectal mucosa. The tube must be inserted into the rectum far enough to prevent leakage of the solution from the rectum.

*14. If the patient complains of cramping, pinch or clamp the tubing for 20 to 30 seconds, then continue allowing solution to flow into the rectum, as tolerated.

*14. Temporarily stopping the flow of solution decreases fluid pressure in the bowel, increasing patient tolerance and comfort.

15. Allow all fluid to enter the bowel (if tolerated). Then clamp the tubing and gently remove the tube from the rectum and anus.

15. The amount of solution tolerated will depend on the patient's condition and the amount of feces and gas in the rectum and sigmoid colon.

*16. Encourage the patient to hold the enema solution in the rectum for 10 to 15 minutes before expelling it (if the patient can tolerate this). If the patient cannot do this, assist the patient to the bedpan, commode, or bathroom.

*16. Retaining the solution for 10 to 15 minutes helps soften the fecal mass and aids bowel emptying.

17. Gather the bag, tubing, and other supplies, and dispose of them in the proper trash container.

17. Proper disposal prevents transfer of microorganisms.

ADULT
NURSING

18. Remove and discard the gloves and wash your hands.

19. Monitor the patient's ability to expel the enema solution.

*20. Observe the character of the expelled feces and enema solution. Ask if the patient also expelled gas.

21. If the patient is on bed rest, provide a basin, soap, water, toilet tissue and towels so the patient can perform hygiene.

22. Document the enema and its results.

18. This helps prevent the spread of microorganisms.

19. Expulsion may take 10 to 15 minutes.

*20. Feces may be hard and formed. An enema aids expulsion of gas, feces, and bacteria.

21. Performing hygiene removes irritants and microorganisms and aids patient comfort.

22. Documentation proves that the procedure was done, assures high-quality care, and provides legal protection.

Applying an abdominal binder

Introduction

An abdominal binder, made of cotton or elasticized flannel, provides external support to the abdomen and its contents. (Procedure steps preceded by an asterisk are especially important.)

Steps

1. Obtain a straight or scultetus (many-tailed) abdominal binder from the supply area.

2. Explain the purpose of the binder and the application procedure to the patient.

*3. Lower the head of the bed so the patient is flat. If the patient cannot tolerate this position, elevate the head of the bed 10 degrees. (The patient's knees can be flexed.) Close the curtain or door.

4. Ask the patient to turn onto the side, away from you, or help the patient into this position.

5. Ask or assist the patient to roll back over onto the folds of the binder.

*6. Pull out the distant folds and smooth the binder.

Rationales

1. Having needed supplies on hand promotes safe, efficient care.

2. Explanations ease patient anxiety and concerns.

*3. Proper patient positioning aids binder application and eases muscle tension. Closing the curtain or door provides privacy.

4. This position permits proper binder placement for application.

5. This puts the patient in the center of the binder.

*6. Smoothing out the binder allows proper application without creases.

ADULT NURSING

*7. For a straight binder, pull the far side to the center of the patient's abdomen and hold it snugly while bringing the near side to the center. Close the pressure-sensitive (Velcro) edges, or close with safety pins. For a scultetus binder, place the lowest tail at the center of the abdomen, using steady pressure. Keep applying pressure on the tail while bringing the next tail from the far side to the center of the abdomen, overlapping the first tail by about one-half. Keep the tension in each tail while continuing to overlap each successive tail to the abdomen, until all tails have been applied. Pin the upper and lower tails to hold them securely.

*7. The binder should be centered over the abdomen and closed snugly but not tightly to provide continuous support to the wound, abdomen, and abdominal contents. Steady pressure helps hold a scultetus binder in place and provides comfort and support to the wound, abdomen, and abdominal contents.

Abdominal binders

An abdominal binder is a rectangular piece of cotton or elasticized flannel used to support the abdominal organs and a large abdominal incision. Abdominal binders come in two styles — scultetus and straight. A scultetus binder (shown at right) has many tails attached to each side of a longer section. A straight binder (shown at left) has long extensions on each side to surround the abdomen.

STRAIGHT BINDER

SCULTETUS BINDER

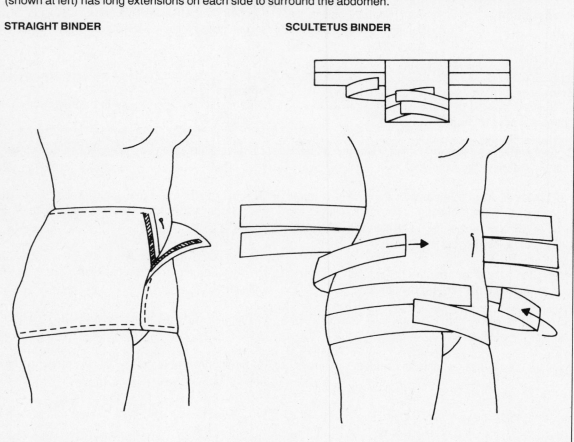

*8. Inspect the binder edges at the patient's chest to ensure that the chest expands fully.

*8. The binder should not impede respiratory function.

*9. Ask the patient if the binder is too tight or too loose.

*9. Proper tension increases patient comfort and provides abdominal support.

10. Raise the head of the bed to the patient's desired level. Open the curtain or door and wash your hands.

10. This bed position promotes patient comfort. Handwashing helps reduce the spread of microorganisms.

11. Document the binder application.

11. Documentation proves that the procedure was done, assures high-quality care, and provides legal protection.

Inserting a rectal tube

Introduction

Inserted into the rectum through the anal sphincter, a rectal tube relieves abdominal distention by removing flatus from the lower bowel. (Procedure steps preceded by an asterisk are especially important.)

Steps

1. To determine the need for a rectal tube, check the patient's condition by assessing for abdominal distention and passage of flatus and evaluating bowel sounds.

Rationales

1. The patient's condition determines the need for a rectal tube. Severe distention and inability to expel flatus indicate the need for a rectal tube.

2. Check the patient's chart for the physician's order for the rectal tube. (However, where this procedure is considered an independent nursing action, a written order may not be needed. In this case, check the nursing procedure manual on the unit.)

2. A physician's order, if required, is the legal basis for the action. The nursing procedure manual provides guidance and authorization for the procedure.

3. Gather needed supplies: rectal tube, water-soluble lubricant, linen-saver pad, clean disposable gloves, and hypoallergenic tape.

3. Having needed supplies on hand promotes safe care.

4. Explain the purpose of the rectal tube and the insertion procedure to the patient.

4. Explanations ease patient anxiety and aid cooperation.

5. Wash your hands. Close the curtain or door. Place the patient in a left side-lying position, or ask the patient to assume this position.

5. Handwashing decreases the spread of microorganisms. Closing the curtain or door provides privacy, which aids patient comfort and dignity. A left side-lying position promotes efficient tube insertion.

6. Place the linen-saver pad under the patient's hips.

6. This ensures a clean surface and prevents soiling of bed linens.

7. Put on the clean disposable gloves.

7. This reduces the spread of microorganisms.

*8. Lubricate the tip of the rectal tube with a water-soluble lubricant.

9. Gently raise the patient's upper buttock to expose the anus.

*10. Ask the patient to breathe slowly and deeply through the mouth.

*11. Insert the lubricated tip of the tube into the anus in an anterior direction toward the umbilicus. Insert it about 6″ (15.2 cm) for an adult or 3″ to 4″ (7.6 to 10.2 cm) for a child.

*12. Tape the tube to the patient's buttocks. Allow the patient to remain on the side or turn onto the back, remaining quiet. Remove the gloves.

13. Explain that the tube should remain in place for 20 to 30 minutes.

14. Document tube insertion, tube removal, and results in the patient's chart.

*8. Lubrication eases tube insertion into the rectum and reduces the risk of injury to the rectal mucosa.

9. The anus should be clearly visible for safe tube insertion.

*10. Deep breathing relaxes the anal sphincter and calms the patient.

*11. The rectal tube should permit passage of flatus but not damage the rectal mucosa. Insertion in an anterior direction conforms to the rectal passageway and reduces the risk of rectal injury. The tube may be inserted further because the rectum usually lacks fluid and pockets of flatus may be higher in the rectum. A plastic bag is attached to the tube to collect flatus or other drainage. If no bag is attached, place the open end of the tube in the linen-saver pad.

*12. Taping aids tube retention in the rectum. Allowing the patient to remain on the side promotes comfort.

13. Longer tube retention may irritate the rectal mucosa.

14. Documentation proves that the procedure was done, assures high-quality care, and provides legal protection.

Removing a rectal tube

Introduction

A rectal tube usually is removed after 20 to 30 minutes to prevent irritation of the rectal mucosa. (Procedure steps preceded by an asterisk are especially important.)

Steps

1. Wash your hands, close the curtain or door, and put on clean disposable gloves.

*2. Raise the patient's buttock to expose the anus. Loosen the tape, then remove the tube carefully. Dry the anal area with tissues. Place the tube in the linen-saver pad. Remove the pad from the bed and take off the gloves. Check the type and amount of drainage (if any) in the bag.

Rationales

1. Washing the hands and putting on gloves decreases the spread of microorganisms. Closing the curtain or door promotes privacy.

*2. Exposing the anus aids safe removal. Cleaning the anal area promotes patient comfort. The bag may contain only flatus or small amounts of liquid stool.

3. Turn the patient onto the back and assess the abdomen to see if distention has lessened.

3. This helps determine the effectiveness of the rectal tube.

4. Ask the patient if gas pains have decreased.

4. The rectal tube may be needed again later if gas pains do not decrease.

5. Dispose of soiled materials in the trash container in the service area. Wash your hands.

5. This prevents the spread of microorganisms.

6. Document the procedure, the type and amount of drainage, passage of flatus, and degree of abdominal distention.

6. Documentation indicates whether the treatment was effective and may reveal the need for reinsertion of the rectal tube, thus assuring high-quality care. It also proves that the procedure was done and provides legal protection.

Listening for bowel sounds

Introduction

By listening for peristaltic movements in selected abdominal areas, the nurse establishes the presence or absence of peristaltic waves—an indicator of bowel function. (Procedure steps preceded by an asterisk are especially important.)

Steps

1. Obtain a stethoscope.

Rationales

1. A stethoscope makes bowel sounds audible.

2. Close the curtain or door.

2. This promotes privacy and prevents patient embarrassment from exposing the abdomen.

3. Expose the entire abdomen.

3. The nurse must listen for bowel sounds over the entire abdomen.

*4. Warm the diaphragm of the stethoscope in your hands.

*4. Abdominal skin is highly sensitive to temperature extremes. The cold metal of the stethoscope could cause patient discomfort.

*5. Apply the diaphragm of the stethoscope to the cecal area of the bowel (right lower quadrant).

*5. Using the diaphragm instead of the bell of the stethoscope provides a wider area over which to listen for bowel sounds.

*6. Listen for bowel sounds in the cecal area for 30 to 60 seconds.

*6. Peristaltic rushes normally occur every 30 to 45 seconds. Bowel sounds may include gurgling or bubbling.

*7. Move the stethoscope to the right upper quadrant (hepatic flexure of the colon) and listen for bowel sounds for 30 to 60 seconds.

*7. Following the same routine each time from the cecal to the sigmoid areas ensures coverage of all bowel areas.

*8. Move the stethoscope to the left upper quadrant (splenic flexure) and listen for 30 to 60 seconds.

*8. The transverse colon curves downward at the splenic area to become the descending colon.

*9. Move the stethoscope to the left lower quadrant (sigmoid area) and listen for bowel sounds for 30 to 60 seconds.

*9. Bowel sounds may be lower pitched and less frequent in the sigmoid area because the fecal mass is firmer here.

*10. Evaluate the quality of bowel sounds in each area.

*10. Low-pitched bowel sounds are normal. High-pitched or squeaky bowel sounds may signify anoxia. Sudden rushes of rumbling or bursts of sound are abnormal. Bowel sounds may occur as often as every 5 to 20 seconds. However, in a patient who is recovering from anesthesia or surgery or whose bowel has been empty for a prolonged period, bowel sounds may be less frequent. Borborygmi (frequent hyperactive sounds) signal increased intestinal motility caused by bowel inflammation, food sensitivity, or excessive laxative use.

*11. When conducting a full abdominal assessment, listen for bowel sounds *after* inspecting the abdomen and *before* percussing or palpating the abdomen.

*11. Percussion or palpation may alter the frequency and characteristics of bowel sounds.

12. Notify the charge nurse if bowel sounds are absent completely or absent in only one quadrant.

12. Absence of bowel sounds signals lack of GI motility or GI function.

13. Document the presence or absence of bowel sounds and the quality of bowel sounds.

13. Documentation proves that the procedure was done, assures high-quality care, and provides legal protection. (If bowel sounds are absent, oral fluids must be withheld.)

Assisting with proctoscopy

Introduction

Proctoscopy—rectal examination with a proctoscope—is done to examine rectal tissues for tumors, ulcerations, or other abnormal conditions or to obtain rectal tissue for biopsy. (Procedure steps preceded by an asterisk are especially important.)

Steps

*1. Assess the patient's vital signs and understanding of upcoming events and the purpose of proctoscopy. Also evaluate the patient's ability to lie on the stomach during the procedure.

Rationales

*1. Assessment data provide information needed for safe care and may reveal the need to modify the procedure.

2. Administer a low enema, such as with a sodium biphosphate-sodium phosphate (Fleet) enema, if ordered. Check the return from the enema.

2. An enema may be needed to empty the rectum for better visualization. Blood may be present in the enema solution or stool.

3. Check the patient's chart for signed informed consent.

3. Signed informed consent may be required by the health care facility (it always is required when a biopsy is to be done).

4. Transport the patient to the treatment room.

4. Special equipment and trays are located in treatment rooms to aid special examinations.

*5. Gather and prepare needed supplies:
• proctoscopy tray containing a proctoscope, sterile drape, sterile gauze squares, lubricant, long cotton-tipped applicators, and sterile gloves
• portable spotlight or other bright light
• suction machine with suction tip
• air insufflator (to force air into the rectum)
• specimen containers with proper labels
• solutions and materials needed to check feces for blood (guaiac test)
• pillow
• adjustable stool for the physician's use (if desired).

*5. Gathering and preparing supplies in advance promotes patient care.

6. Open the proctoscopy tray and supplies, and arrange the items so the physician has easy access to them.

6. This provides optimal aid to the physician, permitting the examination to be completed easily and without delay.

7. Place the patient in the desired position (usually a knee-to-chest position), with a pillow under the abdomen for comfort. If the patient cannot tolerate this position, place in a left side-lying position. Arrange the drape for privacy.

7. The knee-to-chest position allows tissues to fall back by gravity after displacement by air (which is forced into the rectum during the procedure). The drape should have a large opening to allow visualization of the area that will be examined.

*8. As requested, assist as the physician dons sterile gloves, lubricates the finger tip (to examine the rectum digitally), attaches suction tubing to the opening on the proctoscope, checks the proctoscope light, lubricates the proctoscope, and inserts the proctoscope into the anal sphincter and rectum.

*8. Sterile gloves are needed because this procedure is considered aseptic. Suction may be used to empty secretions or feces from the rectum fully. An artificial light is used for visualization. Lubrication aids proctoscope insertion and reduces the risk of injury to the anal sphincter or rectal tissues.

9. During the digital examination, encourage the patient to take deep breaths through the mouth.

9. Deep breaths help calm the patient and relax the anal sphincter.

10. Encourage the patient to continue breathing deeply. Hold the patient's hand for support and offer reassurance.

10. Holding the patient's hand conveys support and understanding. Reassurance promotes continued patient cooperation.

*11. After cotton-tipped applicators have been inserted through the proctoscope to gather fecal specimens, collect them from the physician.

*11. Specimens may be tested for blood during the examination, or they may be sent to the laboratory for definitive analysis.

12. The physician may inflate the rectal area with air. The physician also may use biopsy forceps to secure a small piece of tissue for microscopic examination, then apply pressure to the biopsy site with gauze squares to stop bleeding or oozing. Assess the patient's skin color, respirations, and pulse to evaluate tolerance for the examination.

12. Inflation improves visualization. However, air in the rectum may cause discomfort or pain, necessitating sedation or analgesia. A biopsy may be done to examine tissues for a tumor, determine the type of inflammation or ulceration present, or detect other conditions. The patient may appear pale or flushed from the required body position or discomfort. The pulse and respiratory rates may increase over baseline values.

13. After the physician completes the examination (which takes 5 to 10 minutes), help the patient briefly assume a back-lying, recumbent position.

13. A recumbent position helps stabilize vascular and musculoskeletal tissues.

14. Gather used supplies. Clean and dry reusable supplies, then place them in the central service area for pickup. Discard disposable supplies, then wash your hands.

14. Specialized examination instruments are expensive and can be reused after sterilization. Handwashing prevents the spread of microorganisms.

15. Provide a washcloth, water, soap, and towel for the patient to clean the anal and perineal areas. Help the patient as needed.

15. Hygienic care increases patient comfort.

16. Straighten the furniture in the treatment room.

16. This aids the next examination or treatment.

17. Assist the patient back to the room and to bed.

17. The patient may need to rest because of the general condition or because of discomfort caused by the procedure.

18. Check bowel sounds, and ask if the patient is expelling flatus.

18. Bowel sounds indicate peristalsis. Air in the rectum (caused by proctoscopy) must be expelled.

*19. Check the anal area for signs of bleeding.

*19. Bleeding may result from irritation or injury of hemorrhoids or the rectal mucosa. It should stop promptly.

20. Document the time of proctoscopy, the time any specimens were sent to the laboratory, the patient's tolerance for the examination, and the patient's present condition.

20. Treatments performed and specimens sent to the laboratory must be recorded as part of the treatment plan. Documentation proves that the procedure was done, assures high-quality care, and provides legal protection.

ADULT
NURSING

Drugs used to treat gastrointestinal disorders

This chart presents information about drugs commonly prescribed for gastrointestinal disorders, including the drug action, dosage, and common side effects. Nursing considerations focus on patient comfort and teaching.

DRUG	ACTION	USUAL ADULT DOSAGE	COMMON SIDE EFFECTS	NURSING CONSIDERATIONS
Antidiarrheals				
Camphorated opium tincture (Paregoric)	Slows or blocks intestinal motility to slow transit of bowel contents	10 to 15 drops P.O. after each diarrhea stool, or 5 to 10 ml up to q.i.d.	• Constipation	• This drug contains opium. Observe the patient for side effects or allergic reactions to opium. • Tell the patient to avoid alcohol. • This drug contains alcohol. Dilute with water to make it more palatable.
Diphenoxylate hydrochloride with atropine sulfate (Lomotil)	Slows or blocks intestinal motility to slow transit of bowel contents	2 tablets or 2 tsp of liquid P.O. q.i.d.	• Depression • Euphoria • Restlessness • Headache • Rash • Nausea • Abdominal discomfort • Blurred vision • Dry mouth	• Do not administer to patients with glaucoma. • Observe for fluid and electrolyte imbalances and respiratory depression. • Do not administer to patients receiving monoamine oxidase (MAO) inhibitors because this drug may induce a hypertensive crisis. • Tell the patient to avoid alcohol.
Kaolin and pectin mixture (Kaopectate)	Slows or blocks intestinal motility to slow transit of bowel contents	60 to 120 ml P.O. as needed after diarrhea stool	• Constipation	• Observe for effectiveness.
Loperamide (Imodium)	Slows or blocks intestinal motility to slow transit of bowel contents	2 capsules or 4 tsp of liquid P.O. initially, then 1 capsule or 2 tsp of liquid after each diarrhea stool	• Nausea • Vomiting • Abdominal pain • Abdominal distention • Constipation • Dry mouth	• Observe for fluid and electrolyte imbalances and continued diarrhea.
Anti-ulcer drugs				
Antacids Aluminum hydroxide (Amphojel)	Reduces total acid content in the upper GI tract	5 to 10 ml as suspension q 2 to 4 hours, or 2 tablets P.O. q.i.d.	• Constipation • Abdominal distention	• Instruct the patient to chew tablets before swallowing them. • Give with water. • If the patient is receiving concomitant tetracyclines or quinolones (such as ciprofloxacin), separate administration times by 2 hours.
Calcium carbonate (Alka-2, Trialka, Tums)	Reduces total acid content in the upper GI tract	1- to 4-g tablet P.O. four or more times daily	• Constipation • Distention • Rebound hyperacidity	• Instruct the patient to chew tablets before swallowing them. • If the patient is receiving concomitant tetracyclines or quinolones (such as ciprofloxacin), separate administration times by 2 hours.

(continued)

ADULT NURSING

Drugs used to treat gastrointestinal disorders *(continued)*

DRUG	ACTION	USUAL ADULT DOSAGE	COMMON SIDE EFFECTS	NURSING CONSIDERATIONS
Anti-ulcer drugs *(continued)*				
Magnesium and aluminum hydroxide (Maalox)	Reduces total acid content in the upper GI tract	2 tablets P.O. q.i.d. or as ordered	• Diarrhea • Nausea • Abdominal pain	• Give this drug cautiously to patients receiving tetracyclines because magnesium inhibits tetracycline absorption. • If the patient is receiving concomitant tetracyclines or quinolones (such as ciprofloxacin), separate administration times by 2 hours.
Histamine₂ blockers • Cimetidine (Tagamet), famotidine (Pepcid), nizatidine (Axid), and ranitidine (Zantac)	Blocks histamine action at the cellular level, reducing gastric acid secretion	Cimetidine: 800 mg P.O. h.s. Famotidine: 40 mg P.O. h.s. Nizatidine: 150 mg P.O. h.s. for 8 weeks Ranitidine: 300 mg P.O. h.s. for 8 weeks	• Headache • Dizziness • Insomnia • Constipation or diarrhea • Nausea • Rash	• Observe for relief of gastric discomfort. • Urge the patient to stop smoking. • Instruct the patient to take the drug for the full prescribed course, even if he feels better, to ensure healing.
Laxatives and stool softeners				
Bisacodyl (Dulcolax)	Increases passage and emptying of GI contents by reflex action on the colon	P.O.: 2 tablets (5 mg) daily Rectal: 1 suppository daily as needed (suppository takes effect in 15 minutes to 1 hour)	• Abdominal cramps	• Observe for relief of constipation. • This drug should be used intermittently only.
Docusate sodium (Colace)	Increases water absorption to soften feces for easier passage and emptying of the bowel and rectum	1 capsule t.i.d. or q.i.d.	• Rash • Bitter taste	• Assess the patient for complaints of continued hard stools. • This drug is a stool softener, not a laxative, and is not habit forming.
Magnesium salts (Milk of Magnesia)	Forms hypertonic substance that increases water absorption into the fecal mass for easier passage	15 to 30 ml P.O. in the morning or evening	• Diarrhea • Abdominal pain • Nausea • Vomiting	• Give with water.
Psyllium (Fiberall, Metamucil)	Increases the bulk of the fecal mass	4 to 7 g dissolved in water P.O. one to three times daily	• Abdominal pain • Intestinal obstruction	• Psyllium is a bulk-forming laxative. • Give 8 oz of water after each dose. • Psyllium allergy may occur in people sensitized to inhaled or ingested psyllium. Avoid inhaling airborne dust when administering.

NEUROLOGIC SYSTEM

Anatomy and physiology

I. **Anatomy**
   A. Divisions (by location)
      1. Central nervous system, consisting of the brain and spinal cord
      2. Peripheral nervous system, consisting of the cranial and spinal nerves
   B. Brain
      1. Cerebrum
         a. This is the largest part of the brain
            (1) It is divided into two hemispheres (halves)
            (2) It contains the frontal, temporal, parietal, occipital, and insula (island of Reil)
         b. Furrows separate the cerebral lobes
            (1) The central sulcus separates the frontal and parietal lobes
            (2) The lateral fissure separates the frontal and temporal lobes
            (3) The parieto-occipital fissure separates the parietal and occipital lobes
      2. Brain stem
         a. This structure is located at the base of the brain
         b. It contains the midbrain, pons, medulla oblongata, reticular activating system (RAS), and nuclei (cores) of ten of the twelve cranial nerves
      3. Cerebellum, containing two hemispheres
      4. Basal ganglia
         a. These clusters are located deep within the cerebrum
         b. They contain the caudate nucleus, putamen, globus pallidus, and substantia nigra
      5. Other brain structures: hypothalamus, thalamus, and pituitary gland
   C. Spinal cord
      1. Is located inside the vertebral column for protection
      2. Is a continuation of the medulla oblongata, ending at the level of the second lumbar vertebra
      3. Contains 31 pairs of spinal nerves
         a. These nerves enter or leave the cord through vertebral openings (foramina)
         b. Each nerve has a motor branch (for movement) and a sensory branch (for feeling)
      4. Has a cauda equina (horse's tail) at its end, which contains spinal nerves leaving the cord in the lumbar, sacral, and vertebral areas of the spinal column
   D. Nerves
      1. Include 12 pairs of cranial nerves arising from the undersurface of the brain
      2. Also include 31 pairs of spinal nerves connected to the spinal cord by two roots
         a. The dorsal (posterior) root is made up of sensory fibers that relay sensory messages to the cord
         b. The ventral (anterior) root consists of motor fibers that transmit impulses from the cord to muscles and glands

ADULT
NURSING

Reviewing the neurologic system

This illustration shows the major components of the neurologic system.

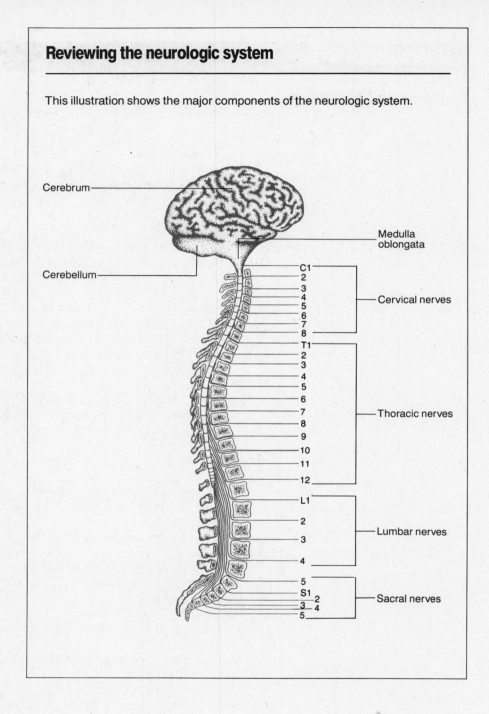

Cerebrum

Cerebellum

Medulla
oblongata

C1
2
3
4
5
6
7
8

Cervical nerves

T1
2
3
4
5
6
7
8
9
10
11
12

Thoracic nerves

L1
2
3
4

Lumbar nerves

5
S1
2
3
4
5

Sacral nerves

E. Neuron
   1. Is a specialized cell that serves as the fundamental unit of the neurologic system
   2. Consists of a cell body, an axon, and a dendrite
   3. Usually has only one axon but more than one dendrite
      a. Axons and dendrites are surrounded by a fatty myelin sheath that insulates and protects them
      b. Gaps in the myelin sheath (nodes of Ranvier) allow passage of impulses between nerve fibers
F. Brain and spinal cord coverings
   1. Outer covering
      a. Cranial bones enclose the brain
      b. Vertebrae enclose the spinal cord
   2. Inner covering (meninges) consisting of three distinct layers: dura mater (outer layer), arachnoid mater (middle layer), and pia mater (inner layer)

II. **Physiology**
   A. Divisions of the neurologic system (by function)
      1. Autonomic nervous system
         a. This division regulates involuntary functions of vital organs
         b. It is subdivided into the sympathetic and parasympathetic nervous systems
            (1) The sympathetic nervous system prepares the body to handle stressful situations (such as by speeding the heart rate and increasing the blood pressure)
            (2) The parasympathetic nervous system helps protect, conserve, and restore bodily resources (such as by slowing the heart rate and dilating vessels)
      2. Somatic nervous system
         a. This division is responsible for all conscious and higher mental processes as well as subconscious and reflex actions
         b. Although activated voluntarily, it also may function independently
   B. Brain: governs all physical and mental functions
      1. Cerebrum
         a. This structure performs sensory and motor functions as well as integrative functions related to mental activities
         b. Each cerebral hemisphere controls the functions of the opposite side of the body
            (1) The left hemisphere controls the right side
            (2) The right hemisphere controls the left side
         c. The frontal lobe controls judgment, abstract thinking, foresight, and some movements
         d. The temporal lobe controls memory, hearing, and some vision
         e. The parietal lobe controls recognition of temperature, pain, pressure, body or limb positions, and body parts
         f. The occipital lobe controls most vision
         g. The insula controls message (stimulus) relays
      2. Brain stem
         a. This structure performs motor, sensory, and reflex functions
         b. The midbrain relays impulses for sight and hearing
         c. The pons (bridge) relays impulses of some sensory and motor nerves

Glossary

Aneurysm: localized ballooning or bulging of the wall of a blood vessel (such as a cerebral aneurysm)

Cerebrovascular accident: injury to brain tissues caused by occlusion from an embolus or cerebrovascular hemorrhage; results in ischemia of the tissues normally perfused by the damaged vessel (also called a stroke)

Concussion: injury caused by a violent blow; brain concussion is characterized by loss of consciousness and increased intracranial pressure

Epilepsy: group of neurologic disorders characterized by recurrent seizures, sensory disturbances, altered sensations, abnormal or repetitive behavior, and loss of consciousness

Intracranial pressure: pressure of the cerebrospinal fluid (which normally measures 140 to 180 cm H_2O or 10 to 15 mm Hg)

Neurologic check: series of assessments of neurologic functions

Reflex: involuntary response to a stimulus

Seizure: sudden involuntary contraction of one or more groups of voluntary muscles; may cause loss of consciousness (also called a convulsion)

Tentorium: fold of tissue covering the cerebral tissues that separate the occipital lobe from the cerebellum

---

    d. The RAS controls wakefulness, attention, and concentration

    e. The medulla oblongata contains major centers for control of breathing, heart rate, vomiting, and hiccoughing

  3. Cerebellum

    a. This structure coordinates muscle movements

    b. It also maintains equilibrium and muscle tone

  4. Basal ganglia: control or aid smooth muscle movements

C. Spinal cord: carries impulses to and from the brain through sensory, motor, and reflex pathways

  1. Sensory (afferent) pathways carry impulses from the cord to the brain

  2. Motor (efferent) pathways carry impulses from the brain to nerves supplying muscle and glands

  3. Reflex pathways form reflex arcs within the spinal cord

    a. Reflexes are involuntary reactions to a stimulus

    b. Reflexes occur almost instantaneously and do not require brain control (see *Tracing the reflex arc*)

D. Neuron

  1. Receives and transmits electrochemical nerve impulses

  2. Is composed of three functional parts

    a. The cell body controls the neuron's metabolism and functions

    b. The axon transmits impulses away from the cell body

    c. The dendrite conducts impulses to the cell body

E. Thalamus: relays sensory impulses to the cerebrum

F. Hypothalamus

  1. Regulates the peripheral autonomic nervous system and endocrine processes

  2. Also regulates such somatic functions as body temperature

G. Pituitary gland

  1. Known as the body's master gland (attached to the hypothalamus)

  2. Controls the thyroid gland, ovaries, testes, adrenal glands, pancreas, and parathyroid glands

H. Meninges

  1. Provide protection, support, nourishment, and blood supply to the brain and spinal cord

Tracing the reflex arc

A reflex arc is a sensory-to-motor transmission path. The knee-jerk reflex involves the following sequence of events:
• The hammer strikes the tendon below the kneecap, which stretches the quadriceps femoris muscle.
• Stretching stimulates peripheral nerves in the muscles, which send impulses through afferent (sensory) nerve fibers to sensory neurons in the dorsal root of the spinal cord.
• The sensory nerve impulse synapses with motor neurons and passes into the ventral root.
• The impulse continues through the spinal nerve, then through the peripheral nerve. It crosses the neuromuscular junction in the quadriceps femoris muscle, where acetylcholine is released.
• Acetylcholine stimulates the muscle to contract, completing the reflex arc.

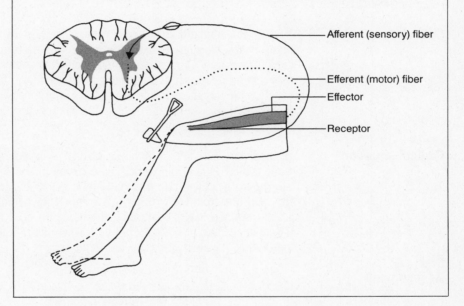

Afferent (sensory) fiber

Efferent (motor) fiber

Effector

Receptor

2. Are composed of three functional layers
   a. The dura mater serves as the inner periosteum of the skull; its inner layer forms a fold called the tentorium, which separates the occipital lobe from the cerebellum
   b. The arachnoid mater helps cushion and protect the brain; its fingerlike projections aid reabsorption of cerebrospinal fluid into the blood stream and into cisterns
   c. The pia mater contains blood vessels; along with the arachnoid mater, it supplies most of the brain's blood supply
I. Nerve pathways
  1. Sensory nerve pathways: control sensations of heat, cold, pain, and pressure
  2. Motor pathways: control movements of muscles, joints, glands, and tissues

J. Nerves
1. Spinal nerves: conduct impulses to the spinal cord from the periphery and conduct impulses from the periphery to the spinal cord
2. Cranial nerves
    a. These nerves control or contribute to such functions as vision, hearing, smell, taste, balance; eye, chewing, shoulder, tongue, and head-turning movements; facial expressions; saliva secretion; and voice production
    b. They also control or contribute to head and face sensations, sensations and movements of certain organs, and movements of the viscera

Head injury and increased intracranial pressure

Overview

Because the cranial cavity is rigid, injury here usually extends inward to the brain tissues, causing the tissues to swell. This, in turn, leads to increased intracranial pressure (ICP) and decreased circulation and perfusion, impairing cellular oxygenation. Increased ICP prevents brain cells from functioning normally; ultimately, it affects the entire body. Besides injury, causes of increased ICP include such conditions as a tumor, cerebrovascular accident, and inflammation or infection of the brain cells or brain coverings.

Clinical situation

Henry Peters, age 19, a warehouse worker, is hit head-on by another vehicle while driving home from work. The collision throws him into the steering wheel, causing his head to strike the windshield. Passersby, fearing the car will catch on fire, pull him from the wreckage. An emergency paramedic team called to the scene finds Mr. Peters confused and holding his head in pain. They take him to the trauma center of a nearby hospital, where he is admitted to the neurosurgical unit with a diagnosis of basal skull fracture.

Assessment

Nursing behaviors	**Nursing rationales**
1. Assess Mr. Peters's level of consciousness.	**1.** Level of consciousness is a major index of cerebral circulation, perfusion, and oxygenation.
2. Assess Mr. Peters's vital signs and temperature.	**2.** Changes in vital signs may indicate the onset of shock. Temperature elevation may signal midbrain involvement.
3. Assess Mr. Peters's ability to move and use his arms and legs normally. Also assess his grip and the strength of his pushing and pulling efforts.	**3.** Ability to move the extremities with normal strength indicates that the motor pathways are intact (whole).
4. Assess Mr. Peters's sensory functions, noting any complaints of numbness, tingling, or a "pins and needles" sensation. Also assess his ability to differentiate sharp and dull pressure.	**4.** If Mr. Peters does not have numbness, tingling, or a "pins and needles" sensation and can differentiate sharp and dull pressure, his sensory pathways are intact.

5. Assess Mr. Peters's pupils for equality, constriction or dilation, and reaction to light. Also check for blurred or double vision.

6. Assess Mr. Peters for headache, noting its onset, type, location, severity, and associated signs and symptoms, such as nausea, vomiting, or photophobia (pain increased by light).

7. Assess Mr. Peters's posture in bed, noting the position of his arms, legs, hands, fingers, and spinal (vertebral) column.

8. Assess Mr. Peters for nausea; vomiting; altered speech or speaking ability; memory changes; and poor orientation to time (such as day), place (such as city), or person (such as his name or his parents' names).

9. Assess Mr. Peters's bowel and bladder continence.

10. Assess Mr. Peters for seizures.

11. Assess Mr. Peters for drainage from the nose or ears. Note whether drainage is clear or bloody.

5. Pupil responses are controlled by the third cranial nerve (oculomotor nerve). Deviations or changes in pupil responses may indicate increased ICP.

6. Headache may signal increased ICP. Headache location and severity help locate the affected brain area.

7. Variations in posture (such as decorticate or decerebrate posture) may indicate which areas of the brain and spinal cord are injured. (For details, see *Decorticate and decerebrate postures,* page 359.)

8. Forceful vomiting may result from increased ICP or injury to the vomiting center in the medulla. Speech, memory, and orientation changes also may reflect increased ICP.

9. Incontinence may result from lack of sphincter tone associated with loss of motor control in the motor area of the cerebral cortex.

10. Head injury may cause seizures.

11. Clear or bloody drainage may indicate skull fracture (with ear drainage) or fracture of the facial or forehead bones (with nasal drainage).

Nursing diagnoses
- Potential for injury related to increased ICP
- Altered peripheral (neurologic) tissue perfusion related to brain injury

Planning and goals
- Mr. Peters will regain his usual neurologic function.
- Mr. Peters's skull fracture will heal without complications or additional trauma.
- Mr. Peters will remain free from lingering headache, vomiting, and other neurologic symptoms.

Implementation

Nursing behaviors
1. Assist in transferring Mr. Peters to the hospital bed and positioning him in low Fowler's position, with the head of the bed elevated 20 to 30 degrees, as ordered. Handle him carefully and gently.

2. Perform all neurologic checks (as described under "Assessment" above and in "Performing neurologic checks," pages 357 to 359).

Nursing rationales
1. Elevating the head of the bed increases venous drainage. Careful, gentle handling reduces the risk of increasing trauma and pain or inducing a seizure.

2. This helps determine Mr. Peters's present condition and reveals any changes from previous neurologic checks.

ADULT NURSING

3. Using a soft, calm voice, explain to Mr. Peters why you cannot give him medicine for his headache at this time.

3. Because analgesics may mask or ease pain, they may cause health team members to misjudge the severity or duration of the patient's headache. Speaking softly and calmly conveys empathy.

4. Place the bed's side rails up before leaving Mr. Peters's room.

4. This promotes patient safety.

5. Close the curtains in Mr. Peters's room.

5. This reduces stimulation which could increase Mr. Peters's headache or cause photophobia.

6. Withhold oral intake, as ordered.

6. Head injury or increased ICP may necessitate surgery. Foods or fluids may increase nausea or vomiting from general or local anesthesia.

7. Maintain I.V. therapy at the ordered rate (usually 50 to 75 ml/hour).

7. I.V. therapy, administered to maintain fluid balance, must be infused slowly to reduce the risk of increasing blood volume (which could increase ICP).

8. Administer steroids and osmotic diuretics, such as mannitol (Osmitrol) or urea (Ureaphil), if ordered.

8. Steroids reduce the inflammatory response and increase microcirculation in the brain. Osmotic diuretics draw interstitial fluid into the bloodstream, reducing cerebral edema and decreasing ICP. (However, because osmotic diuretics may worsen cerebral edema when discontinued, the physician may not order these drugs.)

9. Encourage Mr. Peters to perform deep breathing exercises but to avoid coughing, if possible.

9. Deep breathing increases respiratory gas exchange, which aids cerebral oxygenation, and decreases the risk of pulmonary complications. Coughing increases ICP.

10. Using aseptic technique, change the sterile cotton ball in Mr. Peters's ear (if present), as needed.

10. A sterile cotton ball may be used to absorb drainage from the ear canal (resulting from skull fracture). Aseptic technique avoids the introduction of microorganisms that could cause neurologic infection.

11. Observe Mr. Peters for new or increasing restlessness, confusion, disorientation, and color changes (such as flushing or pallor).

11. Restlessness and pallor signal increased ICP and anoxia. Confusion and disorientation may be associated with increased ICP or trauma.

12. Once Mr. Peters's condition stabilizes, assist him to a bedside chair, when ordered. Stay with him the first time he gets out of bed.

12. When Mr. Peters is stable, the physician will instruct him to sit in a chair to help him regain or maintain muscle strength and to increase his activity and ambulation gradually as his condition improves. The nurse should stay with him the first time he sits up in a chair because positional and circulatory changes may cause a headache.

ADULT
NURSING

13. Prepare Mr. Peters for discharge to the home, as described in steps 14 to 20.

13. Such preparation promotes safe care and reduces patient anxiety.

14. Warn Mr. Peters to avoid becoming constipated and to avoid straining at stool.

14. Straining at stool may increase ICP and cause cranial bleeding.

15. Caution Mr. Peters to avoid coughing or blowing his nose.

15. These actions could increase ICP and cause cranial bleeding.

16. Encourage Mr. Peters to consume a diet high in fluids, fiber, and essential nutrients.

16. Such a diet will help Mr. Peters regain digestive and nutrient functions.

17. Encourage Mr. Peters to ambulate, as ordered or permitted.

17. Ambulation will help Mr. Peters regain muscle strength.

18. Caution Mr. Peters to avoid bending at the waist.

18. Bending at the waist increases ICP.

19. Instruct Mr. Peters to return for medical visits as required.

19. This ensures follow-up evaluation and continuity of care.

20. Instruct Mr. Peters to notify the physician if his headache returns or if he experiences vision or hearing changes, dizziness, or weakness.

20. These symptoms may signal a complication, such as a blood clot or hematoma.

Evaluation (outcomes)

• Mr. Peters regains his usual neurologic functions, as indicated by orientation to time, place, and person, usual level of consciousness (awake and alert), and lack of confusion or dizziness.
• Mr. Peters's skull fracture begins to show callus formation (union) and healing at the time of discharge. (Complete fracture healing will take 3 to 6 months.)
• Mr. Peters is free from lingering headache, nausea, and vomiting at the time of discharge. He receives instructions to consume a regular diet and to increase his intake gradually to 13 8-oz glasses (3,000 ml) of fluid a day.

ADULT NURSING

Cerebrovascular accident

Overview

Cerebrovascular accident (CVA), or stroke, is the most common cerebral circulatory disturbance. It may result from a thrombus (clot) blocking a cerebral artery, an embolus lodged in a cerebral artery, an arterial spasm that blocks circulation temporarily, or a hemorrhage that follows cerebral arterial rupture. Contributing and risk factors for CVA include arteriosclerosis, hypertension, diabetes, cardiac arrhythmias, valvular heart disease, anticoagulant therapy, and heart valve replacement. CVA is a major cause of death among Americans.

Clinical situation

Emily Ryan, age 76, a widow, falls on the sidewalk suddenly while walking to church. She appears unconscious and does not respond to questions from passersby. Her left side is flaccid and loose; her breathing is noisy and irregular. An ambulance takes her to the nearest hospital. After examining her in the emergency department, the physician admits her with a diagnosis of cerebrovascular hemorrhage of the right midcerebral artery. She is transferred to a medical nursing unit.

Assessment

Nursing behaviors	Nursing rationales
1. Assess Mrs. Ryan for a patent airway.	**1.** Respiration depends on an open, unobstructed airway.
2. Assess Mrs. Ryan for tongue position and ability to swallow.	**2.** With CVA, the tongue may fall backward (such as from loss of consciousness), obstructing the airway. Swallowing, necessary to clear oral secretions, may be impossible immediately after a CVA with hemorrhage.
3. Assess Mrs. Ryan's level of consciousness by using a recognized coma scale, such as the Glasgow coma scale (if one is used in your health care facility).	**3.** The Glasgow coma scale, a recognized coma scale, uses numbers to indicate specific determinants of consciousness.
4. Assess Mrs. Ryan's neurologic status by conducting neurologic checks (neurochecks), as described in "Performing neurologic checks," pages 357 to 359.	**4.** Neurologic checks help determine a patient's neurologic status. After a CVA, blood pressure may be low from continued bleeding. The pulse may be rapid, irregular, and thready. Respirations may be irregular and noisy from poor control of secretions; temperature may be subnormal. The skin may appear pale. Arm, leg, facial, cheek, and oral muscles may be weak or paralyzed. Bowel and bladder incontinence may occur; sensory responses may be diminished. The patient may remain unconscious but appear restless, moving only the unaffected arm and leg.
5. Assess Mrs. Ryan for ability to keep her eyes closed. If her eyes are partially open, assess the condition of the conjunctivae. Evaluate her blink reflex by quickly brushing a wisp of cotton over the conjunctivae; lack of blinking signals an absent reflex.	**5.** After a CVA, both eyes may be closed or open partially. If they are open and the blink reflex is absent, the conjunctivae will become dry and the patient will need moisture (such as artificial tears or ointment) to keep the conjunctivae healthy.
6. Assess Mrs. Ryan's position for control of secretions. (Usually, the patient is turned to the affected side every 1 to 2 hours, with brief periods on the unaffected side.) Use caution when positioning paralyzed limbs in a functional (slightly flexed) position.	**6.** A side-lying position promotes gravity drainage of secretions. Positioning Mrs. Ryan on the affected side allows her to use unaffected muscles (when conscious). Turning her every 1 to 2 hours helps prevent pressure ulcers and aids circulation. Maintaining limbs in a functional position permits use of limbs in case contractures develop.

Nursing diagnoses	• Altered peripheral tissue perfusion related to cerebral arterial rupture • Impaired physical mobility related to paralysis
Planning and goals	• Mrs. Ryan will regain and maintain consciousness. • Mrs. Ryan will regain partial or full movement of paralyzed muscles. • Mrs. Ryan will be able to perform her own activities of daily living (ADLs) after rehabilitation. • Mrs. Ryan will regain understandable speech after undergoing speech therapy. • Mrs. Ryan will regain adequate vision using prescribed eyeglasses. • Mrs. Ryan will return to her family and social setting after treatment and rehabilitation.

Implementation

Nursing behaviors	**Nursing rationales**
1. Gently place Mrs. Ryan on her left side, and elevate the head of the bed 20 to 30 degrees.	**1.** Mrs. Ryan's left side is paralyzed and cannot be used. If and when she regains consciousness, she will be able to use her right side. Elevating the head of the bed increases venous return.
2. Suction secretions from Mrs. Ryan's mouth if she cannot swallow.	**2.** Secretions may obstruct the airway unless suctioned or swallowed.
3. Perform all neurologic checks and document results on a flow sheet at the bedside (see "Performing neurologic checks," pages 357 to 359).	**3.** This will help detect changes in Mrs. Ryan's condition.
4. Monitor oxygen administration by nasal cannula, if ordered.	**4.** The physician may order oxygen therapy if blood gas analysis indicates the need.
5. Withhold all oral intake, as ordered.	**5.** Mrs. Ryan's unconscious state precludes oral intake.
6. Maintain I.V. fluid administration at 50 to 75 ml/hour, as ordered.	**6.** Slow infusion is necessary to prevent fluid volume overload, which could cause further bleeding into the brain.
7. Monitor intake and output. Check the position of the urinary catheter and tubing, if present.	**7.** Intake and output records help determine the adequacy of fluid therapy (or establish the need for additional therapy). A urinary catheter may be used until Mrs. Ryan regains voluntary bladder control.
8. Explain care activities to Mrs. Ryan, and talk to her when performing these activities.	**8.** Even though Mrs. Ryan is unconscious, she can hear. Explanations ease anxiety.
9. Place the bed's side rails up before leaving Mrs. Ryan's bedside.	**9.** Side rails will help protect Mrs. Ryan from injury caused by falling from the bed when unattended.

ADULT NURSING

10. Perform passive range-of-motion exercises of the extremities every 4 hours.

10. Passive exercises help preserve muscle strength in a patient who cannot perform active exercises. They also enhance peripheral circulation.

11. Place a roll in Mrs. Ryan's affected hand, or use a splint at the wrist, if ordered.

11. Rolls and splints help prevent flexion contractures (which may develop because flexor muscles are stronger than extensor muscles).

12. Arrange for a consultation with a physical therapist to develop an exercise regimen, if ordered.

12. Mrs. Ryan will need physical therapy to regain mobility and function of paralyzed muscles.

13. Turn and reposition Mrs. Ryan every 2 hours. Allow her to remain on her right side for 15 minutes only.

13. Turning and repositioning promote tissue perfusion. When Mrs. Ryan lies on her right side, she cannot move unaffected tissues; thus, in effect, she is totally paralyzed.

14. Monitor breath sounds in all lung lobes.

14. Audible breath sounds indicate satisfactory respiration. Lack of these sounds may signal atelectasis or pneumonia.

Clinical situation
(continued)

Over the next 6 hours, Mrs. Ryan begins to regain consciousness. She seems frightened and confused until she sees her daughter, Peggy. After Peggy tells her what has happened and informs her that she is in the hospital, Mrs. Ryan becomes calmer. Her left side remains paralyzed and she cannot speak, although she seems to understand explanations. When asked if she has a headache, Mrs. Ryan nods her head slowly as if to say "yes."

The physician arrives to evaluate Mrs. Ryan, then orders a computed tomography (CT) scan of the head to determine the site, cause, and extent of injury. Mrs. Ryan is transported carefully to the radiology department, where the CT scan is performed. When she returns to her room, she seems weak and tired.

Implementation

Nursing behaviors

15. Perform all neurologic checks, and compare findings with past results.

Nursing rationales

15. This may reveal any neurologic changes caused by transportation and examination.

16. Monitor I.V. therapy, intake and output, and urinary catheter status.

16. I.V. therapy will continue until Mrs. Ryan can swallow well enough to avoid choking.

17. Obtain advice from a dietitian about which foods to provide for Mrs. Ryan as she progresses from a soft to a regular diet. Encourage Mrs. Ryan to use utensils to eat.

17. Soft foods are easier to chew and swallow. Mrs. Ryan cannot use a straw for liquids because her facial and oral muscles are paralyzed. However, she may be able to drink and swallow from a glass or cup. She may need tube feedings until she can swallow without choking.

18. Perform oral hygiene every 4 hours.

18. This helps maintain healthy oral tissues.

19. Assist Mrs. Ryan with a bed bath, as necessary.

19. Because Mrs. Ryan can use only one hand, she will need help to wring out and apply soap to the washcloth and to rinse and dry herself.

20. Arrange for a consultation with an occupational therapist, as ordered.

20. An occupational therapist can help Mrs. Ryan learn how to use adaptive utensils for self-care and home maintenance activities.

21. Arrange for a consultation with a speech therapist.

21. Speech commonly is affected by rupture of the midcerebral artery. A speech therapist can help Mrs. Ryan learn to speak again. Mrs. Ryan may need speech therapy for a prolonged period.

22. Remove the urinary catheter, as ordered. When Mrs. Ryan is allowed to get up, place her on a bedpan or help her to a bedside commode. Observe her bowel movements for amount and consistency.

22. Because a urinary catheter commonly causes infection, the catheter will be removed as soon as possible. Observing bowel movements may detect constipation caused by immobility.

23. Encourage Mrs. Ryan to obtain an adequate oral fluid intake, as able. When total fluid intake measures 70 oz (2,000 ml) a day, remove the I.V. line, as ordered.

23. Oral intake helps flush the urinary and gastrointestinal systems, helping to restore or maintain urinary and GI functions.

24. Encourage Mrs. Ryan to ambulate to a chair, as able. When she can move her lower extremities, the physical therapist will develop an exercise regimen and teach her to ambulate in parallel bars or with use of a cane.

24. Motor function may return slowly to the lower limbs, allowing Mrs. Ryan to walk with a limp or staggered gait. Upper limb movement depends on the extent of damage to brain cells caused by the hemorrhage.

25. Encourage Mrs. Ryan's daughter and other family members to attend therapy sessions to learn care activities in preparation for Mrs. Ryan's discharge to the home.

25. Mrs. Ryan will need prolonged rehabilitation and will have to return to the rehabilitation area for continued treatments. If she can regain enough functions to perform her own ADLs, she might be able to return to the home.

26. Complete the continuity-of-care referral for a community health nurse to visit Mrs. Ryan at home. Include instructions on:
• checking breath sounds, blood pressure, pulse rate, respirations, and apical pulse
• monitoring dietary intake and bowel and bladder elimination
• inspecting the skin and assessing for contractures
• teaching Mrs. Ryan how to use a quad cane
• assessing Mrs. Ryan's emotional or psychological status.
   Also include instructions for all medications, if ordered.

26. Referral to a community health nurse helps ensure that Mrs. Ryan receives continued care and monitoring of her progress toward recovery. It also will reveal any need for additional therapy or community services (such as Meals On Wheels or a home care aide).

Evaluation (outcomes)

• Mrs. Ryan regains and maintains consciousness and alertness.
• Mrs. Ryan regains the ability to swallow foods and liquids without choking and can walk with a stagger gait using a quad cane for support. Her left upper extremity remains flaccid and paralyzed, and she cannot use her left hand or fingers.
• Mrs. Ryan can perform some ADLs after rehabilitation. For instance, she can take a shower and dry herself, dress herself with minimal assistance (her daughter has replaced buttons with pressure-sensitive [Velcro] strips), feed herself if the food is cut and containers opened, perform toileting without assistance, and ambulate with a quad cane.
• Mrs. Ryan regains understandable speech sufficient to make her needs known and participate in occasional social conversations.
• Mrs. Ryan obtains new eyeglasses and can read a newspaper and watch television; her blurred vision clears gradually.
• Mrs. Ryan is discharged to live with her daughter temporarily until she is rehabilitated sufficiently to return to her own home.

Epilepsy

Overview

Epilepsy is a chronic neurologic condition characterized by recurrent seizures (convulsions), with loss of consciousness, sensory disturbances, altered sensations, and abnormal or repetitive behavior. The seizures result from excessive, uncontrolled electrical discharge from nerve cells in the cerebral cortex.

Epilepsy may occur at any age. However, it is most common in children and young and middle-aged adults. Causes of epilepsy include cerebral injury, tumor, infection, chemical imbalance, blood vessel disturbance leading to ischemia (lack of oxygenation), and metabolic conditions. However, in most cases, epilepsy has no known cause (idiopathic epilepsy). Although the disorder cannot be cured, seizures usually can be controlled with medications.

Clinical situation

Sherry Miller, age 11, a fifth-grader, falls from a swing in the school yard and strikes her head on a support block. She is treated in the local children's hospital for a skull fracture and an enlarged blood clot (hematoma). The surgeon creates burr holes in her skull to relieve pressure from accumulating fluid. Sherry then is discharged to recover at home.

Ten days after discharge, Sherry has a seizure. She cries out suddenly, makes uncontrolled convulsive movements, and remains unconscious for several moments. Her mother calls 911. An emergency paramedic team arrives and takes Sherry to the children's hospital, where she is readmitted with a diagnosis of epilepsy secondary to head injury. As the physician examines her in the emergency department, she has another seizure. The physician orders an I.V. infusion and medication to control the seizures. After undergoing a computed tomography scan of her head, Sherry is transferred to the neurologic nursing unit.

Assessment

Nursing behaviors

1. Assess Sherry's neurologic status by evaluating her for level of consciousness; vital signs; pupil size, shape, and reaction to light; motor and sensory functions; headache; nausea and vomiting; bowel or bladder incontinence; orientation to time, place, and person; and blurred or double vision.

2. Assess Sherry's physical status for ongoing twitches or jerking movements.

3. Assess Sherry's memory or knowledge of what she was doing just before the seizure began by asking questions worded appropriately for her age and developmental level. (If she is too drowsy to participate, ask her parents these questions.)

4. Assess the I.V. infusion site for signs of redness, edema (swelling), tenderness, and pain.

5. Assess the response of Sherry's parents to her rehospitalization and new diagnosis.

Nursing rationales

1. These assessments, called neurologic checks, yield baseline data about a patient's neurologic condition (see "Performing neurologic checks," pages 357 to 359).

2. This determines if the medication Sherry received is sufficient to control seizures.

3. This helps determine Sherry's or her parents' awareness of what occurred just before the seizure and their knowledge of Sherry's condition. It also helps identify factors that may have triggered the seizure.

4. This helps detect infiltration and determines the status of the infusion.

5. This determines her parents' level of knowledge and understanding about Sherry's current condition.

Nursing diagnoses
- Potential for injury related to seizures
- Knowledge deficit related to newly diagnosed epilepsy

Planning and goals
- Sherry will achieve good control of epilepsy with medications.
- Sherry will remain free from injury if she does have seizures.
- Sherry and her parents will gain knowledge about epilepsy and Sherry's medications.
- Sherry will return to school and social activities without feeling like an outcast.

Implementation

Nursing behaviors

1. Perform neurologic checks every 1 to 2 hours, as ordered. Compare the results with previous findings.

2. Continue the I.V. infusion at the rate ordered (such as 25 to 50 ml/hour). Use a volume-control device for accuracy.

3. Place the bed's side rails up when you are not attending Sherry directly.

4. For the first 2 to 4 hours, visit Sherry's room every 15 to 30 minutes.

Nursing rationales

1. This provides continuous assessment data, allowing comparison of findings over time.

2. The I.V. infusion may be maintained for quick venous access in case Sherry has more seizures.

3. Side rails help prevent injury in case Sherry has a seizure.

4. Frequent visits help the nurse assess Sherry's present condition and her and her parents' responses. Such visits also reassure them of your continued presence.

ADULT
NURSING

5. If Sherry has a seizure, record information about:
• aura (if present)
• level of consciousness during the seizure
• motor activity or movements, including those of the head, limbs, and spinal column
• parts of the body initially involved in the seizure
• eye movements and pupil reactions
• respirations
• skin color changes (if any)
• incontinence
• tonic movements (tense, jerking muscle contractions)
• clonic movements (muscle relaxation)
• length of the seizure
• postseizure state, including level of consciousness, vital signs, drowsiness, speech (whether normal or changed), complaints of nausea and headache, and any injuries, bumps, or bruises.

5. Recording all pertinent data helps the physician identify the type of seizure and the brain area involved.

6. Do not try to force any article between Sherry's teeth during tonic movements. Also, do not try to restrain her convulsive movements.

6. Forcing an article into the mouth could break the teeth. Restraining convulsive movements could cause bone fracture.

7. If Sherry is awake and alert, offer her food and fluids at meal times and regular intervals.

7. Usual patient activities and food intake should be maintained.

8. Administer antiseizure medication, as ordered.

8. Medication may be given orally to help maintain a satisfactory blood drug level.

9. Discontinue the I.V. infusion when ordered.

9. Once Sherry's condition has stabilized, the I.V. infusion will be discontinued.

10. Allow Sherry to play with other patients, as desired.

10. Engaging in normal social activities with her peers will help Sherry feel less isolated and different.

11. Maintain a safe environment by removing sharp or pointed objects from Sherry's immediate area.

11. This helps prevent injury in case of a seizure.

12. Draw the curtains enough to block bright sunlight. Replace any flickering lights, and keep the radio or television at low volume.

12. Bright or flickering lights and loud noise can trigger seizures in some patients.

13. Provide time and opportunity for Sherry and her parents to express their feelings about epilepsy.

13. This will help them sort out their feelings.

14. Emphasize the secondary nature of Sherry's epilepsy.

14. Knowing that epilepsy is secondary to injury might help Sherry and her family accept and cope with it more easily.

15. Instruct Sherry and her parents about medications used to control seizures.

15. Knowledge of the desired effects and side effects of medications is vital to Sherry and her parents. Untoward or toxic side effects of medications may frighten Sherry and her family and jeopardize her health.

16. Teach Sherry and her parents how to recognize signs of an impending seizure (such as aura) and how to provide proper care during and after a seizure.

16. The aura differs for each patient. Teaching about care during and after a seizure helps prevent injury.

17. Teach Sherry and her parents how to obtain an ID card (such as a medical-alert card) and bracelet.

17. Certain organizations can provide ID cards and bracelets for a nominal fee.

18. Teach Sherry and her parents about local, state, and national organizations that help people with epileptic patients and their families.

18. Support can help Sherry and her parents adjust to her condition. Support organizations include the American Epilepsy Society and the Epilepsy Foundation of America.

19. Teach Sherry and her parents how to help her develop regular habits, such as a safe exercise regimen and a regular sleep pattern and diet. Also advise Sherry to avoid exhaustion and highly stressful situations.

19. Establishing regular habits and avoiding exhaustion and stress helps control seizures.

20. Teach Sherry and her parents how she can use prescribed medications, as ordered, and non-expired dated medications. Mention that she should not use medications past their expiration date, and she must not discontinue medications abruptly.

20. To maintain therapeutic blood drug levels, Sherry must take regular doses of full-strength medications on a continuing basis.

21. Advise Sherry and her parents to obtain continuing medical guidance for her.

21. This ensures continuity of care.

22. Prepare Sherry and her parents for discharge after her seizures have been controlled and she has been stabilized on antiseizure medication. (For details on these medications, see *Drugs used to treat neurologic disorders,* pages 370 to 372.)

22. Epilepsy is a chronic condition that can be managed in Sherry's usual surroundings.

23. Complete a continuity-of-care referral for the community nursing association.

23. Such a referral provides for continuity of care after discharge.

Evaluation (outcomes)
- Sherry obtains seizure control through the use of antiseizure medications.
- Sherry remains free from injury during her initial seizures.
- Sherry and her parents can repeat the nurse's explanation of the desired effects and side effects of prescribed medications. They also can identify signs and symptoms of an impending seizure and know how to protect Sherry during and after a seizure.

Brain tumor

Overview

A brain tumor may arise within brain tissues or a cranial nerve (primary tumor), or it may spread to the brain from distant tissues (secondary, or metastatic, tumor). About half of brain tumors are malignant (cancerous). In some cases, the tumor's growth pattern makes complete surgical removal impossible; remaining tumor tissues continue to grow, displacing or destroying brain tissue. Signs and symptoms of a brain tumor result from compression of brain tissue, cranial nerves, and cerebral vessels; cerebral edema; and increased intracranial pressure (ICP). Possible treatments for a brain tumor include surgery, radiation, and chemotherapy.

Clinical situation

Jerry Waterford, a lawyer, age 40, has had a severe, recurring headache that emanates from behind his eyes. His vision is blurred; he vomited recently at his office. He is tense and nervous and angers easily, yelling at his staff and law clerks. His wife, concerned about his headaches and behavior changes, urges him to see the physician. After examining Mr. Waterford, the physician makes a provisional diagnosis of suspected brain tumor and admits him to the hospital for a diagnostic work-up.

Assessment

Nursing behaviors

1. Assess Mr. Waterford's neurologic functions by performing a complete neurologic check (see "Performing neurologic checks," pages 357 to 359). Be sure to assess for possible seizures. Record all findings carefully.

2. Assess Mr. Waterford's ability to walk normally and maintain balance.

3. Assess Mr. Waterford's ability to perform his own activities of daily living.

4. Assess Mr. Waterford's coping behaviors.

5. Assess Mr. Waterford's vision and hearing.

6. Assess Mr. Waterford's family relationships.

7. Assess Mr. Waterford's past medical history.

8. Assess Mr. Waterford's educational level.

Nursing rationales

1. A complete neurologic check with thoroughly documented results yields important baseline data. A seizure or brief loss of consciousness may help confirm the diagnosis.

2. Depending on the brain tumor site, walking ability and balance may be affected.

3. A brain tumor can affect fine motor movements.

4. A tumor in the frontal lobe affects personality and coping.

5. Some brain tumors affect cranial nerve functions.

6. Strong family relationships usually result in strong support for the patient. Family strengths will be important for Mr. Waterford's long-term care.

7. A brain tumor may represent metastasis from a distant tumor site.

8. Some patients may have trouble understanding new or unfamiliar medical terms.

Nursing diagnoses

- Potential for injury related to increased ICP
- Anxiety related to the uncertain diagnosis

Planning and goals

- Mr. Waterford will undergo diagnostic examinations without complications.
- Mr. Waterford will understand his medical diagnosis and participate in treatment decisions.
- Mr. Waterford will achieve brain tumor remission.
- Mr. Waterford will return to his usual roles and responsibilities.

Implementation

Nursing behaviors	Nursing rationales
1. Explain the purpose of assessment and diagnostic procedures to Mr. Waterford, as described in steps 2 and 3.	**1.** Explanations reduce patient anxiety and promote patient cooperation.
2. Explain the purpose of the history and physical examination.	**2.** The history and physical examination yield data about Mr. Waterford's past and present health status.
3. Explain the purpose of the neurologic examination, including: • electroencephalogram (EEG) • brain scans, which may include computed tomography (CT), magnetic resonance imaging (MRI), and positron emission tomography • visual field examination • biopsy.	**3.** The neurologic examination provides baseline data. An EEG, which records electrical brain activity, may detect abnormal brain activity and help locate the tumor site. Brain scans will help localize the tumor and may determine its type. Visual field examination will reveal any pressure on the optic nerve, oculomotor nerves, or other cranial nerves. Biopsy can determine the tumor cell type.

4. Prepare Mr. Waterford for examinations, as follows:
    For an EEG, explain the process of electrode placement and the need to lie completely still during the examination. Have Mr. Waterford wash his hair (or do this for him).
    For a CT scan, no special preparation is needed. Radioisotopes, if used, are administered in the radiology department. The scan will be performed after the radioisotope distributes in the tissues. For an MRI, Mr. Waterford must remove all metallic objects, then go through a metal detector before entering the imaging area to ensure that no metal objects are present. An MRI takes approximately 1 hour.
    For a visual field examination, performed in the ophthalmology department, Mr. Waterford's eyes will be examined by technicians using special machines. He will have to keep his head and eyes still during the examination, as requested by the technician.
    For a biopsy, Mr. Waterford may receive local or general anesthesia.
	4. Preparation increases patient comfort and promotes a safe, efficient examination.
	    Water-soluble jelly is used to attach electrodes to the skull. Washing the hair removes oil, which can interfere with the recording of brain activity. Lying still helps prevent misleading results caused by head movement.
	    Radioisotopes act as markers in the brain, helping to locate abnormal cells. The isotope is excreted in the urine.
	    Metal interferes with the magnet used in MRI and distorts test results. (Patients who are claustrophobic may not be able to have a full-body MRI scan because the opening where the patient lies is narrow and may cause a closed-in feeling.)
	    Visual field examination shows peripheral and central vision areas, possibly revealing areas of blindness or decreased vision.
	    Preoperative preparation is required if the biopsy will be done during surgery (see the "Perioperative nursing" section).

5. Explain and clarify upcoming events to Mr. Waterford (if known).	**5.** Explanations lessen anxiety by replacing the unknown with the known.
6. Provide diversionary materials, as needed.	**6.** The diagnostic period may be long and anxiety-producing. Diversion will help Mr. Waterford cope with delays and uncertainty.

Clinical situation
(continued)

Based on results of the EEG and CT and MRI scans, the physician determines that Mr. Waterford has a malignant astrocytoma in the left and central temporal and frontal lobes. Because of the tumor's location and extension into the pituitary gland, surgery is ruled out. Instead, Mr. Waterford will undergo chemotherapy and radiation therapy (see the "Oncology nursing" section).

While caring for Mr. Waterford during these treatments, the nurse takes measures related to increased ICP (see "Head injury and increased intracranial pressure," pages 338 to 341). Mr. Waterford's prognosis is guarded, pending the effectiveness of treatment in shrinking the tumor, halting its growth, and killing tumor cells. (Also, recurrence is likely with some brain tumors.)

Evaluation (outcomes)

- Mr. Waterford remains free from complications of diagnostic procedures.
- Mr. Waterford understands his medical diagnosis; he and his family participate actively in the treatment regimen.
- Mr. Waterford's tumor enters remission after radiation therapy and chemotherapy.
- Mr. Waterford returns to his law practice after treatment.

Parkinson's disease

Overview

Parkinson's disease, a progressive degenerative disease affecting older adults, is characterized by depletion of the neurotransmitter dopamine in the basal ganglia of the brain. Signs and symptoms include loss of fine motor movement, muscle rigidity, disturbed balance, tremor, difficulty walking, monotonous voice, and masklike facial expression. As Parkinson's disease progresses, it may cause mental deterioration and increasing disability.

Clinical situation

Joseph Jacobs, a retired farmer, age 70, has trouble walking because of increasing stiffness in his legs and knees. He takes short, unsteady steps without bending his knees. Tremors cause constant jerking movements of his fingers and head. His face is blank and expressionless, and he seems unable to smile. When Mr. Jacobs's daughter finally convinces him to get medical help, he passively accompanies his wife and daughter to the family physician. After examining him, the physician diagnoses Parkinson's disease.

Assessment

Nursing behaviors

1. Assess Mr. Jacobs for difficulty rising to a standing position. Evaluate his gait for a forward lean (for balance) and short, rapid, shuffling steps with straight knees and stiff ankles.

2. Assess Mr. Jacobs's entire body for muscle strength, coordinated movements, and muscle rigidity. Note which muscles are affected.

3. Assess Mr. Jacobs for tremor at rest (pill-rolling tremor).

Nursing rationales

1. Gait disturbance results from loss of dopamine, which helps control and coordinate muscles. Mr. Jacobs's gait, called a festinating gait, is characteristic of Parkinson's disease.

2. Parkinson's disease causes muscle stiffness and heaviness. Such changes may be symmetrical, involving corresponding muscles on opposite sides.

3. The typical parkinsonian tremor occurs at rest and worsens with stress and fatigue.

4. Assess Mr. Jacobs's facial expressions and ability to smile, blink his eyelids, whistle, and control salivary secretions.

4. Parkinson's disease causes a blank, masklike expression with limited ability to smile and blink. It also may cause drooling.

5. Assess Mr. Jacobs's posture and ability to stand straight.

5. Parkinson's disease may cause a stooped, forward-leaning posture and the inability to stand up straight.

6. Assess Mr. Jacobs for signs and symptoms associated with Parkinson's disease, such as incontinence, constipation, excessive tearing (lacrimation), and decreased sexual function.

6. These signs and symptoms stem from motor function loss and excessive sympathetic nervous system tone from Parkinson's disease.

7. Assess Mr. Jacobs's emotional responses.

7. Parkinson's disease may cause excessive emotional responses.

Nursing diagnoses
- Potential for injury related to lack of coordinated, controlled movements
- Self-care deficit related to loss of muscle coordination

Planning and goals
- Mr. Jacobs will retain function in unaffected muscles.
- Mr. Jacobs will regain some degree of normal movement in affected muscles by taking medications.
- Mr. Jacobs will retain as much physical mobility as possible by taking medications.
- Mr. Jacobs and his significant others will cope effectively with his chronic condition.

Implementation

Nursing behaviors

1. Teach Mr. Jacobs and his significant others about Parkinson's disease and the need to maintain regular activities and routines.

Nursing rationales

1. Regular activities and routines will help Mr. Jacobs maintain body functions.

2. Administer ordered medications and observe for side effects. For example, levodopa (Dopar) may cause anorexia, nausea, vomiting, foul body odor, postural hypotension, cardiac arrhythmias, and pink to red urine (which turns black when exposed to air). Benztropine mesylate (Cogentin) and trihexyphenidyl (Artane) may cause dry mouth, blurred vision, urine retention, constipation, confusion, and psychotic reactions. Amantadine (Symmetrel) may cause edema of the feet and ankles, confusion, slurred speech, nervousness, dry mouth, nausea, and vomiting.

2. These drugs are used to treat Parkinson's disease. Levodopa crosses the blood-brain barrier and is converted to dopamine by brain cells; it helps counteract dopamine deficiency and reduce muscle rigidity and tremors. Benztropine and trihexyphenidyl have anticholinergic effects that decrease the effects of acetylcholine, reducing muscle rigidity and tremors. Amantadine decreases muscle rigidity, tremors, drooling, and gait disturbances in approximately half of patients with Parkinson's disease.

3. Teach Mr. Jacobs and his significant others about the side effects of medications. (Do not give anticholinergics to a patient with glaucoma.) For more information on medications, see *Drugs used to treat neurologic disorders,* pages 370 to 372.

3. Drug dosages may be adjusted to reduce side effects. However, because of the benefits of these drugs, the physician may ask Mr. Jacobs to tolerate side effects.

4. Administer cool drinks and offer hard candy to Mr. Jacobs, as desired.

4. Cool drinks and hard candy help relieve dry mouth.

ADULT NURSING

5. Arrange for a physical therapy consultation for Mr. Jacobs to ensure appropriate exercise programs.

5. Exercises improve muscle movements and strength.

6. Teach Mr. Jacobs to avoid using methyldopa (Aldomet), monoamine oxidase (MAO) inhibitors, phenothiazines, reserpine (Serpasil), and pyridoxine (vitamin B_6).

6. Methyldopa has parkinsonian effects. MAO inhibitors can cause a hypertensive crisis. Phenothiazines, reserpine, and pyridoxine block the action of levodopa.

7. Teach Mr. Jacobs to maintain bowel regularity by increasing dietary fiber and fluid intake and by using stool softeners or suppositories.

7. Anticholinergic drugs cause constipation.

8. Encourage Mr. Jacobs to ambulate, as able.

8. Ambulation helps maintain strength and mobility.

9. Assist Mr. Jacobs with activities of daily living as needed.

9. This will help Mr. Jacobs conserve strength.

10. Provide time for Mr. Jacobs and his family to discuss their feelings and concerns. Arrange for a consultation with a social worker or mental health worker, if needed.

10. Parkinson's disease is a chronic, progressively debilitating disease that calls for long-term coping. Mr. Jacobs also may need financial help.

11. Discuss ways in which Mr. Jacobs can deal with stress.

11. Managing stress helps reduce or prevent excessive emotional responses.

Evaluation (outcomes)

• Mr. Jacobs retains function in unaffected muscles for an extended period.
• Mr. Jacobs achieves increased muscle strength and easier movements once therapeutic blood drug levels are established.
• Mr. Jacobs and his significant others cope with his chronic condition successfully over time.

Complications of neurologic disorders

This chart presents the most serious or life-threatening complications of neurologic disorders, along with interventions that are crucial to patient safety and comfort.

COMPLICATION	CAUSE	NURSING INTERVENTIONS
Ruptured cerebral aneurysm Localized ballooning and breaking of a blood vessel wall. A berry aneurysm occurs in the circle of Willis in the brain's central posterior portion. Other sites of aneurysm include the anterior cerebral and anterior communicating arteries. Some aneurysms cause no symptoms and are discovered only on autopsy. Others grow and cause signs and symptoms of increased pressure on surrounding structures. 　　Rupture of an aneurysm may be signaled by a sudden sharp pain or popping sensation in the head, followed by nausea, vomiting, change in level of consciousness, weakness, and prostration. Severe neck (nuchal) rigidity occurs, with increased blood pressure and body temperature and gradually decreasing pulse rate.	• Weakness of the blood vessel wall • Sudden severe trauma (such as a blow to the head or a fall) • Increased intracranial pressure	• As appropriate, provide postoperative care after craniotomy, which may be performed if the patient's general health allows. (A silver clip is attached to the neck [beginning] of the aneurysm to stop blood flow to the aneurysm.) For postoperative care see the "Perioperative nursing" section.
Muscle spasticity Spasms of the skeletal muscles characterized by severe muscle flexor activity followed by extensor spasticity. Spasticity can cause severe discomfort and pain. Infection, stress, and metabolic imbalances may exacerbate the condition.	• Damage to nerves supplying or aiding muscle functions, such as from injury to upper motor neurons. Upper motor neuron injury interrupts normal nerve pathways; lack of inhibitory influences makes the nerve respond with intense flexion when stimulated. Even a slight stimulus can cause a severe spastic flexion contraction. • Head injury at birth • Neonatal neurologic trauma with nerve ischemia	• Administer muscle relaxants, as ordered. • Handle the patient gently to reduce the severity of spasticity.
Paralysis Loss of muscle function or sensation. Paralysis can take the form of quadriplegia (paralysis of all four limbs), paraplegia (paralysis of the lower limbs), or hemiplegia (paralysis of one side). Paralyzed muscles lose their mass and become atrophied (shrunken). Flexion contractures develop from lack of active movements and joint extension. Pressure areas develop over bony prominences.	• Damage to nerve or muscle mechanisms	• Help the patient remain as active as possible, such as by encouraging maximal use of a wheel chair, walker, cane, or crutches (depending on the patient's condition). • Assist with or perform activities of daily living, as needed. • Perform range-of-motion exercises. • To prevent constipation, provide a diet high in fiber and at least 100 oz (3,000 ml) of fluid daily. Provide stool softeners and suppositories, as needed. • Use special beds and pads, as ordered and needed, to help prevent pressure areas and pressure ulcers. • Encourage the patient to perform deep breathing exercises and to use an incentive spirometer to avoid respiratory complications. • As appropriate, refer the patient for vocational, educational, and financial support services.

(continued)

ADULT NURSING

Complications of neurologic disorders *(continued)*

COMPLICATION	CAUSE	NURSING INTERVENTIONS
Sensory loss Loss of sensation. Signs and symptoms range from temporary numbness, tingling, and a "pins and needles" sensation to permanent numbness and anesthesia. Lingering numbness can be highly irritating. Because sensory tracts help the central nervous system determine conditions of position, pressure, comfort, and temperature, sensory loss may lead to injury by preventing the patient from sensing heat, cold, or pressure. Sensory loss sometimes involves hearing, sight, smell, taste, and equilibrium.	• Injury to the dorsal horns of the spinal cord or sensory areas of the cerebral cortex (such as from pressure on the nerves or loss of blood supply) • Ruptured (herniated) intervertebral disk • Multiple sclerosis • Amyotrophic lateral sclerosis • Aging	• Include sensory data in each neurologic check, noting any increase or decrease in the affected senses of body areas as well as other patterns that might cause sensory changes. • Perform required nursing care to prevent permanent damage. For instance, periodically change the patient's position to relieve pressure and increase circulation. • Avoid exposure to extreme heat or cold if the patient cannot sense temperature. • Teach the patient how to cope with the specific sensations lost, if the condition is permanent.
Headache Pain in the head. A major complaint of many patients admitted to hospitals, headache may be a symptom of a specific disorder or disease (such as a vascular condition or brain tumor). Posttraumatic or posttreatment headaches can be as debilitating as the original injury or disease.	• Neurologic injury or disease • Medications • The exact causes of migraine, cluster, or tension headaches have not been determined. Tension headaches have been linked with tension and stress. Some patients visit one physician after the other attempting to find the cause of and a cure for headache.	• Maintain a calm, subdued atmosphere to aid relaxation. • Administer prescribed medications. • Apply heat or cold treatments. • Arrange times for scheduled treatments. • Determine the area of the head involved (such as frontal or top), type of pain (such as sharp, dull, or throbbing), onset, duration, severity, and associated signs and symptoms (such as nausea, blurred vision, or nervousness). • Be aware that no treatment is entirely effective for migraine, cluster, or tension headaches, although some treatments relieve pain temporarily. Nonnarcotic analgesics, such as aspirin or acetaminophen, commonly are used for temporary relief. 　To reduce headache frequency, discourage caffeine consumption (caffeine withdrawal can cause headache). • Other treatments may include ergot-containing medications, antihistamines, muscle relaxants, ice applications to the back of the neck, elimination of precipitating foods, and relaxation or biofeedback techniques.
Transient ischemic attack Episode of cerebrovascular insufficiency lasting from a few seconds to 24 hours. A transient ischemic attack (TIA) sometimes precedes rather than follows a neurologic disease.	• Embolism • Partial occlusion of the carotid or cerebral arteries • Atherosclerotic plaques • Pressure changes in blood vessels	• Determine the frequency and duration of TIAs; identify associated signs and symptoms (such as dizziness, visual changes, and headache); and measure the patient's vital signs. • Make sure the patient is referred to the physician to determine the cause of TIAs so that appropriate treatment can begin. For instance, if the carotid artery is occluded, surgical carotid bypass or endarterectomy may be performed, with removal of atherosclerotic plaques to restore circulation. • Treatment may include vasodilator drugs to increase circulation (and possibly avoid the need for cerebral artery surgery) and prevent ischemia from progressing.

Performing neurologic checks

Introduction   Neurologic checks (commonly called neurochecks) are a series of assessments that detect subtle or obvious changes in neurologic function. Each assessment provides specific information about the patient's condition. The series of specific assessments begins with step 5 and ends with step 19 below. (Because all procedure steps are equally important, none is preceded by an asterisk.)

Steps	Rationales
1. Gather needed items: stethoscope, sphygmomanometer, pen light or flashlight, pin, and cotton-tipped applicator.	**1.** Gathering items in advance promotes patient care. (Reflex assessment may be done by other members of the health team.)
2. Take the items to the patient's area and place them on the bedstand.	**2.** Having supplies readily accessible facilitates the procedure.
3. Close the door or draw the curtain around the patient's area. (Draw the curtain slowly to reduce noise.) Avoid bumping the patient's bed. Move quietly and slowly.	**3.** Closing the door or drawing the curtain ensures privacy. Noise is an irritant to the patient with a neurologic problem. Bumping the bed and making loud or sudden movements can startle the patient.
4. Explain to the patient that you are going to do some evaluations that will call for patient cooperation at times.	**4.** Explanation of upcoming events lessens patient anxiety.
5. Begin the specific assessments by evaluating the patient's level of consciousness. To do this, ask the patient his or her name and age, room number, day of the week, month, year, or other questions to evaluate orientation to time, place, and person.	**5.** Level of consciousness is the best index of brain function. *A change in level of consciousness is a major sign of increasing intracranial pressure (ICP).*
6. Measure the patient's blood pressure, pulse rate, respiratory rate, and temperature. Determine pulse pressure by subtracting diastolic pressure from systolic pressure.	**6.** Vital signs changes that may indicate increased ICP include widening of pulse pressure; decreased pulse rate; slow, irregular respirations; and increased temperature (which may be associated with pressure on the hypothalamus).
7. Assess motor functions of the patient's face, arms, and legs as described below: • Ask the patient to grasp or grip, then squeeze, your hands. (Assess both hands at once to compare their strength.) • Ask the patient to push the hand against your hand, or to pull against your finger (or fingers) with one or more fingers. • Put your hands against the bottom of the patient's feet and have the patient push the feet against your hands. Then place your fingers on the patient's toes and ask the patient to hyperextend the toes against backward pressure from your fingers.	**7.** Motor functions (movement) indicate adequacy of tissue perfusion. • A weak grasp or grip may signal injury to or inadequate oxygenation of the brain or spinal cord. • Pushing and pulling ability reflects the patient's circulatory and oxygenation status. • Ability to hyperextend the toes also indicates the adequacy of circulation and oxygenation.

ADULT NURSING

• Ask the patient to flex and extend the forearms and legs by bending and straightening them.

• Evaluate the face and facial expressions by asking the patient to raise the eyebrows together, blink the eyelids, smile and show the teeth, and open the mouth and stick out the tongue.

8. Check the pupils for size, constriction or dilation, and reaction to light. (To check reaction to light, move a pen light or flashlight from the side of the patient's head and shine it briefly into the eye while noting pupil response). Compare the size, shape, and constriction or dilation of the left and right pupils.

9. Assess sensory functions on both sides of the body by using the blunt and sharp ends of a pin on various body parts. First, touch the skin on both sides of the body and limbs with the head of the pin. Then touch these areas with the pin point. Ask if the patient feels a sharp or dull sensation from the pin and whether the sensation is equal on both sides. Ask the patient to describe any numbness or tingling and to point to the affected areas.

10. Observe the position of the patient's arms, legs, head, and spinal column.

11. Assess for double or blurred vision.

12. Check for hearing problems or changes.

13. Observe for changes in behavior, decision making, and judgment.

14. Observe for changes in the ability to speak, enunciate words correctly, and understand speech.

15. Assess for dizziness or ataxia (impaired coordination of movement).

16. Observe for seizures, noting the type of seizure and the body area involved.

17. Determine if the patient has had a headache and if so, ask about its severity, location, frequency, onset (sudden or gradual), changes with activities, accompanying symptoms, and possible precipitating causes.

• Ability to flex and extend the arms and legs reflects motor function and circulatory and oxygenation status.
• Unequal or asymmetrical expressions and movements may help localize a cranial lesion or detect weakness of one or more cranial nerves.

8. Pupil constriction and dilation are controlled by the third cranial nerve (oculomotor nerve). Unequal pupil size or reaction to light may indicate injury or increased pressure on one side. Pupil dilation or slow reaction to light indicates increased ICP and anoxia.

9. Sensations should be equal on both sides. One area or side may have less sensation, numbness, or tingling. With an abnormality localized on one side of the brain, sensory changes or deficits occur on the opposite side of the body.

10. This helps detect an abnormal posture (such as decorticate or decerebrate posture), which may indicate cerebral injury and increased ICP (see *Decorticate and decerebrate postures*).

11. Double or blurred vision indicates increased pressure in the occipital lobe.

12. Hearing problems or changes may indicate temporal lobe involvement.

13. These changes reflect frontal lobe involvement.

14. These changes indicate motor speech impairment.

15. These problems indicate cerebellar involvement or a spinal cord problem.

16. This helps determine the cause of the abnormality or the involved brain area.

17. Headache associated with increased ICP usually is severe and constant; worsens with movement, activities, or noise; and may be accompanied by blurred vision, nausea, vomiting, or dizziness.

Decorticate and decerebrate postures

In *decorticate* posture, the patient lies with the forearms adducted over the thorax (chest), wrists and fingers flexed sharply, hands rotated internally, legs extended, and feet flexed (with toes pointing toward the bed). This posture reflects involvement of the corticospinal nerve pathways. In *decerebrate* posture, the patient lies with arms and forearms extended rigidly and abducted, legs extended rigidly with toes pointing downward and inward, wrists flexed sharply outward, and the vertebral column and back arched upward. This posture reflects involvement of the midbrain and pons.

DECORTICATE POSTURE

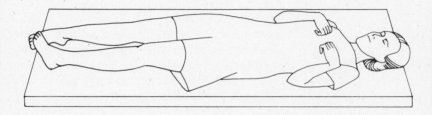

DECEREBRATE POSTURE

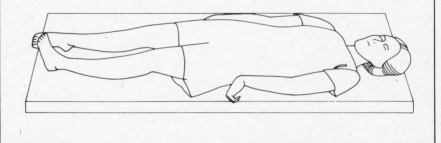

18. Observe for vomiting and nausea. Note the type of vomiting.

18. Increased ICP may cause forceful (projectile) vomiting.

19. Observe for bowel or bladder incontinence.

19. Incontinence may reflect loss of sphincter tone (from motor weakness caused by increased ICP), or it may accompany the clonic phase of a generalized tonic-clonic seizure.

20. Observe for nuchal rigidity (stiff neck) by flexing the patient's head onto the chest. **Caution:** Do not flex the head and neck if these areas are injured.

20. Nuchal rigidity may indicate inflammation or infection, such as meningitis (meningeal inflammation) or encephalitis (brain cell inflammation). Flexing the head and neck in a patient with injury to these areas could exacerbate spinal cord injury.

21. Document all findings.

21. Documentation proves that the procedure was done, assures high-quality care, and provides legal protection.

Placing a patient on a CircOlectric bed

Introduction

The CircOlectric bed is a special bed used to treat patients with paralysis or injury of the head or spinal cord. Controlled electronically, it has two circular frames that can be rotated 210 degrees vertically to move the patient from a back-lying to an abdomen-lying position (see illustration on page 362). The basic procedure described below applies also to placing a patient on a Stryker Wedge Frame bed.

Besides the CircOlectric bed, special beds include the Roto Rest bed, Clinitron bed, and Stryker Wedge Frame bed. These beds turn the patient by rotating the anterior or posterior frames horizontally, in a circular fashion, or from side to side. For instance, the Roto Rest bed, with frames that fit around the body, rotates automatically from side-to-side fourteen times each hour. It is used for severely immobilized patients and those with multiple trauma or spinal cord injury. The Clinitron bed has tiny pellets (ceramic microspheres) that rise to the surface of a fiber sheet by means of a motor and temperature pressure. The pellets massage the body. This bed is used for long-term bedridden patients, such as those with burns or spinal cord injury.

Steps

1. Explain that the patient will be moved to a special bed that will rotate the patient from the abdomen to the back.

2. Gather needed supplies: CircOlectric bed with electrical controls, two canvas sheets with proper laces or ties, two safety belts, arm and head supports, and pillows.

3. Obtain assistance from three other nurses.

4. Shut the door to the room or pull the curtain around the patient area.

5. Explain the transfer technique to the patient, and request that the patient lie quietly during transfer.

6. Place the patient's bed parallel with the CircOlectric bed. Lock the wheels.

7. Move the patient to the CircOlectric bed using the three-person carry technique.

Rationales

1. Explanations reduce patient anxiety.

2. This aids safe care.

3. To ensure safety, three nurses must assist when placing a patient on a CircOlectric bed.

4. This provides privacy for patient transfer.

5. As transfer is about to occur, explanations help reassure the patient. Having the patient lie quietly helps prevent injury.

6. Close parallel bed placement reduces the distance needed for transfer and reduces strain on the nurse's musculoskeletal system. Locking the wheels prevents bed movement during transfer.

7. This technique maintains straight patient alignment.

ADULT
NURSING

8. After the patient is positioned on the CircOlectric bed, place heel pads and arm supports under the patient's heels and arms. Position a foot support properly and place the patient's feet against it.

8. Heel pads, arm supports, and foot supports aid proper positioning and help prevent foot or wrist drop.

9. Apply a safety belt across the patient's waist and lower extremities.

9. This helps prevent accidental falls from the bed.

10. Make sure the electric cord to the bed is unplugged.

10. This prevents accidental turning of the patient.

11. Place a call signal within the patient's reach.

11. This permits the patient to call for assistance.

12. Document placement of the patient on the CircOlectric bed.

12. Documentation proves that the procedure was done, assures high-quality care, and provides legal protection.

Turning a patient on a CircOlectric bed

Introduction

Typically, the patient on a CircOlectric bed cannot move and must be turned to maintain healthy body tissues. The patient usually is turned every 2 to 3 hours from a supine to prone position, or vice versa.

Steps

1. Explain to the patient that he will be turned from the back to the abdomen.

Rationales

1. Explanations ease patient anxiety.

2. Place a pillow over the patient's legs.

2. This provides bulk to help hold the legs during turning and raises the toes off the bed frame when the patient lies on the abdomen.

3. With the help of another nurse or other team member, place the anterior frame on top of the patient so the patient is sandwiched between the frames. Then place the frame through the bed's large rings.

3. This keeps the patient immobilized during turning.

4. Make sure the canvas band supports the patient's head and chin. The band is positioned properly if the patient's head is midline and straight.

4. The canvas band prevents flexion, rotation, or extension of the patient's neck.

5. Secure the anterior frame at the head of the bed with the metal bolt. Tighten the bolt.

5. This prevents the bolt from slipping on the shaft of the metal pin during turning and prevents the patient's weight from loosening the bolts.

6. Place the footboard firmly against the soles of the patient's feet.

6. This prevents the patient from sliding down during turning.

ADULT NURSING

CircOlectric bed

This illustration shows how to move a patient from a supine to prone position in a CircOlectric bed. After applying safety belts and tightening the frames, the nurse slowly rotates the frames in a counterclockwise direction. Then, after lifting the frame, the nurse positions the patient's arms properly.

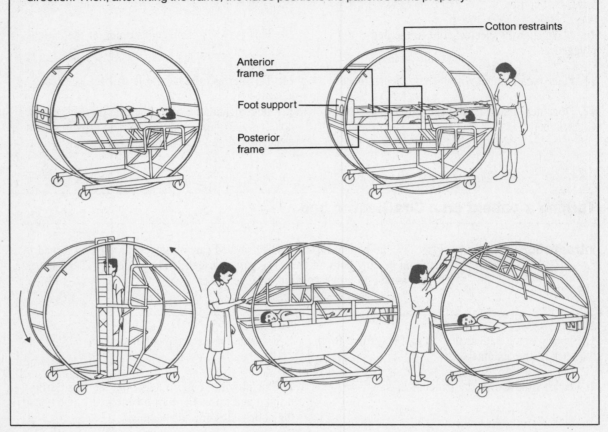

7. Place the patient's arms at the sides or in slings at the side of the frame.

7. This prevents the arms from dropping from the frame during turning.

8. Apply safety belts around both frames and tighten them.

8. Safety belts help prevent the patient from slipping during turning.

9. Clear all equipment from the turning area and plug in the bed's electrical cord.

9. Clearing the area prevents the bed from catching on anything during turning.

10. Tell the patient that you are going to turn the bed.

10. This eases patient anxiety.

11. Rotate the frames in a slow, even, circular movement until the patient is prone.

11. Turning the bed slowly and evenly prevents patient injury. Turning is complete when the patient is in the desired position (supine or prone).

12. Remove the safety belts and loosen the bolts holding the posterior frame. Lift the frame and place it in the support bar of the bed until it locks in place.

12. Raising the frame removes the pressure of the frame from the patient's body, increasing comfort and aiding respiratory effort.

13. Raise the gatch on the posterior frame over the patient's feet.

13. This removes pressure over the patient's heels.

14. Replace the safety belts over the patient's legs and around the waist.

14. This reduces the risk of falling.

15. Place the side boards on the frame and position the patient's arms properly.

15. This permits elbow flexion and arm abduction on the arm boards.

16. Unplug the electrical cord and place the call light within the patient's reach.

16. This promotes safety and allows the patient to call for help.

17. Check the patient's skin for signs of pressure. Massage around bony prominences but never directly over reddened areas.

17. Heat, edema, or red, blue, or white skin discoloration may signify pressure areas. Massage stimulates blood flow. Massaging over reddened areas may increase injury; also, reddened areas may indicate capillary or arterial injury.

18. Observe the patient's head and neck in the canvas ring for proper position.

18. The head and neck should be in a neutral position.

19. Document turning of the patient onto the abdomen and the patient's skin condition.

19. Documentation proves that the procedure was done, assures high-quality care, and provides legal protection.

Turning a patient on a Stryker Wedge Frame bed

Introduction

A double-layered orthopedic bed, the Stryker Wedge Frame bed is used for patients with cervical or thoracic spinal fractures. The frame, which sandwiches the patient between the layers, can be rotated horizontally to a supine or prone position. Arm and head-neck rests serve as frame extensions. The frame can be turned by one nurse without assistance. Its wedge shape angles the upper frame toward the lower side on which the frame turns, preventing the patient from sliding out during turning.

Steps

1. Assemble needed supplies: anterior or posterior Stryker frame, depending on the side to which the patient will be turned (obtained from the bedside); special sheets and ties for the frame; restraining straps; footboards; pillows; and protective skin pads (such as sheepskin pads or incontinence pads).

Rationales

1. Having all needed supplies on hand aids patient care.

2. Obtain help from a second nurse, if institutional policy stipulates that two nurses must be present when turning a bed frame.

2. Institutional policy must be followed to ensure patient safety at all times.

3. Inform the patient of the direction of the turn (such as onto the left or right side).

3. This reduces patient anxiety.

4. Arrange the patient's catheter or drainage tubing safely so the bed frame can be turned without pulling or exerting pressure on the tubing.

4. This helps ensure the safety of the patient and health team members.

5. Make sure the wheels of the frame are locked.

5. This prevents the frame from moving during the turn.

6. Remove bed linens covering the patient; also remove arm boards.

6. Bed linens must be removed so that they do not catch in the turning mechanism; arm boards must be removed so that the bed turns properly.

7. Place a pillow lengthwise over the patient's lower legs.

7. The pillow adds bulk, helping to hold the patient's legs during turning.

8. Place the anterior frame over the patient and tighten the nut at the head of the frame. (When turning a regular frame, tighten the nuts at both ends of the frame.)

8. The nut secures the frame during turning.

9. Make sure the head and chin bands are positioned properly so that they do not obstruct the patient's nose, mouth, or eyes.

9. These bands hold the head and chin when the patient is prone. Obstruction can cause breathing problems.

10. Close the turning ring over the anterior frame and lock it securely. Make sure the nuts are tight.

10. This helps ensure safe turning.

11. Place one restraining strap around the frame and the other around the patient's legs and chest. Buckle the straps securely.

11. Straps help prevent the patient from slipping during turning.

12. Have the patient wrap the arms around the anterior frame (if able). If the patient cannot do this, restrain the arms.

12. Wrapping the arms around the anterior frame or restraining them promotes a secure turn.

13. Remove (pull out) the positive lock pin at the head of the frame.

13. This allows the frame to pivot.

14. Pull out the red turning lock knob on the turning ring.

14. This allows the frame to turn.

15. Grasp the handle on the turning ring. Tell the patient that you will turn the frame on the count of 3.

15. This prepares the patient for the turn.

16. On the count of 3, turn the frame toward you (toward the narrower side of the wedge), using a smooth, gradual motion.

16. A smooth, gradual turn provides security.

ADULT
NURSING

17. Replace the positive lock pin.

17. This stabilizes the frame and prevents it from pivoting.

18. Push in the circular silver lock knob on the turning ring.

18. This opens the turning ring.

19. Open or unscrew the nut and remove the posterior frame.

19. This allows removal of the frame for linen changes and patient care.

20. Place the patient's head in the bands and place the arms on arm boards so the patient is comfortable.

20. This ensures proper alignment.

21. Check the patient's skin for pressure areas. As needed, wash, dry, massage, and cover these areas.

21. This helps maintain skin integrity.

22. Position the catheter or drainage tubing for proper drainage.

22. Gravity aids proper flow.

23. Place the signal cord and button within the patient's easy reach.

23. This allows the patient to call for assistance as needed.

24. Document the bed turning, the patient's response, and the patient's skin condition.

24. Documentation proves that the procedure was done, assures high-quality care, and provides legal protection.

Positioning a patient in bed

Introduction

Changing a patient's position in bed helps maintain integrity of the musculoskeletal, integumentary, and cardiovascular systems and promotes proper body alignment and comfort. (Procedure steps preceded by an asterisk are especially important.)

Steps

1. Gather needed supplies: pillows, blankets or towels (for rolls), and sandbags, as needed. Make sure a footboard is available.

Rationales

1. Having needed supplies on hand promotes patient care.

2. Obtain additional help, as needed.

2. This increases the safety of the patient and health team members.

*3. Inform the patient and helpers which position the patient will assume.

*3. This eases patient anxiety and ensures that all helpers work together.

*4. Raise the bed to a height that allows comfortable positioning for the patient and helpers.

*4. This allows all staff members to use their bodies efficiently, preventing improper body mechanics.

*5. Lower the head of the bed to a flat position.

*5. A flat position allows staff members to adjust the patient's position without working against gravity.

ADULT NURSING

6. Move the patient to the head of the bed.

7. Place the patient in the desired position by following the steps below.

Sims' (semiprone) position:
(a) With the bed flat, turn the patient onto the left or right side, turned partially toward the abdomen.
*(b) Flex the patient's upper and lower arms at the elbows and the upper leg at the knee.
*(c) Place pillows under the upper arm and upper leg; support the elbow and knee well.

*(d) Check the position of the patient's feet and toes; if needed, place a small roll under the ankle. Place a blanket roll or sandbag parallel to the sole of the patient's foot.
*(e) If the patient can respond, ask if the new position is comfortable. Cover the patient with the bed linens.
(f) Place the call light within the patient's reach and raise the bed's side rails.

Prone position:

(a) With an assistant, slide the patient to the side of the mattress.
*(b) Have the nurse nearest the patient push the patient gently to the side as the other nurse pulls the patient toward her self with one hand on the patient's shoulder and the other on the upper hip.
*(c) Continue turning slowly until the patient is lying prone (on the abdomen).
*(d) Gently slide the patient toward the foot of the bed so that the feet extend over the end of the mattress, or place a pillow under the patient's legs so that the feet and toes are off the mattress.
*(e) Place a small pillow under the patient's head and turn the head to one side.

(f) Flex the patient's arms at the elbows and position them comfortably.

*(g) Place a small pillow under the patient's abdomen below the level of the diaphragm.

*(h) If the patient can respond, ask if the position is comfortable.
*(i) Place a call light within easy reach; replace the covers over the patient and put the side rails up.

6. This allows enough room for staff members to position the patient.

7. Position is determined by the patient's condition.

Sims' position is comfortable for most patients.
(a) A left or right side-lying position reduces pressure on many bony prominences.
*(b) Flexion places the joints in a comfortable position and prevents hyperextension.
*(c) Support with pillows helps prevent internal shoulder rotation and hip adduction and helps maintain alignment.
*(d) The toes should not press into the mattress. A roll is used to lift the foot up and keep pressure off the toes. A blanket roll or sandbag helps prevent footdrop.
*(e) Patient input helps ensure comfort. Covers provide privacy and warmth.

*(f) Making the call light accessible and raising the side rails promote patient safety.

A prone position allows joint extension, preventing contractures.
(a) Assistance promotes safe turning onto the abdomen.
*(b) Combined push and pull maneuvers reduce strain on the patient and staff members, easing the turning procedure.

*(c) Slow, gentle handling eases turning pressure.

*(d) Raising the feet off the mattress reduces pressure on the toes and helps prevent footdrop by maintaining a neutral ankle position.

*(e) A pillow provides comfort to the head and face, reduces pressure on the lower ear region, and decreases flexion or hyperextension of the cervical vertebrae.
(f) Flexing the arms and placing them in a comfortable position helps maintain proper body alignment, promotes comfort, and reduces the risk of joint dislocation or shoulder adduction.
*(g) A pillow reduces pressure on the breasts, lumbar vertebrae, and lower back. Placing the pillow below the diaphragm decreases breathing problems.
*(h) Patient input helps ensure comfort.

*(i) These measures promote patient safety and comfort.

Upright position:

(a) If the patient can help, you need not obtain assistance from another nurse. Throughout this procedure, be sure to use proper body mechanics. For instance, stand with your feet parallel to the bed, one foot in front of the other. The bed should be at hip level to minimize strain during lifting. Bend your trunk sufficiently to gain a secure hold on the patient's head and shoulder to prevent strain to your shoulder and back muscles. Keep in mind that small upward moves are safer than one large move—for both the nurse and the patient.
(b) Place the head of the bed flat.

*(c) Remove the pillow from under the patient's head and place it at the head of the mattress.
*(d) Have the patient bend the knees and place the feet flat on the mattress; or bend the knees for the patient.
*(e) Reach under the patient's head with one hand to support the head and neck.
*(f) With the other hand and arm, reach under the axilla to place your hand under the patient's shoulder. Have the patient place a hand on your shoulder if able.

*(g) On the count of three, gently pull the patient upward. (You may need to do this a few times to move the patient up sufficiently.)
(h) Place a pillow under the patient's head and shoulders.
*(i) Elevate the head of the bed as desired; replace the covers and place the call light within easy patient reach.

8. Document patient repositioning or turning, the patient's response, assistance used (if any), and other pertinent observations.

An upright position permits high Fowler's position so the patient can be more active if desired.
(a) When placing a patient upright, your weight shifts from the back foot to the front foot, aiding gravity. Smaller upward moves reduce the risk of muscle and joint strain, which could cause injury to you or patient.

(b) This positions the patient upright without working against gravity.
*(c) The pillow causes friction, increasing the force needed to position the patient upright.
*(d) Bent knees and flat feet reduce friction against the mattress.

*(e) Supporting the head and neck eases patient positioning.
*(f) Placing a hand under the patient's shoulder supports the trunk to position the patient upright. Having the patient place a hand on your shoulder lets your hand and arm serve as a lift for the patient's trunk. (The patient may lift using a trapeze on the bed.)
*(g) Using a countdown prepares the patient for the move so that the patient can help (if able).

(h) A pillow provides comfort and reduces pressure on the occipital area of the head.
*(i) These measures promote safe, comfortable care.

8. Documentation proves that the procedure was done, assures high-quality care, and provides legal protection.

ADULT NURSING

Assisting with lumbar puncture

Introduction   In lumbar puncture, the physician inserts a needle into the subarachnoid space of the spinal column to measure cerebrospinal fluid (CSF) pressure, obtain CSF specimens for examination, or inject a medication or dye.

Steps

1. Gather all needed supplies: lumbar puncture tray containing towels, sponges, spinal needles, antiseptic solution, alcohol swabs, anesthetic agent, syringes, needles, gloves, manometer with three-way stopcock, test tubes, and pressure bandage; and large towels or blankets to place under the patient's side, if needed for proper positioning.

2. Explain the procedure to the patient.

3. Have the patient empty the bladder and bowels.

4. Wash your hands.

5. Help the patient into the preferred position — on the side, with the head and neck flexed onto the chest and knees flexed toward the abdomen (fetal position). As ordered, place a small pillow under the head to maintain proper spinal alignment.

6. Open the lumbar puncture tray. After the physician preps the area with antiseptic, assist in placing a sterile drape over the patient, with the opening over the lumbar area.

7. Hold the patient behind the neck and knees. Instruct the patient to remain still throughout the procedure.

8. Explain that the patient will feel a needle prick as the anesthetic is injected.

9. Hold the top of the manometer, if requested. Once inserted into the subarachnoid space, the needle will be attached to the manometer.

10. Repeat the physician's statement describing the initial pressure measurement (opening pressure and closing pressure measurement). Note CSF color.

Rationales

1. Having all needed supplies on hand promotes a safe, efficient procedure.

2. Explanations ease patient anxiety.

3. This will promote patient comfort during the procedure.

4. This reduces transfer of microorganisms.

5. This position opens the vertebral column, permitting easier access to the desired area.

6. The sterile drape helps maintain a sterile surface during the procedure.

7. Remaining still promotes easier needle insertion and helps prevent the needle from moving after insertion.

8. Anticipatory guidance helps calm the patient.

9. Holding the manometer steady and upright helps ensure correct pressure readings and reduces the risk of needle movement.

10. Opening and closing pressures must be recorded on the patient's chart. Normal CSF appears clear and colorless.

ADULT
NURSING

11. As the physician fills each test tube with CSF, place the tube in the correct container to maintain proper order (tubes #1, #2, and #3). Hold each tube under the stopcock for the physician to fill (this hand should be gloved to prevent contact with any spilled CSF).

11. Maintaining correct order of the CSF tubes is vital for accurate diagnosis. (For instance, if tube #3 appears yellow or contains red blood cells, it may indicate that the patient has suffered a cerebral hemorrhage.)

12. After the tubes have been filled, the closing pressure has been noted, and the physician has removed the manometer and needle, apply a sterile dressing to the needle insertion site and press firmly.

12. Pressure reduces bleeding and CSF loss. Closing pressure should be lower than opening pressure (from CSF withdrawal).

13. Number each tube correctly and attach the proper name labels and requisition forms for the desired examinations.

13. Each tube may undergo different examinations to aid diagnosis.

14. Wash your hands after handling the tubes.

14. This reduces the spread of contaminants or pathogens.

15. Help the patient to a comfortable position, such as a prone position with a pillow under the abdomen.

15. A prone position with a pillow under the abdomen elevates intra-abdominal pressure, increasing pressure on tissues around the spinal column to reduce bleeding or drainage.

16. Enforce bedrest, as ordered, for up to 12 hours.

16. Bedrest reduces the risk of postspinal headache, which can occur if the patient sits upright too soon.

17. Check the patient's vital signs.

17. Lumbar puncture and patient positioning during this procedure may alter vital signs.

18. Administer an analgesic for discomfort, if needed and ordered (unless contraindicated).

18. The procedure and patient positioning may cause discomfort and pain.

19. Encourage the patient to increase fluid intake (unless contraindicated).

19. An increased fluid intake helps replenish CSF levels.

20. Document the procedure, the patient's condition, and the patient's vital signs.

20. Documentation proves that the procedure was done, assures high-quality care, and provides legal protection.

21. Send CSF specimens to the laboratory.

21. Laboratory analysis aids diagnosis.

ADULT NURSING

Drugs used to treat neurologic disorders

This chart presents important information about drugs commonly prescribed for neurologic disorders, including the drug action, dosage, and common side effects. Nursing considerations focus on patient comfort and teaching.

DRUG	ACTION	USUAL ADULT DOSAGE	COMMON SIDE EFFECTS	NURSING CONSIDERATIONS
Anticonvulsants				
Carbamaze-pine (Tegretol)	Reduces polysyn-aptic responses	200 mg/day P.O. in three divided doses; increase dosage to obtain a therapeutic blood level.	• Blood dyscrasias • Nausea • Vomiting • Vertigo • Drowsiness • Skin rash	• Instruct the patient to have regular blood tests (as often as every 10 days initially) because this drug may cause aplastic anemia. • Instruct the patient to take this drug three times daily, as ordered, because it is rapidly metabolized. Stress the importance of taking it as prescribed and not to stop it suddenly. • Teach the patient to take this drug with food to reduce GI upset. • Tell the patient to report fever, sore throat, and unusual bleeding or bruising. • Instruct the patient to store tablets in a cool, dry place (preferably not the bathroom medicine chest).
Diazepam (Valium)	Slows nerve transmission by facilitating the inhibitory neuro-transmitter gamma-aminobutyric acid (GABA)	Variable; in adults, the dosage ranges from 5 to 20 mg	• Vein irritation and tissue sloughing with I.V. infiltration • Drowsiness • Respiratory depression • Headache	• Make sure the needle is in the vein when administering the drug I.V. • Do not store in plastic syringes because the drug can bind to plastic. • Do not mix with other drugs in the I.V. line because this causes precipitate formation.
Ethosuximide (Zarontin)	Slows nerve transmission in the cerebral cortex and basal ganglia to decrease petit mal (absence) seizures	Up to 1 g/day P.O.	• Double vision • Ataxia • Skin rash • Drowsiness • Gastric irritation • Blood dyscrasias	• Give this drug with meals to reduce gastric irritation. • Instruct the patient to have regular blood tests to detect toxic and therapeutic drug effects. • Instruct the patient to report sore throat, fever, and unusual bleeding or bruising.
Parametha-dione (Paradione)	Slows nerve transmission to reduce petit mal (absence) seizures	Individualized; dosage ranges from 900 mg to 2,400 mg/day P.O. t.i.d.	• Bone marrow depression • Photophobia • Nausea • Vomiting	• Advise the patient to wear sunglasses. • Instruct the patient to adhere to the laboratory schedule for blood tests. Frequent testing may be necessary to detect toxicity. • Instruct the patient to report sore throat, fever, and unusual bleeding or bruising.
Phenobarbital sodium (Luminal)	Slows or stops seizures by depressing cortical and subcortical nerve activity	100 to 300 mg/day P.O.	• Drowsiness • Confusion • Blood dyscrasias	• Warn the patient not to stop the drug suddenly because status epilepticus may result. • Warn the patient to avoid driving or operating dangerous machinery while taking this drug. • Teach the patient to discontinue this drug over several days rather than stop it suddenly. • Instruct the patient to have regular blood tests to monitor blood drug levels and detect blood dyscrasias.

Drugs used to treat neurologic disorders (continued)

DRUG	ACTION	USUAL ADULT DOSAGE	COMMON SIDE EFFECTS	NURSING CONSIDERATIONS
Anticonvulsants (continued)				
Phenytoin sodium (Dilantin)	Blocks rapid nerve discharges (probably by inhibiting sodium flux)	300 to 600 mg/day P.O.	• Nystagmus • Double vision (diplopia) • Drowsiness • Coagulation defects • Blood dyscrasias • Hyperplasia of the gums • Hirsutism (hair overgrowth)	• Instruct the patient to take this drug regularly and not to stop taking it abruptly. • Instruct the patient to have regular blood tests to detect toxic and therapeutic effects. • Teach the patient to maintain good oral hygiene because this drug may cause gum hyperplasia. • Warn the patient that this drug may discolor the urine pink, red, or brown. • Give the patient a chance to discuss feelings about hirsutism, if appropriate.
Primidone (Mysoline)	Slows nerve transmission to prevent seizures (is metabolized to phenobarbitol)	125 mg/day P.O.	• Confusion • Drowsiness • Blood dyscrasias • Dizziness • Hyperexcitability	• Warn the patient not to stop the drug abruptly becaue status epilepticus may result. • Teach the patient to adhere to the dosage schedule. • Warn the patient to avoid driving or operating dangerous machinery while taking this drug.
Valproic acid (Depakene)	May facilitate or increase brain levels of GABA	15 mg/kg P.O. divided equally, b.i.d. or t.i.d.	• Gastric irritation • Diarrhea • Nausea • Vomiting • Stomach cramps • Teratogenicity • Alopecia (hair loss) • Pancreatitis	• Do not administer to a patient with hepatic disease. • Instruct the patient to take this drug immediately after meals to decrease gastric irritation. • Teach the patient to swallow tablets whole; crushed tablets may be irritating and have an unpleasant taste. • Warn the patient not to stop the drug abruptly because this may cause seizures.
Antiparkinsonian drugs				
Amantadine hydrochloride (Symmetrel)	Stimulates release of dopamine from basal ganglia cells	100 to 200 mg/day P.O.	• Edema of the feet and ankles • Confusion • Psychosis	• Weigh the patient daily. • Observe for edema. • Observe for confusion or psychotic changes. • Administer after meals. • Warn the patient not to stop taking the drug abruptly because this could cause parkinsonian crisis. • Teach the patient to avoid alcohol. • instruct the patient to rise slowly and avoid sudden position changes because this drug can cause orthostatic hypotension (especially early in the morning).
Bromocriptine mesylate (Parlodel)	Directly stimulates postsynaptic dopamine receptors	1.25 mg P.O. b.i.d., up to 10 mg/day	• Hypotension • Psychosis • Twitching or tics • Cramps • Pleural effusion	• Check vital signs frequently. • Observe the patient for confusion or psychotic changes. • Give with meals.
Levodopa (Dopar)	Acts as a precursor to dopamine (necessary for muscle coordination)	500 mg P.O. q.i.d. initially; increase as needed and tolerated to a maximum of 8 g daily	• Nausea • Vomiting • Postural hypotension • Foul body odor • Urine color changes • Psychosis	• Instruct the patient to rise slowly when standing to avoid dizziness from postural hypotension. • Inform the patient that this drug may discolor the urine pink or red and that the urine may turn black when exposed to air. • Instruct the patient not to take vitamin supplements without the physician's permission.

(continued)

Drugs used to treat neurologic disorders *(continued)*

DRUG	ACTION	USUAL ADULT DOSAGE	COMMON SIDE EFFECTS	NURSING CONSIDERATIONS
Antiparkinsonian drugs *(continued)*				
Trihexyphenidyl (Artane)	Blocks central cholinergic receptors; restores balance of acetylcholine and dopamine in the basal ganglia	6 to 10 mg/day P.O.	• Dry mouth • Blurred vision • Urine retention • Constipation • Confusion	• Instruct the patient to drink cold fluids or suck on sugar-free hard candy to relieve dry mouth. • Monitor bowel and bladder output. • Give stool softeners or suppositories to prevent constipation.
Sedatives				
Alprazolam (Xanax)	A benzodiazepine that facilitates the action of the inhibitoryneurotransmitter GABA	0.25 to 0.5 mg P.O. t.i.d.	• Drowsiness • Headache • Dry mouth • GI discomfort	• Warn the patient to avoid driving or operating heavy equipment until the CNS effects of the drug are known. • Instruct the patient to report side effects, including short-term memory loss. • Instruct the patient to avoid alcohol and CNS depressants and not to take any over-the-counter medication without first checking with the physician. • If the drug will be taken for a prolonged period, instruct the patient not to stop it suddenly, but to consult the physician.
Amobarbital sodium (Amytal Sodium)	Nonspecific cortical depressant; decreases polysynaptic nerve transmission	30 to 50 mg P.O. t.i.d.	• Drowsiness • Blood dyscrasias • Vertigo • Nausea • Diarrhea • Photosensitivity • Drug dependence	• Warn the patient to avoid driving or operating dangerous machinery while taking this drug. • Caution the patient to wear sunglasses in sunlight.
Flurazepam hydrochloride (Dalmane)	A benzodiazepine; facilitates action of GABA	15 to 30 mg P.O. at bedtime	• Nausea • Vomiting • Drowsiness • Uncoordination	• Check the patient during the night to assess the drug's sedative effects. • This drug can cause daytime sedation. • Warn the patient to avoid alcohol because it can cause an interaction even if the drug was taken the previous night. • This drug is more effective if taken for several consecutive days. • Supervise the patient during ambulation.
Glutethimide (Doriden)	General CNS depressant; decreases polysynaptic transmission	250 to 500 mg P.O.	• Pupil dilation • Constipation • Drug dependence • Respiratory depression • Hypotension	• Do not give to patients with glaucoma. • Check vital signs frequently. • This drug is for short-term use only. • Discontinue this drug gradually.
Mephobarbital (Mebaral)	Nonspecific cortical depressant; decreases polysynaptic nerve transmission	30 to 100 mg P.O. up to q.i.d.	• Drowsiness • Blood dyscrasias • Vertigo • Nausea • Diarrhea • Photosensitivity • Drug dependence	• Warn the patient to avoid driving or operating dangerous machinery while taking this drug. • Caution the patient to wear sunglasses in sunlight.

GENITOURINARY SYSTEM

Anatomy and physiology

I. **Anatomy**
   A. Kidneys
      1. These paired structures are located in the retroperitoneal region of the lumbar area
      2. The cortex, the outermost layer, contains the glomeruli
      3. The medulla, the inner layer, contains the pyramids, papillae, and papillary ducts
      4. The kidneys' blood supply comes from renal arteries that branch into five segmental arteries, each supplying a different kidney region
   B. Ureters
      1. These paired structures are fibromuscular tubes
      2. They convey urine from the renal pelvis to the urinary bladder
   C. Urinary bladder
      1. This structure is a hollow sac located in front of and below the peritoneal cavity, behind the pubic bones
      2. It stores urine
   D. Urethra
      1. This structure is located at the neck of the urinary bladder
      2. In the male, it is approximately 8″ (20.3 cm) long
         a. It runs through the penis
         b. Just below the bladder, the urethra passes through the prostrate gland
      3. In the female, the urethra is approximately 2″ (5.1 cm) long
   E. Testes (in the male)
      1. These paired structures are the male gonads
      2. They are enclosed in the scrotum

II. **Physiology**
   A. Kidneys
      1. The kidneys excrete urine, helping to maintain homeostasis
         a. One ureter from each kidney carries urine to the bladder, where it is stored
         b. Urine passes through the urethra for elimination outside the body
         c. Normally, the bladder can retain 300 to 400 ml of urine before bladder distention causes the urge to void
      2. The kidneys filter waste products and return needed materials to the blood
         a. Substances required by the body, such as glucose, electrolytes, and water, are reabsorbed into the bloodstream
         b. Waste products, such as urea and creatinine, are excreted as urine (as are some electrolytes and water)
      3. The kidneys maintain water and electrolyte balance and help maintain acid-base balance; if they cannot perform these functions, death results (unless homeostasis is maintained artificially)

Reviewing the genitourinary system

The first illustration is an anterior view of the genitourinary structures. The second illustration shows the nephron, where the real work of the kidneys takes place.

GENITOURINARY STRUCTURES

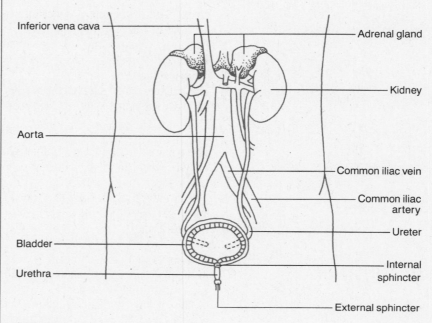

Inferior vena cava

Adrenal gland

Kidney

Aorta

Common iliac vein

Common iliac artery

Ureter

Bladder

Internal sphincter

Urethra

External sphincter

NEPHRON

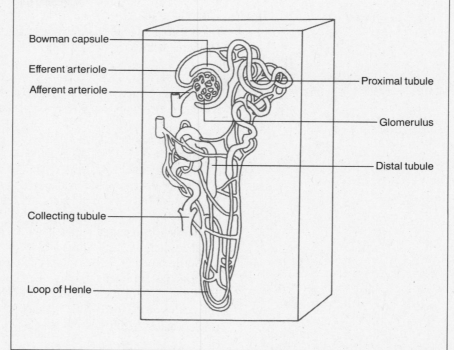

Bowman capsule

Efferent arteriole

Afferent arteriole

Proximal tubule

Glomerulus

Distal tubule

Collecting tubule

Loop of Henle

Glossary

Anuria: inability of the kidneys to secrete adequate urine

Dialysis: procedure in which certain waste products are removed from the blood through an external semipermeable membrane or through the peritoneum; used for some patients with renal dysfunction

Diffusion: process by which molecules and ions move from an area of greater concentration to an area of lesser concentration, causing even particle distribution

Diuresis: increased urinary output

Enuresis: urinary incontinence, especially that occurring during sleep (bed-wetting)

Glomerulus: part of a nephron, made up of capillaries

Hematuria: presence of blood in the urine

Lithiasis: formation of calculi (stones), such as in the kidney

Micturition: urination (voiding)

Nephrectomy: surgical removal of a kidney

Nephron: structural and functional unit of the kidney

Nocturia: excessive urination at night

Oliguria: decreased urinary output

Osmosis: movement of a pure solvent (such as water) across a semipermeable membrane from a solution with lower solute concentration to one with a higher solute concentration

Phimosis: constriction of the foreskin of the penis so that it cannot retract over the glans

Uremia: excessive amounts of urea and other nitrogenous waste products in the blood, causing a toxic condition

---

    4. The kidneys filter blood in cellular structures called nephrons, their functional units

B. Prostate gland (in the male)

    1. The prostate secretes a fluid that mixes with fluid from the seminal vesicles and sperm from the testes

    2. The mixed fluid (semen) is ejaculated through the urethra during coitus

C. Testes (in the male)

    1. The testes produce sperm and testosterone

    2. Sperm is stored at a temperature that is slightly lower than that of the rest of the body

---

Glomerulonephritis

Overview

Acute glomerulonephritis is a bilateral inflammation of the glomeruli that follows a group A beta-hemolytic streptococcal infection (such as strep throat or scarlet fever). Caused by an immune response in the walls of glomerular capillaries, inflammation leads to passage of red blood cells (RBCs) and protein in the urine. Acute glomerulonephritis may resolve without residual kidney damage, or it may progress to a chronic form. Extensive glomerular damage causes chronic renal failure, necessitating dialysis. The disease is most common in children but also affects adults.

Clinical situation

Bonnie Glidden, a receptionist, age 23, has had a headache, malaise, and facial edema and is voiding scanty amounts of rust-colored urine. When she develops lower back discomfort, she goes to the emergency department of the local hospital. The health team discovers she has mild hypertension and tenderness over the costovertebral angle (where the bottom rib joins the vertebrae in the back). Ms. Glidden tells the nurse that she had pharyngitis (sore throat) and a high fever 2 weeks earlier; she did not seek medical treatment and her symptoms resolved within a few days.

Urinalysis reveals a thick sediment of RBCs, leukocytes, and large amounts of protein. Ms. Glidden's blood urea nitrogen (BUN) and serum creatinine levels are elevated and she is slightly anemic. The physician diagnoses acute glomerulone-phritis, then admits her to the hospital for close monitoring and prompt detection and treatment of complications. Her medical orders include bed rest, vital sign checks every 4 hours, daily weight measurement, and careful monitoring of fluid intake and output. She is to receive a low-sodium, low-protein diet.

Assessment

Nursing behaviors

1. Assess Ms. Glidden's urine output, noting the color and amount of urine.

Nursing rationales

1. Fluid replacement is based on the amount of fluid loss. Any decrease in urine output may indicate renal failure. Rusty urine reflects RBCs in the urine.

2. Review urinalysis findings for protein, albumin, and blood cell levels. Note any changes in BUN and creatinine levels.

2. Results of these laboratory tests reflect the adequacy of kidney function.

3. Check vital signs and blood pressure.

3. Vital sign changes may indicate onset of complications. A blood pressure decrease signals a positive response to treatment.

4. Assess Ms. Glidden for peripheral edema, paying close attention to the lower extremities and sacral area.

4. Retained fluid collects in the lowest area—the legs, when Ms. Glidden sits; the sacrum, when she reclines.

Nursing diagnoses
- Activity intolerance related to fatigue caused by kidney dysfunction
- Altered nutrition (less than body requirements) related to protein and sodium restrictions

Planning and goals
- Ms. Glidden's weight and blood pressure will stabilize at preillness levels.
- Ms. Glidden's urine will be free from RBCs and albumin with treatment.
- Ms. Glidden's edema will resolve.
- Ms. Glidden's urine output will be appropriate for her fluid intake.

Implementation

Nursing behaviors

1. Maintain Ms. Glidden on bed rest during the acute illness phase.

Nursing rationales

1. Excessive activity may exacerbate proteinuria and hematuria. Rest promotes diuresis.

2. Provide a high-carbohydrate diet.

2. Carbohydrates provide energy and reduce protein catabolism. (With insufficient carbohydrate intake, protein is broken down, placing added stress on the kidney.)

3. Restrict Ms. Glidden's dietary protein and sodium intake, as ordered.

3. Renal insufficiency may cause nitrogen retention, as shown by elevated BUN levels. Sodium retention contributes to edema and hypertension.

4. Weigh Ms. Glidden daily.

4. Weight measurement helps gauge fluid retention or loss.

Evaluation (outcomes)

- Ms. Glidden's urine output begins to increase within a few days and edema starts to resolve.
- Ms. Glidden's vital signs remain stable and her hypertension subsides.
- Ms. Glidden's weight stabilizes.
- Ms. Glidden's BUN and creatinine levels begin to normalize, indicating improved kidney function.

Benign prostatic hyperplasia

Overview

Benign prostatic hyperplasia (BPH) refers to prostate gland enlargement. As the prostate enlarges, it presses on the urethra, obstructing urine flow from the bladder and causing incomplete bladder emptying or urine retention. Common in men over age 50, the condition causes such signs and symptoms as urinary frequency, nocturia, and a decrease in the size and force of the urine stream.

If the urethra is obstructed, prostatectomy (surgical prostate removal) is necessary. (With a severe obstruction that prevents voiding, a catheter must be inserted until surgery can be performed.) In transurethral prostatic resection (TURP), the most common type of prostatectomy, an endoscopic instrument is inserted through the urethra to remove hyperplastic prostate tissue. Other types of prostatectomies involve an abdominal incision (suprapubic prostatectomy) or perineal incision (perineal prostatectomy). Each procedure entails different nursing care, and may be complicated by the patient's age or coexisting chronic diseases. (For details on prostatectomies, see *Comparing prostatectomy procedures,* page 378.)

Clinical situation

Raymond Boyden, a retired bricklayer, age 69, visits the physician complaining of fatigue from lack of sleep. He states that a few years ago he began to have trouble initiating voiding; when the urine stream finally began, it was small and had little force. He also began to awaken several times during the night to void. Even after voiding, he states, his bladder does not feel empty; consequently, he has terminal dribbling, a condition that he finds distressing. He also confides that he is afraid he might have cancer. After reassuring Mr. Boyden that his symptoms most likely result from BPH, a common benign disorder, the physician orders diagnostic studies to assess his general health and urinary functions.

One month later, Mr. Boyden is admitted to the hospital for a TURP. He arrives on the morning of surgery with all preoperative preparations completed, has surgery under spinal anesthesia without complications, and is transferred to the surgical unit with a three-way catheter connected to continuous bladder irrigation. Urinary drainage is reddish pink with normal saline irrigation running. Because the spinal anesthesia has not worn off completely, a sheet lift transfer is used to move Mr. Boyden from the gurney to his bed. He remains in bed the rest of the day, tolerating a light supper.

Assessment

Nursing behaviors

1. Assess Mr. Boyden for hemorrhage. Note the color of urinary drainage and check for clots.

Nursing rationales

1. A hyperplastic prostate gland is vascular. Bleeding may occur from remaining prostatic tissue. Clots may form and obstruct the urine flow.

Comparing prostatectomy procedures

Surgery currently is the preferred treatment for benign prostatic hyperplasia. The type of procedure performed depends on the degree of glandular enlargement and whether cancer is present.

PROCEDURE	ADVANTAGES	DISADVANTAGES	NURSING CONSIDERATIONS
Transurethral resection (TURP): prostate removal through the urethra	• Avoids surgical incision • Is safer for high-risk patients	• May not prevent future obstruction • May cause retrograde ejaculation (but usually does not impair sexual performance)	• Check for bleeding by monitoring the drainage bag. • Observe for signs of urethral stricture, such as dysuria and a small urine stream.
Suprapubic prostatectomy: prostate removal by means of an abdominal incision, with an approach through the bladder	• Permits exploration to detect cancerous lymph nodes	• Requires a more prolonged convalescence	• Provide care for the suprapubic tube. • Stay alert for signs and symptoms of hemorrhage or shock.
Perineal prostatectomy: prostate removal by means of an incision through the perineum	• Can be used for radical cancer surgery	• Is associated with a higher incidence of impotency (from damage to the pudendal nerve) • Carries a greater infection risk	• Avoid using a rectal thermometer, rectal tube, or enemas. • Use drainage pads, held with a T-binder, to absorb drainage. • Provide a rubber ring to increase patient comfort when sitting.
Retropubic prostatectomy: prostate removal by means of a low abdominal incision, without opening the bladder	• Avoids bladder sphincter damage	• Carries a high risk of hemorrhage	• Check for posturinary leakage after catheter removal. • Stay alert for signs and symptoms of hemorrhage.

2. Assess the catheter drainage and evaluate Mr. Boyden for bladder distention.

2. An obstructed catheter may cause pressure and bleeding from the prostatic capsule. Bladder distention can damage the surgical site and cause marked discomfort.

3. Assess Mr. Boyden for pain. Before administering an analgesic (if needed and prescribed), assess catheter patency.

3. Catheter obstruction may cause pain (from bladder spasms).

4. Assess Mr. Boyden's fluid intake and output. To determine true urine output, subtract the amount of irrigating fluid infused from the total amount of drainage.

4. Irrigating fluid drains continuously from the bladder via the catheter, adding to the total amount collected.

Nursing diagnoses

• Pain (bladder spasms) related to clots in the catheter
• Potential for injury (infection or hemorrhage) related to surgery

Planning and goals

• Mr. Boyden will maintain acceptable urinary elimination.
• Mr. Boyden will remain free from infection and hemorrhage.
• Mr. Boyden will express relief of discomfort.

Implementation

Nursing behaviors	**Nursing rationales**
1. Maintain the urinary drainage tubing to the collection bag without kinks. Position the bag below the bladder level.	**1.** The collection bag system drains by gravity.
2. Maintain continuous bladder irrigation at the rate ordered or at a rate that keeps urine clear, pink, and clot-free.	**2.** Continuous irrigation cleans the bladder and prevents clot formation. If continuous irrigation is not used, small clots will appear and manual irrigation will be needed to keep the catheter patent.
3. Instruct Mr. Boyden to ambulate on the first postoperative day; increase ambulation to short walks, as tolerated. Teach Mr. Boyden to avoid prolonged sitting.	**3.** Ambulation prevents complications of immobility. Sitting increases intra-abdominal pressure, possibly causing discomfort or bleeding.
4. Apply antiembolism stockings, as ordered, while Mr. Boyden is in bed.	**4.** Antiembolism stockings help prevent thrombus formation while Mr. Boyden is immobile.
5. After the catheter is removed, observe the time, amount, and color of each urine voiding.	**5.** Initially, small voidings (15 to 30 ml) are common. The amount of urine eliminated at each voiding will increase gradually, and urine color will change from reddish pink to yellow when the surgical site has healed fully.
6. Provide teaching and emotional support to Mr. Boyden if he experiences urinary frequency, burning, or dribbling.	**6.** These problems may take several weeks or longer to diminish.
7. Encourage Mr. Boyden to eat high-fiber foods to prevent constipation.	**7.** This helps avoid straining to defecate, which may cause hemorrhage.
8. Encourage an oral fluid intake of at least 70 oz (2,000 ml).	**8.** Increased fluid intake helps flush the urinary tract.

Evaluation (outcomes)

• Mr. Boyden maintains drainage of large amounts of clear, pink urine through the continuous irrigation drainage system. The catheter is removed on the second postoperative day.
• Mr. Boyden voids small, frequent amounts of pink urine; initially, he experiences burning on urination.
• Mr. Boyden avoids infection and hemmorrhage.

ADULT NURSING

Kidney or bladder tumor

Overview

A tumor of the kidney—rare and usually malignant—can spread rapidly to the lungs and bones. In many cases, painless hematuria is the first sign. Treatment involves nephrectomy (surgical kidney removal), radiation therapy, or chemotherapy. One type of malignant kidney tumor, Wilms' tumor, occurs in children.

A tumor of the bladder may be benign or cancerous. A cancerous bladder tumor may represent spread of cancer from the colon, prostate, or reproductive tract. Risk factors for bladder cancer include smoking and exposure to such carcinogens as chemicals and dyes. The most common sign of a bladder tumor is gross, painless hematuria; if a urinary tract infection also is present, the patient may experience urinary frequency, urgency, and dysuria. Cystoscopy with a biopsy confirms the diagnosis. Treatment of bladder cancer usually entails complete or partial cystectomy (surgical bladder removal). If a complete cystectomy is done, the patient will need urinary diversion (for details, see *Urinary diversion techniques*).

Clinical situation

Joseph Martinez, age 55, has worked in an ink-manufacturing plant for the last 20 years. Although he has no urinary complaints, a urinalysis ordered during a routine physical examination reveals hematuria. To determine the cause of hematuria, the physician orders ultrasound and radiologic studies, then performs a cystoscopy and biopsy. The biopsy reveals an early-stage cancerous bladder tumor.

Because of the early disease stage, Mr. Martinez's age, and his good overall health, the surgeon decides to perform a radical cystectomy with an ileal conduit. Mr. Martinez arrives at the hospital on the morning of surgery, then has surgery under general endotracheal anesthesia. After a stay in the post-anesthesia care unit, he is transferred to the surgical unit.

Assessment

Nursing behaviors

1. Perform all routine postoperative assessments appropriate for a patient recovering from abdominal surgery: vital signs, fluid intake and output, return of peristalsis, and anesthesia complications. Also assess the incision site.

2. Assess Mr. Martinez's urine output hourly. Promptly report output below 30 ml/hour.

3. Assess Mr. Martinez's urine for color and clarity. With ileal conduit drainage, mucus will appear.

4. Assess the stoma for bleeding and adequate blood supply during every shift.

5. Assess the drainage appliance for leakage and check the skin around the drainage pouch for irritation during every shift.

Nursing rationales

1. Mr. Martinez will have an I.V. line and a nasogastric (NG) tube connected to suction. All oral intake will be withheld. He is recovering from general endotracheal anesthesia and will have an abdominal incision.

2. Urine output below 30 ml/hour may indicate an obstruction, with possible backflow or pressure on the suture lines.

3. Mucus is secreted by the small intestinal lining of the conduit.

4. A change in tissue color from the normal pinkish red to dark purple indicates compromised blood supply.

5. Skin around the stoma may become irritated from contact with urine.

Urinary diversion techniques

Urinary diversion surgery is performed to treat cancer, birth defects, and urinary tract trauma. For permanent diversion, the most common surgeries are ureterostomy and ileal conduit.

TECHNIQUE	DESCRIPTION	NURSING CONSIDERATIONS
Ileal conduit 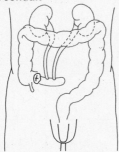	A section of the terminal ileum is isolated and made into a closed tube (conduit), with one end brought through the abdominal wall to form a stoma. The ureters are transplanted into the tube.	• The patient may return from surgery with a catheter in place in the stoma or with a clear, disposable pouch to collect the urine. • Maintain urinary flow to prevent distention and damage to the conduit. • Withhold all oral intake while the nasogastric tube is in place and until peristalsis returns, as ordered. • Urine will contain mucus from the conduit lining. Provide extra fluids to help prevent the mucus from congealing and to promote drainage.
Ureterosigmoidostomy 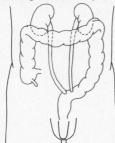	The ureters are brought into the sigmoid colon, allowing urine to drain into the colon and out through the rectum.	• Voiding occurs through the rectum frequently (as often as every 2 hours); voided matter has the consistency of watery diarrhea. • A rectal catheter will be inserted after surgery to prevent reflux into the kidneys. • Monitor serum electrolyte levels because urinary constituents may be reabsorbed by the colon. • Instruct the patient never to wait more than 3 hours before emptying urine from the intestine. • Some patients develop upper urinary tract infections after this procedure from reflux of bacteria from the colon.
Cutaneous ureterostomy 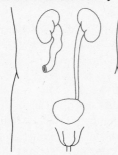	The detached ureter is brought through the abdominal wall and attached to an opening in the skin. This procedure is less extensive than other urinary diversion techniques and is used for high-risk patients with ureteral obstruction.	• The patient wears a urinary appliance immediately after surgery. Care is similar to that required for an ileal conduit.
Continent ileal urinary reservoir (Kock pouch) 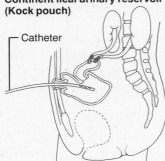 ⌐ Catheter	The ureters are transplanted to an isolated segment of the ileum, in which one-way valves have been created by telescoping the intestine. This segment then becomes a pouch for urine storage. (This procedure also may be done to treat neurogenic bladder.)	• Urine must be drained by a catheter inserted through a nipple valve, which prevents urine leakage. • The pouch must be drained at regular intervals to prevent absorption of urinary products and reflux of urine to the ureters and kidneys. • The patient can use the catheter to empty the urine.

6. Assess Mr. Martinez's learning ability and teaching needs related to caring for the urinary diversion.

6. Mr. Martinez must be able to perform self-care by the time of discharge.

Nursing diagnoses

• Potential ineffective individual coping related to fear of the diagnosis and the impact of surgery
• Knowledge deficit related to management of the urinary diversion

Planning and goals

• Mr. Martinez will recover from surgery without complications.
• Mr. Martinez's urinary diversion apparatus will function without obstruction or other problems.
• Mr. Martinez will demonstrate knowledge of the care required for his urinary diversion.
• Mr. Martinez will discuss his plans to cope with his diagnosis and the impact of surgery on his self-concept.

Implementation

Nursing behaviors

1. Carry out routine postoperative care measures, including maintaining NG tube patency; administering analgesics for pain; encouraging coughing, turning, and deep breathing every 2 hours; maintaining I.V. infusions; and providing oral hygiene.

Nursing rationales

1. Postoperative care for Mr. Martinez resembles that required after any surgery involving an abdominal incision, general anesthesia, and small-bowel resection. Preventing postoperative complications is a priority. (For information on routine postoperative care, see the "Perioperative nursing" section.)

2. Maintain a clear drainage pouch over the stoma to collect urine.

2. The clear pouch allows stoma visualization.

3. Empty the drainage pouch every 2 hours, or when it is one-third to one-half full. Attach the pouch to gravity drainage at night. If a catheter has been inserted into the stoma, attach it to gravity drainage.

3. If the drainage pouch becomes too full, it will pull on the skin or start to leak.

4. Gather needed supplies before changing the appliance. Read and follow the manufacturer's directions. Instruct Mr. Martinez to bend over for a minute to allow the conduit to drain before washing the skin.

4. Having all supplies on hand reduces patient discomfort. The skin must be dry to allow the new appliance to adhere.

5. Change the appliance every 5 to 7 days and apply a skin barrier. Recalibrate the size of the stoma every few weeks for the first few months. If the appliance is permanent, wash it in water and white vinegar and allow it to air dry. A commercial deodorizer may be added to the pouch.

5. The appliance should be changed routinely to prevent leakage and provide skin care. The skin barrier protects skin from direct contact with urine. Stoma size changes during the postoperative period. Vinegar helps control odor.

6. Clean the skin around the stoma when changing the appliance. Remove any adhesive with solvent and wash the skin with soap and water; rinse the skin well and pat dry. Inspect the skin for irritation. Apply new adhesive and skin barrier according to the manufacturer's directions. To absorb urine during the appliance change, place a tampon or piece of gauze at the insertion site.

6. The skin must be kept clean and dry to prevent irritation or breakdown. A soap film may interfere with adherence of the appliance.

7. Begin teaching Mr. Martinez about ostomy care and to involve him in his care. Encourage him to contact the local ostomy association after discharge for support and practical information. Remind him to keep all follow-up medical appointments.

7. Mr. Martinez will perform his own care at home but will need support and additional instructions.

Evaluation (outcomes)

• Mr. Martinez recovers from surgery and anesthesia without complications.
• Mr. Martinez maintains drainage of adequate amounts of urine from his ileal conduit, with large amounts of mucus initially. Urine odor remains normal. The stoma appears red, with no bleeding, and shrinks over the next 6 months.
• Mr. Martinez begins to express his fears that the cancer might return as well as his concern over the self-image changes caused by radical surgery.
• Mr. Martinez begins to empty his appliance and assist with changing it. Before discharge, he changes the appliance himself with supervision and expresses confidence that he can manage this at home.
• Mr. Martinez returns to work and resumes his usual activities within 6 to 8 weeks.

Dialysis

Overview

Dialysis is a procedure that removes fluids and waste products normally excreted by the kidneys. It works on the principles of osmosis and diffusion (for definitions of these terms, see *Glossary*, page 375). Typically, dialysis is ordered for patients with acute or chronic renal failure or toxicity (as from excessive amounts of drugs). Although dialysis does not cure the underlying cause of renal failure, it does sustain the patient's life and prevents damage to other organs until kidney function is restored. (For a patient with chronic renal failure or end-stage renal disease, a kidney transplant may be performed as an alternative to life-long dialysis.)

Types of dialysis include hemodialysis and peritoneal dialysis. Hemodialysis involves an external machine that pumps arterial blood through a coil in a dialysate bath. A membrane allows water and electrolytes to diffuse until the concentrations of blood and dialysate equalize; blood then is pumped back into the venous system. Temporary circulatory access may be gained through an arteriovenous (AV) shunt, an external tube connecting an artery and a vein. (If the shunt is on an arm or leg, never use a tourniquet for venipuncture or a cuff for blood pressure measurement on this extremity.) An alternative technique to gain circulatory access involves fistula creation through anastomosis of an artery to a vein to accommodate the large-bore needles used in long-term hemodialysis. If the patient's blood vessels are not suitable for the fistula, a graft is used to provide a needle insertion site. (For details on AV shunts, see "Caring for an arteriovenous shunt," pages 391 and 392.) The patient on long-term hemodialysis must restrict dietary protein, sodium, potassium, and fluid intake.

In peritoneal dialysis, the peritoneum acts as the diffusing surface. The dialysate fluid is infused into the peritoneal cavity through a catheter and left there for a specified period (called dwell time). Then the dialysate is drained by gravity from the peritoneal cavity through the catheter and back into its original bag, which is retained as a closed system. The dialysis exchange schedule may vary from several times daily to continuous use. The latter method, called continuous ambulatory peritoneal dialysis (CAPD), allows the patient to maintain normal daily activities. CAPD usually does not call for dietary restrictions.

ADULT NURSING

Clinical situation

George Brown, age 42, has had insulin-dependent diabetes mellitus since childhood. Married with two children, he works as a cashier at a local supermarket. For the past 4 years, he has suffered renal insufficiency. During the past week, he has been voiding less than 200 ml of urine daily. His serum potassium level is elevated and he has moderate hypertension.

Drowsy and confused, Mr. Brown is admitted to the hospital with a diagnosis of end-stage renal disease. His treatment plan involves CAPD to control uremia and hypertension. He hopes to return to work soon and manage CAPD without drastic changes in his family life, employment, and life-style.

Assessment

Nursing behaviors	Nursing rationales
1. Assess Mr. Brown's fluid and electrolyte status, measure his weight, and check his vital signs.	**1.** Such complications as dehydration, circulatory collapse, or shock can occur if too much fluid is lost through peritoneal dialysis drainage. Weight change is a good index of fluid loss or retention.
2. Check fluid intake and output, including fluids instilled into and drained from the peritoneal cavity.	**2.** During dialysis, drainage measures approximately 2 liters more than the amount of dialysate infused over a 24-hour period. Fluid output must be monitored to determine if the dialysate solution must be changed.
3. Assess Mr. Brown for anorexia and nausea.	**3.** These problems may result from increased blood urea levels and electrolyte imbalance.
4. Assess Mr. Brown and his family for knowledge about his condition.	**4.** This establishes a baseline for teaching.

Nursing diagnoses

• Knowledge deficit related to home management of CAPD
• Potential for ineffective individual coping related to limitations imposed by end-stage renal disease and its treatment

Planning and goals

• Mr. Brown will regain adequate fluid balance and maintain normal serum electrolyte levels.
• Mr. Brown will remain comfortable during dialysis.
• Mr. Brown will express his concerns about his disease, its treatment, and its impact on his life-style.
• Mr. Brown will demonstrate the ability to perform CAPD himself.

Implementation

Nursing behaviors	Nursing rationales
1. Provide physical comfort measures, such as by providing back care with massage of pressure areas, turning in bed, and allowing Mr. Brown to sit up (if the catheter is implanted surgically).	**1.** Dialysis may cause fatigue because it takes a long time. If Mr. Brown has a trocar (large-bore needle) instead of a catheter, he will be on strict bed rest.
2. Provide psychological support during dialysis by reassuring Mr. Brown, allowing him to express his concerns, and considering his family's needs.	**2.** Such holistic care contributes to Mr. Brown's well-being. By boosting his confidence in the nurse and making him more willing to share his problems, holistic care also increases the nurse's ability to detect any problems.

ADULT
NURSING

3. Maintain the dialysis fluid infusion and drainage, using strict aseptic technique. Do not push in the catheter. If the dialysis fluid does not infuse or drain properly, notify the nurse-manager or physician.

3. Pushing in the catheter introduces bacteria into the peritoneal cavity. The physician may need to reposition the catheter if it does not work properly.

4. Teach Mr. Brown how to perform CAPD himself and discuss any recommended dietary changes. He may need continued teaching on an outpatient basis.

4. Although the patient on CAPD usually can eat a regular diet, some changes (such as eating bran to prevent constipation) may be needed.

5. Consult with the home health care department to plan discharge follow-up care.

5. Tubing must be changed every 4 to 8 weeks. Careful blood chemistry monitoring is needed to determine appropriate therapy.

6. Measure urine output.

6. Urine output reflects kidney function; the kidneys may continue to produce some urine during dialysis.

7. Monitor Mr. Brown for complications. Peritonitis may manifest as abdominal tenderness and rigidity, cloudy dialysate solution, bleeding, respiratory problems, leakage around the catheter, or constipation.

7. Peritonitis is the most common dialysis complication. Minor bleeding is common during the first few dialysis exchanges but should not persist. Respiratory problems may stem from pressure of the fluid on the diaphragm; report this complication if it occurs. Constipation may stem from inactivity, decreased nutrition, and fluid pressure in the abdomen.

Evaluation (outcomes)

• Mr. Brown maintains stable vital signs and his hypertension is controlled without medication.
• Mr. Brown maintains normal electrolyte levels and a stable weight, indicating fluid balance.
• Mr. Brown shows no signs of complications; initial fluid leakage around the catheter stops spontaneously when the insertion site heals.
• Mr. Brown reports that he feels better and has more energy.
• Mr. Brown asks many questions, begins to assist in his dialysis, and expresses concern over his ability to remember all the details of his home health care.
• Mr. Brown expresses concern over changes in his sexual function.

ADULT NURSING

Complications of genitourinary disorders

This chart presents the most serious or life-threatening complications of genitourinary disorders, along with interventions that are crucial to patient safety and comfort.

COMPLICATION	CAUSE	NURSING INTERVENTIONS
Uremia Toxic condition characterized by excessive amounts of urea and other nitrogenous waste products in the blood; causes pathologic changes in many body systems	• Chronic renal failure with nephron dysfunction, causing impaired waste elimination	• Monitor blood urea nitrogen, creatinine, serum electrolyte, and urine specific gravity levels. • Determine the cause of uremia, if possible, and carry out ordered treatments. • Carry out measures to maintain fluid and electrolyte balance and manage anemia, as ordered. • Carry out measures to manage hypertension or cardiovascular problems, such as restricting sodium and fluids or administering antihypertensive medications, as ordered. • Carry out dialysis, if necessary and ordered.
Urine retention Inability to empty the bladder, which becomes increasingly distended	• Surgery • Obstruction, such as from an enlarged prostate • Traumatic injury • Spinal cord injury • Labor and delivery • Fear of pain on voiding • Certain medications	• Assess the patient's bladder for distention by palpating the suprapubic area. • Pour warm water over the perineum to help stimulate voiding. • Administer a warm sitz bath, if ordered. • Instruct a female patient to try a sitting position and a male patient to try a standing position to void. • Notify the physician if nursing measures do not induce voiding. • Administer medications to relax the sphincter, such as bethanechol chloride (Urecholine), as ordered. • Catheterize the patient, if necessary (this procedure requires a physician's order).
Renal failure Inability of the kidneys to maintain normal function	• Kidney infection or inflammation • Obstruction of the upper or lower genitourinary tract • Systemic disease or a toxic condition, such as hypertension, diabetes, or hypercalcemia	• Assess the patient's condition, especially hydration status. • Observe for uremia (as described above). • Monitor serum electrolyte levels. • Restrict fluids, as ordered. • Restrict foods high in potassium, sodium, and phosphorus while providing adequate calories and ensuring good nutrition. • Carry out ordered measures to control hypertension (as described in "Hypertension," page 194).
Renal calculi Formation of calculi ("stones") in the renal pelvis; calculi may contain calcium, uric acid, or other crystalline substances	• Urine supersaturation with crystalloids that do not dissolve readily • Urinary infection causing debris around which a calculus may form • Urinary stasis resulting from immobility or obstruction • Presence of urinary substances that encourage crystal formation (such as urate)	• To prevent calculus formation, provide a high fluid intake (up to 135 oz [4,000 ml daily]) to dilute the urine. • Prevent urinary stasis by maintaining adequate drainage of tubes and catheters. • Strain urine to recover any renal calculi for composition analysis. • Administer analgesics for pain, as ordered. • Prevent urinary tract infection or carry out ordered treatment for infection promptly. • Follow dietary restrictions or administer medications to minimize calculus formation, as ordered. • Be aware that surgery may be necessary if calculi do not pass spontaneously. • Changing urine pH may make some substances more soluble.

Inserting a urinary catheter

Introduction A urinary catheter, inserted through the urethra into the urinary bladder, is used to empty the bladder before surgery, treat incontinence or urine retention, obtain a sterile urine specimen, determine the amount of residual urine, or monitor urine output continuously in a seriously ill patient. An indwelling (Foley) urinary catheter remains in the bladder, held in place by a small balloon inflated with sterile water. (Procedure steps preceded by an asterisk are especially important.)

Steps

1. Assemble needed supplies: a sterile catheter tray, sterile gloves, sterile drapes, lubricant, cleaning solution, cotton balls, forceps, syringe (to fill the balloon), basic specimen container, drainage tubing, tape, blanket, waterproof pad, trash bag, and bath towel. For most adults, a #16 French catheter (straight or with a 5-ml balloon) is adequate.

2. Wash your hands.

3. If the purpose of catheterization is to measure residual urine, have the patient void immediately before catheter insertion.

*4. Provide privacy for the patient and arrange for good lighting.

5. Help the patient to a dorsal recumbent position. With a female, flex the knees and position the feet about 2′ (61 cm) apart. With a male, place in a supine position. Put a waterproof pad under the patient; if necessary, clean the genitals with soap and water.

6. Open the sterile catheter tray and put on sterile gloves. Place sterile drapes over the perineal area or penis. Set up the contents of the sterile catheter tray; check balloon inflation, pour the antiseptic, and lubricate the catheter.

7. Spread the labia or position the penis with your nondominant hand. Identify the meatus (in an uncircumcised male, retract the foreskin). Using cotton balls held by forceps, clean the area with antiseptic (use each cotton ball only once).

Rationales

1. Assembling supplies in advance aids the procedure. Leakage may occur around a catheter that is too small. A catheter that is too large may cause discomfort.

2. This helps prevent the spread of microorganisms.

3. Residual urine (the amount left in the bladder after voiding) should measure less than 100 ml.

*4. Good lighting is necessary to see the urinary meatus, especially in a female patient.

5. The waterproof pad protects the bed. Cleaning the genitals decreases the infection risk.

6. The contents of the sterile tray must be set up while both hands are sterile. Lubricating the catheter reduces tissue trauma.

7. The nondominant hand becomes contaminated by touching the patient; the dominant hand remains sterile. Finding the meatus helps guide catheter insertion.

ADULT NURSING

*8. Using the dominant hand, insert the catheter into the meatus until urine flows; for a female, insert a straight catheter 2″ to 3″ (5.1 to 7.6 cm); for a male, 6″ to 8″ (15.2 to 20.3 cm). With an indwelling catheter, advance it another inch (2.5 cm). Do not use force when advancing the catheter. If you meet resistance, rotate the catheter slightly (for a male, exert slight upward tension on the penis).

*8. Advancing an indwelling catheter an extra inch ensures balloon inflation within the bladder. Rotating the catheter may ease the catheter past the sphincter. Holding the penis with slight tension helps straighten the urethra.

9. Hold the catheter securely while the bladder empties. Collect any needed specimens. Measure drainage accurately. (Most institutional policies limit the amount of urine collected at any one time to 1,000 ml.)

9. Movement during bladder emptying may cause introduction of microorganisms. Sudden release of pressure from a large volume of urine could lead to a hypotensive episode.

*10. Remove a straight catheter. For an indwelling catheter, inflate the balloon with sterile water, according to manufacturer's instructions; after the balloon has been inflated, tug gently on the catheter to check placement.

*10. A straight catheter is not intended for continuous use. The balloon anchors the indwelling catheter in the bladder; resistance is felt with a gentle tug on a properly placed indwelling catheter. Improper balloon inflation can cause discomfort or displacement.

*11. Attach the indwelling catheter to the drainage system (if not connected already). Position the collection bag on the bed frame so the tubing is not kinked and movement of the side rails will not impede gravity drainage. Secure the catheter to the patient's thigh, allowing sufficient slack for leg movement. (In a male patient, the catheter may be attached to the abdomen.)

*11. Proper tubing positioning promotes drainage and prevents urethral trauma.

12. Remove the supplies and make the patient comfortable. Clean and dry the genitals. Remove the gloves and wash your hands.

12. These measures promote patient comfort and reduce the spread of microorganisms.

13. Document the date and time of catheter insertion, the amount of urine removed, urine characteristics, the size of the indwelling catheter and balloon, and the patient's response to the procedure.

13. Documentation proves that the procedure was done, assures high-quality care, and provides legal protection.

Caring for an indwelling urinary catheter

Introduction

Ongoing care for an indwelling urinary catheter centers on avoiding bacterial invasion into the urinary tract via the catheter and on maintaining unobstructed urine drainage.

Steps
1. Maintain a closed drainage system. Do not detach the catheter from the drainage tubing unless ordered to do so specifically.

Rationales
1. A closed system helps prevent entry of microorganisms.

2. Twice a day, clean the patient's genitals with soap and water, then dry the area.

2. This helps eliminate microorganisms that could cause infection.

3. Maintain accurate fluid intake and output records while an indwelling catheter is in place. Encourage the patient to increase fluid intake.

3. Increased fluid intake promotes urine output and helps flush the system.

4. Use sterile technique when irrigating the catheter, and irrigate only when ordered.

4. Irrigation carries the risk of introducing microorganisms.

5. Position the tubing to allow gravity drainage. Keep the collection bag lower than the patient's bladder.

5. Proper positioning promotes gravity drainage.

6. Document catheter care provided.

6. Documentation proves that the procedure was done, assures high-quality care, and provides legal protection.

Removing an indwelling urinary catheter

Introduction

An indwelling urinary catheter must be removed carefully to avoid urethral trauma. This procedure requires a physician's order. (Procedure steps preceded by an asterisk are especially important.)

Steps

1. Deflate the catheter balloon by aspirating the water with a syringe. Slowly remove the catheter, then inspect it. If the catheter is not intact, notify the nurse-manager or physician.

Rationales

1. Using a syringe ensures complete balloon deflation. Removing the catheter slowly ensures removal of the entire intact catheter.

*2. Observe the patient for urine retention or dribbling. Record all voidings.

*2. In some cases, the patient cannot void normally after catheter removal; if this happens, the catheter must be replaced. If the bladder is not emptied completely or if bladder capacity decreases temporarily, the patient may void only small amounts. Output records may be needed for several days if the patient has had urologic surgery or has trouble voiding.

3. Document the procedure.

3. Documentation proves that the procedure was done, assures high-quality care, and provides legal protection.

ADULT NURSING

Caring for a nephrostomy tube

Introduction

A nephrostomy tube provides drainage from the kidney when the ureter is obstructed or damaged. It is inserted directly into the pelvis of the kidney (usually through a stab wound or a small incision in the flank) and held in place with skin sutures. The tube may be temporary or permanent. (Procedure steps preceded by an asterisk are especially important.)

Steps

1. Attach the nephrostomy tube to closed gravity drainage or to a urostomy appliance, if ordered. Maintain the sterility of all equipment.

2. Assess for bleeding at the insertion site.

*3. Maintain unobstructed tube drainage. Observe the setup frequently to make sure the tube is draining. Measure and record the amount of drainage once each shift or more often, as ordered. If the patient has a nephrostomy tube in each kidney, keep separate records for each. Immediately report any drainage failure. Never clamp a nephrostomy tube.

4. Monitor the tube for displacement. If displacement occurs, report it to the surgeon immediately.

*5. Do not irrigate the catheter.

6. Document the care procedure.

Rationales

1. The kidney will drain freely by gravity. Sterility is needed to prevent infection.

2. Bleeding is the major complication of a nephrostomy tube.

*3. Obstructed urine flow increases pressure in the pelvis of the kidney, causing kidney damage. Careful output records help assess kidney function. Separate record-keeping allows documentation of drainage from each tube.

4. A displaced tube must be replaced immediately; otherwise, the opening will contract, making reinsertion difficult.

*5. Irrigation of a nephrostomy tube is done rarely and only by a surgeon.

6. Documentation proves that the procedure was done, assures high-quality care, and provides legal protection.

Applying a condom catheter

Introduction

A condom (external) catheter, worn over the penis, is an alternative to an indwelling catheter for a male patient. Made of soft, pliable material, it usually is connected to a leg bag during the day and to a larger gravity drainage bag at night. A condom catheter is used to keep an incontinent patient dry, simplify his home care, and permit normal social activities by making his incontinence less obvious to others. The condom catheter is less likely than an indwelling urinary catheter to cause urinary tract infection. (Procedure steps preceded by an asterisk are especially important.)

Steps	**Rationales**
1. Explain the procedure to the patient. If he will be applying the catheter himself at home, begin teaching him how to do the procedure.	**1.** Explanations promote patient cooperation. Teaching should begin as soon as the patient is ready.
2. Assemble needed supplies: condom catheter, drainage bag or leg bag, and disposable gloves.	**2.** Assembling supplies in advance promotes good time management and facilitates the procedure. Universal precautions stipulate that the nurse wear gloves to protect against genital secretions.
3. Provide privacy. Wash the patient's genitals with soap and water, then dry thoroughly.	**3.** The penis must be free from urine and secretions to minimize irritation.
*4. Grasp the penis with your nondominant hand, then roll the condom onto the penis with your dominant hand. Leave a space of 1″ to 2″ (2.5 to 5.1 cm) between the tip of the penis and the end of the condom.	***4.** Rolling allows for easier application. Leaving a space permits better urine drainage and reduces irritation.
5. Connect the catheter to the drainage tubing or a leg bag. Avoid kinking or twisting the tubing.	**5.** Kinked or twisted tubing causes urine backflow.
6. Document the procedure, including penis condition and color and adequacy of drainage.	**6.** Documentation proves that the procedure was done, assures high-quality care, and provides legal protection.
7. Remove and reapply the condom catheter daily, carefully inspecting the skin for breakdown.	**7.** Daily inspection helps maintain skin integrity, drainage, and penile circulation.
*8. If signs of skin breakdown or circulatory impairment appear, use an alternate means of urine collection, such as by providing easy access to a urinal.	***8.** Prolonged use of a condom catheter can cause skin excoriation and breakdown.
9. Document condom catheter application.	**9.** Documentation proves that the procedure was done, assures high-quality care, and provides legal protection.

Caring for an arteriovenous shunt

Introduction
An arteriovenous (AV) shunt, provides and maintains circulatory access for hemodialysis. Proper care maintains shunt patency and permits early detection of complications (such as infection, occlusion, and cannula separation). The shunt is created with a loop of pliable plastic (Silastic) tubing that connects an artery to a nearby vein. The loop exits through the skin, forming a closed arc during intervals when dialysis is not used. (Procedure steps preceded by an asterisk are especially important.)

(*Note:* Do not confuse AV shunt care with care required for a newer circulatory access method. This alternative method involves a specially designed double-lumen catheter that is inserted into the jugular or subclavian vein to gain access to the vena cava or right atrium for hemodialysis. The catheter is maintained like any central venous infuser.)

Steps	**Rationales**
*1. Wash your hands and put on clean gloves.	*1. Washing the hands helps prevent the spread of microorganisms. Gloves limit the nurse's exposure to body secretions and reduce the patient's infection risk.
2. Remove the old dressings, beginning at the insertion site and working outward. Put on sterile gloves, then clean the access site.	2. Working from cleaner to more soiled areas promotes asepsis.
*3. Assess for a thrill (a palpable vibration) by palpating lightly over the shunt access site. Also assess for extreme warmth or coolness of the site.	*3. A thrill is normal and indicates that blood is flowing through the shunt. Warmth may signal infection; coolness may signal infiltration.
4. Place sterile dressings over the access site and wrap with soft, stretchy cotton (Kerlix) or a rayon and polyester bandage (Kling). Wrap firmly enough to secure the dressing but not so firmly as to occlude blood flow. Leave a piece of shunt tubing visible.	4. Dressings protect the shunt while allowing visualization of continuous blood flow.
5. Discard used items in the proper trash receptacles.	5. This promotes safe care.
*6. Every 2 hours, assess pulses in the affected extremity. Assess blood flow in the shunt by palpating for a thrill and auscultating for a bruit. Also assess for edema, pain, redness, and drainage.	*6. Frequent assessment helps detect complications and prevent unnecessary loss of the access site as a result of occlusion or infection.
*7. Assess for bleeding or cannula disconnection. Keep a pair of cannula clamps at the bedside at all times and clamp the cannula if it separates.	*7. Separation is a potential shunt complication. Clamping the cannula prevents hemorrhage until a new cannula is inserted.
*8. Do not perform blood pressure assessment or venipuncture on the extremity with the shunt. Teach the patient to avoid tight-fitting clothes, watches, elastic bands or garters, and any other items that could restrict blood flow in the affected extremity.	*8. Restricted blood flow from a blood pressure cuff, venipuncture, or constricting garments could cause clotting and shunt occlusion.
9. Document the status of the affected extremity and the shunt access site as well as blood flow in the shunt.	9. Documentation proves that the procedure was done, assures high-quality care, and provides legal protection.

ADULT
NURSING

Measuring fluid intake and output

Introduction
Measurement of fluid intake and output is crucial for patients with an I.V. line, drainage tube, or catheter as well as those with urologic problems, acute cardiovascular problems, or signs of fluid imbalance (such as edema, poor skin turgor, or reduced urine output). Such measurement yields information that helps manage fluid balance or determine the effects of diuretics or hydration measures.

When measuring fluid intake, include all fluids taken into the body from any source, including the oral route, I.V. route, or a nasogastric (NG) tube. When measuring fluid output, include all fluids leaving the body from all exit sites, including urine, liquid stool, drainage from wounds and tubes, and emesis. (Procedure steps preceded by an asterisk are especially important.)

Measuring fluid intake

Steps

1. Measure and total all of the patient's oral fluid intake during each shift and every 24 hours. Include such substances as water, ice chips, beverages, soups, gelatin, and ice cream. Generally, fluid volume should be recorded according to institutional policy or the volume printed on the container. A graduated flask may be used to measure liquids more accurately. Record semisolid foods according to the percentage of fluid content (following institutional standard portions policy).

*2. Measure the amount of solution administered by NG or gastric tube feedings. If the patient is receiving a continuous drip feeding, record and total the amount in the bag at the beginning of the shift and the amount of any new solution added; then subtract the amount left in the bag at the end of the shift. The result is total intake during that shift. Also record any liquids instilled or mixed with medications.

3. Measure and record all I.V. intake, using the same method as described in step 2.

4. Record any instillation or irrigating fluid if it will drain out with other body fluids. (However, in some cases, the amount of irrigating fluid is subtracted from the total output instead of added as intake.)

Rationales

1. All fluids taken by mouth must be included when measuring oral fluid intake.

*2. Fluid intake must be measured accurately during each shift. Fluid left in the bag at the end of the shift will be counted on the next shift.

3. This helps maintain complete fluid intake monitoring.

4. This ensures accurate data.

ADULT
NURSING

Measuring fluid output

Steps

*1. Put on gloves. Measure liquid output using a graduated container marked clearly for such use. Measure and record output at the end of each shift or more often, if indicated. (In some cases, fluid draining into large collection bottles is monitored by marking the fluid level with the date and time directly on the container; fluid level changes are measured and recorded.)

2. Measure the amount of urine eliminated with each voiding, along with the time of voiding. Measure output from a catheter bag at the end of each shift. (For some patients requiring critical care, urine output measurements may be ordered hourly.)

3. Measure and record the amount and source of drainage from sites other than the kidneys (such as a wound drain, chest tube, or NG tube). Record the amount of drainage from each site separately.

*4. Measure and record any emesis, liquid stools, extreme diaphoresis (sweating), or bleeding. To estimate output from diaphoresis or bleeding, weigh soiled pads and subtract their weight from the dry weight.

5. If the patient is receiving NG or bladder irrigation, calculate true output by subtracting the infused irrigating fluid from the total output. Record only true output (unless the calculations also are included on the intake and output form).

6. Add total input and total output at the end of a 24-hour period (usually the end of the evening or night shift). Report any extreme discrepancy to the nurse-manager or physician.

Rationales

*1. Universal precautions stipulate that gloves should be worn when handling all body secretions. Marking drainage containers promotes easier and more efficient monitoring of fluid output.

2. This provides accurate monitoring of urine output.

3. Recording the drainage from each site separately helps identify the source of any abnormal drainage.

*4. All fluid loss must be measured to ensure accurate output calculation. One milliliter of water weighs 1 g; 1 liter weighs 1 kg (2.2 lb). This method also can be used to estimate urine output in a diaper for an incontinent patient.

5. This recording method avoids the error of counting irrigating fluid as output.

6. If fluid intake and output differ by 1 or 2 liters, the patient may have a fluid imbalance. Any fluid discrepancy must be correlated with body weight gain or loss.

ADULT
NURSING

Measuring urine specific gravity

Introduction

Measuring urine specific gravity (urine dilution or concentration [density]) helps determine a patient's hydration status and kidney function. (Procedure steps preceded by an asterisk are especially important.)

Steps

1. Collect a freshly voided urine specimen, or take urine from the drainage tubing of an indwelling catheter.

2. Place the urine in a test tube, and measure its specific gravity with a urinometer.

*3. Document the reading on the progress notes or flow sheet, indicating the time of measurement.

Rationales

1. Unlike urine in the drainage bag, freshly voided urine or urine from the drainage tubing reflects the patient's current hydration status.

2. The more concentrated the urine, the higher the urinometer will float.

*3. This verifies that the measurement has been done. Pure water has a specific gravity of 1.00. As urine becomes more concentrated, its specific gravity increases. Healthy kidneys concentrate urine during periods of fluid restriction. Specific gravity should measure 1.02 or more in this case.

Applying a T-binder

Introduction

A T-binder, a perineal binder resembling the letter T, holds a perineal dressing in place. A single T-binder is used for a female; a double T-binder (one with two vertical pieces instead of one) is used for a male because it elevates and supports the scrotum. (Procedure steps preceded by an asterisk are especially important.)

Steps

1. Wash your hands and put on gloves.

2. Remove the old T-binder and dressings (if present). Clean the perineum and pat dry. Place new dressings, if needed, to absorb drainage. Place additional absorbent dressings at the bottom of any draining wound.

*3. Obtain a clean T-binder, or reuse the old one if it is not soiled or wet. Position the binder with one crosspiece of the T around the patient's waist. Bring the vertical tail down from the back and between the legs to hold the dressings in place or, in a male, to support the scrotum. For a male, bring one of the tails around on each side of the penis. Adjust for length and attach the tails to the waistband in front with safety pins.

4. Make sure the binder is neither too loose nor too tight. If necessary, readjust for comfort.

5. Document T-binder application and the patient's response.

Rationales

1. Handwashing reduces the spread of microorganisms; gloves protect the nurse from the patient's secretions.

2. Cleanliness promotes comfort and healing. Absorbent dressings are needed where drainage likely will accumulate when the patient sits and walks.

*3. One binder size can be used for any patient. Fold and position any extra material to keep the waistband as smooth as possible.

4. Proper fit is needed to hold the dressings, support the scrotum, and maintain patient comfort.

5. Documentation proves that the procedure was done, assures high-quality care, and provides legal protection.

ADULT NURSING

Drugs used to treat genitourinary disorders

This chart presents information about drugs commonly prescribed for genitourinary disorders, including the drug action, dosage, and common side effects. Nursing considerations focus on patient comfort and teaching.

DRUG	ACTION	USUAL ADULT DOSAGE	COMMON SIDE EFFECTS	NURSING CONSIDERATIONS
Thiazide diuretics				
Chlorothiazide (Diuril), hydro-chlorothiazide (Oretic)	Decrease sodium and water reab-sorption, increas-ing urine output	Chlorothiazide: 500 to 1,000 mg P.O. once or twice daily Hydrochloro-thiazide: 25 to 100 mg P.O. once or twice daily	• Fluid and electrolyte im-balances	• Weigh the patient daily until edema resolves. • Measure fluid intake and output. • Observe urine characteristics. • Assess for edema or signs of congestive heart failure daily. • Measure blood pressure two to four times daily when chlorothiazide therapy begins. • Instruct the patient to take this drug in the morning to avoid nocturia. • Encourage the patient to eat plenty of potas-sium-rich foods. • If the patient also is receiving digitalis, hypo-kalemia may lead to digitalis toxicity.
Loop diuretic				
Furosemide (Lasix)	Inhibits sodium and chloride reab-sorption in the as-cending loop of Henle, causing di-uresis	20 to 80 mg P.O. or I.V. once or twice daily; increase dosage and frequency with hypertensive crisis, pulmo-nary edema, or acute renal failure	• Fluid and electrolyte imbalances, especially hypokalemia • Ototoxicity	• This drug is contraindicated in pregnant pa-tients. • Observe for rapid diuretic effect. • Ototoxicity is more likely with rapid injection. • Weigh the patient daily until edema resolves. • Measure fluid intake and output. • Observe urine characteristics. • Assess for edema or signs of congestive heart failure daily. • Measure blood pressure two to four times daily when furosemide therapy begins. • Instruct the patient to take this drug in the morning to avoid nocturia. • Encourage the patient to eat plenty of potas-sium-rich foods. • If the patient is receiving a digitalis prepara-tion, hypokalemia may cause digitalis toxicity. Monitor serum potassium levels daily.
Potassium-sparing diuretic				
Spironolactone (Aldactone)	Blocks the effects of aldosterone on the renal tubules, increasing sodium and water excre-tion and decreas-ing potassium excretion	25 to 200 mg P.O. daily	• Hyperkale-mia • Dehydration • GI distress	• This drug commonly is given in combination with potassium-losing diuretics. • Do not give concomitant potassium supple-ments. • Instruct the patient not to eat potassium-rich foods or use salt substitutes.
Osmotic agent				
Mannitol (Osmitrol)	Increases osmotic pressure of the glomerular filtrate, reducing water and electrolyte reabsorption in the tubules. Increases blood volume by pulling water from tissues into the bloodstream	50 to 100 g in I.V. solution given over 30 to 60 minutes or in a continu-ous drip at a flow rate that maintains a urine output of 30 to 50 ml/ hour	• Pulmonary edema, if the patient cannot tolerate in-creased blood volume	• Use cautiously in patients with renal impair-ment. • Monitor electrolyte and fluid states closely. • Adminsiter I.V. with an in-line filter; avoid ex-travasation. • Solutions commonly crystallize at room tem-perature. Do not use solutions with crystals. Call the pharmacy for instructions on how to dissolve crystals.

ENDOCRINE SYSTEM

Anatomy and physiology

I. **Anatomy**
    A. The pituitary gland, situated in the sella turcica at the base of the cranium, consists of an anterior lobe and a posterior lobe
    B. The thyroid gland is located in the neck
    C. The parathyroid glands are situated near the thyroid gland
    D. The adrenal glands are found above each kidney
    E. The pancreas is located behind the stomach, between the duodenum and spleen
    F. The gonads consist of the ovaries, located in the pelvic cavity of the female, and the testes, located in the scrotum of the male

II. **Physiology**
    A. Endocrine glands secrete hormones directly into the bloodstream or other body fluids
        1. Each endocrine gland is stimulated to secrete its specific hormone in response to need
        2. Hormones regulate metabolic functions in one of three ways
            a. They control the rates of chemical activities in cells
            b. They alter cell membrane permeability to allow transport of substances across the membrane
            c. They activate specific cell functions, such as growth and reproduction
        3. Hormones may affect almost all body cells, one particular organ, or another gland
        4. Hormone overproduction or underproduction may threaten a person's life (A commercially prepared supplement commonly is administered to treat a hormone deficiency)
    B. The pituitary gland (hypophysis) is called the master gland because it stimulates other glands to secrete hormones
        1. The anterior pituitary lobe secretes hormones that control growth, reproduction, lactation, thyroid, and adrenal functions
            a. Thyroid-stimulating hormone controls thyroid activity
            b. Adrenocorticotropic hormone controls adrenal cortex secretions
        2. The posterior pituitary lobe secretes antidiuretic hormone (ADH) and oxytocin
            a. ADH controls reabsorption of water from the kidney
            b. Oxytocin stimulates uterine contraction and lactation
    C. The thyroid gland secretes several substances
        1. The hormones triiodothyronine and thyroxine regulate metabolism
        2. Calcitonin reduces the serum calcium level by causing calcium to move into the bones
    D. The parathyroid glands secrete parathyroid hormone, which maintains calcium and phosphate homeostasis

Reviewing the endocrine system

The illustrations below show the locations of the endocrine glands in the male and female.

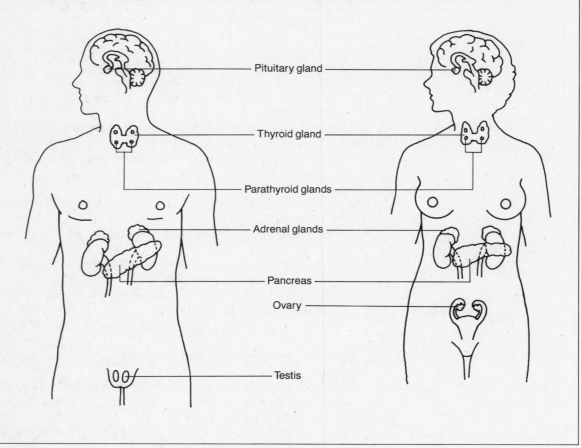

Pituitary gland

Thyroid gland

Parathyroid glands

Adrenal glands

Pancreas

Ovary

Testis

E. The adrenal gland also secretes multiple substances
1. The medulla of the adrenal gland secretes epinephrine, which increases cardiac output and blood pressure
2. The adrenal cortex secretes glucocorticoids and mineralocorticoids
   a. Glucocorticoids (such as cortisol) are essential to survival during stress and play a key role in normal glucose and protein metabolism
   b. Mineralocorticoids (such as aldosterone) promote sodium retention and potassium loss, helping to regulate electrolyte balance
F. The pancreas secretes two pancreatic hormones, insulin and glucagon, which regulate glucose, lipid, and protein metabolism
G. The gonads are the sex glands
1. In the female, the ovaries secrete the hormones estrogen and progesterone
   a. Estrogen is responsible for secondary sex characteristics
   b. Progesterone prepares the uterus for pregnancy and the mammary glands for lactation
2. In the male, the testes secrete testosterone, a hormone needed for the development of masculine characteristics

---

Glossary

Cretinism: severe congenital hypothyroidism caused by lack of thyroid secretion

Endogenous: developing from within the body

Euthyroid goiter: abnormal enlargement of the thyroid gland with normal thyroid hormone levels (also called simple goiter)

Exogenous: developing outside the body

Homeostasis: relatively constant internal body environment

Hormone: chemical substance secreted by an endocrine gland, or the commercially prepared copy of the substance used as a medication

Hyperglycemia: abnormally high blood glucose level

Hypoglycemia: abnormally low blood glucose level

Metabolism: process by which nutrients are oxidized to provide energy for building up, regenerating, and maintaining body functions

Tetany: paroxysmal spasm of the extremities caused by a low serum calcium level

---

Hyperthyroidism

Overview

Commonly called Graves's disease or exophthalmic goiter, hyperthyroidism is characterized by excessive thyroid hormone secretion. It causes an increased metabolic rate, leading to acceleration of all physiologic processes. Signs and symptoms of hyperthyroidism range from nervousness and irritability to tachycardia with cardiac decompensation (heart failure). Other manifestations include an enlarged thyroid gland (toxic goiter) and exophthalmia (bulging of the eyes). Emotional changes, such as depression or euphoria, may occur when thyroid hormones act on the nervous system.

The diagnosis of hyperthyroidism is confirmed by increased levels of the thyroid hormones thyroxine (T_4) and triiodothyronine (T_3) and increased uptake of ^{131}I (radioactive iodine). Treatments include medications that interfere with thyroid hormone production, radioactive iodine (which destroys part of the thyroid gland), and surgical removal of a portion of the thyroid gland.

Clinical situation

Tricia Doyle, age 40, has had a recent unexplained weight loss—despite an increased food intake and insatiable appetite. She has ignored the development of bulging eyes, which make her look startled. She has trouble concentrating on any activity, and her family complains that she has become irritable and suspicious.

When Ms. Doyle develops shortness of breath, a fast pulse, palpitations, and chest pain, she fears she may have a heart problem and decides to go to the medical clinic. In the waiting room, she seems agitated and cannot sit still. She tells the nurse who takes her history that her mother had "the thyroid disease with bulging eyes" and died of cardiac complications. The nurse notes that Ms. Doyle is wearing a light cotton dress despite the cold weather and is quite thin, with flushed skin that feels warm to the touch. Ms. Doyle states that she always feels too warm and perspires constantly; during the health history interview, she frequently wipes perspiration from her forehead. The nurse measures a temperature of 99.2° F (37.3° C), pulse rate of 130 beats/minute, respiratory rate of 26 breaths/minute, and blood pressure of 158/64 mm Hg. After 20 minutes, the nurse rechecks her pulse rate; it is 142 beats/minute.

The physician palpates an enlarged thyroid gland, then orders T_3, T_4, and radioactive iodine uptake tests. The results show elevated levels of all three substances, confirming the diagnosis of hyperthyroidism. Ms. Doyle will undergo outpatient treatment with Lugol's solution (an iodine compound) and propranolol (Inderal; an adrenergic-blocking agent) to reduce thyroid activity temporarily and control the effects of the high metabolic rate.

Assessment

Nursing behaviors	**Nursing rationales**
1. Measure Ms. Doyle's weight.	**1.** Hyperthyroidism causes weight loss despite an increased appetite.
2. Assess Ms. Doyle's blood pressure and pulse rate.	**2.** This yields baseline data. With hyperthyroidism, the pulse rate increases, even at rest, and systolic blood pressure rises.
3. Assess Ms. Doyle's skin for temperature and perspiration.	**3.** Hyperthyroidism causes increased perspiration and heat sensitivity.
4. Assess Ms. Doyle's mental status and behavior.	**4.** Hyperthyroidism may cause personality changes, especially irritability and spontaneous crying episodes.
5. Assess Ms. Doyle for an enlarged thyroid and bulging eyes.	**5.** These are signs of hyperthyroidism.

Nursing diagnoses
- Altered nutrition (less than body requirements) related to increased metabolism
- Anxiety (moderate to severe) related to inability to control the illness

Planning and goals
- Ms. Doyle's nutritional status will improve and she will begin to regain some of the weight she has lost.
- Ms. Doyle will demonstrate the ability to cope with her disease and an understanding of the cause of her emotional instability.
- Ms. Doyle will express relief from discomfort caused by perspiration and heat intolerance.

Implementation

Nursing behaviors	**Nursing rationales**
1. Monitor Ms. Doyle's vital signs and weight on each outpatient visit. Teach her how to monitor her weight at home.	**1.** Tachycardia and hypertension should resolve as her metabolic rate slows. Weight should begin to stabilize.
2. Reassure Ms. Doyle that her emotional symptoms stem from the thyroid disorder and will improve with treatment. Provide support and encouragement for her family.	**2.** Emotional instability can harm one's interactions with family and friends. Ms. Doyle's emotional status should improve when her hormone levels return to normal.
3. Teach Ms. Doyle to eat a diet high in calories and vitamins, adding snacks or carbohydrate supplements if needed.	**3.** The high metabolic rate calls for extra calories.

4. Teach Ms. Doyle to dress comfortably in cool clothing, and suggest that she take cool baths and drink cool fluids for relief. Mention that she will feel more comfortable in a room with a cooler-than-normal temperature.

4. Ms. Doyle's increased metabolic rate and heat production may cause her to feel unbearably warm. She will need explanations and advice.

5. Teach Ms. Doyle to dilute the prescribed iodine solution in fruit juice or water and drink it through a straw.

5. This helps prevent tooth staining from iodine solutions.

6. Teach Ms. Doyle to report any elevated temperature, rapid pulse, confusion, restlessness, or altered level of consciousness.

6. These signs and symptoms represent complications of hyperthyroidism.

7. Inform Ms. Doyle that changes in appearance, appetite, and weight are beyond her control.

7. These changes are caused by thyroid gland dysfunction.

8. Teach Ms. Doyle how to instill eye drops and ophthalmic ointment.

8. These measures help protect against corneal damage from exposure related to exophthalmia.

Evaluation (outcomes)

• Ms. Doyle's thyroid function and metabolic rate return to normal gradually with medication. Propranolol helps to control her tachycardia and hypertension.
• Ms. Doyle's weight stabilizes, although she must eat several snacks and milk shakes daily in addition to extra servings at meals.
• Ms. Doyle has fewer episodes of crying and irritability and her emotional status improves markedly.
• Ms. Doyle's bulging eyes do not improve with treatment. She continues to instill an eye ointment to soothe and protect her eyes.
• Ms. Doyle receives an oral dose of radioactive iodine, which permanently destroys overactive thyroid cells. She remains free from hypothyroidism, the major side effect of excessive thyroid tissue destruction.

Hypothyroidism

Overview

Hypothyroidism refers to inadequate secretion of thyroid hormone to maintain homeostasis. The condition may be present at birth (cretinism) or may develop in adulthood (myxedema). It commonly follows excessive thyroid tissue destruction, such as from surgery or radioactive iodine therapy used to treat hyperthyroidism.

Signs and symptoms of hypothyroidism—nearly the reverse of those of hyperthyroidism—include sensitivity to cold, dry skin and hair, sleepiness, slow pulse, and an abnormally low metabolic rate. The patient typically complains of constipation and feeling cold, and may experience depression and personality changes. Treatment usually involves administration of synthetic levothyroxine (Synthroid) or another thyroid preparation to replace the deficient hormone and restore a normal metabolic state. Replacement therapy must continue lifelong.

Clinical situation   Dorothy Leonard, a secretary, age 52, notices progressively increasing dryness of her skin and hair. Frequently constipated, she has gained 25 lb (11.3 kg) in the last 2 years despite a decreased appetite and food intake. She always feels tired and complains of being cold, even when wearing a sweater—changes she attributes to aging. However, after she falls asleep at work one day, coworkers persuade her to visit the employee health department. The occupational health nurse finds that Ms. Leonard has a slow pulse and a subnormal temperature and responds to questions slowly. After taking a detailed history and conducting a physical assessment, the nurse refers her to her family physician for evaluation.

The physician diagnoses Ms. Leonard's condition as hypothyroidism and prescribes a low dosage of thyroid hormone, admitting her to the hospital for cardiovascular monitoring during initial therapy.

Assessment

Nursing behaviors	**Nursing rationales**
1. Assess Ms. Leonard's vital signs and weight.	**1.** This establishes a baseline for comparison. Severe hypothyroidism typically causes a weight gain and a decreased temperature and pulse rate.
2. Assess Ms. Leonard's cardiac and respiratory status.	**2.** Replacement thyroid hormone increases the metabolism and boosts myocardial oxygen demands, possibly causing angina and arrhythmias.
3. Assess Ms. Leonard's dietary habits.	**3.** She may need to reduce her caloric intake to lose weight. Poor fiber intake may contribute to constipation.
4. Assess Ms. Leonard's bowel and exercise habits.	**4.** Poor bowel habits and lack of exercise may contribute to constipation.
5. Assess Ms. Leonard's understanding of the disease and its treatment.	**5.** Understanding will help her comply with her lifelong therapeutic regimen.
6. Assess Ms. Leonard's skin.	**6.** Dry skin and hair may need special care.

Nursing diagnoses
- Altered nutrition (more than body requirements) related to decreased metabolism
- Knowledge deficit related to lifelong thyroid replacement therapy

Planning and goals
- Ms. Leonard will follow a well-balanced diet and be able to control her weight.
- Ms. Leonard will express an understanding of her medication regimen, including potential side effects (such as tachycardia, palpitations, anxiety, and sleeplessness).
- Ms. Leonard will regain normal bowel function.
- Ms. Leonard will express relief from discomfort caused by cold intolerance.

Implementation

Nursing behaviors	**Nursing rationales**
1. Monitor Ms. Leonard's vital signs and weight.	**1.** Cardiac and respiratory changes may reflect medication side effects or worsening of hypothyroidism.

2. Provide a warm environment with an extra blanket or layer of clothing. Protect Ms. Leonard from exposure to drafts.

2. A person with hypothyroidism feels chilly even in a room that feels warm to others. Extra protection will help Ms. Leonard maintain her body temperature by reducing heat loss.

3. Monitor the effects of medications.

3. Medications, especially central nervous system depressants, must be administered cautiously because Ms. Leonard's depressed metabolic rate may potentiate their effects.

4. Encourage Ms. Leonard to maintain good bowel habits, consume high-fiber foods, maintain a high fluid intake, and exercise, as tolerated.

4. These measures help counter the constipation related to reduced gastrointestinal function (an effect of hypothyroidism).

5. Decrease Ms. Leonard's caloric intake while providing nutritional foods.

5. This promotes good nutritional status and weight loss.

6. Teach Ms. Leonard about her prescribed medication, including both desired effects and side effects.

6. Teaching improves patient compliance and helps ensure that Ms. Leonard can identify and promptly report any side effects or symptoms of recurring hypothyroidism or hyperthyroidism.

Evaluation (outcomes)

• Ms. Leonard's pulse rate returns to normal and she notices a marked energy increase.
• Ms. Leonard has improved bowel function and avoids the need for laxatives.
• Ms. Leonard begins to lose approximately 2 lb (0.9 kg)/month after returning to work, although she does not return to her ideal body weight.

Cushing's syndrome

Overview

Cushing's syndrome results from excessive adrenocortical hormone secretion — usually from a tumor of the adrenal cortex or the anterior pituitary lobe. The disorder sometimes follows exogenous corticosteroid administration to treat an autoimmune or allergic disease. (Such side effects of corticosteroids can be reduced by scheduling alternate-day administration and giving the lowest possible dosage.)

Classic signs of Cushing's syndrome include:
• obesity with fat accumulation in the face, neck, and trunk (called "moon face" or "buffalo hump")
• thin, fragile skin that bruises easily
• muscle wasting
• osteoporosis
• sodium and water retention
• virilization (in females).

Other manifestations include hyperglycemia or diabetes mellitus, mood changes (such as depression), and increased susceptibility to infection. Laboratory studies typically show increased serum sodium, serum glucose, and plasma and urinary cortisol levels. Computed tomography (CT) may reveal a tumor.

Treatment involves eliminating the cause. A pituitary tumor may call for radiation therapy; an adrenal tumor is removed surgically (adrenalectomy). The patient will receive adrenal hormone replacement to treat transient postoperative adrenal insufficiency. After bilateral adrenalectomy, such replacement continues lifelong.

ADULT NURSING

Clinical situation

Jennifer Rodman, age 24, sees her family physician when a cut on her leg becomes infected and does not heal. Markedly obese, she has a round face and protruding abdomen; her arms and legs are thin and covered with bruises. She reports that she has trouble sleeping and fatigues easily. She has not menstruated in several months, and says she is embarrassed by her appearance—especially the facial hair and atrophied breasts.

Suspecting Cushing's syndrome, the physician admits her to the hospital for evaluation and treatment. Laboratory tests confirm the diagnosis.

Assessment

Nursing behaviors	**Nursing rationales**
1. Take a nursing history, focusing on Ms. Rodman's ability to perform activities of daily living (ADLs). Include questions about fatigue, sleep patterns, and the effects of her condition on daily routines.	**1.** Weakness and fatigue typically make performing ADLs difficult.
2. Assess Ms. Rodman's skin for breakdown, bruises, infection, and edema.	**2.** Cushing's syndrome causes easy skin trauma and slow wound healing. Edema may occur with sodium retention.
3. Assess Ms. Rodman's physical appearance and emotional responses to these changes (such as mood and depression level).	**3.** Cushing's syndrome causes mood changes and virilization in females (from excess androgens). Emotional distress and depression are exacerbated by physical changes.
4. Assess Ms. Rodman's vital signs and weight.	**4.** Such baseline data help assess fluid and electrolyte status.

Nursing diagnoses

• Body image disturbance related to changes in physical appearance
• Potential for injury related to altered metabolism and a suppressed inflammatory response

Planning and goals

• Ms. Rodman will demonstrate an increased ability to carry out ADLs.
• Ms. Rodman will avoid new infections or skin breakdown.
• Ms. Rodman will express her feelings about changes in her physical appearance.
• Ms. Rodman will show improved mental function.

Implementation

Nursing behaviors	**Nursing rationales**
1. Monitor Ms. Rodman's vital signs, weight, and serum electrolyte levels.	**1.** An elevated temperature may indicate an infection. Ongoing information about Ms. Rodman's fluid and electrolyte status helps ensure proper care. Hypertension or congestive heart failure are potential disease complications.
2. Encourage Ms. Rodman to alternate moderate activity with planned rest periods.	**2.** Weakness, fatigue, and muscle wasting may impair Ms. Rodman's ability to perform ADLs. However, moderate activity will help prevent complications of immobility. She needs planned rest periods because insomnia contributes to fatigue.

3. Use meticulous skin care, avoiding adhesive tape. Pay extra attention to bony prominences.

3. Ms. Rodman's skin is fragile and easily traumatized. Adhesive tape may tear the skin when removed. Pressure areas need special care to avoid breakdown.

4. Provide a safe environment to prevent falls or injuries. Assist with ambulation, if necessary.

4. A weak patient is at risk for falling or bumping on sharp corners.

5. Protect Ms. Rodman from infection by avoiding exposing her to people with infections. Assess her frequently for signs and symptoms of infection.

5. Cushing's syndrome increases susceptibility to infection.

6. Monitor stools for occult blood. Monitor blood or urine glucose levels.

6. Cushing's syndrome may cause peptic ulcers and diabetes mellitus.

7. Encourage Ms. Rodman to consume a diet high in protein and low in carbohydrates and sodium.

7. Dietary changes may minimize weight gain and edema.

Evaluation (outcomes)

• Ms. Rodman undergoes successful treatment with I.V. antibiotics. The bacterial infection for which she originally sought care resolves.
• Ms. Rodman avoids falls and injuries. Her skin remains intact with no breakdown.
• A CT scan reveals a tumor on the right adrenal gland. It is removed surgically through an abdominal incision; her postoperative care is uneventful.
• Ms. Rodman starts to express her feelings about the disease and resulting physical changes.

Addison's disease

Overview

Addison's disease refers to adrenal hypofunction resulting from bilateral adrenalectomy; adrenal destruction caused by infection, trauma, or atrophy (wasting); or sudden cessation of exogenous adrenocortical hormones. Signs and symptoms, which reflect adrenocortical insufficiency, may include GI symptoms (nausea, vomiting, anorexia, and abdominal pain), muscle weakness, fatigue, low blood pressure, bronze skin pigmentation, sodium and water depletion, and severe chronic dehydration. Laboratory studies confirm the diagnosis.

As Addison's disease progresses, the patient may suffer acute hypotension and addisonian crisis, a life-threatening state of severe adrenocortical insufficiency. A medical emergency, addisonian crisis causes classic signs of shock, which can progress to coma and death. Addisonian crisis commonly stems from stress (such as from surgery). Treatment of this complication focuses on I.V. hydrocortisone administration and fluid replacement with normal saline solution.

Clinical situation

Joe Maguire, a bookkeeper, age 29, has generalized weakness, nausea with occasional vomiting, and weight loss. His friends compliment him on his "great tan" even though he has not been in the sun. Several weeks after noticing these nonspecific symptoms, he has a car accident and requires emergency surgery to repair injuries and control bleeding.

Laboratory tests done before emergency surgery reveal that Mr. Maguire has low serum sodium and glucose levels and a high serum potassium level. His blood pressure measures 96/54 mm Hg. After surgery, in the postanesthesia recovery unit, his blood pressure drops further and he begins to show signs of circulatory collapse and shock. He receives a STAT dose of hydrocortisone I.V.; the primary I.V. solution of 5% dextrose in saline solution is given at a rapid rate. His blood pressure then returns to normal and he emerges from anesthesia without further complications.

The physician diagnoses Addison's disease as the cause of Mr. Maguire's postoperative problems and preaccident symptoms, and updates his orders to include additional doses of I.V. hydrocortisone and change the I.V. fluid from 0.45% to 0.9% (normal) saline solution. To manage Addison's disease, Mr. Maguire's routine postoperative trauma nursing care is modified by the measures described below.

Assessment

Nursing behaviors	Nursing rationales
1. Assess Mr. Maguire's fluid balance. Measure blood pressure and pulse as he lies, then stands.	**1.** A significant blood pressure decrease from a lying to a standing position may reflect inadequate fluid volume.
2. Assess Mr. Maguire's skin turgor and color.	**2.** Skin turgor and color changes may signal decreased blood volume and chronic adrenal insufficiency.
3. Obtain a history of Mr. Maguire's weight loss and any history of weakness, fatigue, or stress.	**3.** The history can help determine the onset of illness.

Nursing diagnoses

• Fluid volume deficit related to inadequate adrenal hormone secretion
• Knowledge deficit related to the need for hormone replacement and dietary modifications

Planning and goals

• Mr. Maguire's fluid and electrolyte balance will improve.
• Mr. Maguire will show improved physiologic responses to the stress of hospitalization and surgery.
• Mr. Maguire will express an understanding of the lifelong hormonal replacement and dietary changes needed to manage Addison's disease.

Implementation

Nursing behaviors	Nursing rationales
1. Monitor Mr. Maguire's weight daily. Observe skin turgor and mucous membranes during each shift. Observe for excessive thirst.	**1.** Weight changes and skin and mucous membrane condition reflect fluid balance. Dehydration signals adrenal insufficiency or inadequate fluid and hormone replacement.
2. Plan a high-sodium diet during periods of GI upset, hot weather, or other stress. Ensure an adequate fluid intake.	**2.** Low adrenocortical hormone levels cause water and sodium loss, calling for fluid and additional sodium replacement.

3. Teach Mr. Maguire how to self-administer replacement hormones, as prescribed. Include written instructions on how to modify the dosage during illness or severe stress.

3. Mr. Maguire will need lifelong adrenal hormone replacement, as well as additional hormones during times of stress. Teaching will improve his therapeutic compliance.

4. Teach Mr. Maguire how to detect and manage early signs of infection and other stressors.

4. Stress management will help prevent an adrenal crisis with vascular collapse.

5. Instruct Mr. Maguire to obtain a medical alert bracelet and to inform other health care providers (such as dentists) of his need for steroid medication.

5. This helps ensure safe health care.

Evaluation (outcomes)

• Mr. Maguire recovers from the motor vehicle accident and surgery without complications.
• Mr. Maguire achieves an improved fluid balance with stable weight, good skin turgor, and no excessive thirst.
• Mr. Maguire identifies sources of stress and begins to plan ways to avoid them.
• Mr. Maguire expresses an understanding of the need for lifelong hormone replacement therapy and the consequences of inadequate replacement.
• Mr. Maguire takes his medication as prescribed and can identify signs and symptoms of overdose and underdose.
• Mr. Maguire obtains a medical alert bracelet and wears it at all times.

Type II diabetes mellitus

Overview

Diabetes mellitus—a group of disorders characterized by glucose intolerance—arises when the body cannot use or produce insulin. The disorder has five main forms:
• Type I—insulin-dependent diabetes mellitus
• Type II—non-insulin-dependent diabetes mellitus
• impaired glucose tolerance
• gestational diabetes mellitus
• diabetes mellitus associated with other conditions or syndromes (such as Cushing's syndrome).
    Type I diabetes mellitus occurs when the pancreas produces insufficient insulin; the patient requires exogenous insulin to control symptoms. This diabetes form may reflect an inherited immune defect coupled with an environmental factor, such as a virus that triggers an autoimmune response. It usually begins in childhood with abrupt onset of polyuria (excessive urine excretion), polydipsia (excessive thirst), and polyphagia (excessive eating). Weight loss and weakness are common. Because carbohydrates cannot be used without insulin, the body breaks down proteins and fats for energy. Metabolism of fatty acids and ketogenic amino acids may cause ketosis, a condition characterized by elevated levels of ketone bodies.

ADULT NURSING

In Type II diabetes mellitus, the pancreas produces some insulin but cells are insulin-insensitive. Major causes include obesity and genetic factors. Typically, Type II diabetes affects overweight adults and goes undetected for many years because symptoms are mild. Once diagnosed, the disease usually can be controlled through diet and exercise. However, some patients may need oral hypoglycemic agents or insulin.

Both Type I and Type II diabetes mellitus carry the risk of long-term complications, including vascular changes in the heart, legs, feet, eyes, kidneys, and nervous system. These complications (which may stem from prolonged hyperglycemia) may have catastrophic consequences, such as gangrene (with subsequent amputation), blindness, and kidney failure.

The diagnosis of diabetes hinges on abnormally high blood glucose levels, as determined from a glucose tolerance test. (For mass screening, the 2-hour postprandial blood glucose test using capillary blood samples is easiest. Urine tests should not be used for diagnosis.) The goal of diabetes management is to control the blood glucose level and delay vascular complications.

Clinical situation

Irene Drake, a waitress, age 48, is 5'3" (160 cm) tall and weighs 170 lb (77.1 kg). The birth weights of her three children averaged 9 lb (4.1 kg). She is in fairly good health. However, she has fatigue and leg cramps, which she blames on extended periods of standing and walking at work. Also, she awakens two or three times at night to void. During a recent gynecologic examination, she complained of vulvar itching.

When a 2-hour postprandial screening test shows that Ms. Drake has an elevated blood glucose level, the physician orders a glucose tolerance test. Results confirm Type II diabetes mellitus. Ms. Drake is to begin a 1,200-calorie weight-reduction diet developed by the American Diabetes Association (ADA). After ruling out heart disease, the physician orders a regular daily exercise program and schedules Ms. Drake for regular clinic visits until the treatment regimen brings her diabetes under control.

Assessment

Nursing behaviors

1. Assess Ms. Drake's skin for signs of infection, including boils and other red, itchy areas (such as from *Candida albicans*).

2. Assess Ms. Drake's weight, blood pressure, and peripheral pulses.

3. Check Ms. Drake's legs and feet for color, nail appearance, pulse strength, and ulcers.

4. Assess Ms. Drake for edema of the extremities and signs of urinary tract infection.

5. Check for signs of peripheral neuropathy, such as tingling, numbness, and decreased sensation (especially of the lower extremities). Assess for dull, aching, or cramping leg pain that worsens at night and subsides with walking.

Nursing rationales

1. Increased skin moisture—particularly between skinfolds in obese patients—and high glucose levels support the growth of microorganisms.

2. These measurements help evaluate her cardiovascular status.

3. Vascular complications of diabetes can cause circulatory compromise.

4. Diabetes may involve the kidneys, causing fluid retention with edema. Urinary tract infection commonly accompanies diabetes.

5. Pain and paresthesias are common symptoms of diabetic neuropathy. Sensation loss can cause both the patient and health care providers to overlook an infection or injury.

Nursing diagnoses
- Knowledge deficit related to diabetes and its management
- Altered nutrition (more than body requirements) related to obesity and the dietary changes needed to control blood glucose levels

Planning and goals
- Ms. Drake will begin to lose weight, following the prescribed therapeutic diet and exercise regimens.
- Ms. Drake's blood glucose levels will stay as close to normal as possible and her carbohydrate metabolism will improve.
- Ms. Drake will perform proper foot care to prevent infection or injury.
- Ms. Drake will avoid, delay, or control long-term complications of diabetes mellitus.
- Ms. Drake will remain free from the acute complication of hyperosmolar nonketotic syndrome (HNKS).

Implementation

Nursing behaviors

1. Begin a teaching program to foster self-care so that Ms. Drake can help control diabetes and its complications. Include such topics as disease pathophysiology, dietary management, her individualized exercise program, urine or blood glucose monitoring, hyperglycemia signs and symptoms, and basic foot care.

2. Monitor Ms. Drake's blood glucose levels. Teach her how to self-monitor capillary or urine glucose levels.

3. Provide the teaching and counseling Ms. Drake needs to follow a weight-reduction meal plan.

4. Encourage daily exercise and physical activity.

5. Teach Ms. Drake to inspect her skin (especially on the feet) regularly for cuts, bruises, dryness, and signs of infection. Encourage her to obtain professional foot care. If she has poor vision, teach a family member to perform skin checks.

Nursing rationales

1. Responsibility for diabetes management lies with the patient. The teaching program should begin at the time of diagnosis and must continue for life.

2. By monitoring blood glucose levels, Ms. Drake can determine if she needs to adjust her diet, exercise, or medication regimen. Many patients with Type II diabetes use urine glucose levels to evaluate diabetes control. During times of stress or illness, blood glucose levels may be used.

3. Ms. Drake needs information about food exchanges and meal planning. Weight reduction and continued therapeutic dietary adjustments may control hyperglycemia, avoiding the need for medication.

4. Exercise and physical activity lower blood glucose and cholesterol levels and increase high-density lipoprotein levels. (Diabetes increases the risk of cardiovascular disease; therefore, some patients need cardiovascular screening before the physician can prescribe exercise.)

5. Detection and early treatment of simple problems may prevent severe complications.

ADULT NURSING

6. Teach Ms. Drake to take such safety measures as removing potential hazards (including throw rugs, slippery floors, and other objects) in both the home and workplace.

7. Monitor Ms. Drake for anxiety, hostility, or denial—behaviors that indicate the need for assistance in coping.

6. Diabetes can lead to retinopathy (which causes decreased vision) and neuropathy (which causes decreased sensation in the lower extremities); these conditions may put Ms. Drake at risk for injury.

7. Such behaviors may arise because diabetes is a chronic disease and Ms. Drake must incorporate diabetes management into her life-style.

Evaluation (outcomes)

• Ms. Drake follows the prescribed 1,200-calorie ADA diet and begins to lose weight.
• Ms. Drake maintains her diet and exercise program.
• Ms. Drake begins to inspect her feet daily.
• Ms. Drake learns how to test her urine for glucose and keeps her appointments for laboratory work.
• Ms. Drake obtains pamphlets and other information from the ADA and reads about diabetes management and complications.
• Ms. Drake returns to her job as a waitress and learns how to follow her diet plan at work.
• Ms. Drake returns to her physician promptly when she notices symptoms of a urinary tract infection. During this visit, her urine tests positive for glucose. After oral antibiotics resolve the infection, her diabetes is controlled.
• Ms. Drake remains free from HNKS.

Complications of endocrine disorders

This chart presents the most serious or life-threatening complications of endocrine disorders, along with interventions that are crucial to patient safety and comfort.

COMPLICATION	CAUSE	NURSING INTERVENTIONS
Adrenal crisis Exacerbation of adrenocortical insufficiency (Addison's disease), causing severe hypotension. A medical emergency, this condition can lead to circulatory collapse, shock, coma, and death.	• Abrupt cessation of exogenous steroids • Overexertion, acute infection, decreased salt intake, or mental or physical stress (such as dehydration or surgery) in a patient with adrenocortical insufficiency	• Emergency treatment focuses on reversing shock. For instance, administer I.V. fluids to increase blood volume and administer I.V. hydrocortisone, as ordered, to compensate for adrenal suppression. • Monitor vital signs. • Place the patient in a recumbent position with legs elevated. • Administer vasopressors, as ordered, if the patient has persistent low blood pressure. • Offer fruit juice and salt broth, when tolerated, to provide sodium and electrolytes. • When the patient regains adequate blood pressure and circulation, carry out measures to treat the condition that precipitated adrenal crisis, as ordered.

Complications of endocrine disorders *(continued)*

COMPLICATION	CAUSE	NURSING INTERVENTIONS
Hypoglycemia (insulin reaction) An acute complication of diabetes mellitus in which the blood glucose level drops below 60 mg/dl. Signs and symptoms include dizziness, irritability, perspiration, and, in some cases, weakness, headache, palpitations, and hunger. Unless treated, hypoglycemia can progress to coma, seizures, and death.	• Insufficient dietary intake • Excessive insulin • Excessive oral hypoglycemic agents • Increased exercise without dietary supplementation	• If the patient is conscious, provide a substance containing a fast-acting simple sugar (such as fruit juice, candy, or regular soda) followed by a complex carbohydrate and a protein (such as crackers and milk). • If the patient is unconscious, administer glucagon parenterally, as ordered. When the patient awakens, provide simple carbohydrates followed by more complex carbohydrates, proteins, and fats. • If the patient does not respond to glucagon, administer concentrated I.V. glucose (50% solution), as ordered. Provide food when the patient can eat. • Record and report hypoglycemia to permit adjustment of the diabetes treatment regimen, if necessary.

Hyperglycemia An acute complication of diabetes mellitus in which the blood glucose level exceeds 300 mg/dl, causing dehydration and electrolyte imbalance (unless treated).
   In Type I diabetes, hyperglycemia occurs as part of diabetic ketoacidosis (DKA). Early signs and symptoms of DKA include increased thirst, increased hunger, and increased urination. Later, the patient may have nausea and vomiting, diminished urination, Kussmaul's respirations, and sweet breath odor. Urine becomes strongly acetone-positive. Drowsiness gradually progresses to coma. Although serious, DKA can be reversed with insulin and I.V. fluids.
   In Type II diabetes, untreated hyperglycemia progresses to hyperosmolar nonketotic syndrome (HNKS). Extreme dehydration and critical illness ensue. (DKA does not occur with Type II diabetes because some insulin is present for carbohydrate metabolism.)
	• Dietary excess
	• Insufficient insulin
	• Influenza, infection, or another condition that increases insulin requirements
	• Emotional stress
		• Hyperglycemia calls for insulin administration and a therapeutic calorie-restricted diet.
		• For DKA, administer short-acting insulin and I.V. fluids, as ordered, to reverse hyperglycemia, dehydration, acidosis, and electrolyte imbalance.
		• For HNKS, administer massive I.V. fluid replacement and small amounts of insulin, as ordered, to reverse metabolic problems.

Thyroid storm (thyrotoxic crisis) A life-threatening complication occurring when large amounts of thyroid hormone enter into the bloodstream, causing a sudden increase in metabolism with a rapid pulse, elevated temperature, and altered mental status. The condition may progress to coma and death.	Thyroidectomy, physical stress (such as surgery, infection, or injury), severe emotional stress, or abrupt withdrawal of antithyroid drugs in a patient with untreated or partially controlled hyperthyroidism	Take measures, as ordered, to control the heart rate and body temperature and to prevent heart failure. For instance, provide a hypothermia blanket to reduce the temperature. Administer oxygen, as ordered, to meet increased metabolic demands. Administer I.V. fluids with glucose, as ordered. Give antithyroid medications (thiamide drugs and iodine), as ordered. Administer propranolol (Inderal) and digitalis to treat cardiac complications, and hydrocortisone to treat shock, as ordered.

Teaching blood glucose self-monitoring

Introduction

By testing a drop of capillary blood, the patient can determine the glucose level at home. This self-care technique, often called self-monitoring of blood glucose (SMBG), helps the patient manage diabetes and determine the insulin requirement. Yielding a direct, immediate measurement, it allows the patient to recognize and manage emergency situations, such as hypoglycemia or illness, as well as make decisions about daily insulin dosage, exercise, and food intake. SMBG is recommended for diabetic patients who use insulin pumps, are pregnant, or are predisposed to hypoglycemia or ketosis. Some patients who do not take insulin or are motivated to maintain careful diabetes control also may use SMBG.

SMBG may involve a reagent strip (which the patient compares to color charts) or an electronic meter (which provides a digital reading). Unlike urine glucose monitoring, blood glucose monitoring does not depend on the renal threshold and reveals low as well as high glucose readings. (Procedure steps preceded by an asterisk are especially important.)

Steps

1. Explain the purpose of SMBG to the patient.

2. Teach the patient how to perform the procedure by following the steps below:
(a) Using a sterile lancet, obtain a drop of blood from the fingertip.
(b) Place the drop of blood on the testing strip. Follow the manufacturer's directions for wiping and timing the strip.
*(c) To use a visual method, compare the color block on the strip to the color chart on the package. (If the strip color appears between the printed colors, you may average a reading between two amounts.)
*(d) To use a meter, check the exact digital reading that appears after the strip is inserted (the color change is measured electronically). Calibrate the machine by comparing the numbers on the bottle with the numbers on the machine.

*3. Instruct the patient to document the results (blood glucose level) along with the date and time. If the patient has signs or symptoms suggesting hyperglycemia or made recent changes in diet, exercise, or insulin dosage, instruct the patient to document this change.

Rationales

1. The patient must assume responsibility for the procedure at home.

2. The patient must follow the steps carefully to ensure an accurate reading.
(a) Sterility prevents infection.

(b) Accuracy of results depends on following directions precisely.

*(c) The reading is an approximation made by determining the color on the chart that most closely matches the color on the strip.

*(d) The meter method may be preferred because it is more accurate. However, this method costs more.

*3. The patient must bring accurate records to the next health care appointment or share them with the visiting nurse to ensure proper diabetes management.

ADULT NURSING

*4. Teach the patient how to apply SMBG results. If insulin dose depends on the blood glucose level, make sure the patient can describe the proper dose to take.

*4. A sliding scale sometimes is used to determine each insulin dose based on the blood glucose level at the time of administration. Some physicians increase or decrease the insulin dose based on SMBG results.

5. Document the content taught and the patient's response to teaching, noting any additional teaching needed.

5. Documentation proves the teaching was done, assures high-quality care, and provides legal protection.

Assisting with the glucose tolerance test

Introduction

The glucose tolerance test is used to diagnose diabetes mellitus. Blood and urine glucose levels are measured while the patient fasts, then at 30-minute, 1-hour, 2-hour, and 3-hour intervals after the patient drinks a high-carbohydrate beverage. Normally, urine is negative for glucose. In a healthy person, the blood glucose level rises slightly 1 hour after drinking the beverage but drops back to normal by the time the 2-hour specimen is collected. With glucose intolerance, such as in diabetes mellitus, the blood glucose level rises faster and higher, becoming elevated at 2 hours and remaining higher longer.

In pregnant and elderly people, normal test results may differ from the usual range. A shortened version of this test commonly is ordered to screen pregnant patients for gestational diabetes. (Procedure steps preceded by an asterisk are especially important.)

Steps

*1. Instruct the patient to eat high-carbohydrate meals for 3 days before the test and to fast overnight on the night before the test. Provide written instructions, if needed. Explain that the patient may need to stop taking such medications as steroids, diuretics, or estrogens for 3 days before the test.

Rationales

*1. Eating high-carbohydrate meals for 3 days before the test helps ensure predictable use of the carbohydrate taken during the test. A fasting blood glucose level helps establish a baseline. These medications may alter glucose metabolism.

2. After fasting blood samples and urine specimens have been obtained, assist the patient to drink the high-carbohydrate beverage, then to rest comfortably while the test is in progress.

2. The sweet drink taken on an empty stomach may cause nausea; a comfortable position may help the patient tolerate the test. If vomiting occurs, the test must be stopped.

3. Reassure the patient as specimens are taken at various intervals. Make sure the patient consumes only water until the test is completed.

3. Activity or eating could alter test results.

4. Document the procedure and the disposition of the samples and specimens.

4. Documentation proves that the procedure was done, assures high-quality care, and provides legal protection.

ADULT NURSING

Assisting with the radioactive iodine uptake test

Introduction

The radioactive iodine (^{131}I) uptake test determines how well the thyroid gland concentrates iodine. It is used in combination with other tests to diagnose thyroid cancer and other thyroid abnormalities, and may be used to determine how much ^{131}I a patient needs to treat a hyperthyroid condition. (Radioactive thyroid studies are contraindicated during pregnancy.)

In the test, the patient receives a small amount (tracer dose) of oral or I.V. ^{131}I. A thyroid scan, which shows iodine uptake in the thyroid, then helps locate and determine the size of a malfunctioning thyroid region. Iodine uptake is measured at varying intervals with an instrument (similar to a Geiger counter) held over the thyroid gland at the anterior neck region. In some cases, urine specimens are collected to determine the amount of iodine excreted. Iodine uptake increases with an overactive thyroid and decreases with an underactive thyroid. (Procedure steps preceded by an asterisk are especially important.)

Steps

*1. Provide reassurance that the test will not cause the patient to become radioactive. Encourage the patient to cooperate with the test.

*2. Instruct the patient to eliminate iodine from the diet for 1 week before the test—for example, by avoiding iodized salt and stopping any iodine-containing medications (including skin antiseptics and multivitamin preparations), as ordered.

3. Ask if the patient uses any iodine-containing substances; note the use of any such substances on the laboratory requisition form. Also note any X-ray studies involving organic iodides as a contrast medium.

4. If urine specimens are needed, ensure accurate collection. (In some cases, all urine for 24 or 48 hours must be saved.)

5. Document the procedure and the disposition of any specimens taken.

Rationales

*1. Although the nurse is not involved with the test directly, these nursing measures may help ensure valid test results.

*2. The thyroid gland responds to small amounts of iodine. Other iodine sources may render test results inaccurate.

3. Iodine-containing substances may alter thyroid function.

4. To determine thyroid iodine uptake, the amount of iodine excreted in the urine is subtracted from the amount administered. Lost urine specimens would alter test results.

5. Documentation proves that the procedure was done, assures high-quality care, and provides legal protection.

ADULT NURSING

Collecting 24-hour urine specimens

Introduction   In this procedure, the nurse collects all urine produced by the kidneys during a 24-hour period. Quantitative tests then are conducted to determine how much of a specific substance (such as a hormone) the patient excretes during a 24-hour period. (Procedure steps preceded by an asterisk are especially important.)

Steps

*1. Obtain a container large enough to hold all urine voided over 24 hours. If a preservative or other chemical is needed, obtain it from the laboratory and add it to the container. If the specimens must be refrigerated, use a specimen refrigerator or keep the container in a basin of ice until the collection is completed.

2. Label the container clearly with the patient's name, along with the date and time when the collection began.

*3. Start the collection by having the patient empty the bladder and discard that urine specimen. Note the exact time of this voiding.

*4. Instruct the patient to collect and save all urine voided for the next 24 hours by voiding into a clean container and pouring the urine into the large collection bottle.

*5. Collect and save the last specimen 24 hours from the time the test began.

6. Document the procedure.

Rationales

*1. Urine must be collected for 24 hours. A preservative or refrigeration may be needed for diagnostic testing. (Refer to laboratory instructions.)

2. This information helps prevent errors.

*3. The collection must consist of urine produced during the specified period. Urine in the bladder at the start of the test was produced before the specified period began.

*4. This instruction is needed because discarding even one specimen during the specified period invalidates the test.

*5. The patient must empty the bladder when the test ends to ensure that all urine produced during the 24-hour period is included.

6. Documentation proves that the procedure was done, assures high-quality care, and provides legal protection.

ADULT NURSING

Drugs used to treat endocrine disorders

This chart presents information about drugs commonly prescribed for endocrine disorders, including the drug action, dosage, and common side effects. Nursing considerations focus on patient comfort and teaching.

DRUG	ACTION	USUAL ADULT DOSAGE	COMMON SIDE EFFECTS	NURSING CONSIDERATIONS
Oral hypoglycemics				
Acetohex-amide (Dymelor)	• Stimulates insulin release from the pancreas • Acts on insulin receptors and cells to increase peripheral glucose use	250 mg to 1 g P.O. in a single daily dose (divided doses may give better glycemic control); may give up to 1.5 g/day in divided doses	• Hypoglycemia • Nausea • Vomiting • Heartburn • Hepatic problems • Epigastric distress • Rash • Weakness	• This drug is less likely than insulin to cause hypoglycemia (although that condition may occur if the patient receives a large dose or decreases food intake). • This drug is contraindicated in patients who are pregnant, allergic to sulfonylureas or thiazides, or have Type I diabetes. • Duration of action is 12 to 24 hours. • Instruct the patient to limit alcohol intake. • Teach the patient that this drug does not cure diabetes. • Help the patient maintain the prescribed diet and exercise program. • Teach the patient not to skip meals. • Observe for hyperglycemia or hypoglycemia. • Warn the patient to avoid alcohol because a mild disulfuram-like reaction may occur.
Chlorprop-amide (Diabinese)	• Stimulates insulin release from the pancreas • Acts on insulin receptors and cells to increase peripheral glucose use	100 to 500 mg/day P.O. (Use divided doses if the patient is receiving 250 mg/day or more.)	• Hypoglycemia • Low serum sodium level • Hypersensitivity • Hepatic problems • Epigastric distress • Rash	• This drug is less likely than insulin to cause hypoglycemia (although this condition may occur if the patient receives a large dose or decreases food intake). • This drug is contraindicated in patients who are pregnant or allergic to sulfonylureas or thiazides. • Duration of action is 1 to 2 days. Prolonged action may cause delayed hypoglycemia. • Teach the patient that this drug does not cure diabetes. • Use cautiously in patients with renal compromise because the drug may accumulate. • Monitor glucose levels. • Help the patient maintain the prescribed diet and exercise program. • Teach the patient not to skip meals. • Observe for hyperglycemia or hypoglycemia. • Warn the patient to avoid alcohol because a disulfuram-like reaction ("chlorpropamide flush") may occur.

Drugs used to treat endocrine disorders *(continued)*

DRUG	ACTION	USUAL ADULT DOSAGE	COMMON SIDE EFFECTS	NURSING CONSIDERATIONS
Oral hypoglycemics *(continued)*				
Glipizide (Glucotrol)	• Stimulates insulin release from the pancreas • Acts on insulin receptors and cells to increase peripheral glucose use	5 mg P.O. in a single daily dose. May increase dosage gradually to a maximum of 40 mg/day. Use divided doses if the daily dose is above 15 mg.	• Hypoglycemia • Hepatic problems • Jaundice • Epigastric distress • Dizziness • Rash	• This drug is less likely than insulin to cause hypoglycemia (although this condition may occur if the patient receives a large dose or decreases food intake). • This drug is contraindicated in patients with ketoacidosis and in those who are allergic to sulfonylureas or thiazides. • This drug is not recommended in pregnant patients. • Duration of action is 12 to 24 hours. • This drug is a second-generation oral hypoglycemic agent and is given in lower dosages than first-generation agents. • Teach the patient that this drug does not cure diabetes. • Help the patient maintain the prescribed diet and exercise program. • Teach the patient not to skip meals. • Observe for hyperglycemia or hypoglycemia.
Glyburide (DiaBeta, Micronase)	• Stimulates insulin release from the pancreas • Acts on insulin receptors and cells to increase peripheral glucose use	2.5 to 5 mg P.O. in a single daily dose	• Hypoglycemia • Hepatic problems • Epigastric distress • Rash	• This drug is less likely than insulin to cause hypoglycemia (although this condition may occur if the patient receives a large dose or decreases food intake). • This drug is contraindicated in patients with ketoacidosis and in those who are allergic to sulfonylureas or thiazides. • Duration of action is 24 hours. • This drug is a second-generation oral hypoglycemic agent and is given in lower dosages than first-generation agents. • Teach the patient that this drug does not cure diabetes. • Help the patient maintain the prescribed diet and exercise program. • Teach the patient not to skip meals. • Observe for hyperglycemia or hypoglycemia.
Tolazamide (Tolinase)	• Stimulates insulin release from the pancreas • Acts on insulin receptors and cells to increase peripheral glucose use	100 to 250 mg P.O. in a single daily dose; may give up to 1 g/day in divided doses	• Hypoglycemia • Rash • Urticaria • Hepatic problems • Epigastric distress	• This drug is less likely than insulin to cause hypoglycemia (although this condition may occur if the patient receives a large dose or decreases food intake). • This drug is contraindicated in patients with Type I diabetes and in those who are allergic to sulfonylureas or thiazides. • This drug is not recommended during pregnancy. • Duration of action is 10 to 16 hours. • Teach the patient that this drug does not cure diabetes. • Help the patient maintain the prescribed diet and exercise program. • Teach the patient not to skip meals. • Observe for hyperglycemia or hypoglycemia. • Warn the patient to avoid alcohol because a disulfuram-like reaction may occur.

(continued)

ADULT NURSING

Drugs used to treat endocrine disorders *(continued)*

DRUG	ACTION	USUAL ADULT DOSAGE	COMMON SIDE EFFECTS	NURSING CONSIDERATIONS
Oral hypoglycemics *(continued)*				
Tolbutamide (Orinase)	● Stimulates insulin release from the pancreas ● Acts on insulin receptors and cells to increase peripheral glucose use	250 mg to 3 g/day P.O. in divided doses	● Hypoglycemia ● Rash ● Hepatic problems ● Epigastric distress	● This drug is less likely than insulin to cause hypoglycemia (although this condition may occur if the patient receives a large dose or decreases food intake). ● This drug is short acting, with a duration of 6 to 12 hours. ● This drug is not recommended during pregnancy. ● Instruct the patient to avoid alcohol because this may cause a disulfuram-like reaction. ● Teach the patient to take the drug as prescribed. ● Teach the patient that this drug does not cure diabetes. ● Watch for drug sensitivity. ● Help the patient maintain the prescribed diet and exercise program. ● Teach the patient not to skip meals. ● Observe for hyperglycemia or hypoglycemia. ● Use cautiously in patients who are allergic to sulfonylureas or thiazides.
Antithyroid drugs				
Thiamide drugs				
Methimazole (Tapazole)	Inhibits thyroid hormone production	● Adults: 15 to 60 mg/day P.O. in divided doses initially, then 5 to 15 mg/day for maintenance ● Children: 0.4 mg/kg/day initially, then 0.2 mg/kg/day for maintenance	● Blood dyscrasias ● Headache ● Dizziness ● Hepatitis	● This drug is contraindicated in lactating patients. ● Use with caution in pregnant patients. ● Euthyroidism (normal thyroid function) may take weeks or months. ● Therapeutic effects occur in 1 to 2 weeks. ● Watch for signs and symptoms of hypothyroidism. ● Teach the patient to report sore throat or mouth sores. ● Instruct the patient to take with meals to avoid GI distress.
Propylthiouracil (PTU)	● Inhibits thyroid hormone production ● Used to treat hyperthyroidism and thyroid storm, before or after radioactive iodine therapy, or as preoperative preparation for thyroidectomy	● Adults: 150 to 300 mg/day P.O. in divided doses initially, then 100 to 150 mg/day in divided doses for maintenance ● Children: dosage depends on age	● Hypothyroidism ● Blood disorders (agranulocytosis is the most severe adverse reaction) ● Skin rash, itching ● Headache ● Nausea ● Hepatitis	● This drug is contraindicated in lactating patients. ● Therapeutic effects occur in 1 to 2 weeks. ● Euthyroidism (normal thyroid function) may take weeks to months. ● This drug may be taken for 1 year or longer. ● Instruct the patient to take with meals to avoid GI distress.

ADULT NURSING

Drugs used to treat endocrine disorders *(continued)*

DRUG	ACTION	USUAL ADULT DOSAGE	COMMON SIDE EFFECTS	NURSING CONSIDERATIONS
Antithyroid drugs *(continued)*				
Iodine preparations				
Strong Iodine Solution, USP (Lugol's solution)	• Blocks thyroid hormone production	2 to 6 drops P.O. t.i.d.	• Nausea • Vomiting • Metallic taste • Tooth discoloration	• Dilute dose in water. • Give after meals. • Warn the patient not to stop taking this drug abruptly. • Store in a dark container.
Potassium iodide solution (SSKI)	• Inhibits thyroid hormone release • Decreases thyroid size and vascularity before thyroidectomy	2 to 6 drops P.O. t.i.d.	• Iodism (metallic taste, burning mouth, hypersalivation, headache) • Hypersensitivity (rash, itching)	• To reduce gastric irritation and prevent tooth staining, dilute the solution in a full glass of fruit juice or milk and have the patient drink it through a straw. • Therapeutic effects appear in 24 hours but may last only a few weeks.
Radioactive iodine (sodium iodide) [131]I	• Destroys thyroid tissue, permanently decreasing thyroid hormone production; used to treat thyroid cancer or hyperthyroidism	For hypothyroidism, 4 to 10 millicuries given in a single P.O. dose (may be repeated in 6 weeks). For thyroid cancer, 50 to 150 millicuries P.O. in a single dose	• Permanent hypothyroidism	• Urine and saliva may be radioactive for up to 6 weeks. Institute precautions as ordered. • Therapeutic effects may be delayed for up to 6 months. In the meantime, the patient typically receives thiamide drugs or propranolol to control symptoms. • This drug is contraindicated in pregnant and lactating patients.
Other medications				
Propranolol (Inderal)	• Blocks sympathetic nervous stimulation in such organs as the heart, helping to control hyperthyroid symptoms (does not affect thyroid function or hormone secretion)	40 to 160 mg/day P.O. in divided doses	• Bradycardia • Hypotension • Bronchospasm	• This drug is discontinued when other treatments control hyperthyroid symptoms.

INTEGUMENTARY SYSTEM

Anatomy and physiology

I.   **Anatomy:** The integumentary system includes the skin and skin appendages
   A. The skin has three layers
      1. The epidermis is the outer layer
         a. Lacking blood vessels of its own, it obtains blood from (and eliminates wastes through) the dermis below
         b. It contains two types of cells
            (1) Melanocytes
            (2) Keratinocytes
      2. The dermis is the middle layer
         a. It is composed of collagen fibers that give strength to the skin
         b. It contains blood vessels, nerves, lymph channels, hair follicles, sweat glands, and sebaceous glands
      3. The subcutaneous layer (hypodermis), composed of fat cells and loose connective tissue, is the innermost layer
   B. Skin appendages include the hair, nails, and three types of glands—apocrine, eccrine, and sebaceous glands

---

Reviewing the integumentary system

This illustration shows the structures of the skin and skin layers.

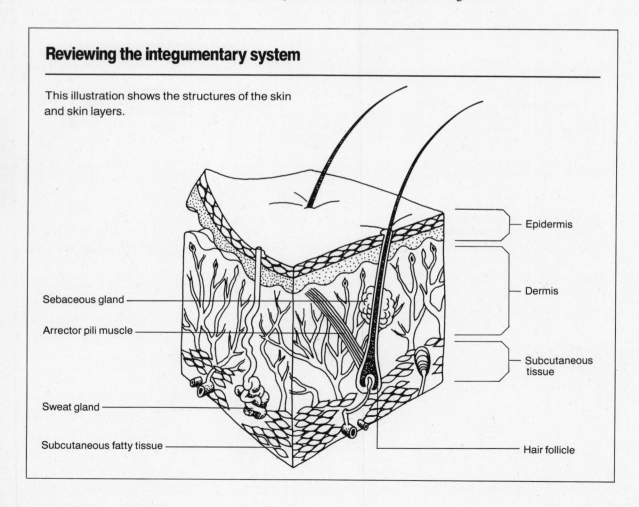

- Sebaceous gland
- Arrector pili muscle
- Sweat gland
- Subcutaneous fatty tissue

- Epidermis
- Dermis
- Subcutaneous tissue
- Hair follicle

Glossary

Alopecia: hair loss
Comedo: blackhead or whitehead containing organisms and skin debris in enlarged skin openings
Ecchymosis: discoloration of a skin area caused by blood extravasation into the subcutaneous tissue
Excoriation: superficial scraping or excavation of the epidermis
Hirsutism: male hair distribution in a woman or child caused by heredity, abnormal adrenal function, or certain medications
Jaundice: yellowish skin discoloration
Keloid: overgrowth of scar tissue at a skin wound site
Malignant melanoma: cancerous skin tumor
Pruritus: itching sensation
Tenting: failure of the skin to return to a normal position immediately after gentle pinching

II. **Physiology**
   A. The skin has important functions
      1. It protects tissues below skin surfaces
      2. It regulates body heat
         a. Vasodilation cools the body
         b. Vasoconstriction keeps heat in the body
      3. It allows sensation so that the body can detect pain, touch, pressure, and temperature
      4. It serves as the site of vitamin D conversion (epidermis)
      5. It provides heat and cold insulation (through fat cells)
      6. It absorbs shocks and insulates the body (hypodermis)
      7. It serves an aesthetic function, giving a person an individual identity
   B. The glands of the skin have distinct functions
      1. The apocrine glands secrete substances that have a distinct odor and bacterial action
      2. The eccrine glands secrete sweat to help regulate body heat
      3. The sebaceous glands secrete sebum into the hair shafts

ADULT
NURSING

Third-degree burn

Overview

Over 2 million Americans suffer burns each year. In 3% to 5% of these cases, the injury is life threatening. Burn injury is the second leading cause of death in young children and the fourth overall cause of accidental death for all ages. (To compare first-degree, second-degree, and third-degree burns, see *Assessing burn injury,* page 422.)

Clinical situation

Colleen Kennedy, a waitress, age 24, suffers severe burns over her arms and chest in a grease fire at the restaurant where she works. She is admitted to the burn unit of a large hospital with third-degree burns over 10% of her body and first- and second-degree burns over 10% of her arms and chest.

Assessing burn injury

Burns are identified by the depth of loss of skin layers or area affected. This chart lists each burn degree with depth of loss and features.

BURN DEGREE	BURN DEPTH	FEATURES
First-degree (superficial)	Epidermal destruction	• Redness • Blanching with pressure • Slight edema • Pain
Second-degree (partial-thickness)	Destruction of the epidermis and part of the dermis	• Blisters • Skin redness with blanching when pressure is applied • Pain
Third-degree (full-thickness)	Destruction of all skin layers and skin appendages	• Charring • Brown, black, or reddish skin appearance • Hard, leathery skin texture • Lack of pain
Fourth-degree	Destruction of all skin layers, skin appendages, muscles, nerves, and bone	• Possible loss of whole body parts or areas

---

Assessment

Nursing behaviors

1. Assess Ms. Kennedy's airway and breathing. Check for smoke marks around her nostrils and mouth.

2. Assess Ms. Kennedy's vital signs, taking her temperature rectally.

3. In conjunction with the physician, assess Ms. Kennedy's skin to determine burn depth and estimate the areas involved.

4. Assess Ms. Kennedy's level of consciousness.

5. Assess Ms. Kennedy for painful sites, noting any complaints of pain.

Nursing rationales

1. Airway patency is crucial to treatment of a burn. Ms. Kennedy may have inhaled toxic substances or smoke from the fire.

2. Vital signs may indicate shock caused by fluid loss or severe sudden injury. (For more information on shock, see the section on "Nursing principles.") Rectal temperature is more accurate than oral temperature.

3. The physician estimates the burn degree and the percentage of total body surface area (TBSA) burned. (For details on evaluating burns, see *Assessing burn injury,* and *Using the rule of nines to determine burn extent.*)

4. Level of consciousness reflects the adequacy of brain perfusion.

5. First- and second-degree burns are painful; third-degree burns are not.

Nursing diagnoses
- Fluid volume deficit related to blood, serum, and electrolyte loss
- Impaired tissue integrity related to third-degree burns

Using the rule of nines to determine burn extent

The rule of nines is used to rapidly estimate the extent of an adult patient's burn injury. This technique divides the body into percentages that equal 100% when totaled. For example, burns affecting both anterior forearms would amount to a 9% burn. The total percentage, a rough estimate of the extent of the patient's burns, is factored into a formula to determine initial fluid replacement needs.

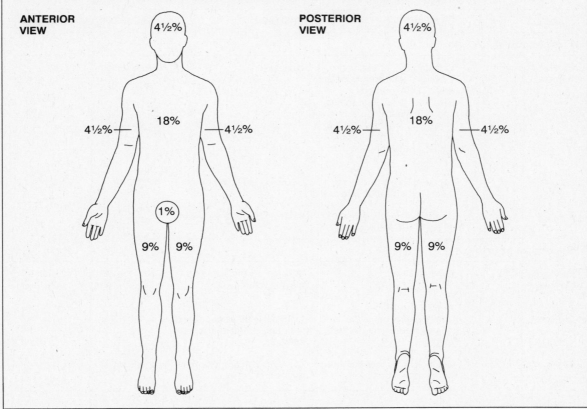

ANTERIOR VIEW

4½%

4½%   18%   4½%

1%

9%   9%

POSTERIOR VIEW

4½%

4½%   18%   4½%

9%   9%

Planning and goals	• Ms. Kennedy will regain skin integrity with treatment.
	• Ms. Kennedy will regain fluid and electrolyte balance with treatment.
	• Ms. Kennedy will remain free from infection in burned areas.
	• Ms. Kennedy will avoid burn complications.
	• Ms. Kennedy will regain a positive body image and self-esteem.

Implementation

Nursing behaviors

1. Assess Ms. Kennedy's vital signs every 15 to 30 minutes.

2. Monitor I.V. therapy closely.

Nursing rationales

1. Vital signs change rapidly during the early postburn period from fluid shifts and possible shock.

2. I.V. therapy is critical after a burn injury. As ordered, administer I.V. fluid according to specific formulas. (For details, see *Fluid replacement formulas for adults with burns,* page 424.)

ADULT NURSING

Fluid replacement formulas for adults with burns

Fluid replacement formulas for burn patients involve crystalloids, colloids, and blood or blood cells. Crystalloids — solutions containing water and electrolytes — restore extracellular fluid volume. Colloids (also called plasma expanders) are protein solutions, such as plasma, plasma protein fraction (Plasmanate), or albumin. Blood and blood cells are given during later resuscitation or during recovery.

FORMULA	CRYSTALLOIDS	COLLOIDS	GLUCOSE IN WATER
First 24 hours			
Parkland (Baxter formula)	Lactated Ringer's solution 4 ml/kg/% total body surface area (TBSA) burned Give one-half of total solution during the first 8 hours, one-quarter during the second 8 hours, and the remaining one-quarter during the third 8 hours.	None given	None given
Brooke	Lactated Ringer's solution; 1.5 ml/kg/% TBSA burned	0.5 ml/kg/% TBSA burned	2,000 ml
Evans	Normal saline solution; 1.0 ml/kg/% TBSA burned	1.0 ml/kg/% TBSA burned	2,000 ml
Second 24 hours			
Parkland (Baxter formula)	None given	20% to 60% of calculated plasma volume	Enough dextrose in water to keep the serum sodium level below 140 mEq/liter
Brooke	One-half to three-quarters of the requirement for the first 24 hours	One-half to three-quarters of the requirement for the first 24 hours	2,000 ml
Evans	One-half of the requirement for the first 24 hours	One-half of the requirement for the first 24 hours	2,000 ml

3. Monitor Ms. Kennedy's urine output by catheter every 30 minutes to 1 hour.

4. Monitor Ms. Kennedy's central venous pressure (CVP).

5. Monitor laboratory results, including serum potassium, serum sodium, and blood urea nitrogen levels.

3. Urine output is a key index of the adequacy of both fluid replacement and renal perfusion.

4. CVP is an important index of fluid balance. Normally, CVP ranges from 5 to 13 cm H_2O. A measurement under 5 cm H_2O indicates insufficient fluid replacement; over 13 cm H_2O, excessive fluid replacement.

5. Close monitoring is crucial to recovery and ongoing care. In a burn patient, cell wall destruction in burned areas causes an above-normal serum potassium level (the normal level ranges from 3.5 to 5 mEq/liter). The serum sodium level may drop from loss in burned areas. Electrolyte balances vary with fluid replacement, fluid and electrolyte shifts into burned areas and, later, fluid return from burned areas into the bloodstream. Burn patients develop negative nitrogen balance during the early post-burn stage.

ADULT NURSING

6. Monitor Ms. Kennedy's fluid intake and output closely.

6. This is necessary because fluid shifts into burned areas in the first 24 to 48 hours after a burn injury, then returns to the bloodstream after 48 to 72 hours. Also, the burn patient risks hypovolemic shock. Urine output, which should measure 30 to 50 ml/ hour, reflects renal perfusion.

7. Administer tetanus antitoxin and tetanus immune globulin, tetanus toxoid, or both, as ordered, during the initial post-burn period.

7. Tetanus antitoxin and immune globulin provide passive immunity (antibodies) against tetanus infection. Tetanus toxoid provides denatured tetanus bacteria that allow the patient to build up active immunity to tetanus.

8. Monitor Ms. Kennedy's level of consciousness every 4 hours, as indicated, until she is stable.

8. Level of consciousness is a key index of cerebral perfusion.

9. Monitor Ms. Kennedy's breath sounds and breathing patterns closely.

9. Breath sounds should be heard clearly in all lobes. Decreased or noisy breath sounds may indicate fluid in the lungs, which could cause pulmonary edema from massive fluid replacement, smoke inhalation, or toxic fume inhalation. Report any breathing pattern changes to the nurse-manager and physician in charge. Oxygen may be ordered to treat an inhalation injury.

10. Monitor nasogastric (NG) tube drainage, if appropriate. Check drainage for blood.

10. An NG tube may be inserted to prevent vomiting (from narcotics or carbon monoxide inhalation) or gastric dilation related to trauma or stress reaction. Bloody drainage may indicate a stress ulcer.

11. Monitor and assist with burn dressing changes and application of topical medication, if ordered.

11. Ms. Kennedy may be in isolation on the burn unit. Silver nitrate, silver sulfadiazine, or mefenide acetate may be applied two or more times daily after she showers, undergoes debridement, or is cleaned in the Hubbard tank.

12. Administer narcotic analgesics every 3 to 4 hours, as ordered, or monitor Ms. Kennedy's use of a patient-controlled analgesia pump with the ordered analgesic.

12. First- and second-degree burns cause intense pain, necessitating analgesia. (As ordered, administer an analgesic about 30 minutes before dressing changes to reduce patient discomfort during this procedure.)

13. Perform active or passive range-of-motion exercises in unaffected joints every 4 to 6 hours. Apply splints to maintain joints in the required positions.

13. These exercises help maintain joint function and muscle strength. Splints keep joints extended or slightly flexed in functional positions. Exercises and splints help prevent flexion contractures (from scar contraction).

14. Monitor Ms. Kennedy's total parenteral nutrition (TPN) intake, if administered. Change the dressing at the catheter insertion site, as required.

14. TPN helps maintain nutrition until the patient can receive oral nourishment. Usually, the dressing at the catheter insertion site must be changed every second or third day.

ADULT NURSING

15. Help feed Ms. Kennedy when she resumes oral intake, if she needs assistance.

15. The burn patient must obtain sufficient calories, proteins, and carbohydrates to restore nutritional balance. Ms. Kennedy may need up to 6,000 calories a day.

16. Monitor Ms. Kennedy's bowel sounds and abdominal girth every 4 hours until she is stable, then every 8 hours, as indicated.

16. Bowel sounds may decrease from lack of oral intake or injury-related stress. They should be audible in all four abdominal quadrants.

17. Monitor Ms. Kennedy's bowel elimination pattern and check her stool for blood. If she is constipated, obtain an order for a suppository.

17. Burn trauma or lack of food intake may cause constipation. Blood in the stool may signal a stress ulcer—a common burn complication. A suppository softens hard stools for easier passage.

18. Prepare Ms. Kennedy for skin grafts. (For more information on preoperative preparation, see the section on "Perioperative nursing.")

18. New skin grows from the skin epidermis and dermis. Skin grafts are needed for third-degree burns that do not heal by granulation tissue because the dermis and epidermis have been destroyed. (For more information on skin grafts, see *Comparing skin grafts*.)

Comparing skin grafts

A skin graft may be named for its depth, source, or shape.

GRAFT	DESCRIPTION
Split-thickness	• Derived from an uninvolved body area (autograft) • May consist of a strip or small pieces of skin (postage-stamp size)
Full-thickness	• Composed of all skin layers
Mesh graft	• Split-thickness graft made into a meshlike graft with a special instrument, then pulled apart to cover a larger burn area
Homograft	• Taken from the skin of a dead person (allograft) • Used temporarily for skin cover
Heterograft	• Made from animal (pig) skin or synthetic material
Autologous cultured human epithelium	• Made from the patient's healthy epidermal cells grown into sheets in a culture flask. The cultured sheets are attached to petrolatum gauze squares and sutured into place over the burned area, then removed in 7 to 10 days.
Tube graft	• Full-thickness graft shaped into a tube, which is moved in stages to other body areas until reaching the area needing the graft

19. Monitor skin graft donor sites for signs of inflammation, infection, and healing.

19. Removal of the top skin layer at the donor site of a split-thickness graft causes marked pain. Expect clear or serosanguineous drainage. The site will be covered with petrolatum (Vaseline) gauze or a clear dressing (Op-Site). In 2 to 3 days, pain decreases and some granulation appears. The site usually closes in 2 weeks.

20. Assist Ms. Kennedy out of bed and during ambulation, when ordered.

20. How soon the patient can get out of bed and ambulate depends on the extent of burn and the patient's overall status. Ambulation helps maintain muscle strength and mass.

21. Listen to Ms. Kennedy as she expresses her concerns, anger, or sadness over her burn scars or disfigurement.

21. By listening, the nurse can determine if Ms. Kennedy's response to her situation is appropriate. If it is not, she may need a referral for counseling.

22. Involve Ms. Kennedy in decision making about her own care, when possible.

22. Active participation in decisions increases the patient's sense of control.

23. Teach Ms. Kennedy about nutrition, or obtain assistance from the dietitian.

23. Ms. Kennedy must increase her intake of carbohydrates, proteins, vitamins, and minerals to restore nutritional balances and regain a positive nitrogen balance. Teaching improves dietary compliance.

Evaluation (outcomes)

• Ms. Kennedy regains skin integrity over third-degree burn sites with topical medication and skin grafts.
• Ms. Kennedy regains fluid and electrolyte balance with I.V. therapy, electrolyte replacement, and proper nutritional intake.
• Ms. Kennedy remains free from infection at burn sites with aseptic technique, sterile dressings, and antibiotic therapy.
• Ms. Kennedy remains free from stress ulcers, contractures, and other burn complications.
• Ms. Kennedy gradually regains a positive body image and self-esteem by expressing her concerns and obtaining counseling.

ADULT NURSING

Complications of burns

This chart presents the most serious or life-threatening complications of burns, along with interventions that are crucial to patient safety and comfort.

COMPLICATION	CAUSE	NURSING INTERVENTIONS
Localized infection of the burn; systemic infection (septicemia) Development of an infection at the burn site or a generalized infection after a burn. Signs and symptoms include high, spiking temperatures; chills; and drainage and pus at the burn site.	*Staphylococcus* or *Pseudomonas* organisms	• Use strict aseptic technique when caring for the burn. • Administer I.V. antibiotics, as ordered, to combat infection. • Administer antipyretic medication (such as acetaminophen), as ordered, to combat fever. • Check vital signs frequently. • Keep the patient's gown and bed linens dry.
Poor body temperature regulation Signs and symptoms include chills followed by high fevers.	High body temperature secondary to an infected burn	• Use strict aseptic technique when providing care for the burn. • Administer I.V. antibiotics, as ordered, to combat infection. • Administer antipyretic medication (such as acetaminophen), as ordered, to combat fever. • Check vital signs frequently. • Keep the patient's gown and bed linens dry.
Electrolyte imbalance Low serum sodium and potassium levels. (For signs and symptoms, see the section on "Fluids and electrolytes.")	Sodium and potassium loss from the burn site	• Monitor serum electrolyte levels closely. • Administer sodium and potassium replacements, as ordered.
Contractures Abnormal joint flexion. This complication manifests as acute joint flexion (bending), preventing full joint extension.	• Lack of proper range-of-motion (ROM) exercises • Scar contraction, which draws joints into acute flexion	• Perform ROM exercises on involved joints, when possible. • Use splints to help maintain arms and legs in a neutral position. • Have the patient exercise while in the Hubbard tank (joints move more easily under water). • Place the patient on a CircOlectric bed to help keep joints extended. • Arrange for a consultation with a physical therapist to develop an exercise regimen.
Stress ulcer Ulcer in the stomach or intestines. Signs and symptoms include bloody emesis, occult blood in stool, and abdominal pain or distention.	Stress related to burn injury	• Check vomitus and stool for blood. • Measure abdominal girth. • Auscultate bowel sounds. • Withhold foods and fluids, as ordered. • Maintain nasogastric tube patency. • Monitor vital signs.

Caring for pressure ulcers

Introduction

Pressure ulcers (ulcerated skin areas) require specialized nursing care—possibly involving multiple treatments. Besides the care described below, such treatments may include magnesium hydroxide (with the ulcer left uncovered), heat lamp treatments, karaya powder, vitamin A & D ointment, povidone-iodine (Betadine), powder with hydrophilic beads that draw drainage from the ulcer to create a clean surface for healing, massage, and special mattresses or bed pads to reduce pressure. To prevent pressure ulcers, the preferred treatment is turning every 2 hours. (Procedure steps preceded by an asterisk are especially important.)

Steps

*1. Gather needed supplies: sterile 4″ × 3″ bandages, sterile basin, hydrogen peroxide, normal saline solution, sterile 50-ml syringe, sterile gloves, plastic or paper bag, karaya pad (Stomadhesive), and linen-saver pad.

*2. Explain to the patient that the sore area will be treated.

3. Close the curtain in the patient's room.

*4. Turn the patient onto the side, if the ulcer is in the sacral area. Otherwise, position the patient so that the ulcer is fully visible.

5. Arrange the supplies on the overbed table.

6. Remove any dressing, check it for drainage, and discard it in the plastic bag. Place this bag in a second bag.

*7. Wash your hands.

8. Open the sterile supplies. Pour half of the saline solution and half of the hydrogen peroxide into the sterile basin.

*9. Assess the condition of the ulcer and any drainage. Place the linen-saver pad under the ulcer site.

*10. Put on the sterile gloves.

Rationales

*1. Ulcer severity may dictate which supplies are needed. (In a stage I ulcer, skin appears red and does not return to its normal color with massage or relief of pressure. In a stage II ulcer, skin is blistered, peeling, or cracked. In a stage III ulcer, skin is broken and loses its full thickness; drainage may appear. A stage IV ulcer is deep and craterlike.)

*2. Explanations reduce patient anxiety.

3. This provides privacy during the procedure.

*4. A side-lying position permits a clear view of an ulcer in the sacral area.

5. Keeping supplies within easy reach facilitates the procedure.

6. The dressing will be full of drainage, which may contain pus.

*7. This reduces the spread of microorganisms.

8. Surgical aseptic technique keeps inner surfaces sterile. Hydrogen peroxide destroys pathogens through its oxidizing action.

*9. Assessment allows comparison with previous data.

*10. This protects the nurse against contamination caused by splashing or drainage.

ADULT NURSING

*11. Draw up the solution into the syringe. Keep the dominant hand sterile for the syringe; use the other hand to hold the emesis basin under the ulcer.

*11. Gently spraying the solution into the ulcer avoids splashing. The emesis basin collects drainage and irrigating solution.

12. Gently flush the ulcer with irrigating solution. Use as much solution as needed to remove all drainage.

12. Removing as much drainage as possible creates a clean surface for tissue regrowth.

13. Remove irrigating fluid in the basin and gently pat the area dry. Note drainage color.

13. Patting dry reduces irritation of tender tissue, which has exposed nerve endings.

*14. Dry the skin around the ulcer thoroughly.

*14. This helps the karaya pad adhere to the site.

15. Remove the gloves. Then remove the adherent covering over the karaya pad to expose the adhesive surface.

15. Gloves must be removed because they would stick to the adhesive surface.

*16. Place the karaya pad over the ulcer site and press the edges firmly against the skin.

*16. Karaya contains an enzyme that promotes ulcer healing.

17. Remove the linen-saver pad and position the patient comfortably on the side.

17. The patient should not lie on the ulcer.

18. Place used supplies in the disposal bag, and place the bag in the trash area of the utility room.

18. Proper disposal helps prevent the spread of microorganisms.

*19. Document the care provided and the condition of the ulcer.

*19. Documentation proves that the procedure was done, assures high-quality care, and provides legal protection.

Drugs used to treat burns

This chart presents information about drugs commonly prescribed for burns, including the drug action, dosage, and common side effects. Nursing considerations focus on patient comfort and teaching.

DRUG	ACTION	USUAL ADULT DOSAGE	COMMON SIDE EFFECTS	NURSING CONSIDERATIONS
Aqueous penicillin	Kills bacteria by preventing synthesis of the cell wall	I.V. dosage varies; 1.2 to 24 million units daily in divided doses q 4 hours	• Nausea • Vomiting • Rash • Allergic reaction (rash)	• Observe for allergic reaction. • Administer all doses on schedule to maintain the proper blood drug level.
Gentamicin (Garamycin)	Kills bacteria by preventing protein synthesis by ribosomes	100,000 U/ml in oral suspension	• Nausea or gastric distress	This drug prevents overgrowth of fungal infections in the mouth or vagina secondary to antibiotic therapy.
Mafenide acetate (Sulfamylon) 5% ointment	Kills bacteria by interfering with cellular metabolism	Apply liberally over the burn.	• Metabolic acidosis • Allergic reaction • Local pain	Warn the patient that this drug causes pain when applied. Administer an analgesic, as ordered, before changing dressings.
Silver nitrate liquid	Denatures proteins causing nonspecific caustic or corrosive action	Apply in wet dressings over the burn.	• Local pain • Permanent silver skin discoloration (with prolonged use)	• Warn the patient that this drug causes pain when applied. Administer an analgesic, as ordered, before changing dressings. • This drug stains all materials on contact.
Topical silver sulfadiazine (Silvadene) ointment 1%	Kills bacteria by causing lysis of the cell wall	Apply liberally over the burn.	• Allergic reaction (rash) • Local pain	• Reassure the patient that the ointment is painless. • Observe for skin rash, which may result from an allergic reaction to sulfa.

IMMUNE SYSTEM

Anatomy and physiology

I. **Anatomy**
  A. The thymus is located in the mediastinum
  B. The spleen is located in the abdomen
  C. The tonsils, situated in the oropharynx, are rounded tissue masses of lymphoid tissue (similar to that of the thymus and spleen)
  D. Lymph nodes are small oval structures distributed throughout the body
  E. Lymphocytes and other cells also are components of the immune system

II. **Physiology**
  A. Immune system components have various functions
    1. The thymus is the site of T-lymphocyte development and maturation
    2. The spleen contains reservoirs of lymphocytes and macrophages that contribute to immunity
    3. Lymph nodes filter foreign material from the lymph and participate in immune cell development
  B. In response to invading antigens (foreign substances, usually proteins that generate an immune reaction), the immune system generates complex interrelated responses
    1. Most antigens are generated from the external environment (exogenous antigens)
      a. However, if the immune system fails to distinguish self from nonself, antigens may arise from within the body (endogenous antigens)
      b. Endogenous antigens are the basis of autoimmune reactions
    2. The body's response to an antigen results from maturation and activation of two types of immunocompetent cells, B lymphocytes and T lymphocytes, which originate from stem cells in the bone marrow
      a. Stem cells become T cells if they migrate to the thymus
      b. They become B cells if they migrate through a specific type of lymphoid tissue in the bone marrow
  C. The immune system defends the body against pathogenic invasion through three types of defenses
    1. Intact skin and mucous membranes represent one type of defense
    2. The two other defenses—humoral and cell-mediated immunity—are specific immune responses that are mobilized when an antigen breaches skin and mucous membrane barriers
      a. In humoral immunity, mature B lymphocytes (plasma cells) form antibodies (proteins called immunoglobulins) that respond to various antigens
        (1) Immunoglobulins involved in humoral immunity include IgM, IgG, IgA, IgD, and IgE
          (a) IgM is the first immunoglobulin produced in response to an antigen
          (b) IgG (gamma globulin), commonly found in the blood and tissues, appears as part of the primary response to antigen after IgM is produced. A major component of the secondary immune response (memory), IgG appears rapidly and is antigen specific

Immune response

The immune system generates two types of immune responses: cell mediated and humoral. The cell mediated response depends on the T lymphocyte (T cell) system; the humoral response, on B lymphocyte (B cell) activity. Below is a diagrammatic representation of both immune responses.

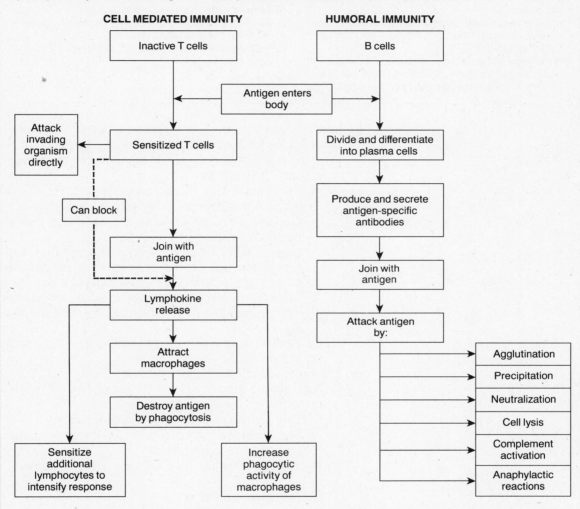

(c) IgA is found in such secretions such as bile, tears, sweat, saliva, and colostrum

(d) IgD, whose specific function is unknown, is found in serum tissue

(e) IgE, involved in hypersensitivity reactions, is responsible for allergic and anaphylactic reactions

(2) B lymphocytes subdivide to form clones, which develop receptors providing an antigen-specific response

(a) Exposure to an antigen induces B lymphocytes to trigger development of memory cells

(b) On the next exposure to the same antigen, a more rapid and powerful response occurs

(c) This is the principle behind many vaccinations

Glossary

Antibody: protein produced by the body to neutralize antigen toxins and inactivate microorganisms

Antigen: foreign substance that induces antibody formation

Immune response: complex series of physiologic events to protect the body from invasion by foreign substances

Immunoglobulin: protein produced by the body in response to antigens, attaching to the antigen, and rendering it easily destroyed by phagocytes

Phagocytosis: ingestion of foreign bodies, cells, or microbes by a phagocyte, a type of white blood cell (WBC)

T lymphocyte: type of lymphocyte that divides rapidly in the presence of infection; primarily responsible for cell-mediated immunity

Virus: minute microorganism that can reproduce only within a cell

  b. In cell-mediated immunity, T lymphocytes become sensitized and attack the invading cells (antigens)
    (1) Types of T lymphocytes include cytotoxic, helper, and suppressor T lymphocytes
      (a) Cytotoxic, or killer, T lymphocytes are effector cells that act directly on invading cells (antigens) by binding to them and releasing toxic substances that change their intracellular environment
      (b) Helper T (CD4 T cell) lymphocytes are regulatory T lymphocytes that stimulate B lymphocytes and probably act as trigger cells for the entire immune system
      (c) Suppressor T lymphocytes regulate the immune response through a negative feedback system, making it self-limiting
    (2) On exposure to an antigen, T lymphocytes increase in number and sensitivity
  c. The immune response also has other components
    (1) Null cells are lymphocytes that are neither B nor T lymphocytes
      (a) They perform without previous sensitization
      (b) They are active in immune surveillance (tumor rejection) and resistance to infection
    (2) Macrophages are white blood cells that perform phagocytosis
      (a) They process antigens
      (b) Then they present the processed antigens to helper T lymphocytes and immature T lymphocytes, which recognize the antigens and cause antibody formation
    (3) Complement consists of enzymes in the bloodstream that are activated in an antigen-antibody reaction
D. Immunity can be passive or active
  1. Passive immunity is acquired when a person receives antibodies from a sensitized person or animal (as in horse serum)
    a. No memory cells develop
    b. Therefore, passive immunity wears off
  2. Active immunity, which can occur naturally or from immunization, results when the body produces antibodies or sensitized lymphocytes on exposure to antigens

Acquired immunodeficiency syndrome

Overview

First recognized as a disease in 1981, acquired immunodeficiency syndrome (AIDS) is a severe immune deficiency that renders its victims unable to fight off life-threatening opportunistic infections and cancers. AIDS results from infection by the human immunodeficiency virus (HIV). The virus enters T lymphocytes, reproducing and damaging the cell. As viral reproduction progresses, immuno-compromise worsens.

Known transmission sources for HIV include the semen, blood, breast milk, and vaginal secretions of infected people. Transmission modes include exposure to infected blood and blood products, sexual contact, transplacental transmission (mother to fetus), perinatal transmission (mother to neonate), and breast-feeding. People at high risk for AIDS include I.V. drug abusers who share needles, sexual partners of infected people, patients who received blood transfusions before screening procedures were developed, and infants born to or breast-fed by infected females.

Clinical effects of HIV infection represent a broad continuum ranging from an asymptomatic HIV-positive state to mild symptoms to the acute problems of severe immune deficiency. The interval between initial HIV infection and the start of active clinical disease may range from 6 to 11 years. Authorities consider clinical disease to be present when the patient develops cancer or a life-threatening infection. The antiviral agent zidovudine (AZT; Retrovir) has proven effective in delaying symptom onset.

Clinical situation

Christine James, age 25, arrives at the health clinic complaining of shortness of breath, a hacking cough, and appetite loss. She has a history of I.V. drug abuse, and reports a weight loss of 15 lb (6.8 kg) over the last several months. Diagnostic tests reveal that she has *Pneumocystis carinii* pneumonia and is HIV-positive. She is admitted to the hospital.

Assessment

Nursing behaviors

1. Assess Ms. James for fatigue, malaise, weakness, anorexia, weight loss, diarrhea, night sweats, pallor, and fever.

2. Observe Ms. James for worsening dyspnea, cyanosis, and pain on breathing.

3. Assess Ms. James for dark purple skin lesions (which may be ulcerated).

4. Inspect Ms. James for herpes lesions.

5. Check Ms. James's mouth for white plaques.

6. Note any complaints of eye pain or inflammation, chest pain, gastric distress, or diarrhea.

Nursing rationales

1. These signs and symptoms reflect decreasing immunocompetence typical in people with AIDS (PWAs).

2. These changes result from lung tissue destruction caused by *P. carinii* pneumonia.

3. Such lesions represent Kaposi's sarcoma, a common cancer in PWAs.

4. All types of herpesviruses commonly occur in PWAs.

5. Many PWAs have monilial infections.

6. These signs and symptoms may reflect cytomegalovirus, a common opportunistic infection.

Diagnosing AIDS

The ELISA test (enzyme-linked immunosorbent assay) and the Western blot assay are screening tests used to diagnose acquired immunodeficiency syndrome (AIDS). The ELISA test detects antibodies to human immunodeficiency virus (HIV) in the blood, indicating HIV infection. This test may yield false positive results. The Western blot assay, a more specific test, is used to confirm positive ELISA results. Because HIV antibodies take an average of 6 to 8 weeks to develop, false negative results can occur with either test. (In some cases, HIV antibodies take 4 months or even longer to develop.)

Depending on the patient's condition, the physician may order any of the following tests to support a diagnosis of AIDS:
- chest X-ray to detect pulmonary disease
- bronchoscopy to confirm *Pneumocystis carinii* pneumonia
- stool culture to check for organisms that commonly cause diarrhea in patients with AIDS
- serum blood tests to check for decreased lymphocyte counts
- tissue biopsy to confirm Kaposi's sarcoma.

---

7. Evaluate Ms. James for neurologic signs and symptoms, such as fever, headache, sweats, stiff neck, and AIDS dementia (forgetfulness and impaired concentration). Assess for spinal cord degeneration and peripheral nerve damage.

7. Neurologic impairment may result from direct HIV invasion into brain cells or from neurologic infection by toxoplasmosis or *Cryptococcus neoformans* organisms.

8. Monitor Ms. James's psychophysiologic responses.

8. PWAs require ongoing observation because immunosuppression makes them vulnerable to multiple organ breakdown.

Nursing diagnoses
- Impaired gas exchange related to respiratory infection
- Altered nutrition (less than body requirements) related to anorexia, weight loss, and GI problems

Planning and goals
- Ms. James will adapt her life-style to better cope with HIV infection.
- Ms. James will maintain adequate oxygenation.
- Ms. James will avoid complications as long as possible.

Implementation

Nursing behaviors
1. If possible, have Ms. James participate in a drug rehabilitation program. Otherwise, teach her never to share needles and syringes with others.

Nursing rationales
1. Drug rehabilitation can help Ms. James stop using drugs and decrease the risk of her spreading HIV through contaminated equipment.

2. Urge Ms. James to abstain from sex. If she cannot do this, teach her about safe sex, such as use of condoms and spermicide for vaginal intercourse or use of condoms and water-soluble lubricant (K-Y jelly) for anal intercourse.

2. Sexual abstinence is the only sure way to prevent HIV transmission through sexual contact. Where abstinence is not realistic, safe sexual practices help reduce the risk of disease spread. Condoms provide barrier protection from transmission through semen. Nonoxynol-9 in spermicide may offer added protection but must be used in conjunction with a condom. Water-based lubricants help prevent condom breakage, whereas oil-based lubricants (such as Vaseline) weaken latex and may cause the condom to break.

3. Administer oxygen and co-trimoxazole (Bactrim), as ordered. Perform chest percussion.

3. Oxygen relieves hypoxemia caused by *P. carinii* pneumonia. The physician also may order co-trimoxazole to treat this infection; side effects include rash, fever, and decreased white blood cell count. (Pentamidine [Pentam], another drug used to treat or prevent *P. carinii* pneumonia, can cause such side effects as fever, sterility, and renal damage.) Chest percussion maintains a patent airway and mobilizes secretions.

4. Give an antiemetic, as ordered, 30 minutes before meals or as needed.

4. Antiemetics decrease nausea and vomiting.

5. Provide small, frequent feedings.

5. Small feedings are more appetizing to an anorectic patient.

6. Encourage Ms. James to perform frequent oral hygiene with a soft toothbrush or cotton swab and to keep her lips moisturized.

6. These measures reduce the risk of infection, refresh the mouth, prevent drying and cracking of the lips, and improve the appetite.

7. Give antidiarrheals, as ordered, to prevent breakdown of perineal skin.

7. Diarrhea commonly results from GI infections and chemotherapy.

8. Turn and reposition Ms. James frequently. Encourage her to ambulate. Balance activity with rest periods.

8. As Ms. James becomes weaker, she is increasingly likely to suffer complications of immobility. Balancing activity with rest periods reduces fatigue.

9. Apply lotion to Ms. James's skin. After bathing or washing her, pat the skin dry, avoiding rubbing.

9. These measures prevent skin dryness, irritation, and breakdown.

10. Protect Ms. James from accidental injury, for instance, by avoiding throw rugs and using a nonskid bath mat.

10. This is needed because Ms. James is weak and cannot recover from balance loss.

Universal blood and body fluid precautions

Because any patient might be infected with the human immunodeficiency virus (HIV), health care workers must use universal precautions to protect their skin and mucous membranes from patients' blood and body fluids. Such precautions include the following:

• Wear gloves when performing any procedure in which you might come into contact with a patient's blood, other body fluids, mucous membranes, skin cuts, or wounds. Also wear gloves when handling soiled items or performing venipunctures or other vascular procedures. After the procedure, remove and discard the gloves.

• To reduce the risk of exposing your mucous membranes to HIV, wear a mask, protective eyewear, face shield, and apron when anticipating blood splashes or droplets generated by contact with a patient's bronchial secretions.

• Consider hand washing a major means of preventing infection spread. Wash your hands immediately if they become contaminated with blood or other body fluids. Also wash them after removing gloves.

• Take precautions to avoid injury from needle sticks and other sharp instruments. Immediately place used needles and other sharp instruments in puncture-proof containers. Do not recap, bend, or remove a needle from the syringe.

ADULT NURSING

Transfusion reactions

Patients with AIDS or various other disorders may require blood transfusions. Types of blood transfusion reactions include allergic reaction, circulatory overload, febrile reaction, hemolytic reaction, and septic reaction.

TYPE OF REACTION	SIGNS AND SYMPTOMS	CAUSE	NURSING INTERVENTIONS
Allergic reaction	Generalized pruritus; urticaria (hives); in some cases, wheezing and anaphylaxis	Sensitivity to donor blood (plasma proteins or antibodies)	• Stop the transfusion and contact the physician or team leader immediately. (Keep the I.V. line open with normal saline solution, but change the tubing. In some cases, the transfusion is allowed to continue at a slower rate.) • Administer antihistamines, as ordered. (Epinephrine [Adrenalin] may be ordered for a severe reaction.)
Circulatory overload	Dyspnea, anxiety, cyanosis, cough, and frothy pink sputum	Pulmonary edema from administration of whole blood or packed cells	• Stop the transfusion and notify the physician immediately. (Keep the I.V. line open with slow infusion of normal saline solution.) • Place the patient in a sitting position with the feet dependent.
Febrile reaction	Fever, chills, hypotension, tachycardia, and nausea	Sensitivity to donor platelets or leukocytes	• Stop the transfusion and contact the physician. (Keep the I.V. line open with normal saline solution, but change the tubing.)
Hemolytic reaction	Headache, chills, low back pain, nausea, chest tightness, tachycardia, hypotension, and hemoglobinuria (red urine)	Hemolysis from incompatibility with donor blood	• Stop the transfusion and notify the physician or team leader immediately. (Keep the I.V. line open with normal saline solution, but change the tubing.) • Monitor vital signs frequently. • Record fluid intake and output. • Administer I.V. colloid and mannitol, as ordered. • Insert an indwelling urinary catheter, as ordered. • Return donor blood to the blood bank.
Septic reaction	Vomiting, chills, high fever, diarrhea, and hypotension	Contamination of transfusion products with bacteria	• Stop the transfusion and notify the physician. (Keep the I.V. line open with normal saline solution, but change the tubing.) • Monitor vital signs. • Administer antibiotics, steroids, and vasopressors, as ordered. • Return donor blood to the blood bank.

11. Support all medical treatments, which may include chemotherapy, antifungal agents, and acyclovir (Zovirax) to treat herpes. The physician probably will prescribe AZT. Blood transfusions may be needed if the patient becomes anemic.

11. Treatment for AIDS depends on the patient's specific problems. AZT prevents HIV replication, delaying disease progression. As appropriate, monitor for side effects of this drug, including bone marrow depression and headache.

12. Listen as Ms. James expresses her concerns and fears.

12. Ms. James will need considerable multidisciplinary support to cope with the many emotional, physical, social, and spiritual concerns and needs that may arise.

Evaluation (outcomes)

• Ms. James is free from respiratory distress.
• Ms. James' weight loss has slowed and her nutritional status has improved.
• Ms. James receives support services through the community AIDS project.

ADULT NURSING

Oncology nursing

Malignant cell development

I.   **Definition**
    A. Cancer is a neoplasm (new tissue growth) characterized by uncontrolled growth of abnormal cells
    B. The term cancer also refers collectively to many different neoplastic diseases, each with specific causes, clinical manifestations, and management

II.   **Contributing factors**
    A. How a normal (benign) cell becomes malignant is not well understood

Mitosis stages

This illustration shows the five stages of mitosis, or normal cell division. Note the disappearance of the nuclear membrane and separation of chromosomes.

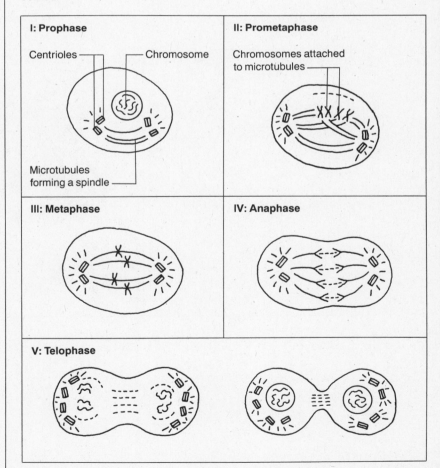

    B. Presumably, many factors contribute to this process, including:
1. exposure to carcinogens (such as viruses, chemicals, hormones, radiation, and irritants)
2. genetic factors
3. obesity
4. diet
5. immune system failure

III. Distinguishing characteristics of cancer cells

    A. A cancer cell differs from a normal cell in that its nucleus is larger and less regular

    B. It divides erratically

    C. Its offspring do not resemble the cells from which they come

    D. Disorderly cell multiplication leads to tumor formation or invasion of healthy tissue (metastasis)

Comparing benign and malignant tumor growth

A benign tumor is localized and well-encapsulated; a malignant tumor lacks a capsule, spreads, and grows irregularly.

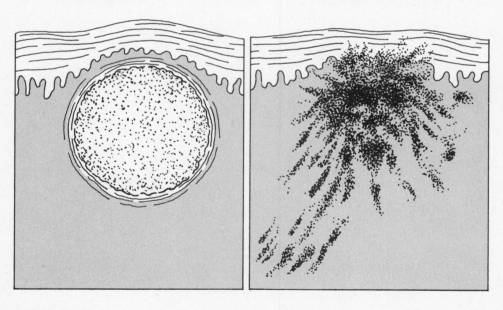

BENIGN TUMOR   MALIGNANT TUMOR

Glossary

Blood-brain barrier: continuous endothelial cell lining in the cerebral vasculature that limits exchange of proteins, ions, and water-soluble drugs but allows transport of lipid-soluble agents
Carcinogen: agent that can cause malignant (cancerous) changes in healthy cells
Cytotoxic: substance that is destructive to cells
Lymphedema: edema caused by obstructed lymphatic drainage
Metastasis: spread of malignant cells to other body regions through the bloodstream or lymphatic system

---

Ovarian cancer and chemotherapy

Overview

Chemotherapy refers to the use of antineoplastic drugs to destroy or prevent the multiplication of malignant cells. Drugs used for chemotherapy typically are cytotoxic, interfering with cell function and reproduction. Acting systemically, they affect benign as well as malignant cells; however, actively dividing cancer cells are the most sensitive to chemotherapy. Side effects of chemotherapy typically involve rapidly multiplying cells, including hair follicles, epithelial cells, and cells of the bone marrow and gastrointestinal tract lining. Each chemotherapeutic drug has specific side effects.

Typically, chemotherapy involves administration of a combination of drugs, possibly in conjunction with other cancer treatments (such as radiation). Usually, the drugs are given I.V. by nurses with advanced skills. Various special-access devices have made chemotherapy more comfortable, convenient, and effective.

Clinical situation

Minnie Jefferson, age 62, has been married for 44 years and has no children. When she experiences abdominal fullness and a decreased appetite, she decides to see her physician. After examining her, the physician refers her to a surgeon, who performs an exploratory laparotomy, including a total abdominal hysterectomy, bilateral salpingo-oophorectomy, omentectomy, and extensive biopsies. Test results confirm a stage IV ovarian cancer.

Four weeks later, Mrs. Jefferson is admitted to the hospital for chemotherapy and evaluation of her recent 15-lb (6.8 kg) weight loss. The admission assessment reveals that she is 5'4" (163 cm) tall and weighs 125 lb (56.7 kg). She states that she usually weighs 140 lb (63.5 kg). Blood studies reveal a hemoglobin level of 10 g/dl and an albumin level of 2.8 g/dl. In the operating room, the physician inserts a central venous catheter for total parenteral nutrition (TPN). After TPN begins, Mrs. Jefferson's nutritional status improves somewhat and the physician allows her to take liquids and other foods, as tolerated, by mouth while TPN continues.

Mrs. Jefferson then starts a chemotherapy regimen that includes cyclophosphamide (Cytoxan), doxorubicin (Adriamycin), and cisplatin (Platinol). After a few weeks, she complains of nausea and a sore mouth. Her hair begins to fall out; however, she seems to accept this change and has brought a wig and several scarves with her.

ADULT NURSING

Assessment

Nursing behaviors

1. Assess Mrs. Jefferson's nutritional status by evaluating her height and weight (comparing it to ideal weight), recent weight changes, laboratory values (hemoglobin, serum albumin, electrolyte, and glucose levels), appetite, and food likes and dislikes.

2. Assess Mrs. Jefferson for nausea and vomiting.

3. Assess Mrs. Jefferson's fluid intake and output.

4. Assess Mrs. Jefferson for edema of the ankles and sacral area.

5. Assess Mrs. Jefferson's oral cavity for pain or burning, color changes, moistness, lesions or ulcers, and saliva appearance. Assess her tolerance for hot, cold, highly seasoned, and acidic foods and beverages.

6. Assess the general condition of Mrs. Jefferson's teeth and the fit of any dentures.

7. Assess Mrs. Jefferson's lips for moistness, color, and cracks.

8. Assess Mrs. Jefferson's usual mouth and denture care regimen, including her oral hygiene routine and frequency of dental visits.

Nursing rationales

1. Assessing nutritional status provides baseline data useful in monitoring Mrs. Jefferson's progress. The cancer patient has increased nutritional needs. TPN may cause hypoglycemia or hyperglycemia.

2. Nausea and vomiting must be controlled to increase Mrs. Jefferson's interest in eating.

3. Nausea and vomiting may alter the fluid balance. Cisplatin can cause renal toxicity.

4. Sometimes associated with cancer, edema may cause a daily weight gain exceeding 3 lb (1.4 kg). In a patient on bed rest, edema may occur in the sacral area.

5. A malnourished patient is at increased risk for stomatitis, a chemotherapy side effect. Stomatitis commonly causes food and beverage intolerance.

6. Poor dental hygiene—especially poorly fitting dentures—may exacerbate stomatitis.

7. Poor nutritional status and lack of fluids may cause dry, cracked lips.

8. This establishes a baseline for patient teaching.

Nursing diagnoses

• Altered nutrition (less than body requirements) related to decreased appetite, stomatitis, cancer, and chemotherapy side effects
• Altered oral mucous membrane related to side effects of chemotherapy

Planning and goals

• Mrs. Jefferson will demonstrate an improved nutritional status.
• Mrs. Jefferson's nausea will be controlled.
• Mrs. Jefferson and her husband will state ways to improve her nutritional status.
• Mrs. Jefferson will be free from signs and symptoms of stomatitis by the time of discharge.
• Mrs. Jefferson and her husband will demonstrate knowledge of a proper mouth care regimen.

Implementation

Nursing behaviors

1. Encourage Mrs. Jefferson to rest before meals.

Nursing rationales

1. Eating meals may tire a cancer patient. Rest may help reduce nausea.

ADULT
NURSING

2. Provide a pleasant mealtime atmosphere.

2. A pleasant atmosphere stimulates the appetite.

3. Arrange to have a nurse, volunteer, family member, or other person stay with Mrs. Jefferson during meals.

3. Companionship during meals promotes eating.

4. Assist Mrs. Jefferson to eat meals.

4. Weakness caused by cancer and poor nutritional status may deter Mrs. Jefferson from eating.

5. Encourage Mrs. Jefferson to eat according to her tolerance.

5. Encouragement may increase her food consumption.

6. Administer antiemetics, as needed and ordered, approximately 30 minutes before meals.

6. Antiemetics reduce nausea.

7. Demonstrate a caring attitude toward Mrs. Jefferson and her husband.

7. This will help Mrs. Jefferson and her husband cope with stress.

8. Encourage Mrs. Jefferson to consume frequent, small amounts of fluids, such as gelatin dessert, flat soda, and electrolyte-rich liquids (for instance, Gatorade or broth)—especially after bouts of nausea and vomiting.

8. Fluids taken frequently in small amounts may eliminate vomiting. Electrolyte-rich liquids help replenish electrolytes lost during vomiting.

9. Instruct Mrs. Jefferson to keep her head elevated for 2 hours after eating.

9. Resting with the head elevated promotes digestion.

10. Maintain fluid intake and output records during every shift.

10. This helps detect fluid imbalance.

11. Weigh Mrs. Jefferson daily (or at least every other day).

11. Weight monitoring helps detect changes in nutritional status.

12. Monitor the TPN infusion and related factors by:
• following prescribed orders
• assessing the central venous catheter site
• changing the dressing at the central venous catheter site, according to institutional policy
• monitoring vital signs every 4 hours
• reporting signs of infection, redness, and tenderness at the catheter site
• reporting a temperature above 100° F (37.8° C).

12. TPN orders must be followed carefully to prevent complications and maintain optimal nutrition. The catheter site requires meticulous care using aseptic technique to prevent infection. The glucose concentration of the TPN solution commonly causes hypoglycemia and hyperglycemia. Vital sign measurements help evaluate Mrs. Jefferson's reaction to the TPN infusion as well as her overall health status. Reporting signs of infection or a temperature over 100° F helps ensure prompt treatment of infection.

13. Monitor laboratory values, such as white blood cell count, and hemoglobin, serum albumin, electrolyte, and glucose levels.

13. This helps detect improvements in nutritional status and possible complications of infection and electrolyte imbalance.

14. Consult a dietitian, as needed.

14. A dietitian can provide expert nutritional support for a cancer patient.

ADULT NURSING

15. Teach Mrs. Jefferson and her family about methods to improve her nutritional status (including TPN). Provide pamphlets on nutrition for cancer patients.

15. Such teaching helps prepare Mrs. Jefferson and her family for her discharge and promotes compliance.

16. Perform oral hygiene before and after meals and after any vomiting. Use such solutions as soda bicarbonate solution (1 tsp in 8 oz water), hydrogen peroxide and normal saline solution (one-fourth hydrogen peroxide to three-fourths normal saline solution), normal saline solution, or normal saline and baking soda (one quart normal saline to 2 tsp baking soda). Avoid commercial mouthwash. Use a soft toothbrush. Have Mrs. Jefferson remove her dentures for at least 8 hours daily.

16. A patient with stomatitis needs scrupulous mouth care to promote healing. Commercial mouthwashes contain alcohol, which could irritate the oral mucosa. A soft toothbrush decreases bleeding. Nighttime denture removal decreases irritation.

17. Assist Mrs. Jefferson to rinse her mouth every 2 hours and as needed.

17. Frequent rinsing removes debris and moistens and soothes the mouth.

18. Administer medications to treat oral infection and relieve discomfort, as ordered.

18. Medications (such as clotrimazole [Mycelex] troche and lidocaine [Xylocaine]) treat fungal infection and relieve pain.

19. Instruct Mrs. Jefferson to avoid foods and beverages that are very hot or cold, highly seasoned, or acidic.

19. These foods and beverages irritate the oral mucosa and cause discomfort.

20. Teach Mrs. Jefferson and her family how to perform oral hygiene.

20. Such teaching prepares Mrs. Jefferson and her family for her discharge.

21. Assist with a referral to social services.

21. Social services can help Mrs. Jefferson and her family make arrangements for a nurse and other home care needs.

Evaluation (outcomes)

- Mrs. Jefferson gains 3 lb (1.4 kg) during hospitalization and has normal hemoglobin, serum albumin, and serum glucose levels by the time of discharge.
- Mrs. Jefferson's nausea is controlled.
- Mrs. Jefferson and her husband state methods to improve her nutritional status.
- Mrs. Jefferson is free from signs of oral stomatitis by the time of discharge.
- Mrs. Jefferson and her husband demonstrate the proper mouth care regimen.

Lung cancer and radiation therapy

Overview

Radiation therapy involves the use of external or internal radiation to destroy or cause decomposition of cancer cells. External radiation is administered by a special machine containing a radiation source; the patient is positioned carefully to ensure that radiation is directed at the tumor site. Treatments usually continue for weeks. Internal radiation involves short-term implantation of a radioactive substance at the cancer site. Typically, the physician inserts needles, catheters, or wires into the patient in the operating room; the radioactive substance is inserted later in the patient's room. Because the patient emits radiation during this treatment, all health team members must use the principles of time, distance, and shielding when providing care.

Actively dividing cancer cells and well-oxygenated tumors are most sensitive to radiation therapy. However, radiation also may damage normal cells—most notably, cells of the skin, bone marrow, and gastrointestinal tract lining. Side effects of radiation relate to the irradiated body area; although most occur at the time of treatment, some may be delayed.

Clinical situation

Joseph Luciani, age 59, is diagnosed with inoperable lung cancer—specifically, small-cell (oat cell) carcinoma. He has no signs of metastasis. A supervisor in a car assembly plant, Mr. Luciani is married, with four grown children who live nearby. He has a 40-year smoking history of one to two packs a day.

One month after diagnosis, Mr. Luciani is hospitalized for radiation therapy; he also is receiving chemotherapy. After radiation therapy begins, he starts to experience anorexia, a persistent cough, and extreme fatigue. Signs of skin irritation appear on his anterior chest. In his left arm, he receives an I.V. infusion of 5% dextrose in 0.45% normal saline solution. Prednisone (Deltasone) 2.5 mg/day and docusate sodium (Colace) 50 mg b.i.d. are the only regular medications prescribed. Mr. Luciani is on a select diet, as tolerated. Nursing notes state that he needs help with bathing, dressing, toileting, and feeding.

Assessment

Nursing behaviors

1. Assess Mr. Luciani's vital signs during every shift.

2. Assess Mr. Luciani's respiratory status during every shift by evaluating his lung sounds. Note the presence, frequency, and productivity of any cough, and assess any sputum for color, amount, and thickness.

3. Assess Mr. Luciani's skin daily for reactions to radiation therapy by checking for such signs as color changes, irritation, scaling, weeping, and itching.

Nursing rationales

1. Changes in vital signs alert the health care team to possible complications of radiation, such as respiratory infection and cardiac changes.

2. Lung cancer commonly alters respiratory status. Respiratory infection (such as pneumonitis) may arise as a complication of radiation therapy. Yellow or green sputum may indicate infection; brown or red sputum, hemorrhage.

3. Skin changes are expected with radiation therapy to the chest. Wet desquamation (scaly weeping) must be detected and treated promptly because it can lead to infection.

ADULT NURSING

4. Assess Mr. Luciani for side effects of radiation therapy, including fatigue, nausea, vomiting, anorexia, and pain and difficulty on swallowing.

4. Side effects of radiation therapy relate to the body region irradiated. Fatigue is common.

5. Assess laboratory results, such as white blood cell (WBC) and red blood cell (RBC) counts and hemoglobin, platelet, and albumin levels.

5. Radiation therapy depresses the hematopoietic system, reducing WBC, RBC, hemoglobin, and platelet levels. Bone marrow depression is a side effect of radiation therapy. A decreased albumin level may indicate altered nutritional status.

6. Assess Mr. Luciani's nutritional status, including his height, weight, appetite, and food tolerance.

6. Anorexia is a common side effect of cancer and radiation therapy.

7. Assess Mr. Luciani for signs and symptoms of dehydration, such as a coated tongue and decreased skin turgor.

7. Anorexia may lead to decreased fluid intake causing dehydration.

8. Assess Mr. Luciani's fluid intake and output during every shift.

8. This helps detect fluid imbalance.

9. Assess the I.V. infusion at least every 4 hours for redness, tenderness, and edema at the site; drip rate and proper fluid infusion; and proper solution, as ordered.

9. This allows prompt detection of phlebitis or infiltration and ensures that the I.V. fluid is infusing as ordered.

10. Assess Mr. Luciani's ability to perform activities of daily living (ADLs).

10. Fatigue is a common side effect of radiation therapy.

11. Assess Mr. Luciani for complications of decreased mobility, such as constipation, skin breakdown, and respiratory infection.

11. Such complications may occur in weakened patients. Detection helps ensure prompt treatment.

12. Assess Mr. Luciani and his family for knowledge of radiation therapy.

12. This establishes a baseline for teaching.

Nursing diagnoses
• Self-care deficit (feeding, bathing, dressing, and toileting) related to extreme fatigue and disease
• Impaired skin integrity related to the effects of radiation therapy

Planning and goals
• Mr. Luciani will experience only minimal changes in skin integrity from radiation therapy.
• Mr. Luciani and his family will describe measures to protect his skin during radiation therapy.
• Mr. Luciani and his family will demonstrate an understanding of the purpose and side effects of radiation therapy.
• Mr. Luciani will participate in ADLs during his hospitalization.

ADULT
NURSING

Implementation

Nursing behaviors

1. Promote rest and sleep.

2. Provide special skin care to the area receiving radiation therapy:
• Do not attempt to remove skin markings.
• Wash gently with mild soap and water. (If skin breakdown appears, do not use soap.)
• Do not use alcohol, oils, creams, deodorant, cologne, powder, or tape on the area.
• Instruct Mr. Luciani to avoid constrictive clothing and irritating fabrics.
• Do not apply heat or cold to the area (such as by using a heating pad, ice pack, or hot water bottle).
• Apply cornstarch to the area, as needed, to help control itching. (However, do not use cornstarch on moist skin.)
• Expose the area to air as often as possible.
• Apply water-based ointment to the area only as ordered.
• Perform special treatments, as ordered, for wet desquamation.

3. Teach Mr. Luciani and his family about protective skin measures.

4. Encourage Mr. Luciani to maintain optimal nutrition by:
• eating a high-protein, high-calorie diet, as tolerated
• consuming food supplements (such as Ensure and instant breakfast formula)
• ensuring pleasant surroundings at mealtime
• avoiding foods that are very hot, very cold, highly seasoned, or acidic
• taking small, frequent feedings, especially of soft, moist foods.

5. Encourage adequate fluid intake.

6. Assist Mr. Luciani with ADLs (bathing, feeding, dressing, and toileting), as needed.

7. Emphasize any progress Mr. Luciani makes with self-care activities.

Nursing rationales

1. Fatigue is a common side effect of radiation therapy.

2. Special skin care reduces irritation. The radiation therapist places indelible ink markings on the patient's body to direct radiation. Oil-based lotions and creams may contain heavy metals, which interfere with X-rays. Moist desquamation may require special treatment to promote healing and prevent infection.

3. Teaching promotes compliance. (Mr. Luciani probably will continue with radiation therapy as an outpatient.)

4. The cancer patient needs optimal nutrition to cope with the disease. Foods that are very hot or cold, highly seasoned, or acidic may exacerbate any esophageal irritation caused by radiation therapy.

5. An anorectic patient is likely to suffer dehydration.

6. A weak, fatigued patient may need such assistance.

7. This will encourage Mr. Luciani to participate in ADLs.

ADULT NURSING

8. Arrange referrals to occupational and physical therapists, as needed.

8. Mr. Luciani may need a referral for assistive devices or exercises to prevent impaired physical mobility.

9. Provide reassurance and support.

9. This may reduce Mr. Luciani's discouragement, and counter any guilt feelings he has about his smoking history.

10. Allay any fears and concerns Mr. Luciani has about radiation therapy.

10. Mr. Luciani may fear radiation effects or incorrectly believe that radiation therapy will make him radioactive.

11. Teach Mr. Luciani and his family about radiation therapy, including:
• its purpose and side effects
• the clicking sound the machine makes during treatment
• the importance of emptying the bowel and bladder before treatment
• the purpose and care of skin markings
• the need to keep scheduled appointments.

11. This will increase patient compliance and relieve concerns.

12. Administer medications, such as stool softeners and antibiotics, as ordered.

12. Stool softeners help prevent constipation caused by decreased mobility. Antibiotics treat any respiratory infection or an infection associated with wet desquamation.

13. Provide Mr. Luciani and his family with pamphlets and information about support groups and resources, such as the American Cancer Society's "I Can Cope" group and the cancer hotline (1-800-4-CANCER).

13. Support and information will help Mr. Luciani and his family understand and better cope with cancer and its treatment.

14. Refer Mr. Luciani to social services, as needed.

14. Mr. Luciani may need a referral for a visiting home care nurse.

Evaluation (outcomes)

• Mr. Luciani experiences only skin redness, dryness, and itching from radiation therapy.
• Mr. Luciani and his family describe skin-protection measures to take during radiation therapy.
• Mr. Luciani and his family show an understanding of the purpose and side effects of radiation therapy.
• Mr. Luciani participates in ADLs while hospitalized.

ADULT
NURSING

Breast cancer and mastectomy

Overview

Breast cancer is the second leading cause of death from cancer among women (it rarely affects males). The disease begins as a lump in the breast, which may go undetected for some time. Because survival hinges largely on early diagnosis, the American Cancer Society encourages women to perform monthly breast self-examination (BSE) starting at age 20, have regular medical examinations, and undergo mammography starting at age 35 to 40.

Researchers have studied many proposed risk factors for breast cancer. The most widely accepted factors include childlessness or first pregnancy after age 35; mother, sister, or daughter with breast cancer; and age over 40.

Several treatment options exist. The trend is toward less radical surgery, such as lumpectomy (followed by radiation therapy) or modified radical mastectomy (possibly followed by chemotherapy). Some women who undergo mastectomy choose breast reconstruction surgery—either at the time of initial surgery or after healing. If breast cancer has metastasized at the time of diagnosis, chemotherapy and hormonal therapy may be the sole treatments.

Clinical situation

Lee Rothchild, age 48, discovers a lump in her left breast. The gynecologist orders a mammogram and performs an ultrasound examination. After reviewing the test results, the gynecologist refers Mrs. Rothchild to a surgeon. An incisional biopsy of the mass, which measures 3 cm, confirms adenocarcinoma.

Mrs. Rothchild undergoes a modified radical mastectomy with removal of axillary lymph nodes. Now, on the third postoperative day, she is recuperating on the surgical unit. The closed-wound drainage system (Hemovac) providing suction to the wound has been removed, she has no complaints of pain, and her vital signs are stable. Nursing notes reveal that Mrs. Rothchild cries often and has trouble accepting the surgery. She states that her husband left her 6 months ago; she has two college-age daughters. Her sister visits daily.

Assessment

Nursing behaviors

1. Assess Mrs. Rothchild's incision site for tenderness, redness, warmth, drainage, and wound approximation.

2. Assess the involved hand and arm for edema, numbness, coolness, decreased or absent pulses, and inability to move the fingers.

3. Assess Mrs. Rothchild's vital signs during each shift.

4. Assess Mrs. Rothchild's ability to perform activities of daily living (ADLs). Determine her hand dominance.

Nursing rationales

1. This yields baseline data for evaluation of healing and allows prompt detection of any infection.

2. This detects any circulatory compromise (from pressure dressings or postoperative edema). Removal of axillary lymph nodes may cause reduced lymphatic drainage and lymphedema.

3. Increased temperature, pulse rate, or respiratory rate may signal infection (such as a wound infection or a respiratory infection).

4. Restricted movement in the operative arm may interfere with Mrs. Rothchild's ability to bathe, eat, dress, and groom herself, especially if surgery involved axillary nodes on the arm of her dominant hand.

5. Assess Mrs. Rothchild's knowledge of her postoperative limitations and restrictions.

5. This provides baseline data. Mrs. Rothchild may have obtained knowledge previously through reading and teaching by health team members. Because some axillary lymph nodes were removed, she must follow hand and arm precautions to prevent infection.

6. Assess Mrs. Rothchild's adaptive responses, such as willingness to participate in self-care and to discuss her feelings and concerns.

6. This helps determine whether Mrs. Rothchild is adapting to her loss in a positive or negative way.

7. Assess Mrs. Rothchild's feelings, concerns, and fears about the loss of her breast and its effect on her role as a woman.

7. Display of inappropriate responses to the loss may indicate the need for referral to a psychiatrist or support group.

8. Assess the family's response to Mrs. Rothchild's surgery.

8. Mrs. Rothchild's sister and daughters may be able to help her to adapt.

9. Assess Mrs. Rothchild's knowledge of postoperative exercises.

9. Because Mrs. Rothchild's surgery involved muscle dissection, she must learn how to perform exercises to ensure maximal range of motion (ROM) of the involved arm.

10. Assess Mrs. Rothchild's knowledge of support resources, such as mastectomy support groups, pamphlets, and the American Cancer Society.

10. Such support resources offer information and support during recovery and after discharge. They also can provide information on breast reconstruction.

11. Assess Mrs. Rothchild's knowledge of BSE technique.

11. Mrs. Rothchild must practice monthly BSE because she is at risk for developing cancer in the other breast.

Nursing diagnoses
- Body image disturbance related to loss of a breast
- Knowledge deficit related to postoperative care and rehabilitation

Planning and goals
- Mrs. Rothchild will remain free from signs and symptoms of infection and lymphedema in the involved arm.
- Mrs. Rothchild will express her feelings, concerns, and fears about the loss of her breast and its effect on her role as a woman.
- Mrs. Rothchild will participate in her care during hospitalization.
- Mrs. Rothchild will demonstrate an understanding of postoperative limitations and restrictions, arm exercises, and BSE.
- Mrs. Rothchild will state the names of support resources for mastectomy patients.

Implementation

Nursing behaviors	Nursing rationales

Nursing behaviors

1. Provide care for the incision:
- Do not change the pressure dressing that was applied in the operating room.
- Inspect the dressing for drainage every 2 to 4 hours.
- Keep the dressing and incision clean and dry.
- After the physician removes the pressure dressing, apply a light dry sterile dressing, if needed.
- After the pressure dressing has been removed, have Mrs. Rothchild shower (as permitted by the physician). Gently clean the incision and pat dry.

2. Elevate the affected arm on pillows to a level above the heart.

3. Assist Mrs. Rothchild to a comfortable position. Provide a small pillow to support the affected side of the chest when she rests.

4. Protect the affected arm from injury by avoiding venipunctures, blood pressure measurements, and injections in that arm and providing a special identification band.

5. Begin an exercise program to restore ROM to the affected arm. However, consult the physician before doing active ROM exercises, and avoid vigorous exercises while Mrs. Rothchild is still hospitalized. Exercises Mrs. Rothchild can perform in the hospital include:
- passive ROM exercises
- squeezing a roll of gauze or a soft ball
- pronating and supinating the hand
- swinging the arm at the side with the back straight
- hairbrushing.

6. Assist Mrs. Rothchild with position changes and ambulation.

7. Teach Mrs. Rothchild postdischarge exercises for the affected arm (with the physician's approval, such exercises can begin approximately 1 week after discharge). These exercises include pendulum swinging, arm raising, rope turning, rope sliding (pulley), and wall hand climbing. (For descriptions and illustrations of some of these exercises, see *Postmastectomy exercises,* page 452.)

Nursing rationales

1. A modified radical mastectomy is an extensive surgical procedure. A pressure dressing, applied to prevent hemorrhage, must be checked frequently. In a patient resting in bed, gravity may cause drainage to be found on the patient's back or bedclothes. Keeping the incision and dressing clean and dry helps prevent bacterial growth in this moist environment. Surgical severing of nerves may alter sensation in the incisional area.

2. Extensive surgery may cause edema in the affected arm; axillary lymph node removal decreases lymphatic drainage. Elevating the arm promotes circulatory return.

3. Mastectomy may impede rest and sleep, especially if the remaining breast is large. A pillow helps restore balance.

4. Lymph nodes filter bacteria. Decreased lymphatic drainage (from axillary lymph node removal) places Mrs. Rothchild at increased risk for infection if the affected arm is injured. An identification band alerts hospital employees that she is at risk from the procedures described.

5. The patient must exercise to regain maximal ROM after modified radical mastectomy with muscle dissection.

6. A mastectomy may alter balance, especially if the remaining breast is large.

7. A modified radical mastectomy is an extensive surgical procedure. Active ROM must not begin until the incision heals. Exercises help restore maximal ROM. (However, because surgery now typically is less radical, less exercise is needed to regain ROM.)

ADULT NURSING

Postmastectomy exercises

After mastectomy, the patient must perform exercises to regain complete range of motion in the affected arm. As appropriate, use the instructions below for patient teaching.

Rope turning. This exercise requires a light rope. Tie one end of the rope around a doorknob, then stand facing the door. Take the free end of the rope in the hand of your affected arm, and place the other hand on your hip. Extend your affected arm and hold it away from your body, nearly parallel with the floor. Then turn the rope, making the widest swings possible. Do this exercise slowly at first, then increase the speed gradually.

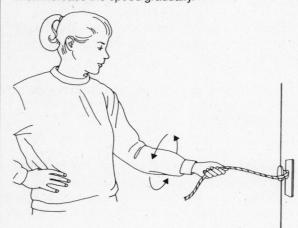

Pendulum swinging. Place your unaffected arm on the back of a chair, then bend forward from the waist. Let your affected arm hang loosely. Begin swinging your arm from left to right (be sure the movement is from your shoulder joint, not your elbow). Next, trace small circles with your arm (again using your shoulder joint). Then, swing in the opposite direction. Finally, swing your arm forward and backward from your shoulder.

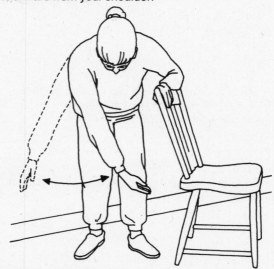

Rope sliding (pulley). This exercise requires a rope and a stationary rod (such as a shower rod or a doorway curtain rod). Toss the rope over the rod. Stand under the rope, then grasp an end in each hand. With your arms extended straight and away from you, pull your left arm up by tugging down with your right arm. Then move your right arm up and your left arm down in a seesaw motion.

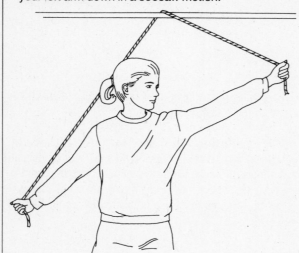

Wall handclimbing. Stand facing the wall, with your feet apart and toes as close to the wall as possible. Bend your elbows slightly, then place your palms on the wall at shoulder level. Work your hands up the wall by flexing your fingers until your arms extend fully. Then work your hands down to the starting point.

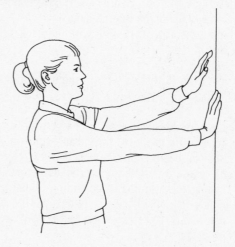

8. Teach Mrs. Rothchild how to care for her incision and improve comfort, such as by:
• observing the incision for redness, increased warmth, drainage, and healing
• reporting fever or signs of infection to the physician
• keeping the incision clean and dry
• using a light dressing only if drainage appears
• showering daily, using mild soap
• using a small pillow to support the chest area during sleep.

8. Teaching helps prevent wound infection, ensures prompt detection and treatment of infection, and promotes comfort.

9. Teach Mrs. Rothchild about arm and hand precautions for the affected arm:
• Avoid injury (including cuts, bruises, insect bites, burns, and hangnails) by using gloves when gardening and a potholder when cooking, and by applying insect repellant.
• Avoid drawing of blood samples from the affected arm.
• Avoid injections and blood pressure measurements involving the affected arm.
• Do not lift heavy objects.
• Apply a lanolin-based hand lotion every day.
• Consider wearing a medical alert bracelet.
• Obtain proper care for cuts, burns, and other wounds.
• Avoid constrictive clothing and jewelry.

9. Such teaching reduces the risk of injury to the affected arm. Axillary lymph node removal increases infection risk. Hand lotion keeps the skin moist and less irritation-prone. A medical alert bracelet alerts health care workers in emergencies.

10. Teach Mrs. Rothchild how to perform BSE.

10. Mrs. Rothchild is at risk for cancer in the remaining breast.

11. Encourage Mrs. Rothchild and her family to express their feelings, concerns, and fears.

11. Expressing feelings, concerns, and fears will reduce stress and provide an opportunity for the nurse to answer questions.

12. Convey a caring attitude toward Mrs. Rothchild and her family by using caring gestures (such as touching and hand-holding), sitting with her, and spending time with her family.

12. A caring attitude makes the patient more comfortable about expressing her feelings and concerns.

13. Encourage Mrs. Rothchild to look at the incision only when she is ready to do so. Support her through the experience. Avoid telling her "it looks good."

13. Mrs. Rothchild should not be forced or encouraged to look at the incision. When she is ready to look, doing so will help her deal with her feelings about the loss of her breast. Telling Mrs. Rothchild that her incision looks good may convey lack of caring.

ADULT NURSING

14. Arrange for Mrs. Rothchild to meet with a mastectomy volunteer. Provide information about support groups and information sources for prostheses, such as the American Cancer Society's "Reach to Recovery" and "I Can Cope" programs and the cancer hotline (1-800-4-CANCER).

14. Meeting people who have been through a similar experience can be comforting. Support groups and other resources are essential to rehabilitation.

Evaluation (outcomes)

• Mrs. Rothchild remains free from signs and symptoms of infection and lymphedema while hospitalized.
• Mrs. Rothchild expresses her feelings, concerns, and fears about the loss of her breast and its effect on her role as a woman (after an initial grieving period).
• Mrs. Rothchild participates in her care while hospitalized.
• Mrs. Rothchild describes her limitations and restrictions, arm exercises, and BSE technique.
• Mrs. Rothchild describes available resources for mastectomy patients.

Complications of chemotherapy

Chemotherapy may cause damage at the injection site and, like any drug, may result in an allergic reaction. This chart reviews these complications. (For details on the side effects of chemotherapeutic drugs and their management, see *Side effects of chemotherapeutic drugs,* pages 465 and 466.)

COMPLICATION	CAUSE	NURSING INTERVENTIONS
Local tissue irritation Burning, inflammation, and phlebitis (venous inflammation) at the I.V. infusion site during or several days after chemotherapy administration.	Irritation from the drug's cytotoxic action	• Monitor the I.V. infusion site. • Report signs and symptoms of tissue irritation.
Extravasation Burning, redness, edema, hyperpigmentation, ulceration, and necrosis at or near the I.V. infusion site. Tissue damage appears within 7 to 10 days of chemotherapy administration and may not heal for months.	Leakage of certain chemotherapeutic agents (called vesicants) into the tissues during administration	• Discontinue the I.V. infusion immediately. • Notify the physician immediately. • Depending on the drug administered, apply ice packs or warm compresses, as ordered. (Local injections of antidotes are available for mechlorethamine [Mustargen] and plant alkaloids.)
Allergic reaction Flushing, urticaria (hives), agitation, dyspnea, facial edema, hypotension, stridor (harsh sound during respiration), and loss of consciousness during chemotherapy administration. Reactions range from mild to severe.	Sensitization to the chemotherapeutic agent	*To help prevent this complication, before chemotherapy:* • assess the patient for allergies, including previous reactions to chemotherapeutic agents • measure vital signs • assess mental status. *If this complication arises during chemotherapy:* • discontinue the I.V. infusion (but keep the I.V. line open) • notify the physician and emergency alert system immediately • monitor vital signs • have an emergency cart brought to the room.

Starting an I.V. line

Introduction   An I.V. line can be used to deliver nutrients, fluids, or electrolytes or to administer I.V. medications. To start an I.V. line, the nurse inserts a needle into a peripheral vein, then connects it to disposable tubing primed with an infusion solution. This procedure calls for sterile technique. (Procedure steps preceded by an asterisk are especially important.)

Steps	Rationales
*1. Check the physician's order for the I.V. solution.	*1. This ensures that the patient receives the correct solution.
2. Gather needed supplies: I.V. pole; infusion pump (if needed); ordered I.V. solution; I.V. administration set (depending on the ordered solution and infusion rate and the need for an infusion pump); clean disposable gloves; tourniquet; antiseptic swab; sterile needle (butterfly, standard needles, angiocatheter); dressing materials, including 2″ × 2″ sterile gauze pads and transparent dressing (Tegaderm); tape; armboard (as needed); and a razor or scissors, as needed.	2. Gathering needed supplies makes the procedure easier and promotes good time management.
*3. Identify the patient using the identification band.	*3. This ensures that the correct patient receives the I.V. solution.
*4. Explain the procedure to the patient.	*4. Explanations help reduce patient anxiety.
5. Assist the patient into a hospital gown.	5. The patient's own nightgown or pajamas may be hard to remove after an I.V. line is started.
6. Wash your hands.	6. This helps prevent the spread of microorganisms.
7. Using sterile technique, expose the entry site on the I.V. bag or bottle. Clamp the I.V. administration set tubing, uncap the spike, and insert the tubing into the entry site on the I.V. bag or bottle. Next, fill the drip chamber half full. Prime the tubing slowly by removing the cap at the end of the tubing and regulating the clamp. Make sure the tubing is free from air bubbles. (If using an infusion pump, consult the manufacturer's instructions.)	7. Sterile technique prevents the spread of microorganisms. Filling the drip chamber only half full allows accurate drop counting. Air in the tubing can cause an air embolus.
8. Place the patient supine or in low Fowler's position.	8. These are comfortable positions that permit easy access to the patient's arms.

9. Select a vein by examining both arms. Adjust the light source, then palpate for a full superficial vein. (Avoid areas of flexion; if possible, use the distal end of the vein.) Next, remove hair at the selected insertion site (if the arm is hairy and if permitted by institutional policy) by shaving a 2″ (5.1 cm) area or using a depilatory agent. If the patient has had a mastectomy with axillary lymph node removal, do not use the affected arm.

9. A full superficial vein permits easier access. Using the elbow or wrist would limit the patient's mobility and cause discomfort. Removing hair helps visualize the vein. (However, shaving the venipuncture site could promote microorganism growth in microabrasions. Instead, hairy areas may be clipped with scissors.) A patient who has undergone axillary lymph node removal is infection-prone because lymph nodes filter bacteria.

10. Apply a tourniquet a few inches above the selected I.V. insertion site.

10. A tourniquet obstructs venous blood return, causing the vein to distend and making it easier to palpate.

11. Instruct the patient to open and close the fist several times. Then palpate the selected vein again.

11. Muscle contractions force blood into the vein.

12. Put on the clean disposable gloves.

12. Gloves protect the nurse from bloodborne infections.

13. Prepare the insertion site by wiping in a circular motion from the site outward. (Use an antiseptic according to institutional policy.) Allow the area to dry.

13. Wiping from the site outward keeps microorganisms away from the insertion site.

14. Hold the skin below the insertion site taut, using the thumb of your nondominant hand.

14. This helps prevent the vein from rolling.

15. Hold the needle in your dominant hand, bevel side up, at a 30- to 45-degree angle. Puncture the skin alongside the vein; then lower the needle, piercing the vein from the side. (As the needle enters the vein, you will feel a pop or note a gentle give.)

15. Proper technique reduces trauma and prevents the needle from going through the other wall of the vein.

*16. Note blood return in the needle. Then advance the needle into the vein. (See the manufacturer's instructions for the specific type of needle used.)

*16. Visualizing blood return helps ensure proper needle placement. Secure needle placement helps prevent infiltration from needle dislodgment.

17. Working quickly, remove the cap from the I.V. tubing and attach the tubing to the needle, using sterile technique.

17. Blood will clot if the step is done too slowly.

18. Release the tourniquet while stabilizing the needle. Open the clamp on the tubing, again working quickly.

18. Quick tourniquet connection and release promote flow of the infusion.

19. Dress the site according to institutional policy. Tape the needle securely.

19. A dressing protects the site from microorganisms. Various dressing techniques can be used. Taping the needle helps prevent damage to the wall of the vein.

20. Remove the gloves.

20. The nurse no longer risks exposure to the patient's blood.

ADULT
NURSING

21. Loop the tubing on the patient's arm and fasten with tape. Use an armboard, if necessary.

21. Looping helps prevent needle dislodgment.

22. Label the tape with the date, time, and needle size and type.

22. The label alerts the nurse to the times for tubing and insertion site changes. I.V. tubing must be changed regularly (for example, every 24 to 48 hours) to decrease contamination by microorganisms.

23. Regulate the flow rate according to the physician's order.

23. This ensures infusion of the I.V. solution as ordered.

24. Return any unused equipment to the supply area and tidy the patient area.

24. The patient area should be left neat to promote safe care.

25. Wash your hands.

25. This deters the spread of microorganisms.

26. Document the time, type of fluid infused, I.V. insertion site, and needle used.

26. Documentation proves that the procedure was done, assures high-quality care, and provides legal protection.

27. Recheck the flow rate and observe the site 30 minutes later.

27. This ensures prompt detection of any infiltration at the site, should the needle become dislodged.

Common I.V. infusion sites on the arm

These illustrations show common I.V. infusion sites on the ventral aspect of the lower arm and the dorsum of the hand.

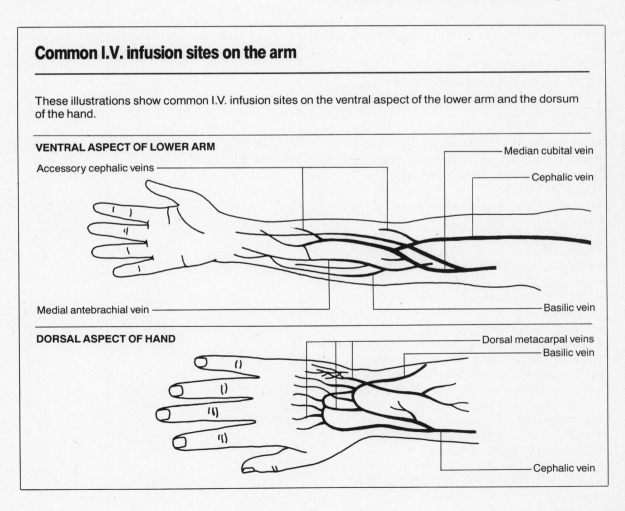

VENTRAL ASPECT OF LOWER ARM

Accessory cephalic veins

Median cubital vein

Cephalic vein

Medial antebrachial vein

Basilic vein

DORSAL ASPECT OF HAND

Dorsal metacarpal veins

Basilic vein

Cephalic vein

Caring for a peripheral venous catheter

Introduction

When caring for a patient receiving an I.V. infusion through a peripheral venous catheter, the nurse must determine if the I.V. solution is infusing as ordered and check for signs of complications. (Procedure steps preceded by an asterisk are especially important.)

Steps

***1.** Assess the I.V. site during every shift. Note any tenderness, redness, burning, warmth, edema, pallor, coolness, or discharge. Also note whether the dressing is clean, dry, and intact.

***2.** Monitor the patient's vital signs at least once every shift.

***3.** Change the I.V. site every 48 to 72 hours, according to institutional policy (see *Starting an I.V. line,* pages 455 to 457).

***4.** Change the I.V. tubing every 24 to 48 hours, according to institutional policy. (This may be done when hanging a new I.V. solution.) Follow these steps:
• Wash your hands.
• Set up the I.V. solution and tubing, using sterile technique (as described in *Starting an I.V. line,* pages 455 to 457).
• Release the tape at the I.V. insertion site.
• Put on clean disposable gloves.
• Lay sterile 2″ × 2″ gauze pads under the needle hub.
• Loosen the cap on the new tubing and set it next to the I.V. site.
• Shut off the I.V. flow.
• Hold the needle hub with your nondominant hand while removing the old tubing with your dominant hand. (A twisting motion may help release the tubing.)
• Remove the cap from the new tubing and insert the tubing securely into the needle hub.
• Open the clamp.
• Dress the site according to institutional policy.
• Remove and discard the gloves.
• Regulate the flow rate.
• Label the tubing with the date and time of the tubing change.

Rationales

***1.** Frequent assessment allows prompt detection of complications or improper infusion administration. Local edema, pallor, and coolness may indicate infiltration. Tenderness, burning, redness, and warmth may signal phlebitis. Tenderness, redness, warmth, and discharge may mean infection. A moist, soiled, loose dressing promotes bacterial growth.

***2.** This allows prompt detection of complications. Fever and chills may indicate infection at the I.V. site or in the bloodstream (septicemia). Increased blood pressure, dyspnea, and neck vein distention may indicate circulatory overload. Decreased blood pressure, rapid and weak pulse, and loss of consciousness may signal air embolism (air in the circulatory system).

***3.** This helps prevent complications.

***4.** Following these steps reduces the risk of bacterial growth in the I.V. tubing.

*5. Monitor the I.V. infusion hourly. Note the amount of solution infusing by observing the timing strip on the I.V. bag or bottle. Also note the drip rate and check the tubing for kinks, obstruction, and air.

*5. Hourly monitoring helps ensure that the I.V. solution is infusing as ordered. Rapid infusion can lead to circulatory overload. Kinks or obstruction in the tubing can interfere with flow; air can cause air embolism.

6. Provide patient teaching, including:
• reason for the I.V. infusion
• what information to report, such as tenderness or burning, the need to change the bag or bottle, and malfunction (such as if the I.V. solution stops running).

6. Knowledge promotes patient compliance and participation in care.

7. Document the type of solution infusing, the flow rate, condition of the insertion site, amount of solution infused during every shift, and the patient's response.

7. Documentation proves that the procedure was done, assures high-quality care, and provides legal protection.

Providing oral hygiene

Introduction

Providing oral hygiene allows removal of plaque and food debris from the patient's teeth and gums, promotes comfort and a positive self-image, and allows the nurse to assess the condition of the mouth and evaluate the patient's oral and dental hygiene practices. The nurse may assist with or provide care for the mouth, teeth, and any dentures. Oral hygiene is especially important for the patient who is undergoing chemotherapy. (Procedure steps preceded by an asterisk are especially important.)

Steps
*1. Wash your hands.

Rationales
*1. This helps prevent the spread of microorganisms.

2. Gather needed supplies: towel, emesis basin, toothbrush or sponge toothbrush (Toothette), toothpaste, dental floss (if available), cup of cool water, mouthwash, denture cup (if needed), denture cleaning agent (if needed), lubricant for the lips (such as petroleum jelly), clean disposable gloves, penlight, tongue blade, and additional supplies if the patient is unconscious (such as a suction catheter with suction apparatus and a bulb syringe).

2. Gathering needed supplies makes the procedure easier and promotes good time management.

3. Place the patient in (or assist the patient to) an appropriate position:
• high Fowler's position, behind the overbed table
• seated in a chair behind the overbed table
• lying on the side, with the head of the bed elevated 30 degrees, if the patient is unconscious (place the emesis basin under the patient's chin).

3. High Fowler's or a sitting position is most comfortable. A side-lying position with the head of the bed elevated 30 degrees helps prevent aspiration in an unconscious patient.

4. Place the towel over the patient's neck area, as needed.

4. The towel protects the patient's gown.

*5. Put on clean disposable gloves.

*5. This helps protect the nurse from microorganisms.

*6. Assess the patient's lips and mouth using a penlight and tongue blade. Note any cracked or dry lips, evaluate the tongue for cracks or a white coating, and note the condition of the teeth.

*6. Assessing the lips and mouth helps detect any complications, such as stomatitis, fungal infection, or dehydration. The condition of the teeth may indicate the need to teach the patient about dental care.

*7. Ask the patient to remove any dentures or, if necessary, remove dentures for the patient, using a rocking motion.

*7. Dentures must be removed to complete the procedure. A rocking motion helps loosen suction, easing denture removal.

*8. Brush the patient's teeth, or encourage the patient to do this, if able. (If the patient is unconscious, insert a padded tongue blade between the molars.) First, moisten the toothbrush with water and apply toothpaste. If the patient has gum or mucous membrane irritation, use a sponge or soft toothbrush, no toothpaste, and normal saline solution or hydrogen peroxide with normal saline. (For details on special oral hygiene solutions, see "Ovarian cancer and chemotherapy," pages 441 to 444.) Move the toothbrush or sponge toothbrush away from the gum line toward the outer and inner tooth surfaces. Next, move it in small circles at the gum line, and finally, move it back and forth on the biting surfaces of the teeth.

*8. Brushing the teeth helps remove plaque and debris from the teeth and gums. A padded tongue blade placed between the molars of an unconscious patient allows brushing. Toothbrush and toothpaste are too harsh for a patient with gum or mucous membrane irritation. Brushing in a circular motion at the gum line stimulates circulation.

9. Brush the tongue, using a gentle motion.

9. This promotes cleanliness. A gentle motion avoids stimulation of the gag reflex.

*10. Rinse the patient's mouth with cool water (to remove the water, use suction, if necessary). If the patient is unconscious, use a bulb syringe.

*10. Cool water is refreshing. A bulb syringe reduces the risk of aspiration in an unconscious patient, who has a decreased gag reflex.

11. Offer mouthwash.

11. Mouthwash helps clean the mouth. Some patients prefer not to use commercial mouthwash. (Do not offer commercial mouthwash to a patient with oral mucosa irritation because its alcohol content could cause further discomfort.)

12. Wipe the patient's mouth with a towel, as needed.

12. This promotes comfort.

13. Apply a lubricant, such as petroleum jelly, to the patient's lips.

13. This helps prevent dry, cracked lips.

*14. Clean any dentures. First, place paper towels in the sink. Then brush all denture surfaces, using a denture cleaning agent, if available. Rinse dentures thoroughly, then replace them in the patient's mouth. If the patient wishes to leave dentures out of the mouth for an extended period (such as overnight), place them in a clearly labeled container with cool water.

*14. Cleaning removes food debris and microorganisms from dentures. Placing paper towels in the sink helps prevent breakage in case dentures are dropped. Returning dentures to the mouth promotes a positive self-image. Placing dentures in a container prevents breakage or loss.

ADULT
NURSING

15. Repeat the oral hygiene procedure at least every morning and evening. With an unconscious patient, repeat every 2 hours.

15. Oral hygiene promotes comfort. An unconscious patient needs more frequent oral hygiene because of mouth breathing, inability to swallow saliva, possible dehydration, and less than optimal nutrition.

16. Document the time the procedure was performed, the condition of the patient's mouth, and any special solution used.

16. Documentation proves that the procedure was done, assures high-quality care, and provides legal protection.

Changing a central line dressing

Introduction

Changing the dressing over a central line reduces the risk of infection at the insertion site. (A central line may be used to deliver nutrients, fluids, electrolytes, or medication.) This procedure, which calls for sterile technique, may be done only by a nurse who has had special preparation in the care of central lines. (Procedure steps preceded by an asterisk are especially important.)

Steps

*1. Review the patient's chart for the date of the last dressing change.

Rationales

*1. The dressing must be changed three times a week or according to institutional policy. If it becomes soiled or loose, it should be changed as needed.

2. Wash your hands.

2. This helps prevent the spread of microorganisms.

3. Identify the patient from the identification band.

3. This ensures that the nurse changes the correct dressing.

4. Gather needed supplies: mask(s) (if required by institutional policy), clean disposable gloves, sterile gloves, cleansing agent (such as normal saline solution or hydrogen peroxide), sterile 2″ × 2″ gauze pads, antimicrobial solution (such as povidine-iodine [Betadine]) or swabs, sterile cotton-tipped applicators (if needed), antimicrobial ointment (such as povidine-iodine ointment), semipermeable transparent dressing materials (such as Tegaderm or Op-Site), and tape.

4. Gathering supplies makes the procedure easier and promotes good time management.

5. Explain the procedure to the patient.

5. Explanations allay patient anxiety.

6. Assist the patient to a supine position, with the head turned away from the insertion site.

6. This position permits maximum access to the insertion site.

7. Put on a mask, if required by institutional policy. (Also assist the patient to put on a mask, if required.)

7. A mask helps prevent contamination of the insertion site.

8. Set up the supplies on the overbed table.

8. This makes the procedure easier.

ADULT NURSING

*9. Put on the clean disposable gloves.

*9. This protects the nurse from bloodborne infections.

*10. Remove the old dressing and discard it properly.

*10. Soiled dressings harbor microorganisms.

11. Remove and discard the clean gloves.

11. Because sterile technique is needed after this point, the nurse must wear sterile gloves after removing the dressing.

12. Wash your hands.

12. This helps prevent the spread of microorganisms.

*13. Put on the sterile gloves.

*13. Sterile technique is needed through step 18.

*14. Clean the insertion site by moistening sterile gauze with a cleaning agent (according to institutional policy), then cleaning a 3″ (7.6 cm) area by working in a circular pattern from the insertion site outward. Do not go back over a previously cleaned area with the same gauze pad. Wipe the catheter gently, using a separate gauze pad. Allow the area to dry.

*14. Cleaning the insertion site removes debris and encrustations. Working from the insertion site outward prevents introduction of microorganisms to the site.

*15. Assess the insertion site for redness, tenderness, increased warmth, and discharge.

*15. These signs and symptoms may indicate infection.

*16. Apply an antimicrobial solution to a 3″ area at the site, working in a circular pattern from the insertion site outward.

*16. Antimicrobial solution helps prevent infection.

*17. Apply antimicrobial ointment to the insertion site.

*17. Antimicrobial ointment helps prevent infection by providing both chemical and mechanical barriers.

*18. Dress the area according to institutional policy. If using a sterile semipermeable transparent dressing (such as Tegaderm or Op-Site), remove the gloves, then carefully mold the dressing around the catheter.

*18. A sterile dressing provides added protection against microorganisms.

19. Remove the gloves and mask.

19. These no longer are needed because the site is covered.

20. Loop the catheter toward the supraclavicular area and fasten it with tape.

20. This prevents pulling on the insertion site.

21. Label the dressing with the date and time of the dressing change. (You may use a small piece of tape for the label.)

21. This alerts the nurse to the time of the next dressing change.

22. Document the date and time of the dressing change and the appearance of the insertion site.

22. Documentation proves that the procedure was done, assures high-quality care, and provides legal protection.

ADULT NURSING

Drugs used to treat cancer

This chart presents information about drugs commonly used to treat cancer (chemotherapeutic drugs), including the drug action and dosage. Dosages are highly variable according to the protocol; a dose may be repeated on a cyclical basis. For information on side effects and nursing considerations, see *Side effects of chemotherapeutic drugs,* pages 465 and 466.

DRUG	ACTION	USUAL ADULT DOSAGE
Alkylating agents		
Busulfan (Myleran)	Alters DNA structure, destroying both resting and dividing cells; nonspecific for cell-cycle phase	4 to 8 mg/day P.O., up to 12 mg
Chlorambucil (Leukeran)	Alters DNA structure, destroying both resting and dividing cells; nonspecific for cell-cycle phase	0.1 to 0.2 mg/kg/day P.O.
Cisplatin (Platinol)	Alters DNA structure, destroying both resting and dividing cells; nonspecific for cell-cycle phase	20 mg/m^2/day I.V. for 5 days
Cyclophosphamide (Cytoxan)	Alters DNA structure, destroying both resting and dividing cells; nonspecific for cell-cycle phase	I.V.: 40 to 50 mg/kg in divided doses over 2 to 5 days P.O.: 1 to 5 mg/kg/day
Dacarbazine (DTIC-Dome)	Alters DNA structure, destroying both resting and dividing cells; nonspecific for cell-cycle phase	2 to 4.5 mg/kg/day I.V. for 10 days
Melphalan (L-phenylalanine mustard, Alkeran)	Alters DNA structure, destroying both resting and dividing cells; nonspecific for cell-cycle phase	6 mg/day P.O. for 2 to 3 weeks
Mechlorethamine (nitrogen mustard, Mustargen)	Alters DNA structure, destroying both resting and dividing cells; nonspecific for cell-cycle phase	0.4 mg/kg I.V. or intracavitary as a single dose or 0.1 to 0.2 mg/kg/day
Streptozocin (Zanosar)	Alters DNA structure, destroying both resting and dividing cells; nonspecific for cell-cycle phase	500 mg/m^2 I.V. daily for 5 days
Thiotepa (triethylene-thiophosphoramide)	Alters DNA structure, destroying both resting and dividing cells; nonspecific for cell-cycle phase	0.2 mg/kg/day I.V., I.M., or intracavitary for 4 to 5 days
Antibiotic antineoplastic agents		
Bleomycin (Blenoxane, BLEO)	Interferes with DNA and RNA synthesis; nonspecific for cell-cycle phase	10 to 20 units/m^2 I.V., I.M., or S.C. weekly or twice weekly
Dactinomycin (actinomycin D, Cosmegen)	Interferes with DNA and RNA synthesis; nonspecific for cell-cycle phase	500 mcg/kg/day I.V. for 5 days
Daunorubicin (Cerubidin)	Interferes with DNA and RNA synthesis; nonspecific for cell-cycle phase	60 mg/m^2/day I.V.
Doxorubicin (Adriamycin)	Interferes with DNA and RNA synthesis; nonspecific for cell-cycle phase	60 to 75 mg/m^2 I.V. as a single dose at 21-day intervals
Mitomycin (Mutamycin)	Interferes with DNA and RNA synthesis; nonspecific for cell-cycle phase	2 mg/m^2/day I.V. for 5 days
Plicamycin, Mithramycin (Mithracin)	Interferes with DNA and RNA synthesis; nonspecific for cell-cycle phase	25 mcg/kg/day I.V. for 1 to 4 days
Procarbazine (Matulane)	Interferes with DNA and RNA synthesis; nonspecific for cell-cycle phase	2 to 4 mg/kg/day P.O.

(continued)

ADULT NURSING

Drugs used to treat cancer *(continued)*

DRUG	ACTION	USUAL ADULT DOSAGE
Antimetabolites		
Cytarabine (cytosine arabinoside, ara-C, Cytosar-U)	Damages cells by depriving them of nutrients essential to their functioning (resembles nutrients needed for cell reproduction); specific for S phase of cell cycle	200 mg/m²/day I.V. or intrathecally for 5 days
fluorouracil (5-FU, Adrucil)	Damages cells by depriving them of nutrients essential to their functioning (resembles nutrients needed for cell reproduction); specific for S phase of cell cycle	12.5 mg/kg/day I.V. for 3 to 5 days; repeated every 4 weeks
Hydroxyurea (Hydrea)	Damages cells by depriving them of nutrients essential to their functioning (resembles nutrients needed for cell reproduction); specific for S phase of cell cycle	20 to 30 mg/kg P.O. daily
Mercaptopurine (6-MP, Purinethol)	Damages cells by depriving them of nutrients essential to their functioning (resembles nutrients needed for cell reproduction); specific for S phase of cell cycle	80 to 100 mg/m²/day P.O.
Methotrexate (MTX, Amethopterin, Folex, Mexate)	Damages cells by depriving them of nutrients essential to their functioning (resembles nutrients needed for cell reproduction); specific for S phase of cell cycle	15 to 30 mg/day P.O., I.V., I.M., or intrathecally for 5 days
Thioguanine (6-TG, Lanvis)	Damages cells by depriving them of nutrients essential to their functioning (resembles nutrients needed for cell reproduction); specific for S phase of cell cycle	2 mg/kg/day P.O.
Hormones		
Adrenocorticosteroid Prednisone (Deltasone)	Suppresses the inflammatory response	2.5 to 15 mg P.O. b.i.d.
Androgen Fluoxymesterone (Halotestin)	Binds to hormone receptor sites, altering cell growth; inhibits RNA synthesis	2 to 10 mg/day P.O.
Estrogen Diethylstilbestrol (DES, Stilphostrol)	Binds to hormone receptor sites, altering cell growth; inhibits RNA synthesis	15 mg/day P.O.
Hormone inhibitors		
Adrenocorticosteroid inhibitor Aminoglutethimide (Cytadren)	Inhibits synthesis of glucocorticoids, mineralocorticoids, and other steroids	250 mg P.O. q.i.d.
Antiestrogen Tamoxifen (Nolvadex)	Blocks estrogen uptake in estrogen-receptor sites, such as in the breast	10 mg P.O. b.i.d.
Progestin Medroxyprogesterone (Provera)	Binds to hormone receptor sites, altering cell growth; inhibits RNA synthesis	5 to 10 mg/day P.O. for 5 to 10 days
Megestrol (Megace)	Binds to hormone receptor sites, altering cell growth; inhibits RNA synthesis	40 mg P.O. q.i.d.

Drugs used to treat cancer *(continued)*

DRUG	ACTION	USUAL ADULT DOSAGE
Nitrosoureas		
Carmustine (BCNU)	Action resembles that of alkylating agents; crosses the blood-brain barrier	75 to 100 mg/m² daily I.V. for 2 days
Lomustine (CCNU)	Action resembles that of alkylating agents; crosses the blood-brain barrier	130 mg/m² P.O.
Semustine (methyl CCNU)	Action resembles that of alkylating agents; crosses the blood-brain barrier	150 to 200 mg/m² P.O.
Plant alkaloids		
Vinblastine (Velban)	Inhibits cell division; specific for M phase of the cell cycle	0.1 or 3.7 mg/m² I.V.
Vincristine (Oncovin)	Inhibits cell division; specific for M phase of the cell cycle	1 to 2 mg/m²/week I.V.

Side effects of chemotherapeutic drugs

Highly toxic, chemotherapeutic agents can cause severe side effects. This chart lists some common side effects of chemotherapeutic drugs by body system, along with related nursing considerations. (For a comprehensive list of the side effects of each drug presented in *Drugs used to treat cancer,* consult a pharmacology reference or drug handbook.)

SIDE EFFECTS	NURSING CONSIDERATIONS
Cardiopulmonary • Edema • Tachycardia • Dyspnea • Wheezing	• Assess vital signs and breathing. • Monitor weight.
Gastrointestinal • Nausea and vomiting • Stomatitis • Diarrhea • Anorexia	• Assess the patient's oral cavity, denture fit, and dental hygiene routine. • Assess the patient's nutritional status and food tolerances. • Assess bowel elimination. • Assess fluid intake and output. • Provide good oral hygiene. Use a soft toothbrush, a special rinse (such as normal saline solution) if the patient has stomatitis, and avoid commercial mouthwash. • Moisten the patient's lips with petroleum jelly. • Administer antiemetics, topical anesthetics, antifungals, and antidiarrheals, as ordered. • Provide dietary adjustments, as needed.
Genitourinary • Hemorrhagic cystitis (urinary urgency, painful urination) • Increased uric acid, blood urea nitrogen, and creatinine levels	• Monitor laboratory results. • Administer I.V. fluids, as ordered. • Encourage fluids (unless contraindicated). • Record fluid intake and output. • Administer allopurinol (Lopurin) and urinary analgesics, as ordered.

(continued)

ADULT NURSING

Side effects of chemotherapeutic drugs *(continued)*

SIDE EFFECTS	NURSING CONSIDERATIONS
Hematopoietic • Bone marrow depression (decreased white and red blood cell counts, decreased hemoglobin and platelet levels)	• Monitor laboratory results. • Assess for infection and bleeding. • Use good hand-washing technique. • Do not expose the patient to visitors or staff with infections. • Use a sponge toothbrush (Toothette) or small toothbrush for mouth care. • Avoid I.M. injections and venipuncture. • Report mild temperature elevations. • Do not administer medications containing aspirin. • Instruct the patient to use an electric razor. • Assist the patient with activities of daily living (ADLs). • Monitor transfusions, as ordered.
Hepatic • Liver enlargement • Jaundice • Weakness	• Report any discomfort over the liver area. • Assess for jaundice. • Assist with ADLs.
Integumentary • Hyperpigmentation • Alopecia • Nail changes • Dermatitis • Acne • Pruritus	• Assess for body-image changes. • Teach the patient ways to deal with alopecia, such as by using wigs, caps, scarves, and cosmetics. Discourage frequent shampooing. • Reassure the patient that hair will grow back slowly (within approximately 2 years) and that nails will regain a normal appearance after chemotherapy ends. Inform the patient that new hair growth may be a different color and texture. • Use mild soap and moisturizing lotion for skin care. • Encourage the patient to use petroleum jelly on the lips. • Provide relief measures for pruritus, including cool compresses or soaks, special bath oils, and medications (such as antihistamines and corticosteroids, as ordered).
Neurologic • Numbness and tingling in the extremities • Loss of fine motor function and deep tendon reflexes • Equilibrium and gait changes	• Assess gait, balance, and coordination. • Teach the patient safety measures. • Assist with ambulation and activities, such as opening packages on trays. • Arrange for a referral for assistive devices.
Reproductive • Possible sterility • Amenorrhea • Irregular menses • Premature menopause • Change in libido • Impotency • Possible fetal abnormalities • Masculinization, feminization, hot flashes, vaginal bleeding, or breast tenderness (with hormone therapy)	• If appropriate, provide information on sperm banks before chemotherapy begins. • Reassure a female patient that normal menses usually resumes after chemotherapy ends. • Advise the patient to continue using contraception. • Encourage the patient to express related concerns.
Eye, ear, nose, and throat • Tinnitus (ringing in the ears) • Hearing loss • Photosensitivity	• Assess the patient's hearing. • Instruct the patient to report tinnitus promptly. • Advise the patient to avoid bright sunlight.

ADULT
NURSING

Psychiatric nursing

Introduction 468

Anxiety disorder 470

Bipolar disorder – manic phase 473

Depression 475

Alcohol abuse 477

Alzheimer's disease 481

Schizophrenia 484

Anorexia nervosa 486

PSYCHIATRIC NURSING

Introduction

This review of psychiatric nursing covers the topics you need to know to achieve success on the NCLEX-PN. Careful study will help prepare you to provide safe, effective care for the psychiatric patients you may encounter in daily practice. Focusing on the psychiatric disorders the nurse is most likely to encounter, this review uses the nursing process framework to present clinical situations. These situations demonstrate important nursing actions based on sound principles — actions you must take to provide safe, effective care.

The disorders covered range from anxiety to schizophrenia. Anxiety — common in many patients — becomes pathologic when it interferes with activities of daily living. A patient with a mood disorder, such as bipolar disorder or depression, may be treated in a psychiatric or general health care setting. Substance abuse may go unnoticed unless the nurse has the skills to recognize signs of abuse and withdrawal and knows how to take an adequate history of substance use. (Questions on substance abuse appear regularly on NCLEX-PN.) Like patients who abuse substances, those with anorexia nervosa are adept at denying their disorder. Nurses who work with older adults inevitably will care for patients suffering from Alzheimer's disease. Nurses working in emergency departments or walk-in clinics typically encounter patients with schizophrenia or other chronic mental disorders as these patients seek help for physical problems or side effects of medications.

When reading this review, you will note that the clinical situations take place mostly in mental health settings. However, keep in mind that patients with psychiatric disorders are just as likely to receive care in other types of health care facilities. You will also find that this review stresses the principles of therapeutic communication described in the section on "Nursing principles" because effective communication is a key nursing tool to reduce patient stress and anxiety. The clinical situations presented here show how to apply the principles of effective communication in patient care.

Glossary

Addiction: psychological or physical dependence on a substance

Affect: outward expression of feelings or emotions

Akathisia: condition characterized by motor restlessness and agitation; a common side effect of antipsychotic medications

Akinesia: condition characterized by muscle paralysis or motor and psychic hypoactivity; a common side effect of antipsychotic medications

Alzheimer's disease: progressive, degenerative brain disease characterized by diffuse atrophy throughout the cerebral cortex, resulting in memory disturbances and personality changes and progressive deterioration to profound dementia

Ambivalence: state in which a person experiences opposing feelings, attitudes, drives, desires, or emotions toward the same object

Anhedonia: profound inability to experience pleasure, characteristic of severe depression or schizophrenia

Anorexia: loss or lack of appetite associated with an underlying illness

Anorexia nervosa: mental disorder characterized by prolonged refusal to eat, leading to emaciation, fear of obesity, and body-image disturbance

Anxiety: state or feeling of agitation, uneasiness, and uncertainty, resulting from the anticipation of some threat or danger. When prolonged, pervasive, and not reality-based, it is pathologic

Aphasia: condition in which language function is defective or absent because of disease of or injury to certain areas of the cerebral cortex. The defect may be sensory or receptive (in which language is not understood) or expressive or motor (in which words cannot be formed or expressed)

Glossary (continued)

Ataxia: condition characterized by impaired muscle coordination

Bulimarexia: cycle of food restriction followed by binging and purging

Bulimia nervosa: mental disorder characterized by episodes of binge eating followed by purging (such as through excessive exercising, vomiting, or use of laxatives or diuretics) and periods of depression and self-deprivation

Compulsion: irresistible, persistent urge to perform an act whose purpose appears irrational or useless

Confirm: to assure the validity of or give approval to

Defense mechanism: unconscious reaction that protects the self from overwhelming anxiety

Delirium: condition characterized by confusion, disorientation, restlessness, altered consciousness, fear, anxiety, incoherence, excitement, and possibly also illusions, hallucinations, or delusions

Delusion: persistent false belief or perception regarding the self or other persons or objects, even though the belief is illogical

Dementia: progressive, organic mental disorder characterized by chronic personality disintegration; confusion; disorientation; stupor; deteriorating intellectual capacity and functioning; and impaired memory, judgment, and impulses

Denial: unconscious defense mechanism in which a person avoids emotional anxiety and conflict by refusing to acknowledge thoughts, feelings, impulses, or external facts that are consciously intolerable

Depression: mood disturbance characterized by feelings of discouragement, sadness, and despair; ranges from normal feelings of sadness to major depression, marked by exaggerated feelings of sadness, melancholy, dejection, hopelessness, worthlessness, emptiness, and sleep and appetite disturbances

Disorientation: inadequate or incorrect perception of place, time, or identity

Displacement: unconscious defense mechanism used to avoid emotional conflict and anxiety by transferring emotions, ideas, or wishes from one object to a less anxiety-producing substitute

Ego: part of the personality that keeps a person reality-oriented and functional

Euphoria: feeling or state of well-being or elation; an exaggerated or abnormal sense of well-being not based in reality, disproportionate to the cause and inappropriate to the situation (as commonly seen in the manic phase of bipolar mood disorder)

Flight of ideas: rapid shift from one idea to another, each idea remaining incomplete

Grief: response to loss or separation, especially the death of a loved one; characterized by mental anguish

Inappropriate affect: expression of feelings or emotions that is inconsistent with the situation

Loose association of ideas: lack of logical connections between similar or simultaneously occurring ideas or perceptions

Mania: mood disorder characterized by expansiveness, extreme excitement and elation, hyperactivity, agitation, hypertalkativeness, flight of ideas, increased psychomotor activity, and fleeting attention; seen in the manic phase of bipolar mood disorder

Mental disorder: clinically significant behavioral or psychological syndrome characterized by signs or symptoms or significant functional impairment

Neologism: new word whose meaning may be known only to the person using it. The creation of neologisms sometimes occurs in schizophrenia

Obsession: recurrent, persistent thought or idea that arises involuntarily despite attempts to ignore or suppress it

Panic attack: acute anxiety reaction typically characterized by palpitations, shortness of breath, dizziness, faintness, profuse sweating, pallor of the face and extremities, and a vague feeling of imminent death

Paranoia: intense, unwarranted belief that one will be harmed

Phobia: irrational, exaggerated fear of a specific object, activity, or situation

Projection: unconscious defense mechanism by which a person attributes unacceptable traits, ideas, or impulses of the self to others or the environment

Rationalization: unconscious defense mechanism in which a person justifies attitudes and actions by applying incorrect reasoning

Reality testing: ability to examine one's behavior and to judge its social acceptability and effectiveness against established norms

Regression: return to an earlier, more primitive form of thought and behavior, as in some mental disorders; a defense mechanism used to protect the self against anxiety

Repression: unconscious defense mechanism in which a person keeps unacceptable thoughts, feelings, ideas, and impulses out of conscious awareness

Self-concept: composite of ideas, feelings, and attitudes a person has about one's own identity, worth, capabilities, and limitations

Self-esteem: satisfaction and confidence in oneself

Tardive dyskinesia: condition characterized by involuntary repetitious movements of the face, limbs, and trunk muscles; an adverse effect of phenothiazine drugs

Validate: to support on a sound basis

Withdrawal: retreat from interpersonal contact and social activities; may become pathologic if it interferes with one's perception of reality and functioning in society (as in schizophrenia)

Withdrawal symptoms: substance-specific physiologic symptoms that follow cessation of regular use of certain psychoactive substances

PSYCHIATRIC NURSING

Anxiety disorder

Overview

Although everyone experiences anxiety from time to time, few people suffer disabling effects. An anxiety disorder occurs when anxiety causes serious impairment. Behaviors seen in anxiety disorder may include obsessions, compulsions, phobias, and anxiety or panic attacks. Physical, cognitive, and emotional signs and symptoms vary. Nursing care aims to reduce the patient's anxiety level and help the patient develop effective coping skills.

Clinical situation

Marvin Dole, age 33, was admitted to the psychiatric unit 3 days ago after a panic anxiety attack at work. He spends up to 6 hours each day straightening his room and the dayroom, and becomes upset when someone makes a mess in either room or when his daily schedule is changed. (His roommate, who suffers from depression, makes no effort to keep his side of the room tidy.)

Mr. Dole tells the nurse that he will not use the elevator because, he states, "elevators are dangerous" and "something awful" will happen if he rides in one. Whenever he sees the elevator, he perspires profusely, complaining that his heart feels as if it will "pound itself out of my body."

Assessment

Nursing behaviors

1. Assess Mr. Dole's anxiety level at each encounter by evaluating his cognitive, emotional, and physical responses.

2. Assess for patterns in Mr. Dole's anxiety level, such as by noting whether his anxiety increases or decreases during certain times of day or is triggered by certain activities or events.

3. Assess Mr. Dole's response to medication (lorazepam [Ativan] 1 mg b.i.d.).

Nursing rationales

1. Frequently assessing Mr. Dole's anxiety level allows appropriate adjustment of nursing care.

2. This will yield information about how often Mr. Dole experiences intolerable amounts of anxiety and how much time he spends trying to control it.

3. If Mr. Dole has side effects, he may be less willing to comply with the medication regimen. (However, some side effects are transient, subsiding as the body adjusts to the medication.) If he develops signs of drug toxicity, withhold the medication and notify the nurse-manager or supervisor.

Nursing diagnoses

• Ineffective individual coping related to limited coping skills
• Altered thought processes related to anxiety that fluctuates from moderate to panic level

Planning and goals

• By the time of discharge, Mr. Dole will spend less than 1 hour each day straightening his room and the dayroom and will sleep 6 continuous hours each night.
• By the time of discharge, Mr. Dole will state two methods to prevent his anxiety from progressing beyond a moderate level.
• By the time of discharge, Mr. Dole will use progressive relaxation when he determines that his anxiety level is moderate.
• By the time of discharge, Mr. Dole will state three reasons for complying with his medication regimen and will state what he should do if he has side effects.

Signs and symptoms of anxiety

This chart presents the typical cognitive, emotional, and physical manifestations of anxiety.

COGNITIVE RESPONSE (THOUGHTS)	EMOTIONAL RESPONSE (FEELINGS)	PHYSICAL RESPONSE (BODILY SENSATIONS)
• Dwelling on the past • Forgetfulness • Inability to concentrate • Poor attention • Poor memory and recall • Poor problem solving	• Apprehensiveness • Easy provocation to tears • Excessive control • Excessive worrying • Feeling of dread or doom • Inflexibility • Irritability • Lack of spontaneity	• Change in eating or sleeping pattern • Fatigue • Inability to relax • Inability to sit still • Increased pulse rate and blood pressure • Increased sweating • Muscle tightness • Nervous, intense speech

Implementation

Nursing behaviors

1. Allow time in Mr. Dole's schedule for compulsive or ritualistic behaviors (such as straightening his room). Plan his daily schedule with him and give him an alarm clock.

2. When Mr. Dole's anxiety level is severe, instruct him to engage in activities involving large muscles, such as walking, cleaning windows, or raking leaves.

3. When Mr. Dole's anxiety level is moderate, assist him with progressive relaxation and help him to express his feelings and thoughts.

4. Teach Mr. Dole to identify times when he should engage in activities to keep his anxiety at or below the moderate level.

5. Teach Mr. Dole about his medication. For instance, make sure he knows its name, dosage, when and how to take it, and what to do if he misses a dose or has side effects. Instruct him to abstain from alcohol or other drugs causing sedation (unless the physician approves). Warn him not to stop taking the medication abruptly.

Nursing rationales

1. Compulsive or ritualistic behavior protects Mr. Dole from overwhelming anxiety. Time for such rituals should be incorporated into the daily routine rather than interrupted because he may become panic stricken if not allowed to complete them. An alarm clock allows Mr. Dole to get up early if he needs to.

2. Such activities help drain off excess energy created by anxiety, eventually reducing anxiety.

3. With moderate anxiety, the patient can make connections between events, if assisted. Progressive relaxation and expression of thoughts and feelings further reduce anxiety and increase one's sense of control.

4. By becoming aware of his anxiety level, Mr. Dole can take steps to control it.

5. Teaching Mr. Dole about his medication will increase his compliance. Most likely, altered brain chemistry contributes to his anxiety; to assure his continued health, he may need to take the medication on a long-term basis to maintain normal brain chemistry. Teaching him to abstain from other CNS depressants helps prevent drug toxicity (CNS depressants potentiate the effects of anxiolytic drugs).

PSYCHIATRIC NURSING

Comparing anxiety levels

Anxiety may be mild, moderate, or severe. When acute, it may take the form of a panic attack. This chart contrasts the behaviors associated with each anxiety level and provides nursing considerations for each.

ANXIETY LEVEL	BEHAVIORS	NURSING CONSIDERATIONS
Mild	• Ability to resolve problems and make decisions without help • Ability to structure one's own time • Alertness • Good memory and recall • Maximal learning • Spontaneous affect	No interventions are needed
Moderate	• Ability to follow a daily routine with minimal assistance • Ability to resolve problems and talk through feelings and thoughts with assistance • "Butterflies" in the stomach • Jitteriness • Pounding heart • Selective inattention (may tune out certain aspects of the environment) • Urinary frequency	Teach relaxation exercises
Severe	• Aimless wandering • Hyperactivity • Increased pulse rate and blood pressure • Marked distractability • Poor concentration • Sense of dread or horror • Short attention span • Narrowed perceptual field	• "Talk" therapy does not help because the patient has poor concentration. • Relaxation exercises are not helpful because the patient cannot concentrate. • Encourage large-muscle activity, such as brisk walking or throwing a ball. • Help the patient perform activities of daily living and follow a daily schedule.
Panic	• Bizarre behavior • Irrational speech or thought patterns • Lack of touch with reality, with hallucinations or delusions	• This is an emergency. The patient needs immediate attention; do not leave alone. • Orient the patient to reality by using simple words and encouraging structured activities or large-muscle activity.

6. Allow Mr. Dole to use the stairway rather than forcing him to use the elevator.

6. Mr. Dole has a phobia of elevators. Forcing him to ride one would cause severe anxiety or a panic attack.

7. If Mr. Dole has a panic attack, administer an anxiolytic drug, as ordered, and remain with him until his anxiety level decreases to at least a moderate level.

7. During a panic attack, a person needs to focus attention. Being alone at this time will increase an already overwhelming anxiety level. By remaining with Mr. Dole until his anxiety level subsides, the nurse can direct his energies to maintain his safety.

Evaluation (outcomes)

• Mr. Dole sleeps 7 hours each night without awakening.
• Mr. Dole spends only 30 minutes each day tidying his part of the room and only 10 minutes tidying the dayroom.
• Mr. Dole can determine when his anxiety rises to a moderate level, and uses progressive relaxation or finds a staff member to talk with when this occurs.
• Mr. Dole states the name, dosage, schedule, and side effects of his medication. He states that if he misses a dose, he will take the regular dose at the next regularly scheduled time.
• Mr. Dole has been free from panic attacks for 5 days.
• Mr. Dole can tolerate riding in the elevator, although he prefers to take the stairs.

PSYCHIATRIC NURSING

Bipolar disorder — manic phase

Overview

Bipolar (manic-depressive) disorder refers to a mood disturbance involving one or more manic phases. Classifications of bipolar disorder include manic, depressed, and mixed (the classification depends on signs and symptoms observed). Usually, bipolar disorder is a chronic condition that can be controlled through careful lifestyle management and medication. Researchers have linked it with brain chemistry imbalance and family history. Women are more likely than men to develop bipolar disorder.

During a manic episode, the patient has boundless energy and euphoria, speaks rapidly, moves quickly from one idea to another (flight of ideas), is intrusive, and becomes irritable if others try to set limits on behavior. Emotions shift rapidly and the patient seldom sleeps more than 3 hours at a time. Weight loss may result from constant activity and inability to sit still long enough to eat a complete meal. During an acute manic episode, physical exhaustion may occur.

Clinical situation

Ida Kern, age 35, is brought to the hospital by her husband because of her disruptive behavior. Mr. Kern states that his wife has not slept for the past 4 days, is alternately irritable and euphoric, and has drained all the money from their bank account "to feed the hungry children of the world." He says she stopped taking lithium carbonate (Lithobid) about 2 weeks ago. Mrs. Kern previously was hospitalized with a diagnosis of bipolar mood disorder — manic phase.

On her way down the hall 2 days after her admission, Mrs. Kern stops the nurse and says, "Good morning, love! Isn't it a glorious day? You look so good! I think I need a haircut. My husband should visit today. I hope breakfast is good." The nurse immediately notes her energy and flight of ideas, sees that her makeup is applied heavily, and notes that she is wearing shoes with 3" (7.6 cm) heels and a low-cut dress with an open side seam extending to midthigh.

When Mrs. Kern stops talking, the nurse reminds her that breakfast is being served. She thanks the nurse for the reminder and proceeds to the dining area, where she quickly consumes a piece of toast and several cups of coffee. She smokes three cigarettes while talking enthusiastically to anyone within earshot. Roaming from table to table, she greets other patients, occasionally snatching and noisily eating food from someone else's tray.

Assessment

Nursing behaviors

1. Assess Mrs. Kern's safety needs, including environmental, sex-related, and physiologic needs.

Nursing rationales

1. During a manic episode, the patient neglects details and risks self-harm from impaired judgment. An increased libido can lead to irresponsible sexual activity. Extended periods of hyperactivity can cause physiologic collapse. The anxiety level usually is severe.

2. Assess Mrs. Kern's activity pattern.

2. This allows the nurse to plan rest periods during relative "down" times.

3. Assess Mrs. Kern's effect on other patients.

3. The nurse must maintain a healing environment for all patients. If Mrs. Kern makes others anxious, she will need constant attention until she has better self-control. If she becomes aggressive, she may need to be confined to her room or placed in seclusion.

4. Assess the effects of medication. The physician has ordered lithium carbonate (Eskalith) 300 mg t.i.d. and perphenazine (Trilafon) 10 mg b.i.d.

4. Lithium toxicity may occur at any time. Until stabilization occurs, blood drug levels should be measured daily, then weekly as Mrs. Kern's manic behaviors decrease. Blood drug levels exceeding 2.0 mEq/liter typically lead to toxicity. Positive effects of lithium take 7 to 10 days to appear after therapy begins. Perphenazine, a neuroleptic drug, commonly is used in conjunction with lithium during this interval to control hyperactivity.

Nursing diagnoses
- Impaired social interaction related to severe anxiety level
- Potential for injury related to impaired judgment

Planning and goals
- Mrs. Kern will adopt appropriate social behaviors, as demonstrated by not taking food from others' trays, wearing more casual makeup and clothing in keeping with the atmosphere on the unit, and not intruding on others' spaces.
- Mrs. Kern will not harm herself or others during her hospital stay.

Implementation

Nursing behaviors

1. Provide Mrs. Kern with a highly structured and predictable environment by following a set routine, minimizing noise, and occupying her with structured activities.

Nursing rationales

1. Structure and consistency reduce the anxiety level and permit rest. A consistent routine decreases the potential for angry outbursts. Noise is highly stimulating and exacerbates hyperactive behavior.

2. If Mrs. Kern cannot sleep at night, allow her to stay up in the dayroom. Provide her with a quiet, structured activity, such as rug hooking, laundry folding, or furniture dusting.

2. During a manic state, a person cannot remain still and quiet. Letting Mrs. Kern stay up in the dayroom permits her roommate to sleep. Providing her with an activity channels her energies into something constructive.

3. Give nighttime sedation, if ordered.

3. This may allow Mrs. Kern to sleep for a few hours.

4. Provide Mrs. Kern with finger foods if she cannot sit down for a meal.

4. This helps maintain nutritional intake.

5. Weigh Mrs. Kern twice a week.

5. This allows the health care team to monitor the adequacy of her food intake.

6. Observe Mrs. Kern for signs and symptoms of lithium toxicity: unsteady gait, excessive urine output, tinnitus, slurred speech, nausea and vomiting, diarrhea, hand tremors, lethargy, and mental confusion. If you suspect toxicity, withhold the medication and notify the nurse-manager or supervisor. Document your observations.

6. Initially, Mrs. Kern's severe anxiety level may prevent her from reporting side effects. Lithium has a narrow therapeutic window (therapeutic levels are close to toxic levels). Lithium toxicity may occur at any time during treatment.

7. Teach Mrs. Kern about the importance of taking her medication regularly and about the side effects.

7. Because of lithium's narrow therapeutic window, Mrs. Kern needs to know the factors that affect the amount of lithium in her body. For instance, excessive sweating, vomiting, diarrhea, and fluid restriction increase lithium concentration, causing toxicity. Excessive fluid intake reduces lithium concentration, leading to return of symptoms. She also must understand that she needs this medication to remain healthy. (The nurse may liken this to a diabetic patient's need for insulin.) Teaching her about side effects will help ensure that she reports them.

Evaluation (outcomes)

• Mrs. Kern can sit down and consume a meal. She no longer wanders about the dining room helping herself to food from others' trays.
• Mrs. Kern sleeps 6 hours a night, between midnight and 6 A.M.
• Mrs. Kern wears casual clothing and more subdued makeup.
• Mrs. Kern interacts appropriately without intruding on others' space.
• Mrs. Kern does not harm herself or others during her hospital stay.
• Mrs. Kern states the name, dosage, and toxic side effects of her medication and states that she understands the importance of remaining on her medication

Depression

Overview

An abnormal elaboration of sadness and grief, depression is the oldest and most often observed human ailment. It ranges from short episodes of sadness to a full-blown illness requiring psychiatric intervention. Common signs and symptoms include sleep and appetite disturbances; feelings of emptiness, unworthiness, and hopelessness; lack of energy; inability to experience pleasure (anhedonia); poor concentration; and thoughts of death. (The illness of depression should not be confused with bipolar disorder, which includes episodes of depression and mania.)

Anyone experiencing depression is at risk for suicide. Many depressed people do not seek treatment, however, because they do not realize the condition is treatable. Typically, pathologic behavior leads to family intervention.

Clinical situation

Doreen Sill, age 45, is admitted to the hospital after a serious suicide attempt. She is diagnosed with major depression. In the past 3 weeks, she has lost 15 lb (6.8 kg).

Three days after Mrs. Sill's admission, the nurse who enters her room at 7:45 A.M. finds she still is in bed and has not begun to get ready for breakfast. When the nurse reminds her that breakfast will be served in 30 minutes, she closes her eyes, sighs, and says softly, "I just want to die." The nurse helps her get up and dress; she slowly follows the nurse's commands. It takes her 10 minutes to remove her nightgown and put on the sweatsuit that the nurse has chosen for her because she cannot decide what to wear.

In the dining room, Mrs. Sill sits motionless in front of the food selected for her. She eats two bites of her scrambled egg, takes one sip of juice, then says in a monotone, "I'm full." After breakfast, Mrs. Sill returns to her room and lays on top of her unmade bed. She remains there for the rest of the morning, not getting up for her scheduled therapies. She makes no effort to respond verbally when someone speaks to her.

Assessment

Nursing behaviors

1. Assess Mrs. Sill's potential for suicide, such as by noting any expressions of a desire not to live and prior suicide attempts.

2. Assess Mrs. Sill's depression level by uncovering such subjective feelings as anhedonia, hopelessness, despair, and low self-esteem and by evaluating such objective data as energy level, sleep pattern, and eating pattern.

3. Assess Mrs. Sill's ability to perform activities of daily living (ADLs).

4. Assess the effects of Mrs. Sill's medication — amitriptyline (Elavil) 150 mg at bedtime and 75 mg at 9 A.M.

Nursing rationales

1. Depression places a person at risk for suicide.

2. Subjective and objective data reflect the level of depression. The more severe the depression, the more assistance the patient needs from the nurse. As depression appears to lift, the person gains the energy to plan and carry out suicide.

3. This helps the nurse determine Mrs. Sill's self-esteem and energy level. Commonly, people with low self-esteem do not groom themselves.

4. In her present condition, Mrs. Sill may be not be aware of or report side effects. Stay especially alert for anticholinergic side effects. Keep in mind that antidepressant medications generally take 2 to 5 weeks to start to relieve depression. The larger bedtime dose takes advantage of the side effect of sedation to promote sleep.

Nursing diagnoses

- Self-care deficit (dressing and grooming) related to lack of energy
- Potential for self-directed violence related to feelings of despair and low self-esteem

Planning and goals

- Mrs. Sill will not attempt suicide while hospitalized.
- Mrs. Sill will demonstrate the ability to feed, dress, and bathe herself by a planned date.
- Mrs. Sill will name at least four people she can call on for help after she is discharged.

Implementation

Nursing behaviors

1. Assist Mrs. Sill with daily grooming and other ADLs, even if she resists or responds negatively to such help, until her energy returns.

2. Do not ask Mrs. Sill to make decisions when she lacks the energy to do so.

3. Escort Mrs. Sill to daily activities. Do not allow her to spend more than 2 daytime hours in bed.

Nursing rationales

1. Assistance conveys that the nurse cares at a time when Mrs. Sill lacks the energy to care for herself. If the nurse fails to help her, she will feel more alone, worthless, and hopeless.

2. Decision making takes energy. Requiring Mrs. Sill to make decisions before she is ready would tax her depleted energies; furthermore, her inability to make even minor decisions would confirm her perception of herself as a failure.

3. Making Mrs. Sill go through the motions of a daily routine can help her regain energy. Making her go to activities reduces her social isolation.

4. Weigh Mrs. Sill twice a week on a set schedule (such as every Tuesday and Saturday).

4. Monitoring weight helps assess the adequacy of food intake. A set schedule promotes a comfortable routine.

5. Check Mrs. Sill's sleeping pattern at the end of each night shift.

5. Depressed people have disturbed sleep patterns. As Mrs. Sill's depression lifts, she will be able to sleep for longer periods at night.

6. Teach Mrs. Sill about her medication, including its name, dosage, when and how to take it, what to do if she misses a dose, how to manage bothersome side effects, and dietary restrictions (if she is receiving a monoamine oxidase inhibitor).

6. Research shows that many depressed people have an imbalance in brain chemistry, which usually can be corrected with proper medication. If Mrs. Sill understands why she must take medication, she is more likely to comply with the regimen.

7. When Mrs. Sill's energy returns, help her identify outside resources she can call on in times of need.

7. This will help Mrs. Sill build a social support system, which can decrease her risk for suicide.

Evaluation (outcomes)

• Mrs. Sill makes no suicide attempts during her hospital stay.
• Mrs. Sill independently performs all self-care activities. Her weight returns to its usual level.
• Mrs. Sill makes two successful home visits and contacts the people she said she could call on in times of need.
• Mrs. Sill states the name, dosage, and side effects of her medication. She states that she will remain on the medication as long as necessary.

Alcohol abuse

Overview

Alcohol abuse, a major public health problem, affects over 10 million Americans. Both a depressant and an irritant, alcohol is associated with such medical problems as gastritis, pancreatitis, esophagitis, chronic obstructive pulmonary disease, cirrhosis, hypertension, and leg and foot ulcers. When consumed even in small quantities by a pregnant woman, it can cause fetal alcohol syndrome.

The causes of alcohol abuse vary, and may include biological, psychological, and social factors. Alcohol abuse typically begins when a person starts consuming alcohol to cope with stress; eventually, the desired result comes about only by increasing alcohol consumption. As tolerance develops, withdrawal symptoms may occur if alcohol is not available.

The alcohol abuser typically uses denial, projection, and rationalization to hide the problem from others, and must abandon these defense mechanisms before treatment can begin. Usually, the alcohol abuser does not see health care workers until related health problems, such as hepatitis or gastritis, develop. The following clinical situation focuses on a patient whose alcoholism surfaces after his admission to a health care facility for acute gastritis.

PSYCHIATRIC NURSING

Clinical situation

Robert Kyle, age 40, a successful realtor, is admitted to the medical unit with a diagnosis of acute gastritis. Ten hours later, the nurse who checks his vital signs sees that he is tremulous, restless, and diaphoretic. His pulse rate is 110 beats/minute and his blood pressure, 180/100 mm Hg. The nurse reports these findings to the nurse-manager, who reveals that Mr. Kyle has a history of alcohol abuse and states that the findings suggest he is experiencing withdrawal. The nurse-manager instructs the nurse to give him his P.R.N. dose of diazepam (Valium).

Over the next 3 days, Mr. Kyle begins to confide in the practical nurse, revealing that he consumes alcohol every day. However, he does not believe his consumption has caused any problems. He says he has a responsible job and gives his wife and children everything they need. Furthermore, he states, his job requires that he drink with prospective clients over lunch. He also reveals that he usually has a drink or two every evening "to unwind" but has not felt drunk for years.

The physician orders Mr. Kyle to abstain from alcohol and cut back on his work load. Mr. Kyle tells the nurse he thinks this order is nonsense. "Except for my stomach pain," he says, "I'm fine. I expect to be around for at least 40 more years."

Assessment

Nursing behaviors

1. Assess Mr. Kyle's physiologic status by measuring his vital signs and weight, checking his orientation level, observing for ascites and esophageal bleeding, and checking laboratory results.

2. Assess Mr. Kyle's history of alcohol and other substance use.

3. Assess Mr. Kyle's readiness to examine his alcohol abuse.

Nursing rationales

1. Monitoring Mr. Kyle's physiologic status helps ensure his safety. Esophageal bleeding and liver cirrhosis are common in long-term alcohol abusers. Once withdrawal begins, it can progress to stage 4. (For details on the stages of alcohol withdrawal, see *Recognizing alcohol withdrawal stages*.)

2. The substance use pattern yields clues to the response to withdrawal. (Withdrawal symptoms occur in direct proportion to the alcohol consumption level.)

3. Mr. Kyle risks death if he does not abstain from or reduce his alcohol consumption.

Nursing diagnoses

• Impaired adjustment related to denial of alcohol abuse
• Noncompliance with the treatment plan related to perceived invulnerability

Planning and goals

• By the time of discharge, Mr. Kyle will be free from complications of gastritis.
• By the time of discharge, Mr. Kyle will talk with the clinical nurse specialist about his alcohol abuse.

Implementation

Nursing behaviors

1. Follow the standards of care for a patient with gastritis. Provide a soft, bland diet. Monitor vital signs every 4 hours. Administer antacids and cimetidine (Tagamet), as ordered. Provide dietary teaching.

Nursing rationales

1. These standards ensure proper care. A soft bland diet decreases irritation of the gastric lining. Monitoring vital signs helps detect signs of internal bleeding and alcohol withdrawal. Antacids decrease irritation from stomach acids. Cimetidine decreases stomach acid production. Dietary teaching helps ensure compliance and good nutrition.

Recognizing alcohol withdrawal stages

This chart reviews the four stages of alcohol withdrawal. Keep in mind that during stages 2 through 4, the patient requires one-on-one care. Use restraints only as a last resort because they may heighten the patient's anxiety and agitation.

WITHDRAWAL STAGE	SIGNS AND SYMPTOMS	ONSET	NURSING INTERVENTIONS
1	• Diaphoresis • Increased blood pressure • Mild tremors • Nausea • Nervousness • Tachycardia	Within 8 hours after the last drink	• Monitor vital signs. • Monitor the patient's behavior carefully. • Seek a physician's order for medication to relieve withdrawal symptoms. • Stay with the patient once withdrawal begins. • Talk to the patient about withdrawal symptoms.
2	• Anorexia • Delusions • Disorientation • Hyperactivity • Increased tremors • Insomnia • Visual hallucinations	8 to 10 hours after the last drink (follows quickly after stage 1)	• Monitor vital signs. • Administer medications, as ordered, to relieve withdrawal symptoms. • Stay with the patient and orient the patient to reality. • Keep the environment free from distractions and unnecessary noise.
3	Same as for stages 1 and 2, plus generalized tonic-clonic seizures and persistent hallucinations	12 to 48 hours after the last drink	• Monitor vital signs. • Stay with the patient. • Institute seizure precautions. • Administer anticonvulsant medications, as ordered. • Offer fluids and light foods, as tolerated, during lucid periods. • Maintain a calm environment.
4	• Delirium tremens • Hallucinations • Sleeplessness • Tachycardia	Within 3 to 5 days after the last drink	• Monitor vital signs. • Stay with the patient. • Maintain a calm environment. • Offer fluids and light foods, as tolerated, during lucid periods.

2. Monitor Mr. Kyle's abdominal girth during every shift.

2. This helps evaluate ascites.

3. Perform the guaiac test on all stools and emesis.

3. This test detects occult blood, which may stem from GI bleeding.

4. Monitor Mr. Kyle's orientation level.

4. This helps detect delirium related to alcohol withdrawal.

5. Consult with the primary care nurse about a referral to the clinical nurse specialist for help in addressing Mr. Kyle's alcohol abuse.

5. The clinical nurse specialist can provide Mr. Kyle with initial assistance and referral to other sources. His denial and sense of invulnerability are defensive and protect him from intolerable anxiety.

6. Attend an in-service program on alcohol abuse and its manifestations.

6. An increased knowledge base helps the nurse provide safe, competent nursing care.

7. Ask Mr. Kyle what it would take to get him to change his alcohol abuse (in other words, his "bottom line").

7. This question plants a seed in Mr. Kyle's mind and challenges his denial indirectly. Most people can identify their bottom line, which serves as a measuring stick.

Evaluation (outcomes)

- Mr. Kyle remains free from complications of gastritis and alcohol withdrawal.
- Mr. Kyle tells the clinical nurse specialist that he will cut back to two drinks daily, although he does not plan to abstain from alcohol.

Signs and symptoms of substance withdrawal

Because nurses are likely to care for patients at risk for substance withdrawal, they must be able to recognize impending withdrawal. This chart shows signs and symptoms of withdrawal from various substances, along with corresponding interventions. (For information on signs and symptoms of alcohol withdrawal, see *Recognizing alcohol withdrawal stages,* page 479.)

DRUG CATEGORY	SIGNS AND SYMPTOMS	NURSING INTERVENTIONS
Opiates (such as morphine, heroin)	• Chills • Dilated pupils • Excessive sweating • Fever • Food craving • Insomnia • Muscle aches • Nausea or vomiting • Runny nose • Yawning • Tachycardia • Tearing of the eyes	• Monitor vital signs. • Stay with the patient. • Offer fluids and light foods, as tolerated. • Provide a soothing, nondistracting environment. • As ordered, wean the patient by administering small doses of the abused opiate. (Methadone [Dolophine] also may be given in some cases.)
Central nervous system stimulants (such as amphetamines, cocaine, crack cocaine)	• Agitation • Disorientation • Fatigue • Insomnia or hypersomnia • Mental depression • Paranoia • Suicidal tendencies	• Promote sleep and rest. • Monitor vital signs. • Stay with a frightened or disoriented patient. • Stay alert for suicidal behavior. Administer an antidepressant, as ordered and needed. • Orient the patient to reality.
Hallucinogens Lysergic acid diethylamide (LSD)	• None known	• If the patient has a "bad trip," stay with and keep the patient oriented to reality.
Phencyclidine (PCP)	• Depression • Food craving • Lethargy	• Monitor vital signs and level of depression. • Ensure the patient's safety.
Cannabis (marijuana)	• Apathy • Lethargy • Memory loss	• Help the patient fill in memory gaps. • Attend to any neglected self-care needs.
Barbiturates (such as pentobarbital [Nembutal]) and anxiolytics (such as diazepam [Valium])	• Anxiety • Coarse tremors of the hands, eyelids, and tongue • Excessive sweating • Generalized tonic-clonic seizures • Insomnia • Irritability • Malaise • Nausea or vomiting • Orthostatic hypotension • Tachycardia	• Monitor vital signs. • Stay with the patient. • Promote rest and sleep. • Offer fluids and light foods, as tolerated. • As ordered, administer medications for weaning (such as progressively smaller dosages of a similar drug). • Take seizure precautions.

Alzheimer's disease

Overview

Affecting mainly older adults, Alzheimer's disease is a serious health problem after age 65. Onset usually is gradual; the most striking early symptom is loss of memory for recent events. As brain impairment continues, signs and symptoms become more dramatic. (For information on the stages of Alzheimer's disease, see *Assessing Alzheimer's disease,* page 482.) Impairment increases as various brain structures deteriorate. Structures associated with higher-level functions (such as thought and memory) deteriorate first. Structures associated with lower-level functions (such as talking and walking) deteriorate last.

Clinical situation

Annette Riley, age 73, was admitted to the nursing home 6 months ago when her family no longer could manage her care at home. A pleasant woman, she is in the second stage of Alzheimer's disease. She believes she is in a foreign country and sometimes calls the nurse by her daughter's name. She wanders around the nursing home, often rummaging through other patients' belongings, then becoming upset when the nurse sets limits on this behavior.

Unless reminded or assisted, Mrs. Riley forgets to brush her teeth and comb her hair. Occasionally, she urinates in the corner of the hall, explaining that she got lost on the way to the "outhouse." Although she wears eyeglasses, she says she does not see well; her hearing also seems poor. The nurse notes that despite a large appetite, Mrs. Riley weighs only 93 lb (42.2 kg). Today, during a bingo game, she puts the bingo pieces in her mouth.

Assessment

Nursing behaviors

1. Assess Mrs. Riley's nutritional, neurologic, and elimination status.

2. Assess Mrs. Riley's mental status, including her memory; orientation to time, place, and person; and problem-solving ability.

3. Assess Mrs. Riley's ability to walk without help.

4. Assess Mrs. Riley's ability to meet her grooming and hygiene needs.

Nursing rationales

1. This yields baseline data that help monitor disease progression and guide nursing interventions.

2. This contributes to baseline data that help monitor disease progression. Assessment of mental status guides nursing interventions. Mrs. Riley's problem-solving ability determines what she can do without assistance.

3. Mrs. Riley's coordination and gait may be impaired, predisposing her to falls that could result in bone fractures or head injury.

4. As Alzheimer's disease progresses, Mrs. Riley will become increasingly unable to perform grooming and hygiene tasks. For instance, she may not remember how to work zippers or buttons and may lack the coordination to put on or take off clothing.

Nursing diagnoses

• Altered thought processes related to inability to organize incoming stimuli
• Potential for injury related to poor judgment and vision

Planning and goals

• Mrs. Riley will be able to perform self-care with assistance.
• Mrs. Riley will remain free from serious injury.

PSYCHIATRIC NURSING

Assessing Alzheimer's disease

Understanding how Alzheimer's disease progresses helps the nurse plan appropriate care and maximize the patient's functional ability. This chart summarizes the stages of disease progression.

STAGE	APPROXIMATE DURATION	SIGNS AND SYMPTOMS	NURSING CONSIDERATIONS
I	2 to 4 years	• "Fishing" for words • Forgetfulness progressing to inability to recall details of recent events • Irritability or apathy • Occasional episodes of getting lost • Periods of disorientation • Significantly impaired reasoning ability and judgment	• The patient typically can manage most daily activities and does not require institutionalization. • The patient senses a decrease in mental faculties and may use denial to cope with this. Do not force the patient to "face the facts."
II	2 to 12 years	• Reduced vision, hearing, and pain sensation • Hyperorality (chewing or tasting anything within reach) • Inability to recognize familiar things (may not recognize own mirror reflection) • Increased aphasia (language defect) • Increased appetite without weight gain • Perserveration (repeating the same word or action over and over) • Seizures • Social inappropriateness, such as poor table manners, personal hygiene, and grooming	• Assist the patient with hygiene and grooming to preserve self-esteem and dignity. • Avoid using puns or jokes because these will confuse the patient. • Call the patient by name rather than "Honey," "Grandma," or another belittling term. • If the patient has trouble walking, accompany the patient on walks several times a day to prevent muscle contractures and other complications of immobility. • Maintain a consistent, calm environment to orient the patient. • Make sure the patient wanders only in safe areas. • Monitor the items the patient places in the mouth. • Maintain the patient on a toileting schedule to minimize incontinence. • Stay with the patient during meals to observe for swallowing problems and assist with table manners.
III	1 year	• Apraxia (inability to perform purposeful movements, even on command) • Bladder and bowel incontinence • Decreased appetite • Disappearance of perseveration and hyperorality • Generalized tonic-clonic seizures • Muteness • Unresponsiveness to verbal and physical stimuli	• Maintain a consistent routine. • Monitor the patient's skin for breakdown and pressure ulcers. • Monitor all body systems carefully for physiologic deterioration. • Perform passive range-of-motion exercises at least 4 times a day to prevent contractures, if the patient is bedridden.

Adapted with permission from R. Charles, M. Truesdell, and E. Wood (1982). Alzheimer's disease: Pathology, progression, and nursing process. *Journal of Gerontological Nursing*, 8(2), pp. 69-73.

Implementation

Nursing behaviors	Nursing rationales
1. Ensure that Mrs. Riley's routines (meals, daily care, bedtime rituals) and activities are highly structured.	**1.** Structured routines and activities help orient the patient and reduce confusion.
2. Assign the same staff consistently to work with Mrs. Riley.	**2.** The patient with Alzheimer's disease has trouble adjusting to new personnel. Seeing the same staff members each day will help keep Mrs. Riley oriented and give her a sense of control.
3. Accompany Mrs. Riley to meals and other activities.	**3.** Mrs. Riley risks choking during meals. By accompanying her, the nurse can prevent this problem while ensuring appropriate table manners and helping her perform simple activities.
4. Have Mrs. Riley wear a small helmet.	**4.** This helps protect her from injury caused by a fall (for instance, from a seizure).
5. Weigh Mrs. Riley every Tuesday and Saturday (or on another schedule with 3-day intervals). If Mrs. Riley loses more than 1 lb (0.5 kg) a week, notify the physician.	**5.** Regular weighing helps monitor the adequacy of food intake. The physician may prescribe a dietary supplement (such as Ensure) to bolster caloric intake if Mrs. Riley loses more than 1 lb (0.5 kg) a week.
6. Escort Mrs. Riley to the bathroom every 2 hours, between 7 A.M. and bedtime.	**6.** Mrs. Riley may be unaware of the urge to urinate or move her bowels, or she may get lost on the way to the bathroom. Escorting her provides routine and maintains her dignity. If she is incontinent and needs to wear protection, refer to the protective garment as a brief or special underwear—never as a diaper.
7. Help Mrs. Riley organize her personal items every day.	**7.** This provides routine and structure, helping to keep her oriented.
8. Provide a safe place in which Mrs. Riley can wander (such as an enclosed patio, a hallway, or a dayroom).	**8.** Wandering is beneficial because it is both a familiar activity (walking) and good exercise. Preventing Mrs. Riley from wandering would cause unnecessary frustration.

Evaluation (outcomes)

- Mrs. Riley dresses herself with assistance.
- Mrs. Riley takes small bites when eating (otherwise, she chokes). She does best with soft foods.
- Mrs. Riley learns the names of the three staff members who care for her most of the time and seldom misidentifies them.
- Mrs. Riley's seizures are under control and she has not suffered a fall in 3 weeks.
- Mrs. Riley spends several hours each day wandering in the hall or in the enclosed patio, where she feeds the squirrels and watches the birds.

PSYCHIATRIC NURSING

Schizophrenia

Overview

Approximately half of the people diagnosed with psychiatric disorders have schizophrenia, a disorder that seriously impairs the ability to function in a socially appropriate manner. Typically, schizophrenia manifests as changes in thinking, perception, emotions (affect), physical activity, and relationships.

Changes in thinking may manifest as delusions and loose associations (illogical flow of ideas). The language may include neologisms, or nonsense words. Changes in thinking also cause inappropriate behavior and limit the ability to perform self-care.

Changes in perception may cause the patient to respond to sensory stimulation that does not exist in the external world. For instance, the patient may hallucinate (see, hear, feel, smell, or taste things that do not exist); be unable to distinguish the self from others; or have disturbed body perception, perceiving a body part as much larger than it is.

Changes in emotions may include flat affect or inappropriate emotions (for instance, hilarity after receiving sad news). Some patients experience intense ambivalence—for example, fearing a relationship yet longing for one at the same time.

Changes in physical activity range from hyperactivity to slow-motion movements. The person may act impulsively if challenged or frustrated, or may assume a fixed posture for a prolonged period.

Changes in relationships manifest as inability to relate well with others. The patient spends much time alone or on the periphery when others gather, keeps relationships superficial to protect against being hurt, and rarely makes or welcomes eye or physical contact.

Clinical situation

Alan Wood, age 49, developed schizophrenia at age 21. Since then, he has been in and out of hospitals. Three months ago, he stopped taking thioridazine (Mellaril), an antipsychotic medication. Just before his most recent hospital admission 4 days ago, he became acutely psychotic. He hears voices (auditory hallucinations) but cannot determine what they are saying. For the last 2 days, he has had delusions, telling staff members he is dead. When they point out that he is alive, he tells them they are wrong.

Mr. Wood has a noticeable body odor. Patches of whiskers dot his face and his clothing is dirty and torn. His speech is hard to follow because his thoughts do not hang together (loose associations). He approaches staff members, then retreats when they turn their attention to him. While using the toilet in the main hall, he often leaves the door open (reflecting social inappropriateness). The physician orders fluphenazine decanoate (Prolixin Decanoate) 50 mg to be administered I.M. every 4 weeks.

Assessment

Nursing behaviors	**Nursing rationales**
1. Assess Mr. Wood's anxiety level.	**1.** The anxiety level guides nursing interventions.
2. Assess Mr. Wood's ability to perform self-care activities, such as hygiene and grooming.	**2.** This yields information about Mr. Wood's functional level. Disturbed thinking and severe anxiety may make self-care difficult.

3. Assess Mr. Wood's response to staff members and other patients, noting his social involvement and eye contact.

3. This provides information about Mr. Wood's interpersonal skills and degree of loneliness.

4. Assess the nature and pattern of Mr. Wood's hallucinations, including any precipitating events.

4. Command hallucinations (for instance, "Kill yourself") place the patient at risk for injury. Identifying precipitating events can reduce or prevent hallucinations.

5. Assess the nature and pattern of Mr. Wood's delusions.

5. Delusions are a response to underlying needs.

Nursing diagnoses
• Sensory-perceptual alterations (auditory) related to failure of the ego to remain reality oriented
• Impaired social interaction related to disturbance in thinking

Planning and goals
• Mr. Wood will stop hallucinating or gain control of hallucinations by the time of discharge.
• Mr. Wood will relate to his primary care nurse and at least two other people in an appropriate way.
• Mr. Wood will be able to perform self-care activities by the time of discharge.
• Mr. Wood will state three reasons why he must keep taking his medication after discharge.

Implementation

Nursing behaviors

1. Provide Mr. Wood with a structured, predictable environment and a written daily schedule. Assign as few staff members as possible to care for him.

Nursing rationales

1. Structure and predictability will help reduce Mr. Wood's anxiety, help him stay oriented to reality, give him a sense of control, and eliminate the need for him to expend energy adjusting to changes (including staff changes).

2. Involve Mr. Wood in small group projects, such as baking, puzzle building, and weeding.

2. This will help build Mr. Wood's social skills, provide a structured activity, give him a sense of accomplishment, and reduce his social isolation.

3. Assist Mr. Wood with his daily care until he can provide such care for himself.

3. Until Mr. Wood's thought processes clear, he will lack the concentration to perform his own care independently. To neglect his care would contribute to his sense of isolation and increase his anxiety.

4. Teach Mr. Wood how to control or stop his hallucinations, such as by singing, humming, talking, engaging in an activity, listening to music, or saying the word "Stop!"

4. These techniques may control or interrupt hallucinations, allowing the patient to remain functional and reality oriented.

5. Do not ask Mr. Wood questions about his hallucinations while they are in progress.

5. Questioning Mr. Wood while he hallucinates would keep him out of touch with reality. Instead, involve him in an activity, such as walking, raking leaves, throwing a ball, or singing.

PSYCHIATRIC NURSING

6. After an episode of hallucinations, allow Mr. Wood to rest.

6. Hallucinations are tiring. Rest restores energy.

7. When Mr. Wood has delusions, divert him to a structured activity. Do not refute the delusion.

7. Delusions are false ideas that do not go away when refuted. Directly refuting a delusion would increase Mr. Wood's anxiety and make him hang on to the delusion even more.

8. Teach Mr. Wood about his new medication, including its name, reason for taking it, reason for I.M. administration, how to deal with side effects, where to get his monthly injection, and whom to call if he has questions. Explain that he may have to take the medication for the rest of his life.

8. For Mr. Wood to live outside a health care facility, he must take the prescribed medication. Teaching will improve his compliance. Liken his need for medication to correct brain chemistry imbalance to the diabetic patient's need for insulin.

Evaluation (outcomes)

• Mr. Wood learns how to interrupt his hallucinations by singing a familiar song.
• Mr. Wood no longer believes he is dead, although he says he is afraid of getting a bad cold that could kill him.
• Mr. Wood showers daily but continues to need help caring for his clothes. He still misses areas on his face when shaving but can shave these areas if someone helps him.
• Mr. Wood talks for short periods with his primary nurse, his roommate, and one other patient. He joins in unit activities, although remaining on the periphery.
• Mr. Wood experiences no side effects of fluphenazine. He states that after discharge, he will visit the clinic on the last Friday of each month for his injection (he lives within walking distance of the clinic).

Anorexia nervosa

Overview

A potentially life-threatening eating disorder, anorexia nervosa most commonly begins at age 12 to 18. It is characterized by refusal to eat, weight loss, excessive exercising, body-image disturbance, and fear of becoming fat. (For theories on the underlying cause of anorexia, see *Theoretical perspectives on anorexia nervosa*.)

Clinical situation

Linda Woszciak, age 15, is admitted to the health care facility by her family physician when her weight drops from 120 lb (54.4 kg) to 80 lb (36.3 kg) over a 4-month period. On admission, her blood pressure measures 90/60 mm Hg; respiratory rate, 20 breaths/minute; pulse rate, 56 beats/minute; and temperature, 96.8° F (36° C). Physical examination reveals poor skin turgor, ankle edema, and pale conjunctivae. She is 5'5" tall (165.8 cm).

Although Linda is quiet during the intake assessment conducted by two staff nurses, she states that she feels very fat. She says she does not want to gain weight because she knows that once she starts to do so, she will not be able to stop until she weighs at least 300 lb. Linda's discharge depends on achieving and maintaining a weight of at least 105 lb (47.6 kg) for at least 1 week.

Theoretical perspectives on anorexia nervosa

The chart below compares various theories on the underlying cause of anorexia nervosa.

THEORY	PROPOSED CAUSE OF ANOREXIA NERVOSA
Psychoanalytic	Rejection of femininity and sexuality, which results from unconscious fears of maturing and becoming an adult woman
Developmental	Unsatisfactory resolution of autonomy issues (food restriction imparts a sense of self-control)
Biologic	Neurochemical brain changes, genetic predisposition, or depression (especially when anorexia nervosa is accompanied by bulimia)
Feminist	Devaluation of self-worth and the body caused by the perception that one does not measure up to cultural (male) expectations for femininity (thinness and passivity)

Assessment

Nursing behaviors

1. Assess Linda's physiologic status.

2. Assess Linda's ability to perform self-care activities.

3. Assess Linda's ability to eat the foods prescribed during the initial refeeding process.

Once Linda attains a weight of at least 90 lb (40.8 kg), also conduct the following assessments:

4. Ask Linda why she thinks she has been hospitalized.

5. Assess Linda's expectations of herself.

6. Assess Linda's self-perception.

Nursing rationales

1. Starvation has compromised Linda's physiologic status, placing her at risk for complications.

2. Linda may need assistance with self-care because of lack of energy caused by being underweight.

3. Linda may have trouble ingesting foods because of her small stomach capacity and fear of becoming fat.

4. Eliciting Linda's perception conveys the nurse's interest in her as a person and allows the nurse to discuss areas of misperception with her.

5. This helps the nurse determine if Linda has reasonable, age-appropriate expectations.

6. If Linda does not adjust her body image to one incorporating an increased weight (105 lb), she will continue to risk disordered eating.

Nursing diagnoses
- Body image disturbance
- Altered growth and development: Failure to attain age-level independence

PSYCHIATRIC NURSING

Planning and goals
- Linda will express acceptance of her body.
- Linda will engage in age-appropriate activities with her peers.

Implementation

Nursing behaviors	**Nursing rationales**
1. Monitor Linda's physiologic status daily, including vital signs, skin turgor, and laboratory results, until her weight reaches at least 90 lb.	**1.** Linda cannot attend to higher-level needs, such as self-esteem and independence, until her physiologic status no longer is compromised. If her weight drops or laboratory results reveal further compromise, notify the nurse-manager and physician immediately to prevent death from an electrolyte imbalance or other complication.
2. Assist Linda with self-care activities, as needed.	**2.** Assistance conveys caring, helps Linda conserve energy, builds her self-esteem, and promotes trust.
3. Stay with Linda as she eats.	**3.** The nurse's presence will deter Linda from disposing of food secretly and provide social stimulation and emotional support.

After Linda reaches 90 lb, carry out the following implementations:

4. Help Linda set attainable daily goals.	**4.** Setting daily goals involves Linda actively in her care, empowers her, and maximizes the benefits of her hospitalization.
5. Have Linda write down her expectations of herself, then determine if each expectation is reasonable.	**5.** This allows Linda to "see" her expectations and possibly to judge them realistically.
6. Every week, use a body-image scale, containing drawings of various body shapes, with Linda. After you both fill out the scale, discuss the drawing she selects to represent her.	**6.** This allows Linda to see her progress toward developing a realistic body image and to compare her self-perceptions with those of another person. The nurse who is comfortable with her own body provides a healthy role model for Linda.

Evaluation (outcomes)
- Linda attains a medically safe weight.
- Linda expresses self-acceptance.
- Linda sets and meets reasonable daily goals and expresses satisfaction with them.
- Linda makes plans to engage in activities with her peers.

Drugs used to treat psychiatric disorders

This chart presents information about drugs commonly prescribed for psychiatric disorders, including the drug action, dosage, and common side effects. Nursing considerations focus on patient comfort and teaching; side effects appear in italicized type in this column.

DRUG AND USUAL ADULT DOSAGE	ACTION	NURSING CONSIDERATIONS AND COMMON SIDE EFFECTS
Antianxiety drugs		
Alprazolam (Xanax): 0.25 mg P.O. b.i.d. or t.i.d. Chlordiazepoxide (Librium): 25 to 100 mg P.O. daily in divided doses Diazepam (Valium): 5 to 40 mg P.O. daily in divided doses Hydroxyzine (Atarax, Vistaril): 50 to 400 mg P.O. daily in divided doses Lorazepam (Ativan): 1 to 6 mg P.O. daily in divided doses	Produces a calming effect by enhancing the action of the inhibitory neurotransmitter gamma-aminobutyric acid (GABA)	• To reduce *daytime sedation,* ask the physician for an order for a smaller dosage and allow the patient to nap during the day until the body adjusts to the medication. • Offer sugar-free drinks and candy to relieve *dry mouth.* • To avoid *orthostatic hypertension,* have the patient rise slowly. • Because of *lethargy* and *drowsiness,* advise the patient to avoid driving or operating heavy machinery.
Antidepressants		
Tricyclics Amitriptyline (Elavil): 75 to 200 mg/day	Elevates the mood by blocking reuptake of norepinephrine and serotonin into central nervous system (CNS) neurons	• Before starting therapy, document the patient's baseline pulse rate, blood pressure, and electrocardiogram (ECG). Monitor these periodically to detect *hypotension* or *arrhythmias.* • This drug is associated with a high incidence of *drowsiness,* especially when therapy begins. Some clinicians prefer to administer the entire daily dose at bedtime to minimize daytime drowsiness. • To reduce *orthostatic hypotension,* instruct the patient to rise slowly when shifting to an upright position. Measure and document the patient's supine and standing blood pressure; withhold the drug and inform the nurse-manager if systolic pressure drops more than 30 mm Hg. • Offer sugar-free drinks and candy to relieve *dry mouth.* • To detect *urine retention,* monitor urine output. Inform the nurse-manager if output is low.
Amoxapine (Asendin): 50 mg P.O. t.i.d.	Elevates the mood by blocking reuptake of norepinephrine and serotonin into CNS neurons; also may block post-synaptic dopamine receptors	• Before starting therapy, document the patient's baseline pulse rate, blood pressure, and ECG. Monitor these periodically to detect *hypotension* or *arrhythmias.* • Use cautiously in patients with Parkinson's disease because the drug may worsen this disorder. • This drug is associated with a high incidence of *drowsiness,* especially when therapy begins. Some clinicians prefer to administer the entire daily dose at bedtime to minimize daytime drowsiness. • To reduce *orthostatic hypotension,* instruct the patient to rise slowly when shifting to an upright position. Measure and document the patient's supine and standing blood pressure; withhold the drug and inform the nurse-manager if systolic pressure drops more than 30 mm Hg. • Offer sugar-free drinks and candy to relieve *dry mouth.* • To detect *urine retention,* monitor urine output. Inform the nurse-manager if output is low.

(continued)

Drugs used to treat psychiatric disorders *(continued)*

DRUG AND USUAL ADULT DOSAGE	ACTION	NURSING CONSIDERATIONS AND COMMON SIDE EFFECTS
Antidepressants *(continued)*		
Desipramine (Norpramine): 100 to 200 mg/day	Elevates the mood by blocking reuptake of norepinephrine and serotonin into CNS neurons	• Before starting therapy, document the patient's baseline pulse rate, blood pressure, and ECG. Monitor these periodically to detect *hypotension* or *arrhythmias*. • This drug is associated with a high incidence of *drowsiness,* especially when therapy begins. Some clinicians prefer to administer the entire daily dose at bedtime to minimize daytime drowsiness. • To reduce *orthostatic hypotension,* instruct the patient to rise slowly when shifting to an upright position. Measure and document the patient's supine and standing blood pressure; withhold the drug and inform the nurse-manager if systolic pressure drops more than 30 mm Hg. • Offer sugar-free drinks and candy to relieve *dry mouth.* • To detect *urine retention,* monitor urine output. Inform the nurse-manager if output is low.
Doxepin (Sinequan): 75 to 150 mg/day	Elevates the mood by blocking reuptake of norepinephrine and serotonin into CNS neurons; also may have anxiolytic effects	• Before starting therapy, document the patient's baseline pulse rate, blood pressure, and ECG. Monitor these periodically to detect *hypotension* or *arrhythmias*. • Some clinicians prefer to administer the entire daily dose at bedtime to minimize daytime *drowsiness*. • This drug is a good choice for anxious patients. • To reduce *orthostatic hypotension,* instruct the patient to rise slowly when shifting to an upright position. Measure and document the patient's supine and standing blood pressure; withhold the drug and inform the nurse-manager if systolic pressure drops more than 30 mm Hg. • Dilute the oral concentrate with juice; do not mix drug with soda because they are incompatible. • Offer sugar-free drinks and candy to relieve *dry mouth.* • To detect *urine retention,* monitor urine output. Inform the nurse-manager if output is low.
Imipramine (Tofranil): 100 to 200 mg/day	Elevates the mood by blocking reuptake of norepinephrine and serotonin into CNS neurons	• Before starting therapy, document the patient's baseline pulse rate, blood pressure, and ECG. Monitor these periodically to detect *hypotension* or *arrhythmias*. • Some clinicians prefer to administer the entire daily dose at bedtime to minimize daytime *drowsiness*. • To reduce *orthostatic hypotension,* instruct the patient to rise slowly when shifting to an upright position. Measure and document the patient's supine and standing blood pressure; withhold the drug and inform the nurse-manager if systolic pressure drops more than 30 mm Hg. • Offer sugar-free drinks and candy to relieve *dry mouth.* • To detect *urine retention,* monitor urine output. Inform the nurse-manager if output is low.
Trimipramine (Surmontil): 75 to 200 mg/day	Elevates the mood by blocking reuptake of norepinephrine and serotonin into CNS neurons	• Before starting therapy, document the patient's baseline pulse rate, blood pressure, and ECG. Monitor these periodically to detect *hypotension* or *arrhythmias*. • To reduce *orthostatic hypotension,* instruct the patient to rise slowly when shifting to an upright position. Measure and document the patient's supine and standing blood pressure; withhold the drug and inform the nurse-manager if systolic pressure drops more than 30 mm Hg. • Instruct the patient to avoid over-the-counter sympathomimetics. • Advise the patient to take drug with food or milk if it causes *GI upset.* • Offer sugar-free drinks and candy to relieve *dry mouth.* • To detect *urine retention,* monitor urine output. Inform the nurse-manager if output is low.

Drugs used to treat psychiatric disorders *(continued)*

DRUG AND USUAL ADULT DOSAGE	ACTION	NURSING CONSIDERATIONS AND COMMON SIDE EFFECTS
Antidepressants *(continued)*		
Monoamine oxidase (MAO) inhibitors Isocarboxazid (Marplan): 10 to 30 mg/day in divided doses	Elevates the mood by increasing levels of CNS catecholamines (by blocking their metabolism by MAO)	• To reduce *orthostatic hypotension,* instruct the patient to rise slowly when shifting to an upright position. Measure and document the patient's supine and standing blood pressure; withhold the drug and inform the nurse-manager if systolic pressure drops more than 30 mm Hg. • Warn the patient to avoid foods high in tyramine or tryptophan (Chianti wine, aged hard cheese, beer, whiskey and other hard liquor aged in wooden casks, avocados, chicken livers, bananas, chocolate, soy sauce, meat tenderizers, salami, bologna, preserved meats), large amounts of caffeine, and self-medication with nonprescription drugs (especially cold, hay fever, and diet preparations) to prevent *hypertensive crisis.* • Offer sugar-free drinks and candy to relieve *dry mouth.* • To detect *urine retention,* monitor urine output. Inform the nurse-manager if output is low. • Advise the patient to avoid driving or operating heavy machinery because this drug causes *drowsiness.*
Phenelzine (Nardil): 15 to 60 mg/day in divided doses	Elevates the mood by increasing levels of CNS catecholamines (by blocking their metabolism by MAO)	• To reduce *orthostatic hypotension,* instruct the patient to rise slowly when shifting to an upright position. Measure and document the patient's supine and standing blood pressure; withhold the drug and inform the nurse-manager if systolic pressure drops more than 30 mm Hg. • Warn the patient to avoid foods high in tyramine or tryptophan (Chianti wine, aged hard cheese, beer, whiskey and other hard liquor aged in wooden casks, avocados, chicken livers, bananas, chocolate, soy sauce, meat tenderizers, salami, bologna, preserved meats), large amounts of caffeine, and self-medication with nonprescription drugs (especially cold, hay fever, and diet preparations) to prevent *hypertensive crisis.* • Offer sugar-free drinks and candy to relieve *dry mouth.* • To detect *urine retention,* monitor urine output. Inform the nurse-manager if output is low. • Advise the patient to avoid driving or operating heavy machinery because this drug causes *drowsiness.*
Tranylcypromine (Parnate): 10 to 20 mg/day in divided doses	Elevates the mood by increasing levels of CNS catecholamines (by blocking their metabolism by MAO)	• To reduce *orthostatic hypotension,* instruct the patient to rise slowly when shifting to an upright position. Measure and document the patient's supine and standing blood pressure; withhold the drug and inform the nurse-manager if systolic pressure drops more than 30 mm Hg. • Warn the patient to avoid foods high in tyramine or tryptophan (Chianti wine, aged hard cheese, beer, whiskey and other hard liquor aged in wooden casks, avocados, chicken livers, bananas, chocolate, soy sauce, meat tenderizers, salami, bologna, preserved meats), large amounts of caffeine, and self-medication with nonprescription drugs (especially cold, hay fever, and diet preparations) to prevent *hypertensive crisis.* • Offer sugar-free drinks and candy to relieve *dry mouth.* • To detect *urine retention,* monitor urine output. Inform the nurse-manager if output is low. • Advise the patient to avoid driving or operating heavy machinery because this drug causes *drowsiness.*

(continued)

PSYCHIATRIC NURSING

Drugs used to treat psychiatric disorders *(continued)*

DRUG AND USUAL ADULT DOSAGE	ACTION	NURSING CONSIDERATIONS AND COMMON SIDE EFFECTS
Antidepressants *(continued)*		
Miscellaneous antidepressants		
Fluoxetine (Prozac): Initially 20 mg/day in the morning, then increase as tolerated	Elevates the mood by blocking reuptake of serotonin into CNS neurons	• To reduce *orthostatic hypotension,* instruct the patient to rise slowly when shifting to an upright position. Measure and document the patient's supine and standing blood pressure; withhold the drug and inform the nurse-manager if systolic pressure drops more than 30 mm Hg. • Avoid administering late in the day or at bedtime because this may cause *insomnia.* If the patient is taking more than 20 mg/day, give divided doses at breakfast and lunch. • Offer sugar-free drinks and candy to relieve *dry mouth.* • To detect *urine retention,* monitor urine output. Inform the nurse-manager if output is low.
Trazodone (Desyrel): 100 to 300 mg/day	Elevates the mood by blocking reuptake of norepinephrine and serotonin into CNS neurons	• To reduce *orthostatic hypotension,* instruct the patient to rise slowly when shifting to an upright position. Measure and document the patient's supine and standing blood pressure; withhold the drug and inform the nurse-manager if systolic pressure drops more than 30 mm Hg. • Offer sugar-free drinks and candy to relieve *dry mouth.* • To detect *urine retention,* monitor urine output. Inform the nurse-manager if output is low. • Advise the patient to avoid driving or operating heavy machinery because this drug causes *drowsiness.*
Antimanic agent		
Lithium carbonate (Eskalith, Lithane, Lithobid, Lithonate, Lithotabs): 1,800 to 2,400 mg during acute mania; 300 to 1,200 mg/day in divided doses for maintenance. Blood levels should be maintained at 0.6 to 1.2 mEq/liter throughout therapy.	Reduces hyperactivity by altering cationic exchange at the sodium-potassium pump	• Emphasize the need for routine blood studies, especially at the start of therapy, to monitor for therapeutic levels and prevent toxicity. • Monitor for excessive *weight gain.* • Offer sugar-free drinks and candy to relieve *dry mouth.* • To relieve *hand tremors,* have the patient perform an activity that controls tremors, such as sewing or writing. • Monitor *diarrhea* for severity. Have the patient wash rectal area as often as needed. Report this side effect to the nurse-manager. • Monitor laboratory results. Report a white blood cell (WBC) count over 11,000/microliter to the nurse-manager. • If signs of toxicity occur, notify the nurse-manager or supervisor and withhold the medication. Signs and symptoms of toxicity include persistent nausea and vomiting, severe diarrhea, ataxia, blurred vision, tinnitus, excessive output of dilute urine, increasing tremors, muscle irritability, mental confusion, nystagmus, and seizures (in order of severity). Document findings. To help prevent toxicity, ensure adequate daily fluid intake. • Advise the patient to avoid driving or operating heavy machinery because this drug causes *drowsiness.*

Drugs used to treat psychiatric disorders *(continued)*

DRUG AND USUAL ADULT DOSAGE	ACTION	NURSING CONSIDERATIONS AND COMMON SIDE EFFECTS
Antipsychotics		
Chlorpromazine (Thorazine): 300 to 1,200 mg/day	Relieves symptoms of psychosis by blocking postsynaptic dopamine receptors in the CNS	• Because this drug is associated with a high incidence of *sedation*, advise the patient to avoid driving or operating heavy machinery. • To reduce *orthostatic hypotension*, instruct the patient to rise slowly when shifting to an upright position. Measure and document the patient's supine and standing blood pressure; withhold the drug and inform the nurse-manager if systolic pressure drops more than 30 mm Hg. • Offer sugar-free drinks and candy to relieve *dry mouth*. • To detect *urine retention*, monitor urine output. Inform the nurse-manager if output is low. • To minimize *weight gain*, monitor food intake, offer low-calorie snacks, and encourage as much physical activity as possible. • To prevent *photosensitivity,* do not allow the patient to sunbathe. Instruct the patient to apply a sunscreen before going outdoors and to wear long-sleeved garments. • Reassure the patient that *blurred vision* decreases after 1 or 2 weeks. Do not ask the patient to perform activities requiring the eyes to accommodate (such as reading or handwork) until this side effect diminishes. • Monitor bowel movements. If *constipation* occurs, document it and ask the nurse-manager about a laxative order. Offer high-fiber foods. • *Akathisia* may occur within the first few weeks of therapy. Signs and symptoms, which usually disappear spontaneously, include restlessness and agitation; inability to sleep or sit down; and fright, anger, terror, or rage. Compare the patient's behavior with his pretherapy behavior to distinguish true akathisia from psychopathology. • *Parkinsonism* may occur during the first few weeks of therapy, usually abating 2 to 3 months after stabilization of the drug regimen. Depending on the severity of symptoms (cogwheel muscular rigidity; stooped posture and shuffling gait; tremor affecting fine motor coordination; masklike expression; and hypersalivation and drooling), the clinician may reduce the dosage, switch to another drug, or prescribe an antiparkinsonian drug. • *Dyskinesia* and *dystonia* may occur suddenly within the first few weeks of therapy but usually abate within 2 weeks. Signs and symptoms include coordinated, involuntary rhythmic movements; uncoordinated, jerking spastic movements of the neck, face, eyes, and muscles; and twisting of the neck. If necessary to manage the patient's reaction, administer an anticholinergic agent, as ordered. • *Tardive dyskinesia* may occur if the patient takes the drug for more than 1 year, especially if the patient is elderly or has brain damage. Signs and symptoms, which may be permanent, include coordinated rhythmic mouth and tongue movements and involuntary sucking, chewing, licking, grimacing, and blinking. Observe the patient for early signs (blinking and fine vermiform tongue movements), and conduct screening tests every 3 months.

(continued)

PSYCHIATRIC NURSING

Drugs used to treat psychiatric disorders *(continued)*

DRUG AND USUAL ADULT DOSAGE	ACTION	NURSING CONSIDERATIONS AND COMMON SIDE EFFECTS
Antipsychotics *(continued)*		
Chlorprothixene (Taractan): 75 to 200 mg/day	Relieves symptoms of psychosis by blocking postsynaptic dopamine receptors in the CNS	• See *Chlorpromazine* for nursing considerations and common side effects.
Fluphenazine decanoate (Prolixin Decanoate): 12.5 to 100 mg I.M. q 1 to 4 weeks Fluphenazine enanthate (Prolixin Enanthate): 12.5 to 100 mg q 1 to 2 weeks Fluphenazine hydrochloride (Prolixin): 2 to 30 mg/day I.M.	Relieves symptoms of psychosis by blocking postsynaptic dopamine receptors in the CNS	• See *Chlorpromazine* for nursing considerations and common side effects.
Haloperidol (Haldol): 2 to 60 mg/day	Relieves symptoms of psychosis by blocking postsynaptic dopamine receptors in the CNS	• See *Chlorpromazine* for nursing considerations and common side effects.
Loxapine succinate (Loxitane): 60 to 100 mg/day	Relieves symptoms of psychosis by blocking postsynaptic dopamine receptors in the CNS	• See *Chlorpromazine* for nursing considerations and common side effects.
Perphenazine (Trilafon): 8 to 64 mg/day	Relieves symptoms of psychosis by blocking postsynaptic dopamine receptors in the CNS	• See *Chlorpromazine* for nursing considerations and common side effects.
Thioridazine (Mellaril): 300 to 800 mg/day	Relieves symptoms of psychosis by blocking postsynaptic dopamine receptors in the CNS	• See *Chlorpromazine* for nursing considerations and common side effects.
Trifluoperazine (Stelazine): 15 to 60 mg/day	Relieves symptoms of psychosis by blocking postsynaptic dopamine receptors in the CNS	• See *Chlorpromazine* for nursing considerations and common side effects.

Drugs used to treat psychiatric disorders *(continued)*

DRUG AND USUAL ADULT DOSAGE	ACTION	NURSING CONSIDERATIONS AND COMMON SIDE EFFECTS
Anticholinergic agents		
Benztropine mesylate (Cogentin): 1 to 4 mg/day	Counters extrapyramidal reactions to antipsychotic drugs by blocking central cholinergic receptors and restoring the balance of acetylcholine and dopamine in the basal ganglia	• Offer sugar-free drinks and candy to relieve *dry mouth*. • Monitor bowel movements. If *constipation* occurs, document it and ask the nurse-manager about a laxative order. Offer high-fiber foods.
Biperiden (Akineton): 2 to 6 mg/day	Counters extrapyramidal reactions to antipsychotic drugs by blocking central cholinergic receptors and restoring the balance of acetylcholine and dopamine in the basal ganglia	• Offer sugar-free drinks and candy to relieve *dry mouth*. • Monitor bowel movements. If *constipation* occurs, document it and ask the nurse-manager about a laxative order. Offer high-fiber foods.
Trihexyphenidyl (Artane): 6 to 10 mg/day	Counters extrapyramidal reactions to antipsychotic drugs by blocking central cholinergic receptors and restoring the balance of acetylcholine and dopamine in the basal ganglia	• Offer sugar-free drinks and candy to relieve *dry mouth*. • Monitor bowel movements. If *constipation* occurs, document it and ask the nurse-manager about a laxative order. Offer high-fiber foods.

PSYCHIATRIC NURSING

Part V

Appendices

Appendices

Appendix 1: Recommended daily dietary allowances 498

Appendix 2: Healthful weights 500

Appendix 3: Sample meal planning exchange lists 501

Appendix 4: Normal values for common laboratory tests 504

Appendix 5: Drug administration, calculations, and equivalents 505

Appendix 6: Precautions to take when administering drugs 507

Appendix 7: NANDA nursing diagnostic categories 508

Appendix 8: NCLEX-PN dates and state boards of nursing 509

Appendix 9: Canadian examination information 512

Appendix 10: Selected references 513

Appendix I: Recommended daily dietary allowances[a]

AGE (YEARS) AND SEX GROUP	WEIGHT[b]		HEIGHT[b]		PROTEIN	FAT-SOLUBLE VITAMINS			
	KG	LB	CM	IN		VITAMIN A	VITAMIN D	VITAMIN E	VITAMIN K
					g	mcg RE[c]	mcg[d]	mg αTE[e]	mcg
Infants									
0.0 to 0.5	6	13	60	24	13	375	7.5	3	5
0.5 to 1.0	9	20	71	28	14	375	10	4	10
Children									
1 to 3	13	29	90	35	16	400	10	6	15
4 to 6	20	44	112	44	24	500	10	7	20
7 to 10	28	62	132	52	28	700	10	7	30
Males									
11 to 14	45	99	157	62	45	1,000	10	10	45
15 to 18	66	145	176	69	59	1,000	10	10	65
19 to 24	72	160	177	70	58	1,000	10	10	70
25 to 50	79	174	176	70	63	1,000	5	10	80
51	77	170	173	68	63	1,000	5	10	80
Females									
11 to 14	46	101	157	62	46	800	10	8	45
15 to 18	55	120	163	64	44	800	10	8	55
19 to 24	58	128	164	65	46	800	10	8	60
25 to 50	63	138	163	64	50	800	5	8	65
51 +	65	143	160	63	50	800	5	8	65
Pregnant					60	800	10	10	65
Lactating									
1st 6 months					65	1,300	10	12	65
2nd 6 months					62	1,200	10	11	65

[a]The allowances, expressed as average daily intakes over time, are intended to provide for individual variations among most normal persons as they live in the United States under usual environmental stresses. Diets should be based on a variety of common foods in order to provide other nutrients for which human requirements have been less well defined.

[b]Weights and heights of Reference Adults are actual medians for the U.S. population of the designated age, as reported by NHANES II. The median weights and heights of those under 19 years of age were taken from Hamill P.V.V., Drizd, T.A., Johnson, C.L., Reed, R.B., Roche, A.F., and Moore, W.M.: Physical growth. National Center for Health Statistics Percentiles. Am J Clin Nutr 32:607,

	WATER-SOLUBLE VITAMINS						MINERALS						
VITAMIN C	THIAMIN	RIBO-FLAVIN	NIACIN	VITAMIN B_6	FOLATE	VITAMIN B_{12}	CALCIUM	PHOS-PHORUS	MAGNE-NESIUM	IRON	ZINC	IODINE	SELE-NIUM
← mg →			mg NE[f]	mg	← mcg →		← mg →					← mcg →	
30	0.3	0.4	5	0.3	25	0.3	400	300	40	6	5	40	10
35	0.4	0.5	6	0.6	35	0.5	600	500	60	10	5	50	15
40	0.7	0.8	9	1.0	50	0.7	800	800	80	10	10	70	20
45	0.9	1.1	12	1.1	75	1.0	800	800	120	10	10	90	20
45	1.0	1.2	13	1.4	100	1.4	800	800	170	10	10	120	30
50	1.3	1.5	17	1.7	150	2.0	1,200	1,200	270	12	15	150	40
60	1.5	1.8	20	2.0	200	2.0	1,200	1,200	400	12	15	150	50
60	1.5	1.7	19	2.0	200	2.0	1,200	1,200	350	10	15	150	70
60	1.5	1.7	19	2.0	200	2.0	800	800	350	10	15	150	70
60	1.2	1.4	15	2.0	200	2.0	800	800	350	10	15	150	70
50	1.1	1.3	15	1.4	150	2.0	1,200	1,200	280	15	12	150	45
60	1.1	1.3	15	1.5	180	2.0	1,200	1,200	300	15	12	150	50
60	1.1	1.3	15	1.6	180	2.0	1,200	1,200	280	15	12	150	55
60	1.1	1.3	15	1.6	180	2.0	800	800	280	15	12	150	55
60	1.0	1.2	13	1.6	180	2.0	800	800	280	10	12	150	55
70	1.5	1.6	17	2.2	400	2.2	1,200	1,200	300	30	15	175	65
95	1.6	1.8	20	2.1	280	2.6	1,200	1,200	355	15	19	200	75
90	1.6	1.7	20	2.1	260	2.6	1,200	1,200	340	15	16	200	75

1979. The use of these figures does not imply that the height-to-weight ratios are ideal.
[c] Retinol equivalents. 1 retinol equivalent = 1 mcg retinol or 6 mcg β-carotene.
[d] As cholecalciferol. 10 mcg cholecalciferol = 400 IU of vitamin D.
[e] α-Tocopherol equivalents. 1 mg d-α tocopherol = 1 α-TE.

[f] 1 NE (niacin equivalent) is equal to 1 mg of niacin or 60 mg of dietary tryptophan.

APPENDICES

Appendix 2: Healthful weights

Excess or inadequate weight increases the risk of developing heart problems. A healthful weight depends on how much of the weight is fat, where the fat is located, and whether the person has weight-related problems or a family history of such problems.

The chart below lists weight ranges for men and women that are accepted as standards for good health. These 1990 standards allow more latitude in weight range than previous standards.

	WEIGHT IN POUNDS	
HEIGHT	AGE 19 TO 34	AGE 35 AND OVER
5'0"	97 to 128	108 to 138
5'1"	101 to 132	111 to 143
5'2"	104 to 137	115 to 148
5'3"	107 to 141	119 to 152
5'4"	111 to 146	122 to 157
5'5"	114 to 150	126 to 162
5'6"	118 to 155	130 to 167
5'7"	121 to 160	134 to 172
5'8"	125 to 164	138 to 178
5'9"	129 to 169	142 to 183
5'10"	132 to 174	146 to 188
5'11"	136 to 179	151 to 194
6'0"	140 to 184	155 to 199
6'1"	144 to 189	159 to 205
6'2"	148 to 195	164 to 210

Source: U.S. Department of Agriculture, Department of Health and Human Services. 1990. *Nutrition and your health: Dietary guidelines for Americans,* (3rd ed.), Washington, D.C.

Appendix 3: Sample meal planning exchange lists

The following material has been modified from *Exchange Lists for Meal Planning,* which is the basis of a meal planning system designed by a committee of the American Diabetes Association and the American Dietetic Association. Although designed primarily for people with diabetes and others who must follow special diets, the exchange lists are based on principles of good nutrition that apply to everyone.

List 1: Starch and bread exchanges

One exchange contains approximately 15 g carbohydrate, 3 g protein, a trace of fat, and 80 calories. Here are some of the types and amounts of breads, cereals, starchy vegetables, and prepared foods to use for one bread exchange.

Cereals, grains, and pastas

Bran cereal, concentrated	⅓ cup
Bran cereal, flaked	½ cup
Bulgur, cooked	½ cup
Cooked cereal	½ cup
Cornmeal, dry	2½ tbs
Grits, cooked	½ cup
Other ready-to-eat unsweetened cereal	¾ cup
Pasta, cooked	½ cup
Puffed cereal	1½ cup
Rice (white or brown), cooked	⅓ cup
Shredded wheat	½ cup
Wheat germ	3 tbs

Dried beans, peas, and lentils

Baked beans	¼ cup
Beans and peas, cooked	⅓ cup
Lentils, cooked	⅓ cup

Starchy vegetables

Corn	½ cup
Corn on cob, 6″	1
Lima beans	½ cup
Peas, green (canned or frozen)	½ cup
Plantain	½ cup
Potato, baked	1 small
Potato, mashed	½ cup
Squash, winter (acorn or butternut)	1 cup
Yam or sweet potato, plain	⅓ cup

Bread

Bagel	½
Bread sticks, 4″ × ½″	2
Croutons, low-fat	1 cup
English muffin	½
Frankfurter or hamburger bun	½
Pita, 6″	½
Plain roll, small	1
Raisin bread (unfrosted)	1 slice
Rye or pumpernickel bread	1 slice
Tortilla, 6″	1
White bread (including French and Italian)	1 slice
Whole wheat bread	1 slice

Crackers and snacks

Animal crackers	8
Graham crackers, 2½″ square	3
Matzo	¾ oz
Melba toast	5 slices
Oyster crackers	24
Popcorn (popped, no fat added)	3 cups
Pretzels	¾ oz
Rye wafers, 2″ × 3½″	4
Saltines	6
Whole wheat crackers (no fat added)	¾ oz

Starch foods prepared with fat

Biscuit, 2½″ across	1
Chow mein noodles	½ cup
Corn bread, 2″ cube	1
Crackers, round butter type	6
French fried potatoes, 2″ to 3½″	10
Muffin, plain, small	1
Pancakes, 4″ across	2
Stuffing, bread	¼ cup
Taco shell, 6″ across	2
Waffle, 4½″ square	1
Whole wheat crackers (fat added)	4 to 6

List 2a: Meat exchanges — Lean meat and substitutes

One lean meat exchange has 7 g protein, 3 g fat, and 55 calories. Here are the types and amounts of lean meat and other protein-rich foods to use for one low-fat meat exchange.

Beef: USDA Select or Choice grades of lean beef, such as chipped beef, flank steak, tenderloin, round (bottom, top), sirloin — 1 oz

Pork: Fresh, canned, cured, or boiled ham; Canadian bacon; tenderloin — 1 oz

Veal: All cuts of veal except for ground or cubed cutlets, such as chops and roasts — 1 oz

Poultry: Chicken, turkey, cornish hen (without skin) — 1 oz

Fish: Any frozen or fresh fish — 1 oz
Crab, lobster, scallops, shrimp, clams (fresh or canned in water) — 2 oz

Oysters	6 medium
Tuna, canned	¼ cup
Herring, uncreamed or smoked	1 oz
Sardines, canned	2 medium

Wild game: Venison, rabbit, squirrel; pheasant, duck, goose (without skin) — 1 oz

Cheese: Any cottage cheese — ¼ cup
Grated Parmesan — 2 tbs
Diet cheeses — 1 oz

Other: Luncheon meat, 95% fat-free — 1½ oz
Egg substitutes — ½ cup
Egg whites — 3 whites

(continued)

Appendix 3: Sample meal planning exchange lists *(continued)*

List 2b: Meat exchanges — Medium-fat meat and substitutes

One medium-fat meat exchange has 7 g protein, 5 g fat, and 75 calories. Here are the types and amounts of medium-fat meat and other protein-rich foods to use for one medium-fat meat exchange.

Beef: All ground beef, roast (rib, chuck, rump), steak, meatloaf	1 oz	**Cheese:** Skim or part-skim cheeses	
Pork: Loin roast, chops, cutlets	1 oz	Ricotta	¼ cup
Lamb: Chops, leg, roast	1 oz	Mozzarella	1 oz
Veal: Cutlet (ground, cubed, unbreaded)	1 oz	Diet cheeses	1 oz
Poultry: Chicken (with skin), domestic duck or goose (well drained), ground turkey	1 oz	**Other:** Luncheon meat, 86% fat free	1 oz
		Egg (high in cholesterol; limit 3 per week)	1
Fish: Tuna (canned in oil, drained)	¼ cup	Egg substitute	¼ cup
Salmon (canned)	¼ cup	Tofu (2½″ cube)	4 oz
		Liver, heart, kidney, sweetbreads (high in cholesterol)	1 oz

List 2c: Meat exchanges — High-fat meat and substitutes

One high-fat meat exchange has 7 g protein, 8 g fat, and 100 calories. Here are the types and amounts of high-fat meat and other protein-rich foods to use for one high-fat meat exchange. Note that these items should be used only three times per week.

Beef: Most USDA prime cuts, such as ribs, corned beef	1 oz	**Other:** Luncheon meat, such as bologna, salami, pimento loaf	1 oz
Lamb: Patties (ground lamb)	1 oz	Sausage (Polish, Italian, or smoked)	1 oz
Pork: Spare ribs, ground pork, sausage (patty or link)	1 oz	Knockwurst or bratwurst	1 oz
		Frankfurter (turkey or chicken)	1 frank
Cheese: All regular cheeses, such as American, Blue, Cheddar, Monterey Jack, Swiss	1 oz	Peanut butter	1 tbs

List 3: Vegetable exchanges

One vegetable exchange has about 5 g carbohydrate, 2 g protein, and 25 calories. Here are the vegetables to use for one vegetable exchange. (One exchange is ½ cup. For starchy vegetables, see the starch and bread exchange list.)

Artichoke (½ medium)	Celery	Leeks	Sauerkraut
Asparagus	Chinese cabbage	Lettuce (Iceburg, Romaine)	Spinach, cooked
Beans (green, Italian, wax)	Cucumber		Summer squash
Bean sprouts	Eggplant	Mushrooms	Tomato (1 large)
Beets	Endive	Okra	Tomato juice
Broccoli	Escarole	Onions	Turnips
Brussels sprouts	Green pepper	Pea pods	Vegetable juice
Cabbage, cooked	Greens (collard, mustard, turnip)	Radish	Water chestnuts
Carrots		Rutabaga	Zucchini, cooked
Cauliflower			

List 4: Fruit exchanges

One fruit exchange has 15 g carbohydrate and 60 calories. Here are the types and amounts of fruits to use for one fruit exchange. Unless otherwise noted, the serving size for one exchange is ½ cup for fresh fruit or fruit juice and ¼ cup for dried fruit.

Apple, raw	1 small	Cherries	12
Apple juice, cider	½ cup	Dates, dried	2½ medium
Applesauce, unsweetened	½ cup	Figs, dried	1½
Apricots, canned	4 halves	Figs, fresh	2
Apricots, dried	7 halves	Grapefruit, medium	½
Apricots, medium, raw	4	Grapefruit juice	½ cup
Banana (9″)	½	Grape juice	⅓ cup
Berries		Grapes, small	15
Blackberries	¾ cup	Kiwi, large	1
Blueberries	¾ cup	Mandarin oranges	¾ cup
Raspberries	1 cup	Mango, small	½
Strawberries	1¼ cup		

Appendix 3: Sample meal planning exchange lists (continued)

List 4: Fruit exchanges (continued)

Melon		Pear	1 small
Cantaloupe	⅓ small	Pears, canned	½ cup
Honeydew	⅛ medium	Persimmon (native), medium	2
Watermelon	1¼ cup	Pineapple	¾ cup
Nectarine (2½″)	1	Pineapple juice	½ cup
Orange (2½″)	1	Plums, medium	2
Orange juice	½ cup	Prune juice	⅓ cup
Papaya	1 cup	Prunes, dried, medium	3
Peach (2¾″)	1	Raisins	2 tbs
Peaches, canned	½ cup	Tangerine (2½″)	2

List 5: Milk exchanges

One milk exchange has 12 g carbohydrate, 8 g protein, and varying amounts of fat and calories. Very low-fat milk contains trace amounts of fat and about 90 calories; low-fat milk, about 5 g fat and 120 calories; whole milk, about 8 g fat and 150 calories. Whole milk contains more than 3¼% butterfat; try to limit choices from this group. Here are the types and amounts of milk or milk products to use for one milk exchange.

Skim and very low-fat milk		**Low-fat milk**	
Skim milk	1 cup	2% milk	1 cup
½% or 1% low-fat milk	1 cup	Yogurt, plain low-fat (with added nonfat milk solids)	1 cup
Dry nonfat milk	⅓ cup	**Whole milk**	
Evaporated skim milk	½ cup	Whole milk	1 cup
Buttermilk, low-fat	1 cup	Evaporated whole milk	½ cup
Yogurt, plain, nonfat	1 cup	Yogurt (whole, plain)	1 cup

List 6: Fat exchanges

One fat exchange has 5 g fat and 45 calories. Here are the types and amounts of fat-containing foods to use for one fat exchange. Everyone should modify fat intake by eating unsaturated fats instead of saturated fats.

Unsaturated fats		**Salad dressing:**	
Avocado	⅛ medium	Mayonnaise type	2 tsp
Margarine, diet	1 tbs	Mayonnaise type, reduced-calorie	1 tbs
Mayonnaise	1 tsp	Oil variety	1 tbs
Mayonnaise, reduced-calorie	1 tbs	Reduced-calorie	2 tbs
Nuts and seeds:		**Saturated fats**	
Almonds, dry roasted	6 whole	Bacon	1 slice
Cashews, dry roasted	1 tbs	Butter	1 tsp
Pecans	2 whole	Chitterlings	½ oz
Peanuts	20 small or 10 large	Coconut, shredded	2 tbs
		Coffee whitener, liquid	2 tbs
Pine nuts, sunflower seeds (without shells)	1 tbs	Coffee whitener, powder	4 tsp
Pumpkin seeds	2 tsp	Cream (light, coffee, table)	2 tbs
Oil (corn, cottonseed, olive, peanut, safflower, soybean, sunflower)	1 tsp	Cream, heavy	1 tbs
		Cream, sour	2 tbs
Olives	10 small or 5 large	Cream cheese	1 tbs
		Salt pork	¼ oz

APPENDICES

Appendix 4: Normal values for common laboratory tests

TEST	NORMAL VALUES
Electrolyte levels	
Sodium	135 to 145 mEq/liter
Potassium	3.5 to 5 mEq/liter
Calcium	4.5 to 5.8 mEq/liter or 9 to 10.5 mg/dl
Arterial blood gas levels	
pH	7.35 to 7.45
PaO_2	80 to 100 mm Hg
$PaCO_2$	35 to 45 mm Hg
Serum bicarbonate	21 to 29 mEq/liter
Oxygen saturation	95% to 100%
Complete blood count	
Red blood cell count	4.2 to 6 million/mm^3
Hemoglobin level	12 to 18 g/dl
White blood cell count	5,000 to 10,000/mm^3
Platelet count	150,000 to 400,000/mm^3
Erythrocyte sedimentation rate	1 to 20 mm/hour
Prothrombin time	11 to 12.5 seconds
Partial thromboplastin time	30 to 40 seconds
Other blood tests	
Fasting plasma glucose test	80 to 120 mg/dl
Serum cholesterol level	150 to 250 mg/dl
Renal function tests	
Blood urea nitrogen	8 to 20 mg/dl
Creatinine level	0.8 to 1.5 mg/dl
Liver function tests	
Total protein	6 to 8 g/dl
Albumin-globulin ratio	Albumin—3.5 to 5.5 g/dl
	Globulin—2.5 to 3.5 g/dl
	Ratio—1.5:1 to 2.5:1
Serum alanine aminotransferase	5 to 35 U/ml
Serum aspartate aminotransferase	5 to 40 U/ml
Lactic dehydrogenase	200 to 450 U/ml
Alkaline phosphatase	1.5 to 4 Bodansky units or 3 to 13 King-Armstrong units
Serum bilirubin	Less than 1 mg/dl
Prothrombin time	11 to 12.5 seconds or 100%
Clotting time	6 to 17 minutes
Partial thromboplastin time	30 to 40 seconds

Appendix 5: Drug administration, calculations, and equivalents

Drug administration

When administering any drug, remember to use the five rights:

1. right client   2. right drug   3. right dose   4. right route   5. right time

Calculations

The proportion method
A proportion is made up of two ratios, each indicating the relationship one quantity has to the other. It can be written as whole units or as a fraction:

$$A{:}B = C{:}D$$
$$2{:}3 = 4{:}6$$

$$\frac{A}{B} = \frac{C}{D}$$

$$\frac{2}{3} = \frac{4}{6}$$

The first and fourth terms (A and D) are called the extremes, and the second and third terms (B and C) are called the means. The product of the means equals the product of the extremes.

$$A{:}B = C{:}D \qquad \frac{A}{B} = \frac{C}{D}$$

$$2{:}3 = 4{:}6 \qquad \frac{2}{3} = \frac{4}{6}$$

$$2 \times 6 = 3 \times 4 \qquad 2 \times 6 = 3 \times 4$$

$$12 = 12 \qquad 12 = 12$$

The proportion method can be helpful when one of your terms is unknown *(x)*.
- Keep the unknown quantity on the left, the known on the right.
- Solve the proportion by equating the product of the means to the product of the extremes.
- For the value of *x*, simply divide the numerical value of the product containing the *x* into the product on the right of the equation.

Example: $2{:}x = 4{:}6$
or

Unknown		Known
$\dfrac{2}{x}$	$=$	$\dfrac{4}{6}$

$$4x = 2 \times 6$$

$$4x = 12$$

$$x = 3$$

(continued)

*From *Administering Medications*. Nursing Photobooks Series. Springhouse, Pa.: Springhouse Corp., 1981.

Appendix 5: Drug administration, calculations, and equivalents (continued)

Calculations (continued)

You can prove your answer when the problem is solved by substituting it in place of the x:

$$\frac{2}{3} = \frac{4}{6}$$

$$4 \times 3 = 2 \times 6$$

$$12 = 12$$

When using the proportion method to solve medication problems, be sure the ratios are expressed in the same units of measure.

Formulas for calculations

To calculate the number of doses in a specified amount of medicine:

$$\text{Number of doses} = \frac{\text{Total amount}}{\text{Size of dose}}$$

To calculate the size of each dose, given a specified amount of medication and the number of doses it contains:

$$\text{Size of dose} = \frac{\text{Total amount}}{\text{Number of doses}}$$

To calculate the amount of a medicine, given the number of doses it contains and the size of each dose:

$$\text{Total amount} = \text{Number of doses} \times \text{size of dose}$$

Short formula for determining rate of I.V. solution infusion:

$$\frac{\text{Volume of solution}}{\text{Time interval in minutes}} \times \text{Drop factor} = \text{Drops/minute}$$

Equivalents

Metric weight equivalents
1 kg = 1,000 g
1 g = 1,000 mg
1 mg = 0.001 g
1 mcg or g = 0.001 mg

Conversions
1 oz = 30 g
1 lb = 453.6 g
2.2 lb = 1 kg

Metric volume equivalents
1 liter = 1,000 ml
1 deciliter = 100 ml

Liquid measures

	Household		Apothecary		Metric
1 teaspoonful	=	1 fluidram	=	4 or 5 ml
1 tablespoonful	=	4 fluidrams	=	15 or 16 ml
2 tablespoonfuls	=	1 fluid ounce	=	30 ml
1 measuring cupful	=	8 fluid ounces	=	240 ml
1 pint	=	16 fluid ounces	=	500 ml
1 quart	=	32 fluid ounces	=	1,000 ml

Note: Although the fluidram is about 4 ml, in prescriptions it is considered equivalent to the teaspoon (which is 5 ml).

Temperature conversion

Centigrade to Fahrenheit
$$(°C \times \tfrac{9}{5}) + 32 = °F$$

Fahrenheit to Centigrade
$$(°F - 32) \times \tfrac{5}{9} = °C$$

*From *Nursing88 Drug Handbook*. Springhouse, Pa.: Springhouse Corp., 1988.

Appendix 6: Precautions to take when administering drugs

To ensure proper drug administration, follow these guidelines:

● Before administering any drug, make sure you understand the drug's action, dosage range, and purpose.

● Compare the name of the drug with the drug listed on the patient's medication administration record (MAR) to make sure you are administering the correct drug. (Some drugs have similar names or spellings.)

● Check the patient's chart for the day of administration. Also check the hour (A.M. or P.M.) or number of times per day to be administered.

● Check the drug label three times: before removing the drug from the shelf or drawer, when you have the drug in hand, and after taking the required dose from the bottle, package, envelope, or unit-dose packet.

● Before administering the drug, ask the patient to state his or her name, then compare the stated name with the name on the patient's identification bracelet and the name on the drug record or card.

● Before administering such drugs as propranolol (Inderal) or digitalis, collect appropriate data—for example, by measuring the patient's blood pressure and pulse or respiratory rate. (Restrictions regarding drug administration usually are listed on the MAR or a card.)

● Prepare drugs away from patients and other personnel to avoid distractions and possible drug loss to unauthorized personnel.

● When preparing a dose from a bottle, pour the required number of tablets or capsules into the lid of the bottle, then transfer them to a paper drug cup. Do not touch tablets with your fingers.

● When preparing a dose from a unit-dose packet, tear off the required number of individual dose packets and place them in a paper cup.

● When administering a liquid, remove the cap and place it upside down on a countertop to avoid contamination. Hold the bottle in your dominant hand for greater control, with the label facing your palm to prevent soiling. Hold the drug glass or cup at eye level, with your thumbnail on the line of the desired milliliters. Then pour the desired amount of drug, wipe off any drops from the neck of the bottle, and replace the lid carefully.

● When administering a unit-dose packet, open the packet only at the patient's bedside, after rechecking the drug label. Do not touch tablets with your fingers.

● Assist the patient to a position that allows easy drug administration.

● As appropriate, offer water to help the patient swallow the drug.

● Stay with the patient until all drugs have been swallowed.

● Do not leave drugs at the patient's bedside, except when ordered to do so specifically (such as with antacids).

● Administer drugs within 15 minutes of the ordered time.

● Record the drug administration on the patient's MAR.

● Keep in mind that elderly patients typically require smaller dosages, may have unusual drug reactions (such as confusion or restlessness), and may forget to take ordered drugs.

Appendix 7: NANDA nursing diagnostic categories

The nursing diagnoses below were adopted at the 9th National Conference of the North American Nursing Diagnosis Association, 1990. They are classified according to M. Gordon (1989), *Manual of nursing diagnoses, 1988-89.**

I. Health perception-health management pattern
Altered health maintenance
Noncompliance (specify)
Potential for infection
Potential for injury
Potential for trauma
Potential for poisoning
Potential for suffocation
Health-seeking behaviors (specify)

II. Nutritional-metabolic pattern
Altered nutrition: potential for more than body requirements
Altered nutrition: more than body requirements
Altered nutrition: less than body requirements
Ineffective breast-feeding
Potential for aspiration
Impaired swallowing
Altered oral mucous membrane
Potential fluid volume deficit
Fluid volume deficit
Fluid volume excess
Potential impaired skin integrity
Impaired skin integrity
Impaired tissue integrity
Potential altered body temperature
Ineffective thermoregulation
Hyperthermia
Hypothermia

III. Elimination pattern
Constipation
Perceived constipation
Colonic constipation
Diarrhea
Bowel incontinence
Altered urinary elimination
Functional incontinence
Reflex incontinence
Stress incontinence
Urge incontinence
Total incontinence
Urine retention

IV. Activity-exercise pattern
Potential activity intolerance
Activity intolerance
Impaired physical mobility
Potential for disuse syndrome
Fatigue
Bathing-hygiene self-care deficit
Feeding self-care deficit
Toileting self-care deficit
Diversional activity deficit
Impaired home maintenance management
Ineffective airway clearance
Ineffective breathing pattern
Impaired gas exchange
Decreased cardiac output
Altered (specify type) tissue perfusion (renal, cerebral, cardiopulmonary, gastrointestinal, peripheral)

Dysreflexia
Altered growth and development

V. Sleep-rest pattern
Sleep pattern disturbance

VI. Cognitive-perceptual pattern
Pain
Chronic pain
Sensory-perceptual alterations (specify) (visual, auditory, kinesthetic, gustatory, tactile, olfactory)
Unilateral neglect
Knowledge deficit (specify)
Altered thought processes
Decisional conflict (specify)

VII. Self-perception/self-concept pattern
Fear
Anxiety
Hopelessness
Powerlessness
Body image disturbance
Personal identity disturbance
Self-esteem disturbance
Chronic low self-esteem
Situational low self-esteem

VIII. Role-relationship pattern
Anticipatory grieving
Dysfunctional grieving
Altered role performance
Social isolation
Impaired social interaction
Altered family processes
Potential altered parenting
Altered parenting
Parental role conflict
Impaired verbal communication
Potential for violence: self-directed or directed at others

IX. Sexuality-reproductive pattern
Sexual dysfunction
Altered sexuality patterns
Rape-trauma syndrome
Rape-trauma syndrome: compound reaction
Rape-trauma syndrome: silent reaction

X. Coping-stress tolerance pattern
Ineffective individual coping
Defensive coping
Ineffective denial
Impaired adjustment
Post-trauma response
Family coping: potential for growth
Ineffective family coping: compromised
Ineffective family coping: disabling

XI. Value-belief pattern
Spiritual distress (distress of the human spirit)

---

*The nursing diagnoses *Altered protection* and *Effective breast-feeding* were added by NANDA in 1990.

Appendix 8: NCLEX-PN dates and state boards of nursing

NCLEX-PN dates

1992:	April 15 and October 21	**1996:**	April 17 and October 16
1993:	April 14 and October 13	**1997:**	April 16 and October 9
1994:	April 13 and October 12	**1998:**	April 7 and October 20
1995:	April 12 and October 24	**1999:**	April 14 and October 13

State boards of nursing

Alabama
Board of Nursing
500 E. Blvd., Suite 203
Montgomery, AL 36117
(205) 261-4060

Alaska
Board of Nursing
Division of Occup. Lisc.
P.O. Box D
Juneau, AK 99811
(907) 465-2544

Arizona
Board of Nursing
2001 West Camelback Road
Suite 350
Phoenix, AZ 85015
(602) 255-5092

Arkansas
Board of Nursing
1123 So. University Avenue
Suite 800
Little Rock, AR 72204
(501) 371-2751

California
Board of Nursing
1030 13th Street
Suite 200
Sacramento, CA 95814
(916) 322-3350

Colorado
Board of Nursing
1560 Broadway
Suite 670
Denver, CO 80202
(303) 894-2430

Connecticut
Dept. of Nurse Licensure
150 Washington Street
Hartford, CT 06106
(203) 566-1032

Delaware
Board of Nursing
Margaret O'Neill Building
Box 1401
Dover, DE 19901
(302) 736-4522

District of Columbia
Board of Nursing
614 H Street NW, 923
Washington, DC 20001
(202) 727-7468

Florida
Board of Nursing
111 E. Coastline Drive
Suite 516
Jacksonville, FL 32202
(904) 359-6331

Georgia
Board of Nursing
166 Pryor Street SW
Suite 400
Atlanta, GA 30303
(404) 656-3943

Hawaii
Board of Nursing
Box 3469
Honolulu, HI 96801
(808) 548-4100

Idaho
Board of Nursing
280 N. 8th Street
Suite 210
Boise, ID 83720
(208) 334-3110

Illinois
Dept. of Professional Regulation
320 W. Washington Street
Springfield, IL 62786
(217) 785-0800

Indiana
State Board of Nursing
One American Square,
Suite 1020
Box 82067
Indianapolis, IN 46282
(317) 232-2960

Iowa
Board of Nursing
1223 E. Court Avenue
Des Moines, IA 50319
(515) 281-3255

(continued)

APPENDICES

Appendix 8: NCLEX-PN dates and state boards of nursing *(continued)*

Kansas
Board of Nursing
900 S.W. Jackson, Suite 551-S
Topeka, KS 66612
(913) 296-4929

Kentucky
Board of Nursing
4010 DuPont Circle
Suite 430
Louisville, KY 40207
(502) 897-5143

Louisiana
Board of Nursing
150 Baronne Street
Room 907
New Orleans, LA 70112
(504) 568-5464

Maine
Board of Nursing
35 Anthony Avenue
State House Station 158
Augusta, ME 04333
(207) 289-5324

Maryland
Board of Nursing
4201 Patterson
Baltimore, MD 21215
(301) 764-4747

Massachusetts
Board of Nursing
100 Cambridge Street
Room 1519
Boston, MA 02202
(617) 727-9961

Michigan
Board of Nursing
P.O. Box 30018
Lansing, MI 48909
(517) 373-1600

Minnesota
Board of Nursing
2700 University Avenue W
Suite 108
St. Paul, MN 55114
(612) 642-0567

Mississippi
Board of Nursing
239 N. Lamar, Suite 401
Jackson, MS 39201
(601) 359-6170

Missouri
Board of Nursing
3524 N. Ten Mile Drive
P.O. Box 656
Jefferson City, MO 65102
(314) 751-0681

Montana
Board of Nursing
111 N. Jackson
Helena, MT 59620
(406) 444-4279

Nebraska
Board of Nursing
P. O. Box 95007
Lincoln, NE 68509
(402) 471-2115

Nevada
Board of Nursing
1281 Terminal Way
Suite 116
Reno, NV 89502
(702) 786-2778

New Hampshire
Board of Nursing
6 Hazel Drive
Concord, NH 03301
(603) 271-2323

New Jersey
Board of Nursing
1100 Raymond Boulevard
Room 508
Newark, NJ 07102
(201) 648-2490

New Mexico
Board of Nursing
4253 Montgomery NE
Suite 130
Albuquerque, NM 87109
(505) 841-8340

New York
Board of Nursing
Cultural Education Center
Albany, NY 12230
(518) 474-3843

North Carolina
Board of Nursing
P.O. Box 2129
Raleigh, NC 27602
(919) 782-3211

North Dakota
Board of Nursing
919 S. 7th Street
Suite 504
Bismarck, ND 58504
(701) 224-2974

Ohio
Board of Nursing
7 S. High Street 17th Floor
Columbus, OH 43266
(614) 466-3947

Appendix 8: NCLEX-PN dates and state boards of nursing *(continued)*

Oklahoma
Board of Nursing
2915 Classen Boulevard, 524
Oklahoma City, OK 73106
(405) 525-2076

Oregon
Board of Nursing
10455 SW Canyon Road
Suite 200
Beaverton, OR 97005
(503) 644-2767

Pennsylvania
Board of Nursing
Box 2649
Harrisburg, PA 17105
(717) 783-7142

Puerto Rico
Board of Nursing
Call Box 10200
San Juan, PR 00908
(809) 725-8161

Rhode Island
Board of Nursing
3 Capitol Hill
Room 104
Providence, RI 02908
(401) 277-2827

South Carolina
Board of Nursing
220 Executive Center Drive
Columbia, SC 29210
(803) 731-1648

South Dakota
Board of Nursing
304 S. Phillips Avenue
Suite 205
Sioux Falls, SD 57102
(605) 335-4973

Tennessee
Board of Nursing
283 Plus Park Boulevard
Nashville, TN 37247
(615) 367-6232

Texas
Board of Nursing
P.O. Box 140466
Austin, TX 78714
(512) 835-4880

Utah
Board of Nursing
160 E. 300 South
Box 45802
Salt Lake City, UT 84145
(801) 530-6628

Vermont
Board of Nursing
26 Terrace Street
Montpelier, VT 05602
(802) 828-2363

Virginia
Board of Nursing
1601 Rolling Hills Drive
Richmond, VA 23229
(804) 662-9909

Washington
Board of Nursing
P.O. Box 1099
Olympia, WA 98507
(206) 753-2206

West Virginia
Board of Nursing
922 Quarrier Street
Room 309
Charleston, WV 25301
(304) 348-3596

Wisconsin
Board of Nursing
P.O. Box 8935
Madison, WI 53708
(608) 266-3735

Wyoming
Board of Nursing
2301 Central Avenue, 3rd Fl.
Cheyenne, WY 82002
(307) 777-7601

Appendix 9: Canadian examination information

Examination dates (all provinces except Quebec)

1992: March 20, June 26, October 23
1993: March 26, June 25, October 22
1994: March 18, June 24, October 28

(**Note:** Quebec administers a different examination whose results are not recognized by other Canadian provinces. For information, contact the Quebec Association for Nursing Assistants at the address or telephone number below.)

Provincial nursing assistant-practical nurse associations

Alberta
Professional Council of
  Registered Nursing Assistants
10604-170th Street
Edmonton, Alberta
T5S 1P3
(403) 484-8886

British Columbia
British Columbia Council of
  Licensed Practical Nurses
205-4430 Halifax Street
Burnaby, British Columbia
V5C 5R4
(604) 660-5750

Manitoba
Manitoba Association of
  Licensed Practical Nurses
P.O. Box 249, Transcana
615 Kernaghan Avenue
Winnipeg, Manitoba
R2C 2Z4
(204) 222-6743

New Brunswick
Association of New Brunswick
Registered Nursing Assistants
384 Smythe Street
Fredericton, New Brunswick
E3B 3E4
(506) 453-0747

Newfoundland
Council for Nursing Assistants
LeMarchant Medical Centre
195 LeMarchant Road
St. John's, Newfoundland
A1C 2H5
(709) 579-3843

Northwest Territories
Certification and Student
  Assistance Division
Department of Education
Government of the Northwest
  Territories
Yellowknife, Northwest Territories
X1A 2L9
(403) 873-7669

Nova Scotia
Board of Registration of
  Nursing Assistants of Nova
  Scotia
2021 Brunswick Street
Suite 404
Halifax, Nova Scotia
B3K 2Y5
(902) 423-8517

Ontario
College of Nurses of Ontario
101 Davenport Road
Toronto, Ontario
M5R 3P1
(416) 928-0900

Prince Edward Island
Prince Edward Island Nursing
  Assistants' Registration Board
P.O. Box 3235
Charlottetown, Prince Edward
  Island
C1A 7N9
(902) 566-1512

Quebec
Association for Nursing
  Assistants
531 Sherbrooke Street East
Montreal, Quebec
H2L 1K2
(514) 282-9511

Saskatchewan
Saskatchewan Association of
  Certified Nursing Assistants
2310 Smith Street
Regina, Saskatchewan
S4P 2P6
(306) 525-1436

Yukon
Registrar of Nursing Assistants
Justice Service Division
Consumer Services
P.O. Box 2703
Whitehorse, Yukon
Y1A 2C6
(403) 6676-5811

Appendix 10: Selected references

Auvenshine, M.A., and Enriquez, M.G. (1990). *Comprehensive maternity nursing: Perinatal and women's health* (2nd ed.). Boston: Jones and Barlett.

Bobak, I.M., and Jensen, M.D. (1987). *Essentials of maternity nursing* (2nd ed.). St. Louis: C.V. Mosby.

Centers for Disease Control (1989). Guidelines for prevention of transmission of human immunodeficiency virus and hepatitis B to health-care and public-safety workers. *Morbidity and mortality weekly report,* 38 (s-6).

Dorland, I., and Newman, W.A. (1988). Dorland's illustrated medical dictionary (27th ed.). Philadelphia: W.B. Saunders.

Groenwald, S.L., et al. (1990). *Cancer nursing: Principles and practice* (2nd ed.). Boston: Jones and Bartlett.

Kane, M., and Colton, D. (1988). *Job analysis of newly licensed practical/vocational nurses, 1986-1987*. Chicago: National Council of State Boards of Nursing, Inc.

Ladewig, P.A., London, M.C., and Olds, S.B. (1986). *Essentials of maternal-newborn nursing*. Menlo Park: Addison-Wesley.

National Council of State Boards of Nursing (1989). *Test plan for the National Council Licensure Examination for Practical Nurses*. Chicago: National Council of State Boards of Nursing, Inc.

Porth, C.M. (1990). *Pathophysiology: Concepts of altered health states* (3rd ed.). Philadelphia: J.B. Lippincott.

Potter, P.A., and Perry, A.G. (1990). *Basic nursing theory and practice,* No. 2. St. Louis: Mosby-Yearbook.

Rice, J., and Skelley, E.G. (1988). *Medications and mathematics for the nurse* (6th ed.). Albany, N.Y.: Delmar Publishers.

Smith, A.J., and Johnson, J.Y. (1990). *Nurses' guide to clinical procedures,* Philadelphia: J.B. Lippincott.

Sorensen, K.C., and Luckmann, J. (1986). *Basic nursing: A psychophysiologic approach* (2nd ed.). Philadelphia: W.B. Saunders.

Thompson, J.M., McFarland, G.K., Hirsch, J.E., Tucker, S.M., and Bowers, A.C. (1989). *Mosby's Manual of Clinical Nursing* (2nd ed.). St. Louis: C.V. Mosby.

Thompson, E.D. (1987). *Pediatric nursing: An introductory text* (5th ed.). Philadelphia: W.B. Saunders.

Timby, B.K. (1989). *Clinical nursing procedures.* Philadelphia: J.B. Lippincott.

Part VI

Practice test

Be sure you have:

   • Provided ALL information on the answer sheet

• Enclosed a postal money order or certified check for $15 (U.S. Dollars) payable to "NLN Test Service"

   • Printed your return address on the envelope and affixed sufficient postage.

From: _____

_____

_____

_____

_____

National League for Nursing
NLN Test Service
350 Hudson Street
New York, NY 10014

Part VI

Practice test

Introduction 516

Sample computer report for the NLN Practice Test for PN Licensure 519

NLN Practice Test for PN Licensure 521

PRACTICE
TEST

Introduction

Purpose of the Practice Test

The National Council Licensure Examination for Practical Nurses (NCLEX-PN) is administered by state boards of nursing as part of the process used to determine whether practical-nurse candidates meet licensure requirements. The examination measures a candidate's ability to practice safely and effectively as a practical nurse in an entry-level position. It is designed to test the practical application of knowledge and skills in health care situations that commonly occur in entry-level nursing practice.

The National League for Nursing (NLN) has developed the NLN Practice Test for PN Licensure to assess your nursing ability, skill, and knowledge as you prepare to take NCLEX-PN. The test also can be used for review by nurses returning to active practice after an absence and by graduates of foreign nursing schools who wish to obtain credentials to practice in the United States.

To develop national norms, the questions on the Practice Test were administered to graduating seniors in practical nursing education programs. The norm sample for the pilot test included students representing a broad geographic distribution as well as the various types of nursing education programs in the United States.

When you send your answer sheet to the NLN for scoring, you will receive an individualized report of your strengths and weaknesses based on how you answered the test questions. Your performance will be measured against the performance of the norm sample. The report you receive will include an analysis of test questions and rationales for correct answers. For areas in which your performance was weak, the report will include suggested references to help you focus your review efforts. You also will receive a prediction of your performance on NCLEX-PN.

Understanding the content frameworks

In the report you receive, the information reflecting your test scores will be presented according to the content frameworks of the NCLEX-PN test plan, which measures your knowledge of four elements of the nursing process and four areas of client needs. As with NCLEX-PN, the number of questions for each content area varies. Nursing behaviors included in the nursing process are (1) collecting data, (2) planning, (3) implementing, and (4) evaluating. Client needs include (1) a safe, effective care environment; (2) physiologic integrity; (3) psychosocial integrity; and (4) health promotion and maintenance.

Entering personal data on the answer sheet

Your answer sheet, located inside the envelope in the back of this book, will be read by an electronic scanner and scored by a computer. Please use a #2 (soft black lead) pencil to enter information on the answer sheet and to answer Practice Test questions.

Enter your name and address carefully; whatever information you provide will appear on your score report. If you mistakenly darken the wrong circle for one of the letters in your name, the misspelled name will appear on your score report—even if you have printed your name correctly. Once you have completed the answer sheet, double-check that you have darkened the correct circles below each number and letter. Do not make any stray marks on the pages because the scanner might misinterpret these and "read" them as the answer to a question. This could cause errors in predicting your success and reporting your strengths and weaknesses. If you wish to correct any identification information or change a response to a question, erase carefully and completely.

Your answer sheet provides essential personal data needed to process your test results. In the area labeled "Name," print your last name, first name, and middle initial in the boxes directly below the words "Last Name," "First Name," and "MI." Even if there are not enough boxes for all the letters in your name, do not extend a name from one section into another. Darken the appropriate circles in the columns below each letter. For example, if your last name begins with the letter "B," completely darken the circle containing the letter "B" in the column directly below the box where you have printed the "B." If your name has a space or hyphen, fill in the blank circle in the appropriate column.

In the area labeled "Social Security Number," print your Social Security number in the boxes provided, then darken the appropriately numbered circle in the column below each number. If you do not have a Social Security number, leave these boxes blank.

In the area labeled "Address," print, in the boxes provided, the address to which you want your test results sent. If you live outside the United States, leave the state and ZIP code boxes blank; print the name of your country on the last blank line, including any country mailing code. Failure to provide an accurate and legible address will delay receipt of your test results.

Please respond to the questions in the boxes at the bottom of the page by darkening the appropriate circle or filling in the blank spaces.

Taking the Practice Test

The NLN Practice Test for PN Licensure is based on the same question-and-response format used in NCLEX-PN. It presents a hypothetical clinical situation containing essential background information in paragraph form. Each multiple-choice question that follows poses a problem to be solved. You must select the correct response from the four choices presented. Like NCLEX-PN, the Practice Test does not include any deliberately misleading questions. Only one correct answer choice is given for each question, although a quick glance at a question may not reveal the answer immediately.

Make sure you understand the information in the clinical situation before attempting to answer a question. Read the question carefully and select the single best answer. In some cases, each of the four answer choices might be appropriate nursing behaviors; however, the question will ask which is the most important one or the one to do first.

If you do not know the answer to a particular question, mark it in the test book and go back to it later. Instead of guessing randomly, try to eliminate one—or preferably two—of the possible responses, then choose what seems like the best answer from the remaining choices. Because your test results are based on the number of correct responses, your best strategy is to answer every question. The prediction of your success on NCLEX-PN and the feedback in your test reports will be more accurate and complete if you answer every question—even if you need to spend a bit more time at the end of the test than you intended to at first.

The procedure for recording answer choices for the Practice Test differs from that of NCLEX-PN. On NCLEX-PN, you will mark your answers in the test booklet just next to your answer choice; the entire booklet will be sent in for scoring. The Practice Test, in contrast, uses an answer sheet that is separate from the test booklet; return only this answer sheet

for scoring. Make sure the number of the question you are working on in your test booklet matches the number on your answer sheet.

You must use a #2 pencil to mark your answers. To answer each question, completely fill in the appropriate circle for each item number. Pressing firmly on the pencil, darken the circle that contains the number representing your answer choice. Make sure to darken only one circle for each question. Do not use X's or check marks. Here's an example of how to fill in your answer choice.

Sample question

1. Which of the following can the nurse expect to see in a client after prolonged administration of glucocorticoids?
- ○ **1.** Hypotension.
- ○ **2.** Hypoglycemia.
- ○ **3.** Hirsutism.
- ○ **4.** Protein synthesis.

The correct answer is 3. Darken the entire circle containing the number 3.

Correct mark

When taking the Practice Test, you'll find it helpful to simulate test-taking conditions as nearly as possible. The Practice Test consists of 120 items, for which you should allow approximately 2 hours of uninterrupted time, or two sessions of 1 hour each. If you choose to take the test in two sessions, we recommend that you stop your first session after item #60. Have several sharpened #2 pencils and an eraser handy, as well as a piece of scrap paper on which to make notes and calculations. (No scrap paper will be allowed when you take NCLEX-PN, although space for notes will be provided in the exam book.)

A few reminders:
- Read each question carefully.
- Choose the best answer from the four possible choices.
- Darken only one circle for each question.
- Answer each question.

Returning the answer sheet for scoring

After you have completed all 120 questions on the Practice Test and have filled in the data accurately on the front and back of the answer sheet, mail the answer sheet with a postal money order or bank check in the amount of $15 (U.S. currency only) in the envelope provided. Please make sure to affix adequate postage. **Failing to enclose the correct amount, using any envelope other than the one provided, or affixing insufficient postage on the envelope will cause a significant delay in the return of your individualized report.**

When we receive your answer sheet at our scoring center in New York City, we will score your test, prepare your report, and have the results in the mail to you within 10 working days. (For a sample report, see *Sample computer report for the NLN Practice Test for PN Licensure,* pages 519 and 520.)

Using your individualized test results
The report you receive will include a prediction of your success on NCLEX-PN and detailed, customized analysis of your strengths and weaknesses in the skills and knowledge areas measured by NCLEX-PN. The report will allow you to design an effective, efficient review plan. Questions on both the Practice Test and NCLEX-PN focus on practical application of nursing principles rather than recall of facts. Therefore, if you plan to conduct a study and review after taking the test, focus on the broad areas reported on your performance profile rather than on specific items.

Sample Computer Report for the

NLN PRACTICE TEST FOR PN LICENSURE

PERFORMANCE REPORT FOR:

JOAN A. DOE   REPORT DATE: 01/14/93
405 BACKROAD DRIVE
ANYTOWN MN 36091   191-20-1234

OVERALL PERFORMANCE AND PREDICTION OF SUCCESS ON NCLEX-PN

YOU ANSWERED CORRECTLY 85 (70%) OF THE 121 ITEMS IN THE TEST. OVERALL,
YOU SCORED HIGHER THAN 71% OF THE STUDENTS IN THE NORMS GROUP, WHICH CONSISTED
OF 2,650 STUDENTS PREPARING TO TAKE NCLEX-PN FOR THE 1ST TIME.   BASED ON YOUR
PERFORMANCE, YOU HAVE A BETTER THAN AVERAGE CHANCE OF PASSING NCLEX-PN.
PLEASE USE THE PERFORMANCE PROFILE, ANALYSIS OF INCORRECT RESPONSES, AND ITEM
RATIONALES TO IDENTIFY ANY WEAK AREAS FOR SUBSEQUENT REVIEW.

PERFORMANCE PROFILE

YOUR TOTAL SCORE IS REPORTED IN TWO WAYS: BY THE FOUR CATEGORIES OF NURSING
PROCESS, AND BY THE FOUR CATEGORIES OF CLIENT NEEDS

NURSING PROCESS	YOU ANSWERED CORRECTLY:	PERCENTILE RANKING
COLLECTING DATA.....	24 OF 36 (66%)	74
PLANNING............	19 OF 24 (78%)	79
IMPLEMENTING........	26 OF 38 (69%)	71
EVALUATING..........	16 OF 23 (67%)	63
TOTAL	85 OF 121 (70%)	71

CLIENT NEEDS		
SAFE, EFFECTIVE CARE ENVIRONMENT...	19 OF 30 (63%)	74
PHYSIOLOGICAL INTEGRITY..........	42 OF 56 (75%)	61
PSYCHOSOCIAL INTEGRITY..........	6 OF 8 (75%)	79
HEALTH PROMOTION & MAINTENANCE......	18 OF 27 (67%)	73
TOTAL	85 OF 121 (70%)	71

NLN PRACTICE TEST FOR PN LICENSURE

```
-----------------------------------
ANALYSIS OF INCORRECT RESPONSES                        JOAN A. DOE
-----------------------------------                    191-20-1234        01/14/93
```

ITEM NO.	CORRECT RESP.	YOUR RESP.	RATIONALE FOR CORRECT RESPONSE	REASON YOUR RESPONSE WAS WRONG
12	3	1	VITAMIN K1 ADMINISTERED TO THE NEWBORN PROMOTES BLOOD CLOTTING.	VITAMIN K1 IS NOT RELATED TO THE DEVELOPMENT OF HYPERBILIRUBINEMIA.
29	4	2	QUICK MOVEMENT OF THE HEAD CAN RESULT IN STRESS ON THE STITCHES AFTER CATARACT SURGERY.	IMMEDIATELY POST-OP, PREVENTING INJURY TO THE OPERATIVE SITE HAS A HIGHER PRIORITY THAN ASSESSING APPROPRIATE AFFECT.
104	2	4	THE NURSE FOCUSES ON PROBABLE PATIENT CONCERNS, WITHOUT SUGGESTING ANY TOPIC, SPECIFIC FEELING OR JUDGEMENT, WHICH LEAVES THE PATIENT FREE TO RESPOND IN ANY WAY THE PATIENT WISHES.	BY TELLING THE PATIENT HOW SHE SHOULD FEEL, THE NURSE BLOCKS THE PATIENT FROM EXPRESSING HER CONCERNS.
145	1	3	MILK AND MILK PRODUCTS ARE POOR SOURCES OF IRON.	RAISINS ARE A GOOD SOURCE OF IRON.
192	2	3	AFTER A CRANIOTOMY, THE PATIENT'S POSITION SHOULD BE CHANGED EVERY 2 HOURS.	EXCESSIVE FLUID INTAKE MAY EXACERBATE THE PULMONARY CONDITION.

```
-----------------------------------
SUGGESTED REFERENCES FOR REVIEW
-----------------------------------
```

TITLE	AUTHOR	PUBLISHER
INTRODUCTORY MEDICAL-SURGICAL NURSING (4TH EDITION)	SCHERER	J. B. LIPPINCOTT, 1986
ESSENTIALS OF MEDICAL-SURGICAL NURSING (2ND EDITION)	KEANE	W. B. SAUNDERS, 1986

NLN Practice Test for PN Licensure

Mrs. Jean Larson, age 55, goes to the physician after discovering a lump in her left breast. On examination, the physician notes enlargement of her left axillary lymph nodes. A mammogram is scheduled.

1. Mrs. Larson asks the practical nurse, "What is a mammogram?" Which response by the practical nurse would be correct?
   1. "It is a noninvasive X-ray that reveals areas of abnormal density."
   2. "It is a procedure requiring injection of an opaque substance that will outline the tumors."
   3. "It is an infrared picture showing hot spots that indicate hyperplasia."
   4. "It is similar to an ultrasound that projects darkened areas of overgrowth on the printout."

After the mammogram, Mrs. Larson is admitted to the hospital. She is scheduled for a frozen section biopsy and possible mastectomy.

2. Although the physician has explained the operative procedure, Mrs. Larson asks the practical nurse, "What is a frozen section?" The practical nurse's explanation should include which of these statements?
   1. "The tissue removed will be frozen and quickly submerged in a dye to outline abnormal cells."
   2. "The tissue is excised using cryosurgery and then centrifuged to spin off frozen malignant cells."
   3. "The pathology procedure identifies types of microscopic cells present in frozen tissue."
   4. "After the frozen tissue is removed, acidic solution is placed on frozen tissue to destroy normal cells."

3. Mrs. Larson says to the practical nurse, "The doctor told me I have a tumor, so why do I need to have a frozen section biopsy? Can't the tumor just be removed?" Which of these explanations is best?
   1. "It is the protocol of the American Medical Society to include biopsy as a precautionary measure."
   2. "Results of the biopsy will guide the surgeon as to the type of surgery needed."
   3. "Surgeons do biopsies in all instances because of the high incidence of litigation."

4. "Hospital quality assurance guidelines include this type of biopsy as essential."

4. Mrs. Larson has problems understanding the surgeon's instructions. Which of these explanations describes the most likely cause of her difficulty?
   1. Mrs. Larson lacks knowledge of anatomy and physiology.
   2. Mrs. Larson lacks interest in details.
   3. Mrs. Larson's level of anxiety is high.
   4. Mrs. Larson has a low level of mental ability.

5. Before surgery, skin preparation is ordered for Mrs. Larson primarily for which purpose?
   1. To improve visualization of surgical landmarks.
   2. To reduce the number of bacteria at the site of surgery.
   3. To promote adherence of the surgical tape.
   4. To prevent a reaction to the adhesive on the tape.

A left radical mastectomy with lymph node dissection is performed. Mrs. Larson is taken to the recovery room with a transfusion of whole blood.

6. Which finding would indicate that a hemolytic reaction is occurring?
   1. Low back pain.
   2. Positive Homan's sign.
   3. Hyperreflexia.
   4. Hematemesis.

After Mrs. Larson's condition stabilizes and the blood transfusion is completed, she is transferred to her room. She has a wound drain attached to a portable suction apparatus (Hemovac) and an I.V. infusion.

7. Mrs. Larson has an I.V. order for 1,000 ml of 5% dextrose and water q8h. The I.V. drop factor is 20 gtt/ml. The practical nurse should regulate the flow of the solution at the rate of about how many drops per minute?
   1. 30
   2. 40
   3. 50
   4. 60

8. Which finding would indicate that Mrs. Larson's I.V. infusion has infiltrated?
   1. The flow of fluid in the drip chamber has come to a halt.
   2. There is redness along the vein from the needle site upward.
   3. Puffiness occurs proximal to the insertion site.
   4. A backflow of blood is in the tubing.

9. Because a Hemovac is attached to Mrs. Larson's wound catheter, which of these measures should the practical nurse take?
   1. Clamping the wound catheter when emptying the chamber.
   2. Flushing the chamber with sterile saline solution if it appears clogged.
   3. Applying gentle pressure around the wound catheter to facilitate drainage.
   4. Informing the charge nurse if the chamber fills rapidly.

10. Postoperatively, Mrs. Larson is encouraged to move her legs. Contraction of the leg muscles will prevent which of these complications?
    1. Pleurisy.
    2. Portal hypertension.
    3. Hypostatic pneumonia.
    4. Pulmonary emboli.

11. Which of these findings indicates that Mrs. Larson has accepted the alteration to her body?
    1. She is anxious to be discharged.
    2. She asks when her sutures will be removed.
    3. She sits at the edge of the bed when the physician removes her bulky dressing.
    4. She looks at the incision when the dressing is being changed.

12. Because Mrs. Larson's lymph nodes have been removed, which of these instructions should she receive?
    1. "You should wear an elastic sleeve on your left arm and keep the arm covered at all times."
    2. "Your left arm should not be used for drawing blood or taking blood pressure."
    3. "You should avoid sleeping on your left side or putting any pressure on your left arm."
    4. "Your left arm should be elevated or kept in a sling most of the day."

Mrs. Leah Jacob, age 72, is admitted to a one-day surgery facility for a cataract extraction of her right eye. An antibiotic ointment and mydriatic eyedrops are ordered.

13. Which of these symptoms indicates a cataract?
    1. Loss of peripheral vision.
    2. Tunnel vision.
    3. Double vision.
    4. Blurred vision.

14. When administering the prescribed antibiotic ointment for Mrs. Jacob, the practical nurse should apply the ointment
    1. over the entire sclera.
    2. over the entire eye socket.
    3. along the inner surface of the lower lid.
    4. along the eyelashes.

15. Mydriatic eyedrops are prescribed for Mrs. Jacob for which purpose?
    1. To numb the eyeball.
    2. To make the cornea more visible.
    3. To constrict the lens.
    4. To dilate the pupil.

Mrs. Jacob has the cataract extracted. She is brought to the recovery area.

16. During the postoperative period, Mrs. Jacob should be observed for which symptom of a complication of cataract surgery?
    1. Twitching of the eyelid.
    2. Tearing of the eye.
    3. Itching of the eye.
    4. Sharp pain in the eye.

17. While being prepared for discharge, Mrs. Jacob receives instructions on self-care. Which statement by Mrs. Jacob indicates that she understands the instructions?
    1. "I will cover my mouth when I cough."
    2. "I will get someone to pick up any heavy object from the floor."
    3. "I will practice the Valsalva maneuver daily."
    4. "I will sleep on two pillows."

18. During a follow-up visit to the physician's office, Mrs. Jacob receives instructions about temporary eyeglasses that will be prescribed for her. Which statement by Mrs. Jacob indicates that she understands the instructions?
1. "I will move about with care at first, as the glasses will not correct my depth perception."
2. "The glasses will help my astigmatism."
3. "I will wear the glasses after the sun goes down to improve my vision."
4. "The glasses will improve my peripheral distortions."

John Hall, age 5, is admitted to the hospital for an elective tonsillectomy and adenoidectomy.

19. All of the following observations are made during John's admission. The practical nurse should be sure to obtain more information about which one?
1. John is chewing on his fingernails.
2. John is clutching a ragged teddy bear.
3. John is avoiding eye contact with the nurse.
4. John is sneezing frequently.

20. John needs more preoperative teaching if he makes which comment?
1. "I will wake up in another room and then come back to my room."
2. "I will see Mom and Dad after the operation."
3. "I can have my favorite ice cream after I wake up."
4. "I will feel sleepy for a while after the operation."

21. During the preoperative period, which of these assessments of John is essential?
1. Examining him for loose teeth.
2. Comparing his apical and radial pulse rates.
3. Checking the function of his facial nerve.
4. Determining the range of motion of his head and neck.

John has the surgery and returns to his room.

22. Until John awakens fully, he should be maintained in which position?
1. Trendelenburg.
2. Supine.
3. Recumbent.
4. Semi-prone.

23. During the early postoperative period, John should be observed closely for which behavior?
1. Frequent swallowing.
2. Intermittent moaning.
3. Incontinence.
4. Lethargy.

Mrs. Laura Olsen, age 58, is admitted to the hospital for surgery with a diagnosis of cholelithiasis.

24. Which of these signs is associated with cholelithiasis?
1. Projectile vomiting.
2. Continuous hiccups.
3. Intermittent diarrhea.
4. Clay-colored stools.

25. When taking a nursing history for Mrs. Olsen, which of these questions relating to cholelithiasis would be appropriate for the practical nurse to ask?
1. "Do you have less discomfort when you sleep in semi-Fowler's position?"
2. "Do you get heartburn after a spicy meal?"
3. "Do you have an intolerance to fatty foods?"
4. "Do you have less flatus after taking an antacid?"

26. Before surgery, Mrs. Olsen receives phytonadione (vitamin K_1) I.M. for which purpose?
1. To improve the clotting ability of the blood.
2. To promote healing of connective tissue.
3. To reduce the dosage of the preoperative medication.
4. To attempt to dissolve the calculi.

A cholecystectomy with choledochostomy is performed. Mrs. Olsen returns to her unit with a T-tube and nasogastric tube in place. Her postoperative orders include meperidine hydrochloride (Demerol).

27. On the evening of Mrs. Olsen's surgery, she receives 50 mg Demerol. Two hours later, she complains of incisional pain. Which of these actions should the practical nurse take?
1. Obtain an order for a heating pad to be held against her abdomen.
2. Repeat the Demerol dose.
3. Turn her onto either side and place pillows behind her back.
4. Give her 25 mg Demerol.

PRACTICE TEST

28. To prevent Mrs. Olsen from developing hypostatic pneumonia, the practical nurse should take which action during the immediate postoperative period?
1. Splint Mrs. Olsen's incisional area while she breathes deeply.
2. Have Mrs. Olsen blow into a spirometer q.i.d.
3. Encourage Mrs. Olsen to exhale through pursed lips.
4. Support Mrs. Olsen in an orthopneic position.

29. The primary purpose of the T-tube for Mrs. Olsen is to
1. maintain a patent common bile duct.
2. allow deep wound healing to occur initially.
3. regulate the flow of drainage from the gallbladder bed.
4. prevent the backflow of bile.

30. Which measure should the practical nurse take regarding Mrs. Olsen's T-tube?
1. Irrigate it periodically.
2. Connect it to a straight drainage system.
3. Attach it to a low-suction apparatus.
4. Aspirate it at least four times a day.

31. Which measure would be most therapeutic in preventing Mrs. Olsen from developing thrombophlebitis in the calves?
1. Obtain an order for the use of antiembolic stockings during most of the day.
2. Maintain the knee gatch of her bed in a slightly elevated position while she is in bed.
3. Support her legs so that they are higher than her heart.
4. Encourage her to exercise her lower extremities every hour during the day.

32. Which finding would indicate that Mrs. Olsen is ready for removal of the nasogastric tube?
1. She does not complain of feeling nauseated.
2. She belches after taking a sip of clear fluids.
3. Drainage from her stomach has diminished in volume.
4. She has been passing gas rectally.

Mr. George Trent, age 65, is a homeless man who is brought to the emergency department after falling down a flight of stairs. X-rays show no evidence of fractures. Before transfer to a home for the elderly, Mr. Trent undergoes a thorough medical examination, including a tuberculin test.

33. Mr. Trent has a positive reaction to purified protein derivative (PPD). This means that he
1. has been exposed to tubercle bacilli.
2. has active tuberculosis.
3. has stimulated dormant calcified tuberculin cells.
4. lacks antibodies to fight the tubercle bacillus.

34. Mr. Trent should be observed for an early sign of tuberculosis, which is
1. petechiae.
2. a dry, hacking cough.
3. enlarged lymph nodes.
4. night sweats.

35. Which factor most likely would contribute to Mr. Trent's developing tuberculosis?
1. A smoking habit of 20 years' duration.
2. A history of drinking cocktails before dinner.
3. A cold, damp environment.
4. Close contact with an infected person.

36. Which test would confirm whether Mr. Trent has tuberculosis?
1. Acid-fast sputum test.
2. Tine test.
3. Mantoux test.
4. Australian antigen test.

Isoniazid (INH) and rifampin (Rifadin) are ordered for Mr. Trent.

37. Which comment by Mr. Trent indicates that he understands the instructions about INH and Rifadin?
1. "I will take the medication until I regain my strength."
2. "I will take the medication as prescribed for about a year."
3. "I will take the medication with a citrus juice."
4. "I will take the medication until my white blood cell count is normal."

38. Pyridoxine (vitamin B_6) is prescribed for Mr. Trent to counteract the side effects of INH, which include
1. rectal pruritus.
2. alopecia.
3. peripheral neuritis.
4. diarrhea.

Ira Feld, age 3, is admitted to the hospital with status asthmaticus. He receives aminophylline (aminophylline injection) I.V.

39. Ira is given aminophylline injection I.V. for what purpose?
    1. To increase urine output.
    2. To stimulate peripheral reflexes.
    3. To relax smooth muscles.
    4. To produce a histamine.

40. While Ira is in severe respiratory distress, he should be maintained in which of these positions?
    1. Sitting upright.
    2. Side-lying.
    3. Supine.
    4. Prone.

41. Mrs. Feld is crying outside Ira's room. Which comment by the practical nurse would be appropriate at this time?
    1. "This must be upsetting for you."
    2. "Talking to the doctor will help."
    3. "Most mothers feel this way."
    4. "Come talk with other parents in the waiting room."

Mrs. Maria Garcia is in the thirty-sixth week of gestation and has insulin-dependent diabetes mellitus (Type I). She has a cesarean birth and delivers a girl.

42. Baby Girl Garcia's 5-minute Apgar score is 9. She will need to be
    1. suctioned at regular intervals.
    2. kept in a warm environment.
    3. prepared for I.V. fluid administration.
    4. given oxygen by mask.

43. After Baby Girl Garcia's birth, which action takes priority?
    1. Monitor her hematocrit.
    2. Test her blood sugar level frequently.
    3. Check her Moro reflex at frequent intervals.
    4. Measure her urine output.

44. The practical nurse should expect an infant born of a diabetic mother to
    1. have hypertonia.
    2. be hyperactive.
    3. be fat.
    4. have scaly skin.

Mrs. Charlene Blair, age 76, is overweight and has had osteoarthritis in her knees and hips for the past 20 years. Periodically, she sees the physicians at her health maintenance organization (HMO), who prescribe ibuprofen (Motrin) for her.

45. Mrs. Blair asks the practical nurse, "What is the cause of osteoarthritis?" The practical nurse's response should include which statement?
    1. It is an acquired autoimmune disease.
    2. It is an effect of the process of aging.
    3. It is the result of an infectious process.
    4. It is a disorder of calcium metabolism.

46. Mrs. Blair complains of stiffness in her lower extremities. Which measure should she be advised to carry out?
    1. "Place your weight on the balls of your feet when walking."
    2. "Wear elastic bandages on your legs."
    3. "Stay off your feet as much as possible."
    4. "Extend and flex your feet frequently."

47. Besides complaints of joint stiffness, the practical nurse would expect Mrs. Blair to have which sign related to osteoarthritis of her knees?
    1. Enlargement of the joints.
    2. Swelling of soft tissue surrounding the joints.
    3. Atrophy of the muscles adjacent to the joints.
    4. Erythema around the joints.

48. On a subsequent visit to the HMO, Mrs. Blair is accompanied by her daughter. Because her daughter plans to have her mother visit with her, she asks the practical nurse for instructions in caring for her. The practical nurse should instruct Mrs. Blair's daughter to give Motrin to her mother
    1. with food.
    2. an hour before meals.
    3. with a glass of juice.
    4. whenever she feels pain.

PRACTICE TEST

49. Mrs. Blair enjoys all of the following activities. Which one is most therapeutic for her arthritis?
    1. Playing the piano.
    2. Riding a stationary bicycle.
    3. Doing exercise to music.
    4. Baking a batch of bread twice a week.

50. At a staff conference concerning Mrs. Blair's progress, two members of the nursing staff state that lately Mrs. Blair looks at them intently when being questioned and answers inappropriately at times. On the basis of these data, Mrs. Blair should be evaluated for a possible
    1. hearing loss.
    2. perceptual defect.
    3. shortened attention span.
    4. cerebral oxygen deficit.

Mr. William Maxwell, age 68, is admitted to the hospital for evaluation and management of insulin-dependent (type I) diabetes mellitus. His orders include isophane (NPH) insulin suspension to be administered at 7:30 AM q.d.

51. Which symptoms indicate diabetes mellitus?
    1. Oliguria and hyperthermia.
    2. Diarrhea and clammy skin.
    3. Tremors and tachycardia.
    4. Fatigue and hunger.

52. When preparing to administer the NPH insulin, the practical nurse should take which action?
    1. Rotate the vial between the hands.
    2. Warm the vial to room temperature under the hot water tap.
    3. Invert the vial for a few minutes.
    4. Aspirate the contents without injecting air into the vial.

53. The sites for insulin injection should be rotated to prevent
    1. peripheral neuropathy.
    2. abscess formation.
    3. hemolysis.
    4. lipodystrophy.

54. Within 30 minutes after administration of NPH insulin, which goal should take priority in Mr. Maxwell's care?
    1. To test his urine for sugar.
    2. To observe him for a skin reaction.
    3. To check his injection site for absorption.
    4. To tell him to eat his breakfast.

55. To prevent a hypoglycemic reaction at the peak effect of NPH insulin, the practical nurse must instruct Mr. Maxwell to take nourishment at which time?
    1. Midmorning.
    2. Late afternoon.
    3. Bedtime.
    4. Midnight.

Before Mr. Maxwell is discharged, he receives instructions on his dietary exchange list and exercise regimen.

56. Mr. Maxwell should be taught that a symptom of hypoglycemia is
    1. pruritus.
    2. tinnitus.
    3. hypertension.
    4. confusion.

57. Before doing strenuous exercise, Mr. Maxwell must plan to
    1. give himself extra insulin.
    2. have a carbohydrate food.
    3. rest for an hour.
    4. stretch and bend for 10 minutes.

58. Which dietary instruction is essential to give Mr. Maxwell?
    1. "When you skip a meal, reduce your insulin."
    2. "Substitute 1 ounce of fat for 2 ounces of protein."
    3. "Eat your meals and snacks on schedule."
    4. "Use artificial sweeteners in your food instead of consuming complex sugars."

59. Mr. Maxwell seems anxious while receiving instructions in self-care. He says to the practical nurse, "It's no use. I can't be cured, so what's the sense in you telling me all that nonsense?" After acknowledging his distress, which response by the practical nurse would be appropriate?
    1. "You must not become discouraged and tense because this will only aggravate your condition."
    2. "Just take one step at a time. None of us knows what will happen to us from day to day."
    3. "While it's true that you'll have to modify your life-style, the quality of your life doesn't have to diminish."
    4. "You need not feel so negative about the future. We are trying to help you care for yourself more easily."

Several weeks later, Mr. Maxwell is admitted to the hospital with ketoacidosis.

60. Which behavior most likely has contributed to Mr. Maxwell's developing ketoacidosis?
    1. He has been increasing his daily walking exercise.
    2. He neglected to take his insulin.
    3. He did not maintain his diet.
    4. He has been working 8 hours a day.

61. When a patient is to receive rapid-acting insulin, the practical nurse should expect the physician to prescribe which type of insulin?
    1. Isophane (NPH) insulin.
    2. Protamine zinc (PZI) insulin.
    3. Insulin injection (Regular Insulin).
    4. Zinc suspension (Lente) insulin.

62. Mr. Maxwell receives instructions on how to use the dietary exchange list. He would show that he understands these instructions if he exchanges which of these foods for 1 ounce of meat?
    1. ¼ cup cottage cheese.
    2. 1 slice bacon.
    3. 1 cup whole milk.
    4. ½ avocado.

Miss Jeanette Cleary, age 17, comes to the antepartal clinic for the first time when she is 6 months pregnant. She receives dietary instructions.

63. Jeanette is instructed to eat foods **high** in complete protein. Jeanette would show that she understands these instructions if she selects which food?
    1. Eggs.
    2. Gelatin dessert.
    3. Spaghetti.
    4. Baked beans.

64. Jeanette receives instructions about foods containing high amounts of calcium. She would show that she understands these instructions if she selects which food as **highest** in calcium?
    1. Liver.
    2. Yogurt.
    3. Bran muffin.
    4. Fresh spinach.

Jeanette's pregnancy progresses well. At term, she is admitted to the hospital and delivers a baby girl. Baby Girl Cleary will be bottle-fed; she is transferred to the newborn nursery. Jeanette is transferred to the recovery room.

65. Shortly after Baby Girl Cleary's birth, silver nitrate 1% is instilled into her eyes to prevent
    1. ophthalmia neonatorum.
    2. retrolental fibroplasia.
    3. corneal keratitis.
    4. acute uveitis.

66. At 2 hours postpartum, Jeanette is being assessed for readiness for transfer to the postpartum unit from the recovery room. Which observation by the practical nurse calls for immediate nursing intervention?
    1. Temperature of 99.8° F (37.7° C) and pulse rate of 70.
    2. Breasts soft and nontender and colostrum present.
    3. Uterine fundus soft and located at the umbilicus, left of midline.
    4. Moderate lochia rubra containing small clots.

Jeanette and her baby are to be discharged. The practical nurse has a discharge conference with Jeanette to plan her home care.

67. Which suggestion would be appropriate to include in the discussion with Jeanette?
    1. "Manually express milk from your breasts if they are uncomfortable."
    2. "Apply ice packs to your breasts if they become engorged."
    3. "Massage your uterine fundus to relieve afterpains."
    4. "Remain in bed for 1 or 2 days if your lochia increases or if you pass clots."

Mrs. Doris Kinder, age 78, develops cystitis. The physician orders phenazopyridine hydrochloride (Pyridium). Mrs. Kinder and her husband live in an extended-care facility.

68. Which symptom is associated with cystitis?
    1. Polyuria.
    2. Oliguria.
    3. Nocturia.
    4. Dysuria.

69. Mrs. Kinder tells the practical nurse, "My husband and I have lived together for 60 years. I just don't know why I always get cystitis and he doesn't." Which statement should the practical nurse include when responding?
1. The female urethra is shorter and closer to the rectum than the male urethra.
2. Males have a greater resistance to enterococcic organisms than females.
3. The sphincter of the female meatus does not contract as tightly as the sphincter of the male.
4. Males do not irritate the meatus with toilet tissue as do females.

70. Because Mrs. Kinder has cystitis, which goal takes priority?
1. To increase the alkalinity of her urine.
2. To maintain a balanced intake and output.
3. To provide her with instructions on perineal hygiene.
4. To screen her urine for sedimentation.

71. Which complication is most likely to occur if cystitis is **not** treated?
1. Pyelonephritis.
2. Polycystic kidney disease.
3. Glomerulonephritis.
4. Renal calculi.

72. Which explanation about Pyridium should the nurse share with Mrs. Kinder?
1. "Pyridium stains can be removed with a bleaching product."
2. "Pyridium should be taken on an empty stomach."
3. "Pyridium is more effective when taken with a carbonated beverage."
4. "Pyridium should be withheld if the urine becomes deep amber."

Miss Lona Santana, age 21, is diagnosed with gonorrhea.

73. Because of Miss Santana's diagnosis, she should be assessed for which of the following?
1. Lower abdominal pain.
2. Muscle rigidity.
3. Unsteady gait.
4. Reddish rash on the inner thighs.

74. Miss Santana should be taught that if gonorrhea is **not** treated, the disease most likely will result in
1. endometriosis.
2. infertility.
3. more frequent menstrual periods.
4. prolapsed uterus.

75. The physician prescribes ceftriaxone sodium (Rocephin) I.M. for Miss Santana. Which action should the practical nurse take when administering Rocephin?
1. Inject the medication slowly, taking up to 5 minutes.
2. Weigh Miss Santana before administering the medication.
3. Withhold the medication if Miss Santana has an allergy to penicillin.
4. Dilute the medication with hypotonic solution to prevent abscess formation.

76. To prevent reinfection, Miss Santana receives instructions. Which statement by Miss Santana indicates that she understands the instructions?
1. "I will douche with an alkaline solution after sexual intercourse."
2. "I will send my partner in for treatment before having sexual intercourse."
3. "I will be fitted for an intrauterine device before having sexual intercourse."
4. "I will have my partner wash his genitalia before having sexual intercourse."

Mr. Donald Auger, age 60, is admitted to a coronary intensive care unit with symptoms of myocardial infarction. A *stat* dose of morphine sulfate is ordered.

77. The practical nurse should expect Mr. Auger to have which symptom associated with a myocardial infarction?
1. A sharp stabbing pain on inspiration.
2. A viselike pain in the lower part of the sternum.
3. A feeling of fullness in the lower thorax, with episodes of heartburn.
4. Pain in the heart region, with an increased bounding heart beat.

78. Mr. Auger is to receive 8 mg morphine sulfate; the ampule contains 15 mg/ml. The practical nurse should administer approximately which amount?
1. 0.5 ml.
2. 0.7 ml.
3. 1.0 ml.
4. 1.5 ml.

Studies confirm that Mr. Auger has had a myocardial infarction. The physician orders heparin sodium.

79. The practical nurse should observe Mr. Auger for a side effect of heparin sodium, which is
1. leukoplasia.
2. leukocytosis.
3. thrombophlebitis.
4. thrombocytopenia.

80. To counteract the side effects of heparin sodium, which of these medications should be readily available?
1. Calcium gluconate.
2. Protamine sulfate.
3. Chlorambucil (Leukeran).
4. Lithium carbonate (Lithane).

81. The practical nurse believes Mr. Auger is denying the seriousness of his condition. Which of Mr. Auger's behaviors supports this belief?
1. He refuses to eat solid food.
2. He says that tea made from heart-shaped leaves is good for heart disease.
3. He expects to return to his job within 2 weeks.
4. He is planning to do an oil painting for his daughter.

82. Mr. Auger is instructed about warfarin sodium (Coumadin), which the physician has prescribed for him. Which statement by Mr. Auger indicates that he needs further instruction?
1. "I will use an electric razor for shaving."
2. "I will need periodic blood coagulation tests."
3. "I will expect my urine to be dark brown."
4. "I will check my skin to see if I'm bruising more easily."

83. Mr. Auger receives appropriate instructions in preparation for discharge. Which statement by Mr. Auger indicates that he understands the instructions?
1. "I will stop walking when my pulse rate is 80 beats/minute or higher."
2. "I will wait about 1 hour after my meals before walking."
3. "I will use a ramp to walk the four steps into my house."
4. "I will walk for 10 minutes every 2 hours while I am awake."

Mrs. Susan Stallon, age 30, is a multigravida who is admitted to the hospital at term in labor. She is 4 cm dilated.

84. On admission, Mrs. Stallon's urine is tested for protein. The purpose of this action is to determine if Mrs. Stallon has a sign of
1. pregnancy-induced hypertension.
2. ketoacidosis.
3. placenta previa.
4. gestational diabetes.

85. To prevent Mrs. Stallon from developing a urinary tract infection, which action should the practical nurse take?
1. Provide Mrs. Stallon with ice chips.
2. Encourage Mrs. Stallon to void frequently.
3. Test Mrs. Stallon's urine for glycosuria.
4. Give Mrs. Stallon frequent perineal care.

86. Mrs. Stallon is uncomfortable and requests something for pain. The practical nurse should explain that pain medication is **not** administered in early labor because it is likely to
1. produce sudden tears in her perineum.
2. suppress her baby's sucking reflex.
3. slow her uterine contractions.
4. interfere with her ability to cooperate.

87. Mrs. Stallon's membranes rupture. Which action is most important for the practical nurse to take initially?
1. Check Mrs. Stallon's fetal heart tones.
2. Turn Mrs. Stallon onto her left side.
3. Take Mrs. Stallon's blood pressure.
4. Check to see if Mrs. Stallon has an order for oxytocin (Pitocin).

PRACTICE TEST

88. Mrs. Stallon is 8 cm dilated. After noting that she bears down when having a contraction, the practical nurse teaches her to avoid bearing down. Which observation at the time of her next contraction indicates that the teaching was effective?
1. Mrs. Stallon pants while breathing.
2. Mrs. Stallon holds her breath.
3. Mrs. Stallon holds on firmly to the side rails.
4. Mrs. Stallon maintains a back-lying position.

Mrs. Stallon's labor progresses. She is accompanied by her husband when transferred to the delivery room, where she delivers a boy.

89. During the first hour after Mrs. Stallon delivers her son, which action would best promote early parent-infant bonding?
1. Allow the parents to interact with the infant.
2. Have the parents describe their fears related to parenting.
3. Explain to the parents the care that the infant will need when discharged.
4. Encourage the parents to describe their experience in caring for an infant.

Baby Boy Stallon is transferred to the newborn nursery. Mrs. Stallon is transferred to the postpartum area after a brief stay in the recovery room.

90. Which finding, observed when Baby Boy Stallon is 8 hours old, indicates that his condition is satisfactory?
1. Axillary temperature of 94.6° F (34.8° C).
2. Apical pulse rate of 124 beats/minute.
3. Slight yellowish tinge to his sclera.
4. Respirations audible on expiration.

91. On the first postpartum day, the practical nurse should examine Mrs. Stallon's perineal pad and expect to see
1. lochia alba.
2. lochia serosa.
3. lochia rubra.
4. no lochia.

92. On the third postpartum day, Mrs. Stallon is being discharged. The practical nurse is in the room when Mrs. Stallon begins to cry. Mrs. Stallon denies she has pain. On the basis of this information, which action should the practical nurse take first?
1. Stay with Mrs. Stallon.
2. Leave Mrs. Stallon alone for a while.
3. Report Mrs. Stallon's behavior to the charge nurse.
4. Attempt to obtain an order for a sedative for Mrs. Stallon.

Ms. Flora Dixon, age 19, visits the physician's office complaining of feeling tired. A battery of laboratory tests reveals that Ms. Dixon has iron-deficiency anemia.

93. Considering Ms. Dixon's diagnosis of iron-deficiency anemia, which complaint is she most likely to express?
1. "My skin feels warm."
2. "I get short of breath."
3. "My tongue is swollen."
4. "I have lost my sense of smell."

94. Ms. Dixon experiences episodes of feeling dizzy and faint. Which goal should be included in her care for such an episode?
1. To lie down until the feeling passes.
2. To do breathing exercises whenever it happens.
3. To drink highly sweetened beverages whenever it occurs.
4. To rise slowly from a lying or sitting position to a standing position.

Ms. Dixon receives a *stat* dose of iron dextran injection (Imferon) I.M. as well as a prescription for ferrous gluconate (Fergon).

95. When administering Imferon to Ms. Dixon, the practical nurse should take which action?
1. Ask Ms. Dixon if she drinks alcoholic beverages.
2. Find out if Ms. Dixon is allergic to fish oil.
3. Give the medication by the Z-track method.
4. Use a 1″, 25-gauge needle to inject the medication into the vastus dorsalis.

96. Ms. Dixon has difficulty swallowing pills. The physician prescribes Liquid Fergon for her. How should she be given the Fergon?
    1. Undiluted, with a dropper onto her tongue.
    2. Undiluted, from a teaspoon.
    3. Diluted with milk, in a glass.
    4. Diluted with water, through a straw.

97. Which symptom is most likely to occur as a side effect of Fergon?
    1. Tinnitus.
    2. Ataxia.
    3. Blurred vision.
    4. Black stools.

98. Ms. Dixon is taught to eat foods with a **high** iron content. Ms. Dixon understands the instructions if she selects which snack?
    1. 1 cup of popcorn.
    2. ½ cup of raisins.
    3. ½ cup of blueberries.
    4. 1 cup of hot chocolate.

Mr. Zakaria Smith, age 58, arrives at the clinic with intermittent bouts of diarrhea and constipation. He is scheduled for a sigmoidoscopy and a barium enema.

99. The primary purpose of a sigmoidoscopy is to
    1. dilate the colon.
    2. inspect the intestinal mucosa.
    3. cauterize ruptured vessels of the colon.
    4. obtain a tissue biopsy of the intestine.

100. After the sigmoidoscopy, the practical nurse should observe Mr. Smith for which possible complication?
    1. Muscle atony of the colon.
    2. Fissure of the anal sphincter.
    3. Perforation of the intestinal wall.
    4. Hyperactivity of the intestinal tract.

101. Mr. Smith receives instructions in preparation for a barium enema. Which statement by Mr. Smith indicates that he understands the instructions?

1. "I will need to cleanse my bowels with laxatives and enemas before the test."
2. "I will be given a muscle relaxant during the test."
3. "I will need to drink an opaque substance during the test."
4. "I will need to be on a diet free of red meat for 3 days before the test."

The physician diagnoses rectal cancer. Mr. Smith is admitted to the hospital for an abdominoperineal resection. Before surgery, he is placed on a low-residue diet and neomycin sulfate (Mycifradin) P.O. An I.V. pyelogram (IVP) is ordered.

102. Mr. Smith is receiving Mycifradin for what purpose?
    1. To promote healing of the suture line after surgery.
    2. To reduce the bacterial count in the colon before surgery.
    3. To promote coagulation of blood during surgery.
    4. To reduce gas accumulation in the large bowel after surgery.

103. The I.V. pyelogram is ordered for Mr. Smith for what purpose?
    1. To determine the glomerular filtration rate.
    2. To detect any infection in the ureters.
    3. To detect abnormalities in the urinary system.
    4. To determine his bladder capacity.

104. Mr. Smith has been on a low-residue diet. Now he is on a liquid diet for 24 hours before surgery. What is the purpose of his liquid diet?
    1. To eliminate stress in the diseased bowel.
    2. To empty the bowel of fecal material.
    3. To reduce bowel motility.
    4. To lessen pain in the diseased bowel.

105. During the preoperative period, the practical nurse must help Mr. Smith make an easier adjustment to which change?
    1. His urine output.
    2. His eating habits.
    3. His physical activity.
    4. His body image.

Mr. Smith has an abdominoperineal resection and a permanent colostomy in the descending colon. After a brief stay in the recovery room, he returns to his unit. His orders include I.V. therapy, a nasogastric tube attached to low intermittent suction, and an indwelling urethral catheter to straight drainage.

106. Mr. Smith has an I.V. fluid order of 1,000 ml of 5% dextrose in water every 8 hours. The I.V. setup delivers 20 gtt/ml. Approximately how many drops should be administered every minute?
    1. 27
    2. 35
    3. 42
    4. 50

107. Eight hours after Mr. Smith's surgery, the practical nurse notices that the drainage from his nasogastric tube has stopped. Which action should the practical nurse take first?
    1. Irrigate the tubing.
    2. Have Mr. Smith sit upright.
    3. Check the tubing for kinks.
    4. Turn the suction to constant.

108. Two hours after surgery, the practical nurse notes that Mr. Smith's perineal dressing is saturated with serosanguineous drainage. The practical nurse should suspect the drainage most likely results from
    1. an abrupt movement.
    2. a slipped suture.
    3. a Penrose drain.
    4. a displaced urinary catheter.

109. Which observation indicates that Mr. Smith's peristaltic activity has returned?
    1. He is belching.
    2. He is hungry.
    3. He is passing flatus.
    4. He is thirsty.

Mrs. Marsha Webb, age 21, gravida 1, para O, is admitted to the hospital in labor. Her husband is with her. She states that her due date was last week and that she is having moderate contractions every 4 minutes. Assessment data indicate that her cervix is 3 cm dilated and 100% effaced, membranes are intact, and bloody show is present.

110. While listening to fetal heart tones, the practical nurse counts 90 beats in the lower right quadrant. Which action would be most appropriate to take initially?
    1. Report the fetal heart rate to the charge nurse.
    2. Record the findings.
    3. Compare the finding with the previous fetal heart rate.
    4. Change Mrs. Webb's position.

111. Mrs. Webb's membranes rupture. The practical nurse notices that the umbilical cord is protruding from the vagina. Besides notifying the charge nurse, which action is essential for the practical nurse to take?
    1. Encourage Mrs. Webb to breathe deeply.
    2. Turn Mrs. Webb onto her left side.
    3. Place Mrs. Webb in a deep Trendelenburg position.
    4. Place sterile pads under Mrs. Webb's buttocks.

Mrs. Webb is transferred to the delivery room for a cesarean birth under general anesthesia.

112. After delivery, oxytocin (Pitocin) is added to Mrs. Webb's I.V. infusion for what purpose?
    1. To increase her lochial flow.
    2. To reduce her afterpains.
    3. To keep her uterus contracted.
    4. To prevent uterine infection.

Mr. Keel Nelson, age 64, has a rectal examination in his physician's office. The examination reveals that he has an enlarged prostate. He is scheduled for a cystoscopic procedure and receives instructions about the procedure.

113. Which statement by Mr. Nelson indicates that he understands the instructions about cystoscopy?
    1. "I will be given a radiopaque dye intravenously."
    2. "I will have an instrument inserted into my bladder through my urethra."
    3. "I will be anesthetized during the procedure."
    4. "I will be required to drink plenty of fluids before the procedure."

Mr. Nelson is admitted to the hospital and has a transurethral prostatic resection (TUR) for benign prostatic hyperplasia. He returns to his unit after a brief stay in the recovery room. His orders include propantheline bromide (Pro-Banthine) and an indwelling urethral catheter.

114. Because Mr. Nelson has had a TUR, during the immediate postoperative period the practical nurse should expect him to have
1. discomfort when urinating.
2. a distended bladder.
3. a neurogenic bladder
4. bloody urinary drainage.

115. Several hours later, Mr. Nelson complains of bladder spasms. Which action should the practical nurse take initially?
1. Determine if clots are obstructing the catheter.
2. Support Mr. Nelson in a side-lying position.
3. Administer the ordered Pro-Banthine.
4. Check if Mr. Nelson has an order for pain medication.

Mona Parks, age 15, is a sexually active high school student. She goes to the Woman's Center to get information about contraceptive methods.

116. Mona should be advised against using oral contraceptives if she has a history of which condition?
1. Cystitis.
2. Thrombophlebitis.
3. Venereal disease.
4. Pelvic inflammatory disease.

117. The practical nurse should inform Mona that a possible side effect of oral contraceptives is
1. breast tenderness.
2. hot flashes.
3. urinary frequency.
4. ringing in the ears.

The last section of the test consists of individual items.

118. A patient receives instructions about oral tetracycline hydrochloride (Achromycin). Which statement by the patient indicates an understanding of the instructions?
1. "I will take the medication until I feel better."
2. "I will take the medication with at least 6 oz of orange juice."
3. "If I miss a dose of the medication, I will take two doses at the next scheduled time."
4. "I will take the medication with food if I develop nausea."

119. Alcohol withdrawal manifests as which of these signs or symptoms?
1. Hyporeflexia.
2. Agitation.
3. Drowsiness.
4. Confabulation.

120. A patient's history includes all of the following information. Which statement most likely relates to the development of a peptic ulcer?
1. He is recovering from second- and third-degree burns over the anterior half of his body.
2. He operated a photocopy machine 8 hours a day, five days a week.
3. He is a vegetarian.
4. He has a family history of psoriasis.

This is the end of the test.
Before sending in your answer sheet, make certain that you have:
• completely darkened the answer choice you selected for each question
• erased all stray or accidental marks on your answer sheet
• filled in all the information requested on your answer sheet.

Index

A

Abdominal binder, 323-325, 324*i*
Abduction pillow, 250, 251
Abruptio placentae, 123*t*
ACE inhibitors, 205*t*
Acetaminophen, 281*t*
Acetaminophen poisoning, 163-165
Acetohexamide, 416*t*
Acetylcysteine, 164, 237*t*
Acetylsalicylic acid, 274*t*
Acid-base balance, 74-78
Acidosis
  metabolic, 76-78
  respiratory, 75-77
Acquired immunodeficiency syndrome, 435-438
Actinomycin D, 463*t*
Active transport, 79
Activities of daily living, 66-67, 346
Acute lymphocytic leukemia, 166-168
Addiction, 468
Addison's disease, 405-407
ADH. *See* Antidiuretic hormone.
Adhesions, 70
ADLs. *See* Activities of daily living.
Adolescent
  physical-social development, 35
  scoliosis in, 175-177
Adrenal crisis, 410*t*
Adrenalectomy, 403
Adrenal glands, 397, 398
Adrenalin, 72, 235*t*
Adrenal tumor, 403
Adrenocorticosteroid, 464*t*
Adrenocorticosteroid inhibitor, 464*t*
Adrenocorticotropic hormone, 397, 403
Adriamycin, 463*t*
Adrucil, 464*t*
Advil, 276*t*
Aerolate, 236*t*
Affect, 468
Aging, physical-social changes in, 36-37
Agnosia, 82
Agranulocytosis, 151
AIDS. *See* Acquired immunodeficiency syndrome.
Akathisia, 468
Akinesia, 468
Akineton, 495*t*
Alcohol abuse, 477-480, 479*t*
Aldactone, 396*t*
Aldomet, 204*t*
Alkalosis
  metabolic, 76, 78
  respiratory, 76, 77
Alka-2, 332*t*
Alkeran, 463*t*
Alkylating agents, 463*t*
ALL. *See* Acute lymphocytic leukemia.
Allopurinol, 168
Alopecia, 421
Alprazolam, 372*t,* 489*t*
Atenolol, 204*t*
Aluminum hydroxide, 331*t*
Alupent, 235*t*

Alzheimer's disease, 468, 481, 482*t,* 483
Amantadine hydrochloride, 353, 371*t*
Ambivalence, 468
Ambulation, 85
  aids for, 272-273
  postoperative, 103*t*
American Cancer Society, 448, 449, 454
American Diabetes Association, 408
American Heart Association, 200
Amethopterin, 464*t*
Aminoglutethimide, 464*t*
Aminophyllin, 235*t*
Amitriptyline, 489*t*
Amobarbital sodium, 372*t*
Amoxapine, 489*t*
Amphojel, 331*t*
Amytal Sodium, 372*t*
Anacin-3, 281*t*
Anaphylactic shock, 70-73
Anaprox, 277*t*
Androgen, 464*t*
Anesthesia, 82
Aneurysm, 336
Angina pectoris, 190
Anhedonia, 468
Anions, 79
Anorexia, 468
Anorexia nervosa, 468, 486-488, 487*t*
Anoxia, 82
Ansaid, 275*t*
Antacids, 290, 331-332*t*
Antepartal period, 111
Antiadrenergic agents, 204-205*t*
Antianxiety drugs, 489*t*
Antiarrhythmics, 203*t*
Antibiotic antineoplastic agents, 463*t*
Antibiotics, 173
Antibody, 434
Anticholinergics, 291
Anticoagulants, 207*t*
Anticonvulsants, 370-371*t*
Antidepressants, 489-492*t*
Antidiarrheals, 331*t*
Antidiuretic hormone, 397
Antiembolism stockings, 379
Antiestrogens, 464*t*
Antigens, 432, 434
Antihistamines, 72, 236*t*
Antihypertensives, 203-204*t*
Anti-inflammatory agents, 255, 275-277*t,* 291
Antimanic agent, 492*t*
Antimetabolites, 464*t*
Antiparkinsonian drugs, 371-372*t*
Antipsychotics, 493-496*t*
Antistreptolysin O titer, 151
Antithyroid drugs, 418-419*t*
Antituberculars, 237*t*
Anti-ulcer drugs, 331-332*t*
Anuria, 375
Anxiety disorder, 468, 470-472, 471*t,* 472*t*
Aortic valve, 151

Apgar score, 132*t*
Aphasia, 83, 468
Apocrine glands, 420, 421
Aqueous penicillin, 431*t*
Ara-C, 464*t*
Artane, 353, 372*t,* 495*t*
Arterial blood gases, 210
Arteriosclerosis, 195-196
Arteriovenous shunt, 383, 391-392
Arthritis, 240, 256-261, 257*t*
Arthropan, 274*t*
Ascites, 151
Asendin, 489*t*
Asepsis, medical, 219
Aspirin, 172, 255, 274*t*
Assault, 43
Atarax, 489*t*
Ataxia, 469
Atelectasis, 220*t*
Atenolol, 204
Ativan, 489*t*
Atrial septal defect, 151, 154*i*
Autoimmune disease, 240
Autonomic nervous system, 335
AV shunt. *See* Arteriovenous shunt.
Axid, 332*t*
AZT, 435, 438

B

Baclofen, 277*t*
Bactrim, 437
Balanced-suspension traction, 245, 269-271
Ballottement, 114
Basal ganglia, 333
Battery, 43
BCNU, 465*t*
Beds, types of, 360-367
Benadryl, 72, 236*t*
Benign prostatic hyperplasia, 377-379
Benign tumor, 440*i*
Benztropine mesylate, 353, 495*t*
Beta blockers, 204*t*
Betadine, 144, 178
Biopsy, 351, 380
Biperiden, 495*t*
Bipolar disorder, manic phase, 473-475
Bisacodyl, 332*t*
Bladder exstrophy, 136*t*
Bladder tumor, 380, 382-383
Blenoxane, 463*t*
BLEO, 463*t*
Bleomycin, 463*t*
Blood-brain barrier, 441
Blood buffers, 75
Blood glucose levels, 173-175, 408, 409
  self-monitoring of, 412-413
Blood pressure, 190, 194
Blood vessels, 186
B lymphocytes, 432, 433
Body image disturbance, 487-488
Bone marrow, aspiration and biopsy of, 178-179
Bones, 238, 239*i,* 261*t*
Bottle-feeding, 142-143*t*

Bowel obstruction, 292-296, 299*t*
Bowel perforation, 299*t*
Bowel sounds, 251, 292, 327-328
Brain, 333, 335
Brain stem, 333, 335-336
Brain tumor, 350-354
BRAT diet, 153
Braxton-Hicks contractions, 114
Breast cancer, 449-451, 452*i*, 453-454
Breast-feeding, 139-142
Breast reconstruction surgery, 449
Breast self-examination, 449
Brethine, 235*t*
Bretylium, 203*t*
Bretylol, 203*t*
Bromocriptine mesylate, 371*t*
Brompheniramine, 72
Bronchi, 208
Bronchodilators, 163, 235-236*t*
Bronchoscopy, 210
Bronkosol, 235*t*
Brudzinski's sign, 151
Buffers, 75
Bulimarexia, 469
Bulimia nervosa, 469
Buprenex, 281*t*
Buprenorphine, 281*t*
Burns, 421-427, 422*t*, 423*i*, 424*t*, 426*t*, 428*t*
Bursae, 240
Busulfan, 463*t*
Butorphanol, 281*t*

C

CAD. *See* Coronary artery disease.
Calcitonin, 397
Calcium, 79-82
Calcium blockers, 206*t*
Calcium carbonate, 332*t*
Callus, 240
Calories, 52
Camphorated opium tincture, 331*t*
Canadian nursing assistant and practical nurse associations, 512
Canadian registration and licensure exam dates, 512
Cancer
    AIDS and, 435
    breast, 449-451, 452*i*, 453-454
    colon, 296-298
    complications of chemotherapy, 454*t*
    drugs for, 463-465*t*
    leukemia, 166-168
    lung, 213-215, 445-448
    malignant cell development, 439-440
    ovarian, 441-444
    side effects of drugs for, 465-466*t*
    See also Oncologic disorders.
Cane, 255, 272-273
Cantor tube, 303-306
CAPD. *See* Continuous ambulatory peritoneal dialysis.
Capillaries, 186, 189
Capillary refill, 263

Capoten, 205*t*
Captopril, 205*t*
Carbamazepine, 370*t*
Carbohydrates, 52, 60*t*
Carcinogen, 441
Cardiac arrest, 197*t*
Cardiac arrhythmias, 197*t*
Cardiac catheterization, 157
Cardiac conduction, 189*i*, 189-190
Cardiac output, 190
Cardiogenic shock, 71, 73
Cardiopulmonary resuscitation, 200, 201*i*
Cardiovascular disorders
    arteriosclerosis, 195-196
    complications of, 197*t*
    congestive heart failure, 191-192
    diet for, 56-57
    drugs for, 203-207*t*
    hypertension, 194-195
    myocardial infarction, 192-194
    nursing procedures for, 198-200, 201*i*, 202
Cardiovascular system
    anatomy, 186, 187-189*i*, 189-190
    glossary, 190
    postoperative complications, 105*t*
Cardizem, 206*t*
Carisoprodol, 278*t*
Carmustine, 465*t*
Cartilage, 240
Cast, 240
    application of, 264-266
    care of, 241-244
    removal of, 267
    skin care after removal, 268
Catapres, 204*t*
Catheter, 231*i*, 250, 378, 387-392, 458-459
Cations, 78
Cauda equina, 333
CCNU, 465*t*
Central line dressing, 461-462
Central venous pressure, 424
Cerebellum, 333, 336
Cerebrovascular accident, 190, 197*t*, 336, 341-346
Cerebrum, 333, 335
Cerubidin, 463*t*
Cervical lacerations, 129, 131
Chadwick's sign, 114
Charcoal, 164
Chemotherapy, 151
    complications of, 454*t*
    drugs for, 463-465*t*
    for leukemia, 167-168
    for ovarian cancer, 441-444
    side effects of, 465-466*t*
Chest drainage, 223*i*
Chest retraction, 151
Chest tube, 222, 224
CHF. *See* Congestive heart failure.

Children
    acetaminophen poisoning in, 163-165
    bone marrow aspiration or biopsy in, 178-179
    Croupette care of, 177-178
    diabetes mellitus in, 173-175
    immunization schedule, 159*t*
    laryngotracheobronchitis in, 162-163
    leukemia in, 166-168
    nephrosis in, 169-171
    physical-social development, 33-34
    poisoning in, 165*t*
    rheumatic fever in, 171-173, 172*t*
Chlorambucil, 463*t*
Chlordiazepoxide, 489*t*
Chlorothiazide, 396*t*
Chlorpromazine, 493*t*
Chlorpropamide, 416*t*
Chlorprothixene, 494*t*
Chlorzoxazone, 278*t*
Cholecystitis, 285
Cholecystokinin, 286
Choledocholithiasis, 285
Choline magnesium trisalicylate, 274*t*
Choline salicylate, 274*t*
Chronic obstructive pulmonary disease, 216-217
Chvostek's sign, 82
Chyme, 286
Cimetidine, 255, 332*t*
CircOlectric bed, 360-363, 362*i*
Circulatory system, 188*i*
Cirrhosis, 285
Cisplatin, 463*t*
Cleft lip, 136*t*
Cleft palate, 136*t*
Clinitron bed, 360
Clinoril, 277*t*
Clitoris, 108
Clonidine, 204*t*
Clubfoot, 136*t*
Coarctation of aorta, 151, 154*i*
Codeine sulfate, 279*t*
Cogentin, 353, 495*t*
Colace, 332*t*
Cold application, 90
Colon cancer, 296-298
Colostomy care, 317-321
Colostrum, 113, 140
Comedo, 421
Communication, 45, 46-49*t*
Compartment syndrome, 262*t*
Complete blood count, 126
Compulsion, 469
Computed tomography scan, 344, 351
Concussion, 336
Condom catheter, 390-391
Condoms, 436
Congenital abnormalities, 136-137*t*
Congestive heart failure, 191-192
Constipation, 293, 299*t*
Continent ileal urinary reservoir, 381*i*

Continuous ambulatory peritoneal dialysis, 383-385
Contractures, 70, 428*t*
Convulsion. *See* seizure.
Cooley's anemia, 115
COPD. *See* Chronic obstructive pulmonary disease.
Coronary artery disease, 190
Corpus luteum, 117
Corticosteroids, 73, 163, 281*t*, 403
Cosmegen, 463*t*
Co-trimoxazole, 437
Coughing exercises, 224-225
Coumadin, 207*t*
CPR. *See* Cardiopulmonary resuscitation.
Cranial bones, 335
Cretinism, 399, 401
Crohn's disease, 292
Croup, 162-163
Croupette, 163, 177-178
Crowning, 130
Crutches, 272-273
CT scan. *See* Computed tomography scan.
Curative surgery, 100
Cushing's syndrome, 403-405
Cutaneous ureterostomy, 381*i*
CVA. *See* Cerebrovascular accident.
Cyclobenzaprine, 278*t*
Cyclophosphamide, 463*t*
Cystectomy, 380
Cystoscopy, 380
Cytadren, 464*t*
Cytarabine, 464*t*
Cytosar-U, 464*t*
Cytosine arabinoside, 464*t*
Cytotoxin, 441
Cytoxan, 463*t*

D

Dacarbazine, 463*t*
Dactinomycin, 463*t*
Dalmane, 372*t*
Dantrium, 278*t*
Dantrolene, 278*t*
Darvocet, 280*t*
Darvon, 280*t*
Datril, 281*t*
Daunorubicin, 463*t*
Decerebrate posture, 359*i*
Decorticate posture, 359*i*
Deep-breathing exercises, 224-225, 251
Defecation, 287
Defense mechanism, 469
Delirium, 469
Deltasone, 168, 281*t*, 464*t*
Delusion, 469
Dementia, 469
Demerol, 279*t*
Denial, 469
Depakene, 371*t*
Depression, 138*t*, 469, 475-477
Dermis, 420
DES, 464*t*
Desipramine, 490*t*
Desyrel, 492*t*
Development, 30-37
DiaBeta, 417*t*

Diabetes mellitus
    dialysis for, 383-385
    diet for, 57-58, 501-503*t*
    glucose tolerance test for, 173-175, 413
    insulin-dependent, 173-175, 383-385, 407-408
    non-insulin-dependent, 407-410
Diabetic ketoacidosis, 173
Diabinese, 416*t*
Diagnostic surgery, 100
Dialysis, 375, 383-385
Diarrhea, 150-153
Diastasis recti abdominus, 113
Diazepam, 278*t*, 370*t*, 489*t*
Diclofenac, 275*t*
Diet, 53-54, 62-63*t*
    BRAT, 153
    for diabetes, 408
    exchange, 65*t*, 501-503*t*
    fat-modified, 64*t*
    for renal disease, 58-59
    sodium-restricted, 64*t*
    See also Food groups; Nutrition.
Diethylstilbestrol, 464*t*
Diffusion, 79, 375
Diflunisal, 275*t*
Digestion, 284-287
Digitalis, 192
Digoxin, 157, 206*t*
Dilantin, 371*t*
Dilaudid, 279*t*
Diltiazem, 206*t*
Dimetane, 72
Diphenhydramine hydrochloride, 72, 236*t*
Diphenoxylate hydrochloride, 331*t*
Disalcid, 274*t*
Disopyramide, 203*t*
Disorientation, 469
Displacement, 469
Diuresis, 375
Diuretics, 157, 192, 203-204*t*, 340, 396*t*
Diuril, 396*t*
Documentation, 44-45
Docusate sodium, 332*t*
Dolobid, 275*t*
Dopamine, 73, 352
Dopar, 353, 371*t*
Doriden, 372*t*
Double lumen catheter, 392
Doxepin, 490*t*
Doxorubicin, 463*t*
Drainage systems, 223*i*
Dressing
    changing over central line, 461-462
    pressure, 88
    sterile, 86
    wet-to-dry, 88-89
Drug administration
    calculations and equivalents for, 505-506*t*
    precautions, 509
DTIC-Dome, 463*t*
Dulcolax, 332*t*
Dunlop's traction, 245
Duodenal ulcer, 288

Duodenum, 286
Dwell time, 383
Dymelor, 416*t*
Dyspnea, 210
Dystocia, 134*t*

E

Ecchymosis, 421
Eccrine glands, 420, 421
EDC. *See* Expected date of confinement.
Edema, 126, 156, 169-171, 198, 212-213, 442
Ego, 469
Elastic stockings, 202
Elavil, 489*t*
Elective surgery, 100
Electrocardiogram, 190, 199-200
Electroencephalogram, 351
Electrolytes, 53, 78-79
    imbalances of, 79-82, 428*t*
    movement of, 79
Elimination, 287
ELISA test, 436
Elixophyllin, 236*t*
Embryo, 111
Emergency surgery, 100
Enalapril, 205*t*
Endocrine disorders
    Addison's disease, 405-407
    complications of, 410-411*t*
    Cushing's syndrome, 403-405
    drugs for, 416-419*t*
    hyperthyroidism, 399-401
    hypothyroidism, 401-403
    non-insulin-dependent diabetes mellitus, 407-410
    nursing procedures for, 412-415
Endocrine system
    anatomy, 397, 398*i*
    glossary, 399
    physiology, 397-398
Enema, 321-323
Enterogastrone, 285
Enterokinase, 286
Enuresis, 375
Enzymes, 285-286
Epidermis, 420
Epilepsy, 336, 346-349
Epinephrine, 72, 73, 235*t*, 398
Episiotomy, 131
Epispadias, 136*t*
Ergonovine maleate, 148*t*
Ergotrate, 148*t*
Eskalith, 474, 492*t*
Esophagus, 282, 284
Estrogen, 117, 398, 464*t*
Ethambutol, 237*t*
Ethosuximide, 370*t*
Euphoria, 469
Euthyroid goiter, 399
Excedrin, 281*t*
Excoriation, 421
Excretion, 287
Exercises
    range of motion, 252, 451
    stair climbing, 273
Exophthalmia, 399
Expected date of confinement, 124

i refers to an illustration; *t* refers to a table.

F

Fallopian tubes, 108
Famotidine, 255, 332*t*
Fat embolism, 262*t*
Fats (lipids), 53
Feldene, 255, 277*t*
Female reproductive system, 108, 109*i*, 110
Femoral neck, fracture of, 247, 248*i*, 249-253
Femur, fracture of, 244-247, 269-271
Fenoprofen, 275*t*
Fetal distress, 134*t*
Fetal heart tones, 114, 134
Fetus, 111
    development of, 122*i*
    monitoring of, 125
Fiberall, 332*t*
Fibula, fracture of, 241-244
5-fluorouracil, 464*t*
5-FU, 464*t*
Flatulence, 285
Flexeril, 278*t*
Flight of ideas, 469
Fluid replacement formulas, 424*t*
Fluids, 53, 78
    imbalance of, 79-80
    intake and output, measurement of, 393-394
    movement of, 79
Fluoxetine, 492*t*
Fluoxymesterone, 464*t*
Fluphenazine decanoate, 494*t*
Fluphenazine enanthate, 494*t*
Fluphenazine hydrochloride, 494*t*
Flurazepam hydrochloride, 372*t*
Flurbiprofen, 275*t*
Folex, 168, 464*t*
Foley catheter, 250
Follicle-stimulating hormone, 117
Food groups, 54, 62*t*
Forceps, 131
Formula, infant, 142*t*
Fracture, 240
    of femoral neck, 247, 248*i*, 249-253
    of femur, 244-247, 269-271
    intracapsular, 247
    of tibia and fibula, 241-244
Frontal occipital circumference, 159
FSH. *See* Follicle-stimulating hormone.
Fundal height, 112
Furosemide, 157, 204*t*, 396*t*

G

Gaits, 272
Gallbladder, 284, 288
Gamma globulin, 432
Gangrene, 197*t*
Garamycin, 431*t*
Gastric inhibitory peptide, 286
Gastric juice, 285
Gastric ulcer, 288
Gastrin, 285
Gastroenteritis, 150, 152-153

Gastrointestinal disorders
    colon cancer, 296-298
    complications of, 299*t*
    drugs for, 331-332*t*
    nursing procedures for, 300-330
    small intestine obstruction, 292-296
    ulcers, 288-291
Gastrointestinal system
    anatomy, 282, 283*i*, 284
    glossary, 285
    physiology, 284-288
    postoperative complications of, 105*t*
Gastrointestinal tube, maintenance of, 305
Gastrostomy tube feedings, 310-311
Genitourinary disorders
    benign prostatic hyperplasia, 377-379, 378*t*
    complications of, 386*t*
    dialysis for, 383-385
    drugs for, 396*t*
    glomerulonephritis, 375-377
    kidney or bladder tumor, 380, 381*i*, 382-383
    nursing procedures for, 387-395
Genitourinary system
    anatomy, 373, 374*i*
    glossary, 375
    physiology, 373, 375
    postoperative complications of, 105*t*
Gentamicin, 431*t*
Glasgow Coma Scale, 342
Glipizide, 417*t*
Glomerulonephritis, 375-377
Glomerulus, 375
Glucagon, 151, 398
Glucocorticoids, 398
Glucose tolerance test, 173-175, 408, 409, 413
Glucotrol, 417*t*
Glutethimide, 372*t*
Glyburide, 417*t*
Glycogen, 287
Gonads, 397, 398
Goodell's sign, 114
Granulomas, 70
Grave's disease, 399-401
Gravida, 112
Great vessels, transposition of, 151, 155*i*
Grief, 49, 50*t*, 167, 469
Guaiac test, 168
Guanethidine, 205*t*

H

Haldol, 494*t*
Haloperidol, 494*t*
Halotestin, 464*t*
Hand washing, 94
Headache, 339, 356*t*
Head injury, 338-341
Health history, 37-39
Heart, 186, 187*i*
Heart defects
    acyanotic, 154*t*
    cyanotic, 155*t*

Heart disease, congenital, 153, 154-155*t*, 156-157, 158*t*
Heat application, 90
Heat lamp, 91
Hegar's sign, 114
Hematuria, 375
Hemianopsia, 82
Hemiplegia, 82
Hemodialysis, 383
Hemorrhage
    GI tract, 299*t*
    intrapartal, 133*t*
    postpartal, 138*t*
Hemostats, 222
Hemothorax, 210
Heparin sodium, 207*t*
Hepatitis, 285
Hepatotoxicity, 151
Hep-Lock, 207*t*
Hernia, 70, 136*t*
Hip
    congenital dislocation of, 136*t*
    fractures of, 247, 248*i*, 249-253
Hirsutism, 421
Histamine blockers, 332*t*
HIV. *See* Human immunodeficiency virus.
Hormone inhibitors, 464*t*
Hormones, 397-399
    in cancer therapy, 464*t*
    menstrual cycle and, 117
    pregnancy and, 113
Human immunodeficiency virus, 435
Human needs, 29-30
Hydrea, 464*t*
Hydrochloric acid, 285
Hydrochlorothiazide, 203*t*, 396*t*
HydroDIURIL, 203*t*
Hydromorphone hydrochloride, 279*t*
Hydroxyurea, 464*t*
Hydroxyzine hydrochloride, 236*t*, 489*t*
Hydroxyzine pamoate, 236*t*
Hypercalcemia, 80-82
Hyperglycemia, 151, 174, 399, 411*t*
Hyperkalemia, 80, 81
Hypernatremia, 79-81
Hyperosmolar nonketotic syndrome, 409
Hypertension, 194-195
Hyperthyroidism, 399-401
Hypertonic diarrhea, 151
Hypervolemia, 79
Hypoalbuminemia, 151
Hypocalcemia, 80, 82
Hypodermis, 420
Hypoglycemia, 151, 174, 399, 411*t*
Hypokalemia, 80, 81
Hyponatremia, 79-81
Hypothalamus, 336
Hypothyroidism, 401-403
Hypotonic diarrhea, 151
Hypovolemia, 79
Hypovolemic shock, 71, 73
Hypoxia, 210

I

Ibuprofen, 255, 276*t*
ICP. *See* Increased intracranial pressure.

Ileal conduit, 381*i*
Ileostomy care, 314-316
Imipramine, 490*t*
Immobility, 82-84
Immune response, 432, 433*i*, 434
Immune system
   anatomy, 432
     glossary, 434
     physiology, 432-434, 433*i*
Immunity, 434
Immunization schedule, 159*t*
Immunoglobulins, 432-434
Imodium, 331*t*
Imperforate anus, 137*t*
Inappropriate affect, 469
Incentive spirometry, 228
Incontinence, 359
Increased intracranial pressure, 338-341
Inderal, 204*t*, 419*t*
Indocin, 276*t*
Indomethacin, 276*t*
Induction chemotherapy, 151
Indwelling urinary catheter, 388-389
Infant
   bottle-feeding, 142-143*t*
   breast-feeding, 139-142
   congenital heart defects in, 153, 154-155*t*, 156-157, 158*t*
   gastroenteritis in, 150, 152-153
   immunization schedule, 159*t*
   meningitis in, 158-161, 161*i*
   physical and social development, 30-32
Infection
   from burns, 428*t*
   of wound or joint, 261*t*
Inflammation, 68-70
Informed consent, 44
INH, 237*t*
Insulin, 398
   self-administration of, 179
Insulin-dependent diabetes mellitus, 173-175, 383-385, 407-408
Integumentary disorders
   complications of, 428*t*
   drugs for, 431*t*
   nursing procedures for, 429-430
   third-degree burn, 421-427, 422*t*, 423*i*, 424*t*, 426*t*
Integumentary system
   anatomy, 420, 420*i*
   glossary, 421
   physiology, 421
   postoperative complications, 106*t*
Intermittent claudication, 190
Intermittent positive-pressure breathing, 227
Intracranial pressure, 159, 336, 338-341
Intraoperative period, 101
Intrapartal period, 111, 124
Intravenous therapy, 294, 298
   for burns, 423, 424*t*
   starting I.V. line for, 455-457, 457*i*
Intrinsic factor, 285
Intropin, 73
Iodine uptake, 414
Ipecac, 163, 164

IPPB. *See* Intermittent positive-pressure breathing.
Iron-deficiency anemia, 55-56
Irrigating solution, 319
Ischemia, 190, 192
Ismelin, 205*t*
Isocarboxazid, 491*t*
Isoetharine, 235*t*
Isolation, 160
Isoniazid, 237*t*
Isoptin, 206*t*
Isotonic diarrhea, 151

J

Jaundice, 421
Jejunal tube feedings, 311-312
Jejunostomy tube feedings, 310-311
Jejunum, 286
Joints, 239

K

Kaolin and pectin, 331*t*
Kaopectate, 331*t*
Kaposi's sarcoma, 435
Karaya, 315
Kayexalate, 81
Keloids, 70, 421
Kernig's sign, 151
Ketoacidosis, 151
Ketoprofen, 276*t*
Ketosis, 407
Kidney buffers, 75
Kidneys, 373, 375
Kidney tumor, 380, 382-383
Kock pouch, 314, 381*i*
Kyphosis, 151

L

Labia majora, 108
Labia minora, 108
Labor
   complications of, 133-134*t*
   first stage, 124-129
   second stage, 130-131
   third and fourth stages, 131-133, 135
   transitional phase, 129
   warning signs of, 121
Laboratory tests, normal values for, 504*t*
Lactase, 286
Lactation, 139-142
Laniazid, 237*t*
Lanoxin, 157, 206*t*
Lanvis, 464*t*
Large intestine, 282, 284, 287
Laryngotracheobronchitis, 162-163
Larynx, 208
Lasix, 157, 204*t*, 396*t*
Laxatives, 332*t*
Legal principles, 42-45
Let-down reflex, 141
Leukemia, 166-168
Leukeran, 463*t*
Leukocytosis, 151
Levodopa, 353, 371*t*
Levo-Dromoran, 279*t*
Levorphanol, 279*t*
Levothyroxine, 401
LH. *See* Luteinizing hormone.

Librium, 489*t*
Lidocaine, 203*t*
Ligaments, 239
Lightening, 112, 121
Linea nigra, 113
Lioresal, 277*t*
Lipase, 285
Lipoatrophy, 151
Lisinopril, 205*t*
Lithane, 492*t*
Lithiasis, 375
Lithium carbonate, 474, 475, 492*t*
Lithobid, 492*t*
Lithonate, 492*t*
Lithotabs, 492*t*
Liver, 284, 287-288
Lobar pneumonia, 210-211
Lochia, 135
Lomotil, 331*t*
Lomustine, 465*t*
Loop colostomy, 317
Loop diuretic, 396*t*
Loose association of ideas, 469
Loperamide, 331*t*
Lopurin, 168
Lorazepam, 489*t*
Lordosis, 151
Loxapine succinate, 494*t*
Loxitane, 494*t*
L-phenylalanine mustard, 463*t*
Lugol's solution, 419*t*
Lumbar puncture, 159, 168, 368-369
Luminal, 370*t*
Lumpectomy, 449
Lung abscess, 220*t*
Lung cancer, 213-215, 445-448
Lung resection, 215*t*
Lungs, 208
Luteinizing hormone, 117
Lymphedema, 441
Lymph nodes, 432
Lymphocytes, 432

M

Maalox, 332*t*
Macrophages, 434
Mafenide acetate, 431*t*
Magnesium and aluminum hydroxide, 332*t*
Magnesium salts, 332*t*
Magnesium sulfate, 148*t*
Magnetic resonance imaging, 351
Maintenance chemotherapy, 151
Malignant cell development, 439-440
Malignant melanoma, 421
Malignant tumor, 440*i*
Maltase, 286
Mammography, 449
Mania, 469
Manic episode, 473-475
Mannitol, 396*t*
MAO inhibitors, 354, 491*t*
Marplan, 491*t*
Maslow, A.H., 29
Mastectomy, 449-451, 452*i*, 453-454
Maternal assessment, 145
Matulane, 463*t*
Mebaral, 372*t*
Mechanical ventilator, 233-234
Mechlorethamine, 463*t*
Meclofenamate, 276*t*

Meclomen, 276t
Mediastinal shift, 220t
Mediastinum, 210
Medipren, 276t
Medroxyprogesterone, 464t
Megace, 464t
Megakaryocyte, 240
Megestrol, 464t
Melanotropin, 113
Mellaril, 494t
Melphalan, 463t
Meninges, 151, 335, 336-337
Meningitis, 158-161, 161i
Menstrual cycle, 110, 117i
Mental disorder, 469
Meperidine hydrochloride, 279t
Mephobarbital, 372t
Mercaptopurine, 464t
Metabolic acidosis, 76-78
Metabolic alkalosis, 76, 78
Metabolism, 399
Metamucil, 332t
Metaproterenol sulfate, 235t
Metastasis, 441
Methergine, 148t
Methimazole, 418t
Methocarbamol, 278t
Methotrexate, 168, 464t
Methyl CCNU, 465t
Methyldopa, 204t, 354
Methylergonovine maleate, 148t
Mexate, 464t
Micronase, 417t
Micronutrients, 53
Micturition, 375
Milk of Magnesia, 332t
Milk production, 141
Miller-Abbott tube, 302-303, 306
Milwaukee brace, 175, 176i
Mineralocorticoids, 398
Minerals, 61t
Mithracin, 463t
Mithramycin, 463t
Mitomycin, 463t
Mitosis, 439i
Mitral valve, 151
Mixed agonists-antagonists, 280t
Modified Jones criteria, 172t
Modified radical mastectomy, 449
Mons pubis, 108
Morphine sulfate, 280t
Motrin, 255, 276t
Mouth, 282, 284
MRI. See Magnetic resonance imaging.
MTX, 464t
Mucolytic agents, 237t
Mucomyst, 164, 237t
Mucus, 285
Muscle relaxants, 277-279t
Muscles, 238i, 238-239
Muscle spasticity, 355t
Musculoskeletal disorders
    complications of, 261-262t
    drugs for, 274-281t
    nursing procedures for, 241-253,
        248i, 263-273
    osteoarthritis, 253-256
    rheumatoid arthritis, 256-261,
        257t

Musculoskeletal system
    anatomy, 238-239i, 238-240
    glossary, 240
    physiology, 240
Mustargen, 463t
Mutamycin, 463t
Myambutol, 237t
Mycobacterium tuberculosis, 217
Myleran, 463t
Myocardial infarction, 192-194
Myocardium, 190
Mysoline, 371t
Myxedema, 401

N
Nalfon, 275t
NANDA nursing diagnostic categories, 508t
Naprosyn, 276t
Naproxen, 276t
Naproxen sodium, 277t
Narcotic analgesics, 252, 259, 279-280t
Nardil, 491t
Nasogastric tube, 297
    drainage from, 293, 425
    feeding through, 307-310
    insertion of, 300-301
    removal of, 306
National Council Licensure Examination for Practical Nurses. See NCLEX-PN.
NCLEX-PN
    dates for, 20, 511
    preparation for, 23-25
    test plan, 20-23
Nebulizer, 163
Necrosis, 190, 192
Needs, human, 29-30
Negligence, 42-43
Neologism, 469
Neoplasm, 439
Nephrectomy, 375
Nephron, 375
Nephrosis, 169-171
Nephrostomy tube care, 390
Nerve palsy, 262t
Nerve pathways, 337
Nerves, 333, 338
Neurogenic shock, 71, 73
Neurologic check, 336, 342, 347, 357-359
Neurologic disorders
    brain tumor, 350-354
    cerebrovascular accident, 341-346
    complications of, 355-356t
    drugs for, 370-372t
    epilepsy, 346-349
    head injury and increased intracranial pressure, 338-341
    nursing procedures for, 357-369, 359i, 360i
Neurologic examination, 351
Neurologic system
    anatomy, 333, 334i, 335
    glossary, 336
    physiology, 335-338
    postoperative complications, 106t
Neuron, 335, 336
Neurovascular check, 240, 263-264

Newborn, 111, 131-132
    abnormalities of, 136-137t
    assessment of, 145-146
    bathing of, 147
    bottle-feeding, 142-143t
    breast-feeding, 139-142
    reflexes of, 146
Nifedipine, 206t
Nipple care, 141
Nipride, 73
Nitro-Bid, 206t
Nitrogen mustard, 463t
Nitroglycerin, 206t
Nitrosoureas, 465t
Nizatidine, 332t
Nocturia, 375
Nolvadex, 464t
Non-insulin-dependent diabetes mellitus, 407-410
Nonnarcotic analgesics, 281t
Norflex, 279t
Norpace, 203t
Norpramin, 490t
NPH insulin, 179
Nuchal rigidity, 151, 359
Nuclease, 286
Null cells, 434
Numorphan, 280t
Nurse practice act, 42
Nutrients, 51-53
Nutrition, 51-55
    cardiovascular disease and, 56-57
    concepts of, 60-65t
    deficiencies in, 55-56
    diabetes mellitus and, 57-58
    renal disease and, 58-59

O
Obsession, 469
Obstipation, 293
Oliguria, 375
Oncologic disorders
    breast cancer and mastectomy, 449-451, 452i, 453-454
    complications of chemotherapy, 454t
    drugs for, 463-465t
    glossary, 441
    lung cancer and radiation therapy, 445-448
    malignant cell development, 439i, 439-440, 440i
    nursing procedures for, 455-462, 457i
    ovarian cancer and chemotherapy, 441-444
    side effects of drugs for, 465-466t
Oncovin, 465t
Opisthotonos, 151
Oral hygiene, 444, 459-461
Oral hypoglycemics, 416-418t
Oretic, 396t
Organic nitrate, 206t
Orinase, 418t
Orphenadrine, 279t
Orthopnea, 210
Orudis, 276t
Osmitrol, 396t
Osmosis, 79, 375

Osmotic diuretics, 340, 396*t*
Osteoarthritis, 240, 253-256
Osteomyelitis, 240
Osteoporosis, 56
Ostomy, 380, 381*i*, 382-383
Ovarian cancer, 441-444
Ovaries, 110, 397, 398
Oxycodone, 280*t*
Oxygen, 177, 437
    administration of, 228-229
Oxygen saturation, 151
Oxytocic medications, 131, 148*t*
Oxytocin, 148*t*, 397

P

Palliative surgery, 100
Panadol, 281*t*
Pancreas, 284, 397, 398
Pancreatitis, 285
Panic attack, 469
Paracentesis, 312-314
Paradione, 370*t*
Parafon Forte, 278*t*
Paralysis, 355*t*
Paralytic lieus, 299*t*
Paramethadione, 370*t*
Paranoia, 469
Paraplegia, 82
Para status, 112
Parathyroid glands, 397
Parathyroid hormone, 397
Paregoric, 331*t*
Parental maladaption, 138*t*
Parkinson's disease, 352-354
Parlodel, 371*t*
Parnate, 491*t*
Parotid glands, 284, 288
Paroxysmal nocturnal dyspnea, 210
Patent ductus arteriosus, 151, 154*i*
Patient-controlled analgesia pump,
    252
PBZ, 236*t*
Pelvis, 110
PEM. *See* Protein-energy malnutri-
    tion.
Penicillin, 173
Pentazocine, 281*t*
Pepcid, 255, 332*t*
Pepsin, 285
Peptic ulcer, 288
Percocet-5, 280*t*
Percodan, 280*t*
Perineal lacerations, 131
Perineal prostatectomy, 377, 378*t*
Perineum, 108, 143-144
Peripheral venous catheter, 458-459
Peritoneal dialysis, 383
Peritonitis, 285, 299*t*, 385
Perphenazine, 474, 494*t*
Phagocytosis, 434
Pharynx, 208
Phenelzine, 491*t*
Phenergan, 236*t*
Phenobarbital sodium, 370*t*
Phenothiazines, 354
Phenytoin sodium, 371*t*
Phimosis, 375
Phobia, 469
Physical assessment, 39-41
Physical-motor development, 30-37

Piroxicam, 255, 277*t*
Pitocin, 148*t*
Pituitary gland, 336, 397
Pituitary tumor, 403
Placenta previa, 123*t*
Plant alkaloids, 465*t*
Platelet count, 166, 167
Platinol, 463*t*
Pleural effusion, 220*t*
Plicamycin, 463*t*
Pneumocystis carinii pneumonia,
    435, 437
Pneumonia, 210-211
Pneumothorax, 221*t*
Poisoning, 165*t*
Polyphagia, 407
Polyuria, 407
Positions, for patient in bed, 365-
    367
Positron emission tomography, 351
Postanesthesia recovery area, 101-
    102
Postmastectomy exercises, 452*i*
Postoperative period, 101-105, 103-
    106*t*
Postpartum depression, 138*t*
Postpartum period, 111, 137
    bottle-feeding during, 142-143*t*
    breast-feeding during, 139-142
    complications during, 138*t*
    maternal assessment, 145
    newborn assessment, 145-146
    nursing procedures for, 143-147
Postural drainage, 225-226
Posture, 339
Potassium, 79-81
    sources of, 65*t*
Potassium iodide solution, 419*t*
Potassium-sparing diuretic, 396*t*
Povidone-iodine, 144, 178
Prednisone, 168, 170, 281*t*, 464*t*
Pregnancy
    complications of, 123*t*
    drugs used during, 148*t*
    first trimester, 111-116
    second trimester, 118-120
    signs of, 114
    tests during, 115
    third trimester, 120-122
Prenatal period. *See* Pregnancy.
Preoperative care, 98-100
Prepuce, 108
Pressure ulcers, 429-430
Primidone, 371*t*
Privacy, patient's right to, 43
Procainamide, 203*t*
Procarbazine, 463*t*
Procardia, 206*t*
Proctoscopy, 328-330
Progesterone, 117, 398
Progestin, 464*t*
Projection, 469
Prolixin Decanoate, 494*t*
Prolixin Enanthate, 494*t*
Promethazine hydrochloride, 236*t*
Pronestyl, 203*t*
Propoxyphene, 280*t*

Propranolol, 204*t*, 419*t*
Proprioceptive loss, 83
Propylthiouracil, 418*t*
Prostatectomy, 377, 378*t*
Prostate gland, 377-379
Protein, 52-53
Protein-energy malnutrition, 55
Provera, 464*t*
Prozac, 492*t*
Pruritus, 421
Psychiatric disorders
    alcohol abuse, 477-480, 479*t*
    Alzheimer's disease, 481, 482*t*,
        483
    anorexia nervosa, 486-488, 487*t*
    anxiety disorder, 470-472, 471*t*,
        472*t*
    bipolar disorder—manic phase,
        473-475
    depression, 475-477
    drugs for, 489-497*t*
    glossary, 468-469
    schizophrenia, 484-486
    substance withdrawal, 480*t*
Psyllium, 332*t*
PTU, 418*t*
Ptyalin, 284, 285
Pulmonary edema, 198, 212-213
Pulmonary embolism, 221*t*
Pulse, 190
Pupil responses, 339
Purinethol, 464*t*
Pyridoxine, 354
PZB, 236

Q

Quadriplegia, 82
Quinidex, 203*t*
Quinidine sulfate, 203*t*

R

Radiation therapy, 445-448
Radioactive iodine, 419*t*
Radioactive iodine uptake test, 414
Radioisotopes, 351
Ranitidine, 332*t*
Rationalization, 469
Raynaud's phenomenon, 256
RDAs. *See* Recommended dietary
    allowances.
Reality testing, 469
Recommended dietary allowances,
    51, 498-499*t*
Rectal tube insertion, 325-327
Red blood cells, 166, 375
Reflex arcs, 336, 337*i*
Reflexes, 336
    newborn, 146
    nursing, 141
Regression, 469
Rehabilitation, 66-68
Reinduction chemotherapy, 151
Renal calculi, 386*t*
Renal disease, 58-59
Renal failure, 386*t*
Repression, 469
Reserpine, 205*t*, 354
Respiratory acidosis, 75-77
Respiratory alkalosis, 76, 77
Respiratory buffers, 75

Respiratory disorders
  chronic obstructive pulmonary disease, 216-217
  complications of, 220-221t
  drugs for, 235-237t
  lobar pneumonia, 210-211
  lung cancer, 213-215
  nursing procedures for, 222, 223i, 224-234, 231i
  pulmonary edema, 212-213
  pulmonary tuberculosis, 217-219
Respiratory failure, 221t
Respiratory syncytial virus, 151
Respiratory system
  anatomy, 208, 209i
  glossary, 210
  physiology, 208
  postoperative complications, 106t
Retrovir, 435
Retropubic prostatectomy, 378t
Rheumatic fever, 171-173, 172t
Rheumatoid arthritis, 240, 256-261, 257t
Rifadin, 237t
Rifampin, 237t
Robaxin, 278t
Rotating tourniquets, 198
Roto Rest bed, 360
Rufen, 276t
Rule of nines, 423i
Ruptured cerebral aneurysm, 355t

S

Salicylates, 274t
Saliva, 284
Salivary glands, 284, 288
Salsalate, 274t
Schizophrenia, 484-486
Scoliosis, 175-177
Sebaceous glands, 420, 421
Secretin, 285, 286
Sedatives, 372t
Seizure, 336, 346-349
Self-concept, 469
Self-esteem, 469
Semustine, 465t
Sensory loss, 356t
Septic shock, 71, 73-74
Serpasil, 205t
Sexually transmitted diseases, 115
Shaving, surgical preparation and, 95
Shock, 70-74, 190
SIADH. See Syndrome of inappropriate antidiuretic hormone.
Sickle-cell disease, 115
Sigmoid colostomy irrigation, 318-321
Silvadene, 431t
Silver nitrate, 132, 431t
Silver sulfadiazine, 431t
Sims' position, 366
Sinequan, 490t
Sitz bath, 144
6-MP, 464t
6-TG, 464t
Skeletal traction, 244-247

Skin, 420i, 420-421
Skin appendages, 420
Skin color, 263
Skin grafts, 426t
Skin temperature, 263
Skin traction, 244
Skin turgor, 292
Sling, 268-269
Small intestine, 282, 286-287
  obstruction of, 292-296
Social-play development, 30-37
Sodium, 79-81
Sodium nitroprusside, 73
Sodium polystyrene sulfonate, 81
Soma, 278t
Somatic nervous system, 335
Somatostatin, 286
Sonogram, 114
Specimen collection
  midstream urine, 92, 170
  sputum, 92
  stool, 93, 152
  24-hour urine specimen, 415
  wound drainage, 93
Spina bifida, 137t
Spinal cord, 333, 336
Spirometer, 228
Spironolactone, 396t
Spleen, 432
Spontaneous abortion, 123t
Sputum color, 251
SSKI, 419t
Stadol, 281t
Staple removal, 89
State boards of nursing, 509-511
Stelazine, 494t
Steroids
  for increased intracranial pressure, 340
  for nephrosis, 169
  for neurogenic shock, 73
Stilphostrol, 464t
Stoma, 316, 318
Stomach, 282, 285
Stool softeners, 332t
Streptozocin, 465t
Stress ulcer, 288, 428t
Striae gravidarum, 113
Strictures, 70
Stridor, 151
Stroke, 341-346
Strong Iodine Solution, 419t
Stryker Wedge Frame bed, 363-365
Subcutaneous nodules, 151
Sublingual glands, 284, 288
Substance withdrawal, 480t
Sucrase, 286
Suction catheter, 231i
Sulfamylon, 431t
Sulindac, 277t
Suprapubic prostatectomy, 377, 378t
Surgery, 100
Surmontil, 490t
Suture removal, 89
Sydenham's chorea, 173
Symmetrel, 353, 371t
Syndrome of inappropriate antidiuretic hormone, 151

Synovial fluid analysis, 258
Synovium, 239-240
Synthroid, 401

T

Tachycardia, 156
Tachypnea, 156
Tagamet, 255, 332t
Talacen, 281t
Talwin, 281t
Tamoxifen, 464t
Tapazole, 418t
Taractan, 494t
Tardive dyskinesia, 469
T-binder, 395
Tegretol, 370t
Tendons, 239
Tenesmus, 285
Tenormin, 204, 204t
Tenting, 421
Tentorium, 336
Terbutaline, 235t
Testes, 373, 397, 398
Testosterone, 398
Tetanus prophylaxis, 425
Tetany, 399
Tetrad spell, 151
Tetralogy of Fallot, 151, 155i
Thalamus, 336
Theo-Dur, 236t
Theophylline, 236t
Therapeutic communication, 45, 46-49t
Thiazide diuretics, 396t
Thioguanine, 464t
Thioridazine, 494t
Thiotepa, 463t
Thoracentesis, 210, 229-230
Thoracic cavity, 208
Thoracotomy, 210
Thorazine, 493t
Thrombocytopenia, 151
Thymus, 432
Thyroid gland, 397
Thyroid-stimulating hormone, 397, 401
Thyroid storm, 411t
Thyroxine, 397
Tibia, fracture of, 241-244
T lymphocytes, 432-434
Tofranil, 490t
Tolazamide, 417t
Tolbutamide, 418t
Tolectin, 277t
Tolinase, 417t
Tolmetin sodium, 277t
Tonsils, 432
Torts, 42-43
Total parenteral nutrition, 425, 441, 443
Tourniquets, rotating, 198
Toxic goiter, 399
Trachea, 208
Tracheal suctioning, 230-232, 231i
Tracheostomy care, 232-233
Traction, 240
  for femur fracture, 244-247
Transfusion reactions, 438t

Transient ischemic attack, 190, 356*t*
Transurethral prostatic resection, 377, 378*t*
Transverse colostomy care, 317-318
Tranylcypromine, 491*t*
Trazodone, 492*t*
Tremors, 352
Trendar, 276*t*
Trendelenburg's position, 226
Trialka, 332*t*
Tricuspid atresia, 155*i*
Tricyclics, 489-490*t*
Triethylenethiophosphoramide, 463*t*
Trifluoperazine, 494*t*
Trihexyphenidyl, 353, 372*t*, 495*t*
Triiodothyronine, 397
Trilafon, 474, 494*t*
Trilisate, 274*t*
Trimester, 111
Trimipramine, 490*t*
Tripelennamine citrate, 236*t*
Tripelennamine hydrochloride, 236*t*
Truncus arteriosus, 155*i*
Tube feedings, 307-312
Tuberculosis, 217-219
Tumors, 350-354, 380, 382-383, 403, 440*i*
Tums, 332*t*
TURP. *See* Transurethral prostatic resection.
Tylenol, 163-165, 281*t*
Tylox, 280*t*

U

UCG. *See* Urinary chorionic gonadotropin test.
Ulcers, 167, 288-291, 428*t*, 429-430
Umbilical cord prolapse, 133*t*
Universal precautions, 437
Uremia, 375, 386*t*
Ureterosigmoidostomy, 381*i*
Ureters, 373
Urethra, 373
Urethral orifice, 108
Urinary bladder, 373
Urinary catheter, 387-389
Urinary chorionic gonadotropin test, 115
Urinary diversion, 380, 381*i*
Urine elimination
  pregnancy and, 113
  prostate gland and problems with, 377
  protein in, 375
Urine retention, 386*t*
Urine specific gravity, 170, 394-395
Urine specimen, 24-hour, 415
USP, 419*t*
USRDAs. *See* U.S. Recommended Dietary Allowances.
U.S. Recommended Dietary Allowances, 51
Uterine contractions, 111, 114, 134
Uterus, 110

V

Vagina, 110
Validate, 469
Valium, 278*t*, 370*t*, 489*t*
Valproic acid, 371*t*
Valsalva's maneuver, 190
Vasoconstriction, 421
Vasodilation, 421
Vasodilators, 73, 192
Vasopressors, 73
Vasotec, 205*t*
Veins, 186
Velban, 465*t*
Ventilation, 208, 233-234
Ventricular rupture, 197*t*
Ventricular septal defect, 151, 154*i*
Ventriculoperitoneal shunt, 160, 161*i*
Verapamil, 206*t*
Vertebrae, 335
Vinblastine, 465*t*
Vincristine, 465*t*
Virus, 434
Vistaril, 236*t*, 489*t*
Visual field examination, 351
Vitamins, 60-61*t*, 148*t*
Voltaren, 275*t*

WXYZ

Walker, 272-273
Warfarin sodium, 207*t*
Weights, healthful, 500*t*
Western blot assay, 436
White blood cells, 166-168
Wilms' tumor, 380
Withdrawal, 469, 479*t*, 480*t*
Wound irrigation, 87
Xanax, 372*t*, 489*t*
Xylocaine, 203*t*
Zanosar, 463*t*
Zantac, 332*t*
Zarontin, 370*t*
Zestril, 205*t*
Zidovudine, 435

i refers to an illustration; *t* refers to a table.